THE ENCYCLOPEDIA OF

ARTHRITIS

Second Edition

THE ENCYCLOPEDIA OF

ARTHRITIS

Second Edition

Guy Taylor, M.D.
C. Michael Stein, M.D.

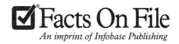

Facts On File
An imprint of Infobase Publishing

The Encyclopedia of Arthritis, Second Edition

Copyright © 2011, 2004 by C. Michael Stein and Guy Taylor

Facts On File
An imprint of Infobase Publishing, Inc.
132 West 31st Street
New York NY 10001

Library of Congress Cataloging-in-Publication

Taylor, Guy, M.D.
The encyclopedia of arthritis / Guy Taylor, C. Michael Stein . — 2nd ed.
p. cm.
Includes bibliographical references and index.
ISBN-13: 978-0-8160-7767-0 (hardcover : alk. paper)
ISBN-10: 0-8160-7767-3 (hardcover : alk. paper)
1. Arthritis—Encyclopedias. I. Stein, C. Michael (Charles Michael) II. Title.
RC933.T29 2009
616.7'22003—dc22   2010012573

Text and cover design by Cathy Rincon
Composition by Hermitage Publishing Services
Cover printed by Sheridan Books, Ann Arbor, Mich.
Book printed and bound by Sheridan Books, Ann Arbor, Mich.
Date printed: October 2010

Printed in the United States of America

10 9 8 7 6 5 4 3 2 1

This book is printed on acid-free paper.

CONTENTS

PREFACE

This book is intended to provide educational information to the public about arthritis and related illnesses. It is not intended to substitute for any aspect of medical care. The authors have made every effort to provide information that is up-to-date, accurate, and useful. However, the diagnosis and treatment of the various conditions described and the monitoring of patients must be performed by their physicians. Readers should use the knowledge gained to work with their physicians to optimize their medical care and should not alter their medical care based on information provided in this book.

INTRODUCTION

Arthritis and related conditions affect millions of people and cause pain, disability, and, for some conditions, increased mortality. Arthritis is difficult to understand because there are hundreds of different arthritis-related conditions and many different treatments for them. It is difficult to obtain accurate, unbiased information because much of the popular literature focuses on miracle cures. This book sets out to provide concise and accurate information about a wide range of arthritis-related topics and to act as a comprehensive resource for patients with arthritis, their families, and anyone interested in understanding musculoskeletal illness.

The late 1980s and the 1990s were times of great excitement in rheumatological research as new messengers that directed and controlled the immune response were discovered. The initial discovery of interleukin-1 as a pro-inflammatory cytokine that upregulated inflammatory mechanisms became a bewildering array of molecules, each with a range of different actions. For years it seemed that these discoveries, interesting though they were, did nothing to improve treatment for patients suffering from inflammatory rheumatic conditions. The new millennium has changed all that. Starting with the use of TNF antagonists for rheumatoid arthritis, researchers have explored using many protein molecules or "antibodies" to interfere with very specific disease processes, sometimes with astonishing success. While inflammatory diseases remain the main target for this "biological" treatment, it has extended to include noninflammatory diseases such as osteoporosis. This revision has been necessary to reflect this growing form of therapy. There have also been new discoveries that have led to drugs being withdrawn and these are discussed.

A new section deals with risk factors and preventive measures for specific diseases. While many autoimmune rheumatic conditions are not preventable to any great extent other than by adhering to the old adage to "choose one's parents carefully," this section emphasizes such preventive or ameliorating strategies as do exist. Conditions are presented alphabetically, but conditions that cause problems predominantly in one part of the body are also listed under that body part, e.g., knee or foot. The authors have endeavored to provide evidence-based information on treatment wherever possible. That means that the recommendations have been studied in clinical trials and shown to be effective. This information is not possible for all treatments or conditions, and this is discussed where it is pertinent.

Small-capital terms for arthritis and related conditions in each section are cross-referenced in the main text of entries. Drug names in small-capital letters are further detailed in Appendix I. Finally, terms in small capitals relating to laboratory and diagnostic tests are expanded upon in Appendix II. Occasionally, a reference to Appendix I or to Appendix II appears following a term in the main text.

ENTRIES A TO Z

Achilles tendon This powerful tendon, sometimes called the *heel cord,* attaches the two major calf muscles (gastrocnemius and soleus) to the calcaneum (heel bone) and transmits the propulsive forces needed for walking, running, and jumping. The tendon is composed of spirals of collagen that are wrapped into bundles forming a thick cord that is both strong and able to stretch. Because of the property of viscoelasticity, a sudden rapid muscle contraction will find the tendon relatively stiff while slower contractions allow greater stretch. With repeated stretching, the tendon becomes more flexible. Although this applies to all ages, maximum flexibility does slowly decrease with increasing age.

Symptoms and Diagnostic Path

The frequency of Achilles tendon injuries appears to be increasing, with about 8 percent of top-level runners having some Achilles problem each year.

Rupture of the Achilles tendon The ability of tendons to stretch and become more elastic during use is the rationale for warming up before participating in sports. The typical Achilles tendon rupture happens when a relatively untrained middle-aged athlete plays a sport such as tennis and makes a sudden forward movement. The rapid stretch of a relatively stiff tendon can cause it to rupture and the athlete feels sudden pain, as if kicked on the back of the leg. He or she is unable to walk or stand on tiptoes and may hear a pop as the tendon snaps. The midtendon rupture of the Achilles is unusual for a tendon. Like most tendons the Achilles is nearly twice as strong as the muscles it joins. Because of this, tendons normally tear in the area where they join onto their muscle since this is the weakest part. Therefore, for the midtendon to rupture there is usually a preexisting abnormality

that has weakened it. The tendon may have been damaged by previous trauma, TENDINITIS, long-term corticosteroid use, local steroid injections into or around the tendon, and other chronic medical illnesses such as kidney failure. A few cases of tendon rupture have been described in people taking quinolone antibiotics, for example ofloxacin (see DRUG-INDUCED RHEUMATIC DISEASE). The treatment of a ruptured Achilles tendon can be either conservative, with the leg immobilized in a plaster cast for about six weeks, or surgical, with open repair of the tendon again followed by immobilization for about six weeks. Surgical repair decreases the risk that the tendon will rupture again from 10 percent to 2 percent. However, surgery may not always be the best option, particularly if the person has other medical problems or is not athletic and is therefore less likely to stress the tendon in the future.

Other conditions affecting the Achilles tendon Inflammation of the tendon at the point where it joins bone is called enthesitis and is common in ANKYLOSING SPONDYLITIS and Reiter's syndrome. Treatment includes an orthotic shoe insert or a special shoe designed to raise the heel, rest, ice, local corticosteroid injection, and NSAIDs followed by rehabilitation stretches.

Inflammation of the Achilles tendon (tendinitis) occurs particularly in long-distance runners and athletes involved in jumping sports or in those using unsuitable footwear or having a biomechanical problem. All these will place unusual or abnormal stresses on the tendon. The statins (cholesterol-lowering drugs) and quinolone antibiotics occasionally cause tendinitis, and in a few cases the initial presentation is with rupture. Tendinitis causes pain in the area around the tendon, particularly when it is stretched during activities such as walking or running. The tendon is often visibly enlarged, warm, and very tender to the touch. It can be very difficult to decide whether the inflammation is mostly in the tendon or around it (peritendinitis), and both are often present. Sometimes the tendinitis occurs because of a partial tendon rupture, and ultrasound or MRI scanning is excellent at showing this.

Treatment Options and Outlook

The treatment of Achilles tendinitis is similar to that of enthesitis except that local steroid injections into the tendon are avoided because they may weaken the tendon and increase the chance that it will rupture. Surgery to remove surrounding inflamed tissue and chalky material from within the tendon where it has degenerated is performed if conservative treatment fails. This is successful in 80 percent of competitive athletes.

Studies on athletes have shown that the presence of minor abnormalities on ultrasound scanning of their Achilles tendons predicts a higher risk of injury during the following season. Stretching and eccentric exercise are widely believed to be the best rehabilitation exercise for muscles and tendons. A study was therefore done on professional soccer players to see if stretching and eccentric training would reduce the frequency of injury in those with ultrasound abnormalities in their Achilles. Unfortunately this was not the case, perhaps because these athletes had some minor biomechanical problem that continued to put them at risk.

If the person's shoes or biomechanics of walking or running are faulty, the condition may be corrected with appropriate shoes. Bursae between the skin and tendon and between the tendon and underlying bone can become inflamed (see BURSITIS) and cause symptoms similar to tendinitis. The treatment of bursitis around the Achilles tendon is similar to that of tendinitis.

Risk Factors and Preventive Measures

The risk factors for both tendonitis and rupture are increasing age, a sudden increase in the training load, or biomechanical factors such as weight, gait, shoes, and training surface. The drugs discussed above are rare causes but important to recognize. Obviously these should not be used again. A grad-

ual warm-up before training or competition and also a gradual increase in training load have both been shown to reduce the frequency of Achilles tendon injuries. While stretching makes physiological sense and is widely practiced, it has not been shown to reduce the injury rate in athletes. The study of soccer players discussed above was particularly disappointing as it included eccentric strengthening, widely believed to be beneficial. However, the causes of significant Achilles tendon problems are likely to be multifactorial, and it may be difficult to show that a single intervention works for a large group of people. Other common-sense precautions include dressing appropriately for cold weather, avoiding hard surfaces for training, and correcting biomechanical problems if possible. Running shoes do deteriorate with use, and it has been suggested that they be replaced about every 600 kilometers, but this has not been proven to reduce injuries.

acne arthralgia Severe acne that causes cysts and nodules on the buttocks, thighs, and upper arms as well as in areas more usually affected by acne can be associated with attacks of arthralgia and myalgia that can last several weeks or months. Joint problems related to acne are rare and occur most often in adolescent males. In addition to arthralgia and myalgia, fever, loss of weight, and arthritis can occur. The cause of this illness is not known, but it may be a reaction to the bacteria that cause acne. Treatment of the arthralgia is symptomatic with NSAIDs and is combined with treatment to control the acne. This can include long-term antibiotic treatment, often with a tetracycline type of antibiotic, topical creams, retinoids, or in females, drugs that block their male hormones (androgens) that stimulate acne. Severe acne is occasionally complicated by the SAPHO SYNDROME.

acquired immunodeficiency syndrome (AIDS) See HUMAN IMMUNODEFICIENCY VIRUS.

acromegaly A syndrome due to excessive formation of growth hormone (GH) by a tumor in the pituitary gland and characterized by coarse facial features, enlargement of hands and feet, headache, sweating, neuropathy, SLEEP APNEA, and musculoskeletal symptoms. Acromegaly affects 40 to 60 people per million population.

An adenoma (a benign tumor) of the pituitary gland that produces GH is the cause of acromegaly in 99 percent of patients. Other rare causes include tumors of the gut, pancreas, and lung that produce GH.

Symptoms and Diagnostic Path

Acromegaly results in gigantism if it develops in children before puberty. More commonly, however, it develops slowly between the ages of 20 and 40 years. Symptoms may be due to either excessive production of GH or pressure effects caused by the adenoma itself. GH causes enlargement of the soft tissues, resulting in a characteristic coarse facial appearance with an enlarged jaw and tongue, separation of the teeth, and large hands and feet. Because of this, unrelated patients with acromegaly are said to look more like each other than like any of their family members. Internal organs such as the heart, liver, and kidneys also enlarge. Hypertension (30 percent) and diabetes (20 percent) are common. If the adenoma in the pituitary enlarges, it can cause pressure effects in the brain. The optic nerves that run from the eye to the brain pass very close to the pituitary gland. If the adenoma presses on an optic nerve, it can cause partial blindness. The tumor can also affect normal pituitary tissue and cause reduced production of some hormones, for example gonadotrophins (hormones that regulate the release of sex hormones) and increased production of others, for example prolactin, a hormone that regulates the secretion of breast milk.

Musculoskeletal symptoms Bone and joint problems develop in at least 50 percent of patients with acromegaly. Initially the cartilage in the joints increases in amount, and the capsule of the joint and the ligaments close to it soften and thicken, resulting in hypermobility. Later degenerative changes develop in joints perhaps because of the altered biomechanics caused by the changes in cartilage and soft tissues. The arthritis associated with acromegaly causes pain, stiffness, and reduced range of movement, as happens in OSTEOARTHRITIS

of any cause. The fingers, spine, and knees are commonly involved, and the shoulders, elbows, and ankles are affected more frequently than occurs in the usual type of osteoarthritis. OSTEOPOROSIS may develop because of reduced sex hormone production as well as increased loss of calcium in the urine. When the median nerve reaches the wrist it passes through a tunnel of relatively fixed size, the carpal tunnel. In acromegaly, the tissues around this tunnel often thicken, causing compression of the nerve and giving rise to symptoms of CARPAL TUNNEL SYNDROME. Similarly, other nerves that run through narrow channels can become trapped by soft tissue, resulting in neuropathy.

Premature coronary artery disease, heart failure, and sleep apnea all contribute to the increased mortality rate in people with acromegaly. The mortality rate in untreated acromegaly is twice that of the general population. However, if treatment is successful in reducing GH levels in the blood to less than 5 mU/L, there is no increased risk of death. The concentration of calcium in the blood is elevated (hypercalcemia) in 5 percent of patients, and the increased excretion of calcium in the urine can increase the risk of developing kidney stones. The osteoarthritis that often accompanies acromegaly may cause considerable pain and disability, and there is an increased risk of CALCIUM PYROPHOSPHATE DIHYDRATE DEPOSITION DISEASE, or pseudogout. A large pituitary tumor can cause permanent loss of vision, particularly peripheral vision.

The characteristic appearance of the face and hands usually prompts the diagnosis. X-rays can support the diagnosis, showing characteristic *tufting* of the bones at the ends of the fingers. Other X-ray changes include widened joint spaces (because of the increased amount of cartilage) and typical changes of osteoarthritis. They include the formation of osteophytes sometimes occurring in joints such as shoulders and elbows, which are not usually affected by osteoarthritis. In the spine the X-rays have an appearance similar to that of DISH. Blood tests showing elevated levels of GH or somatomedin C are useful for making the diagnosis. Abnormalities of other pituitary hormones such as prolactin or gonadotrophins may be found but are not specific. An MRI scan is useful because the pituitary adenoma can often be seen. Eye tests may show loss of peripheral vision that the patient had not noticed.

Treatment Options and Outlook

The aim of treatment is to relieve symptoms of acromegaly, reduce GH levels to less than 5 mU/L, treat the local pressure effects of the tumor, and maintain normal pituitary function. The treatment of choice, transsphenoidal surgery, achieves a cure rate of between 40 and 90 percent. Radiotherapy may be used to treat the tumor in patients who are not healthy enough to undergo surgery or those who choose not to have it. After treatment with radiotherapy the GH levels decline slowly over a few years, and with time there is an increased chance that production of other pituitary hormones will also decline.

Treatment of acromegaly with drugs such as octreotide and bromocriptine decreases GH production. These drugs are used when GH levels remain raised after surgery or radiotherapy or sometimes as the only therapy in elderly patients who prefer not to undergo surgery or radiotherapy. Joint symptoms are treated with analgesics, NSAIDs, and physical therapy as appropriate. Surgical removal of large osteophytes is sometimes helpful, and total joint replacement may become necessary if a hip or knee joint is badly affected. The symptoms caused by carpal tunnel syndrome improve with adequate control of GH levels, but those caused by arthritis do not.

Risk Factors and Preventive Measures

There are no known specific risk factors or preventive measures for acromegaly.

acupuncture People with arthritis frequently use complementary and alternative therapies such as acupuncture, an ancient Chinese art that seeks to correct imbalances in the flow of energy by selecting appropriate acupuncture points for stimulation. Such stimulation often involves the puncturing of the skin with needles. However, practitioners can also use needle manipulation, heat, pressure, suction, and electrical current to stimulate the chosen points. The concept of yin and yang is the most important theory in traditional Chinese medicine.

It claims that all things have two aspects, yin and yang, that are at the same time both opposite and dependent on each other. They are in a constant state of change and balance. Disease results from loss of this balance, and treatment is directed at restoring it. Qi (chi) is the life force that governs the functions of the organs and flows through meridians or channels to all parts of the body. Pain results from disturbances of this flow. Several types of acupuncture practice may be found in the Western world.

- Traditional Chinese acupuncture is based on traditional diagnoses and aims at restoring yin and yang and normal qi flow.

- Cookbook acupuncture consists of techniques borrowed from Chinese acupuncture but used to treat disorders based on a Western medical diagnosis. An example is the commonly used auricular acupuncture to help with smoking cessation. A small but increasing number of Western medical practitioners are using this type of acupuncture as well as trigger point acupuncture.

- Trigger point acupuncture is used to relieve musculoskeletal pain. The trigger points so often found in FIBROMYALGIA have been scientifically studied in the West only in the past 70 years. As long ago as 600 B.C. the Chinese were inserting needles into these *ah shi* (ah yes) points.

- Scientific acupuncture is based on modern scientific interpretations of the physiological effects of traditional methods.

The insertion of the needles is not particularly painful. However, for maximum benefit a needling sensation should be felt. This is variously described as dull, aching, heavy, sore, distending, or warm, and it may travel away from the needle site. Patients may feel relaxed afterward and can get quite drowsy and occasionally euphoric, presumably as a result of endorphin release. An average treatment involves five to 10 sessions, and most acupuncturists continue treatment until the patient is cured or no further improvement occurs.

Determining if acupuncture is useful for the treatment of arthritis has been difficult. Clinical trials examining the effectiveness of acupuncture for the treatment of rheumatological problems have been criticized because the number of patients studied was often small and because it was difficult to control for a placebo effect occurring in response to the needles (see CLINICAL TRIAL). Some studies have tried to overcome this criticism by using needles to stimulate sham or placebo points that should not result in benefits and then comparing these results with those of active acupuncture. There has, however, been disagreement whether a nonacupuncture type of treatment or acupuncture at a sham point is the most appropriate control group.

There are few well-designed studies, and some have shown a small improvement in pain in patients with OSTEOARTHRITIS and fibromyalgia. Several trials have shown modest benefits in treating particularly troublesome joints in RHEUMATOID ARTHRITIS. The risks from acupuncture are small, provided that needles are adequately sterilized and are not inserted into a nerve, vital organ, or artery. Puncture of the lung (pneumothorax), transmission of HEPATITIS B or HEPATITIS C, nerve damage, infectious arthritis, and bleeding are uncommon complications. In Western countries, between 5 and 10 percent of patients will have a minor adverse reaction to acupuncture and one to three in 1,000 will have a serious adverse reaction.

adult-onset Still's disease   See JUVENILE IDIOPATHIC ARTHRITIS.

Alexander technique   This technique was developed by an actor, F. M. Alexander, to improve his voice. He believed that the way we breathe affects the function of our bodies and that the relationship between the head, neck, and upper body are the primary controls of posture. Abnormal posture causes abnormal muscular tension in one muscle group and can adversely affect the whole body. Treatment with the Alexander technique usually involves individual or group lessons during which a teacher observes the posture and tension in a student. The teacher then explains, using touch and instructions, more efficient posture, movement, and breathing.

This is an educational process teaching students better movement patterns to practice at home or work rather than a treatment given to a client. In the United Kingdom, the National Health Service has used it for BACK PAIN, repetitive strain injury, stuttering, voice loss, and balance problems, including Parkinson's disease in which a controlled study has shown modest benefit. Anecdotal evidence suggests that many students rapidly feel lighter and move more easily. The widespread use by schools of music, voice, dance, and drama demonstrates considerable acceptance of its efficacy. Despite this, there is minimal scientific evaluation of the Alexander technique. Also, it cannot overcome structural abnormalities, thereby limiting its usefulness in people with significant arthritis.

alkaptonuria (ochronosis)   This rare, inherited deficiency of the enzyme homogentisic acid oxidase results in homogentisic acid reaching high levels in the body. This acid is excreted in the urine, which will then turn black if left to stand for a while because the acid oxidizes. The diagnosis of alkaptonuria is suspected if a person gives a history of passing dark urine or of urine that becomes dark after standing for a while. Pigmented or dark-colored deposits of homogentisic acid collect in tissues such as cartilage that are rich in collagen, an important component of joints and soft tissues. These pigmented deposits are called ochronosis. In early adult life, blue or black darkening of the ears or nose may occur. Homogentisic acid is also deposited in the cartilage of large joints such as the knees, resulting in osteoarthritis. It affects the cartilaginous discs between vertebrae, resulting in pain and stiffness of the spine. On X-ray these intervertebral discs are often heavily calcified. There is no specific treatment for the arthritis associated with alkaptonuria. High doses of vitamin C may slow the accumulation of pigment in tissues, but the effects of this treatment on the long-term arthritis problems are not known.

amyloidosis   A rare group of illnesses caused by an insoluble protein complex (amyloid) being deposited between the cells of internal organs and eventually impairing their function. Amyloidosis can rarely cause arthritis but is more often a complication of long-standing inflammatory arthritis.

Although amyloid was first described 150 years ago by the famous German pathologist R. Virchow, the proteins involved have been well characterized only in the last 30 years. The types of amyloid are named *A* for amyloidosis, followed by a letter or abbreviated name that represents the type of amyloid protein. Three main types of amyloid protein cause different types of amyloidosis. In addition, there are also rare hereditary forms of amyloidosis and associations with rare diseases such as FAMILIAL MEDITERRANEAN FEVER.

1. In AA amyloidosis, a protein called serum amyloid A (SAA) is produced as part of the immune response to chronic inflammation. The condition is therefore sometimes called secondary amyloidosis. This used to be a common complication of chronic infections such as tuberculosis. However, with the development of more effective antibiotics, it now usually results from long-standing inflammatory arthritis such as RHEUMATOID ARTHRITIS and ANKYLOSING SPONDYLITIS and a chronic inflammatory disease, familial Mediterranean fever. Genetic factors probably affect how often amyloidosis complicates chronic arthritis. For example, in Scandinavian countries, amyloidosis complicating rheumatoid arthritis, although uncommon, occurs significantly more often than in the United States.

2. AL amyloidosis is sometimes called primary amyloidosis. It can be thought of as a type of malignancy of blood cells (plasma cells) that overproduce an amyloid protein composed of the light (L) chains of an immunoglobulin protein. AL amyloid may also occur in patients with a type of cancer called multiple myeloma that affects the plasma cells of the bone marrow. It can occur in people with benign monoclonal gammopathy and sometimes occurs in the absence of any associated illness. In all these conditions, a type of white blood cell called plasma cells have escaped from their normal control mechanisms and produce increased amounts of the amyloid proteins.

3. $A\beta_2M$ amyloidosis, or beta$_2$-microglobulin amyloidosis, is the third type and is sometimes called dialysis-associated amyloidosis. It occurs in patients who have received hemodialysis for a long time (see DIALYSIS) and can be detected in most patients after 15 years of dialysis.

Symptoms and Diagnostic Path

AA amyloidosis may not cause any symptoms and is sometimes diagnosed only after protein has been found in the urine and investigated. The amount of protein in the urine is often small initially, but it can increase and result in nephrotic syndrome. This may progress to kidney failure. Amyloid protein can be deposited in many tissues, including the heart, but heart failure is rare.

In AL amyloidosis the abnormal protein is deposited in greater quantities in organs such as the heart, liver, and tongue. Nephrotic syndrome and heart failure are common and usually have a poor outcome. The liver may enlarge, and gastrointestinal involvement can lead to poor absorption of nutrients and GI bleeding. Arthritis occurs in less than 5 percent of patients and usually affects shoulders, knees, wrists, metacarpophalangeal (MCP) joints, and proximal interphalangeal (PIP) joints. Amyloid can deposit in the soft tissues of the wrist and cause CARPAL TUNNEL SYNDROME.

Patients on long-term dialysis who have beta$_2$-microglobulin amyloidosis develop arthritis, tendinitis, and carpal tunnel syndrome as well as destructive bony cysts that can sometimes cause fractures.

Biopsy of either an affected organ (e.g., heart or kidney) or of more easily accessible tissues (rectum or subcutaneous fat) will show the amyloid in approximately 80 percent of patients. Aspiration of fat, a test that involves drawing a small amount of abdominal fat into a syringe, is often the most convenient way to obtain a tissue sample. The type of amyloid protein can be determined by staining the tissue with dyes that are specific for the different types of protein. If the heart is affected, echocardiography (an ultrasound of the heart) may show thickening of the walls of the ventricles and reduced contractility of the heart. Nuclear medicine scans using various radiolabeled molecules have been useful when defining the extent of the disease and its response to treatment. However, they are not used in routine clinical care. If myeloma is suspected, examination of the bone marrow will show increased numbers of plasma cells.

Treatment Options and Outlook

Complications caused by amyloidosis such as heart and kidney failure are treated in the usual manner. Treatment of amyloidosis itself is directed at reducing the production of amyloid protein so that less is de posited in the tissues. A lot of research has been directed toward developing methods to remove amyloid protein from tissues, but this is not currently possible. In AA disease, the most important aspect of treatment is to suppress the inflammation or, in chronic infections, to eliminate its cause. If AA amyloidosis is caused by chronic inflammatory arthritis, CORTICOSTEROIDS and drugs that suppress the immune system are often used to control the inflammation. AL amyloidosis associated with myeloma or a monoclonal gammopathy is usually treated with a combination of an anticancer drug, such as melphalan, and prednisone. Some patients with AL amyloidosis have been treated with bone marrow transplantation. COLCHICINE may be helpful for patients with amyloidosis associated with familial Mediterranean fever. In patients with beta$_2$-microglobulin amyloidosis, renal transplantation enables them to stop hemodialysis and can improve the symptoms.

Risk Factors and Preventive Measures

Chronic inflammation of any cause is the risk factor for AA amyloidosis, and obviously kidney failure is the risk factor for hemodialysis-associated amyloidosis. Kidney transplant where available will prevent the latter, although newer techniques in dialysis are being worked on to try to prevent it. Excellent treatment of inflammatory disease will prevent AA amyloidosis, which has become much rarer with better antibiotic treatment of infectious diseases. It is expected to become even less frequent with the better control of inflammation in diseases such as rheumatoid arthritis that has been possible over the last 10 years, but the actual frequency is difficult to know as it is often unrecognized in these patients.

ANA   See ANTINUCLEAR ANTIBODY in Appendix II.

ANCA   See ANTINEUTROPHIL CYTOPLASMIC ANTIBODY in Appendix II.

angiokeratoma corporis diffusum   A rare hereditary condition usually associated with a group of genetic conditions known as lysosomal storage diseases, for example Fabry's disease. Angiokeratomas are small vascular lesions composed of one or more dilated blood vessels lying under the skin associated with the proliferation of connective tissue cells. Affected children often have a degenerative arthritis affecting their distal interphalangeal joints and characteristic dark red skin lesions are present. They also get episodic burning pain in the fingers and toes that is not due to the arthritis. Other manifestations include premature vascular disease, kidney failure, corneal opacities, and diarrhea. The diagnosis is made by biopsy of affected tissue, for example skin, liver, or bone marrow.

ankylosing spondylitis (AS)   A chronic inflammatory arthritis that predominantly affects the spine. It has a strong genetic component, and over 95 percent of AS patients who are of Caucasian extraction have a gene called HLA-B27. The disease affects mainly young men and has a male to female ratio of 5:1. The frequency of AS in women may be underestimated because they develop milder disease. Symptoms almost always start before the age of 40 years, usually in the 20- to 30-year age range. AS affects approximately 0.5–1 percent of people in the U.S.

The association of AS with the HLA-B27 gene was first described in the early 1970s and stimulated considerable research into the causes of AS and associated SPONDYLOARTHROPATHIES. The HLA-B antigens are molecules that human cells express on their surface. In Caucasian populations, approximately 10 percent of people have the HLA-B27 gene. The frequency of this gene varies widely in other populations. It almost never occurs in the black African population living south of the Sahara Desert but is found in as many as 50 percent of Haida Indians in Canada. Generally AS is common where the gene HLA-B27 is common and rare where HLA-B27 is rare. Experimental evidence also suggests that the HLA-B27 molecule carries a particular predisposition for AS. Experiments transferring the human HLA-B27 gene to rodents resulted in their developing an AS-like illness.

One role of the HLA molecules is to carry small peptide antigens processed in the cell to the surface where they can be recognized by a subgroup of lymphocytes called CD8+ T cells. Less than 2 percent of all people with HLA-B27 have AS. However, in families of patients with AS, nearly 20 percent of people who carry HLA-B27 will develop AS. These findings suggest that other genetic factors in addition to HLA-B27 are important. Environmental factors may be needed to activate the disease in people who carry the gene. HLA-B antigens are expressed on all cells in the body, so it is not clear why the spine is particularly affected by AS. One popular theory is that of molecular mimicry. Simply put, this theory suggests that an immune response is started against an infecting bacterium and that the response continues because antigenic determinants (small parts of an organism or other structure recognized by the immune system) are shared between the bacterium and the HLA-B27 molecule. Some bacteria and the HLA-B27 molecule do have identical antigenic determinants. That is, they look alike to the immune system. The related diseases REACTIVE ARTHRITIS and Reiter's syndrome are known to occur after infection with such organisms. This lends support to the theory that AS has a similar trigger. However, we still do not understand exactly why AS develops.

Symptoms and Diagnostic Path

Inflammation typically affects the large sacroiliac (SI) joints at the base of the spine and the small joints between vertebral bodies and between ribs and vertebral bodies (spondylitis). This leads to pain and stiffness, which is most severe in the mornings and tends to improve with exercise. The lower back and neck are affected more than other parts of the spine. In many people this stiffness can progress to complete loss of movement as ligaments and joints are gradually replaced by bone and fuse (ankylosis). This process takes many years, and the rate at which it occurs varies in different people. Ankylosing spondylitis can also affect the peripheral joints, usually large joints such as the hips, knees, and

shoulders. The hips are more likely to be involved if the disease starts before the age of 20. If hip arthritis does not occur in the first 10 years after diagnosis, it is unlikely to do so.

Enthesitis, or inflammation where tendons or ligaments join onto bone, is a hallmark of this disease. This occurs particularly at the heel where the ACHILLES TENDON joins the calcaneus (heel bone), in the lower pelvis where the inner thigh muscles attach, and along the spine and the breastbone where the ribs join. Involvement of the joints where the ribs meet the breastbone and spine can cause severe chest pain and difficulty in breathing. Many patients have had tests performed to exclude a myocardial infarction (heart attack) or lung disease as a cause of unexplained chest pain before the diagnosis of AS was made. In teenagers a variant of AS occurs. In this condition, enthesitis is the most common manifestation. The clinical presentation of enthesitis and arthritis in a teenager is sometimes called the SEA (seronegative enthesitis and arthropathy) syndrome. Not all teenagers with the SEA syndrome develop the adult form of AS. In many with SEA, the arthritis lasts for a few months or years and then disappears.

In many patients, fusion of the joints in the spinal column causes increasing stiffness and eventually a stooped posture that is typical of AS. Restricted movement in the neck makes it difficult for patients with AS to turn their heads. As a consequence, activities such as reversing a car become difficult. Stiffness and restricted movement in the hips and knees can cause these joints to become permanently flexed, making walking difficult. Fusion of the rib joints reduces the ability of the chest to expand when a deep breath is taken. Reduced lung expansion can cause recurrent chest infections and shortness of breath when the patient exercises. Scarring of the upper lobes of the lungs may develop late in the disease and can become infected with organisms that do not usually affect healthy lungs (opportunistic infection).

Patients with AS can also develop several medical problems that are unrelated to their joints. Eye inflammation is common, and anterior uveitis or iritis occurs in 25 percent of patients (see EYE PROBLEMS). Usually this presents with pain in one eye, blurred vision, discomfort in bright light (photophobia), and increased redness and watering of the eye. Attacks of iritis or uveitis usually subside within a few months but may recur later in either eye. The eye inflammation in AS seldom causes permanent loss of vision, but if treatment is delayed it can.

A number of cardiovascular complications may occur and are thought to be caused by chronic inflammation. Why the heart is a specific target in AS is not known. Cardiovascular complications include the following conditions:

- Inflammation of the first part of the aorta that originates from the left ventricle (aortitis)
- Leaking of the aortic valve (aortic regurgitation), causing blood to flow back into the left ventricle after it has been pumped out
- Heart block, in which electrical impulses fail to pass normally through specialized conducting tissue from the upper chambers of the heart, the atria, to the lower chambers, the ventricles that pump blood
- Enlargement of the heart
- Pericarditis (inflammation of the lining layers around the heart)

Aortic regurgitation and heart block are the most common cardiovascular complications. These are more likely to occur in patients who have had AS for many years with involvement of peripheral joints such as the wrists, shoulders, or knees.

Spinal fracture can occur after relatively minor trauma because the spine is rigid and less flexible. OSTEOPOROSIS is common and may occur early in the disease, suggesting that it results from the inflammatory process rather than immobility. AMYLOIDOSIS, glomerulonephritis caused by deposition of immunoglobulin IgA, and cauda equina syndrome are rare complications. In the cauda equina syndrome, the fluid-filled membranes at the lower end of the spinal cord enlarge. This causes pressure and damage to the lower spinal nerves, particularly those supplying function to the bladder and bowels.

AS is often not diagnosed for several years after the onset of symptoms, especially in women. This is because the onset of back pain and stiffness is gradual and in a young person is often ascribed to back strain. Women develop AS less often than men and therefore the diagnosis may not be considered in women.

A history of back pain with unusual morning stiffness and signs of enthesitis or arthritis that affects large joints in a young adult should suggest the diagnosis of AS. X-ray evidence of inflammation of the sacroiliac joints is required to make a definite diagnosis of AS. However, it is important to recognize that X-ray changes can take up to 10 years to develop. Therefore, in early disease, the X-rays can be normal. X-rays of the SI joints are difficult to interpret in teenagers and young adults. Radioisotope bone scans can show increased uptake in the SI joints in the early stages of disease before X-ray changes are visible.

CT scans are both sensitive in that they show changes fairly early on and highly specific in showing changes that only AS or related diseases could cause. These include apparent widening of the joint, erosions in the joint surface, increased density of the underlying bone, and the initially very fine bridges of bone growing across the joint. Their major disadvantage is exposure of the reproductive organs to significant radiation, especially in patients who are usually of a childbearing age. MRI scans are even more sensitive to the early inflammatory changes showing an appearance generally referred to as bone edema. As cartilage and bone are black on an MRI scan, however, it is much more difficult to see the erosions or bony bridging than it is on CT. But because there is no exposure to radiation, MRI has become the tool of choice for diagnosing suspected AS. Inflammatory markers in the blood such as ESR and CRP are helpful but may not always be raised in people with mild disease. Tests for RHEUMATOID FACTOR and ANTINUCLEAR ANTIBODIES are negative (hence the historical term of seronegative arthritis). The presence of HLA-B27 increases the likelihood of the diagnosis of AS in patients of Caucasian extraction. However, because approximately 10 percent of healthy people have the HLA-B27 gene, this test is most helpful as supporting evidence when the patient has features typical of AS and is of very limited utility in those with poorly characterized back pain.

Treatment Options and Outlook

The aims of treatment are relief of symptoms (pain and stiffness), improvement in flexibility, and maintenance of posture, thus enabling the individual to continue his or her occupation and partake in leisure activities. Longer term goals include prevention of joint damage and of spinal fusion, minimization of non-joint complications such as eye and heart problems, and prevention of the complications of a stiff spine should this occur. Crucial to achieving these aims is early diagnosis and patient education. Self-care through stretches, exercises, and appropriate knowledge and use of medications is essential for a good outcome. Learning a routine of stretches and exercises under the supervision of a physical therapist is very useful. Swimming is an excellent exercise for patients with AS because it exercises the heart and lungs and puts many joints through a wide range of motion.

For most people with mild AS physical therapy, NSAIDs and occasional analgesics are sufficient. Patients with more severe disease require more aggressive treatment with drugs that attempt to control inflammation or slow down the progression of disease. Most patients with established disease and fused joints or deformity will benefit from occupational therapy, including assessment for work environment alteration or use of ASSISTIVE DEVICES.

Many NSAIDs are used to treat AS. PHENYLBUTAZONE is an NSAID that has a reputation among older rheumatologists for being particularly effective in controlling the symptoms of AS. Because it has a relatively high incidence of side effects, including potentially devastating bone marrow damage, it is no longer available in many countries, and we would not advocate its use. In surveys of AS patients, INDOMETHACIN was the preferred NSAID, but it too has a high incidence of side effects, including central nervous system effects such as dizziness. In a properly controlled study this preference was no longer apparent. NAPROXEN was the next most preferred NSAID in the patient survey and would be a good starting point. It is likely that all the NSAIDs will have some effect on AS and that some patients will respond better to one than another for reasons we cannot yet explain. They do need to be used at full dosage in

AS. Two weeks of regular use is the minimum time period to see if they are going to be effective. There is some evidence that COX-2 inhibitors have similar efficacy, but they have no advantage, and there are concerns about their long-term cardiovascular safety. NSAIDs have been shown to slow the progression of joint damage when used regularly over a two-year period. However, daily use over a prolonged period increases the risk of side effects, and, if there is difficulty controlling symptoms, a second line drug should probably be used.

SULFASALAZINE is the traditional second line drug with the best evidence supporting its use in AS. It is most effective in those patients with involved joints outside the spine such as knees and ankles and has very little effect on spinal disease. AZATHIOPRINE and METHOTREXATE are used in severe AS, but there is little evidence of their efficacy. Some patients will respond but many will not. Treatment trials should be limited to three to four months at adequate dose, and the treatment stopped if there is no response. CORTICOSTEROIDS should only be used for local injection into inflamed joints or entheses, in which situation they are often very effective. THALIDOMIDE has shown some promise, but the side effect rate is high, and good controlled studies still need to be done. The BISPHOSPHONATE drug, PAMIDRONATE, improves symptoms and function in patients taking NSAIDs to a modest degree. High doses are required. Radiotherapy was used in the 1930s for spinal disease with good responses but stopped when it was discovered that these patients had an increased risk of getting leukemia. These days, radiotherapy can still be used occasionally in small doses to treat local problems such as refractory Achilles tendinitis that has not responded to all other treatment.

TUMOR NECROSIS FACTOR ANTAGONISTS (TNF antagonists) have radically altered the management of severe and refractory AS. There are three agents currently in use: INFLIXIMAB, ADALIMUMAB, and ETANERCEPT (see tumor necrosis factor antagonists for more detailed discussion). They are all effective in AS, and there are no comparisons between them. About 80 percent of AS patients treated with TNF antagonists, i.e., those with the most active disease, will respond to some extent. Unlike with other DMARDs, the response is often rapid, with some patients who were struggling to dress themselves going back to a physical job two days after their first infusion of infliximab. The beneficial effect does not appear to wear off although the longest formal study of this is currently three years. The incidence of HLA-B27-related eye inflammation is also reduced, and there is some evidence that patients who do not respond to the initial TNF antagonist may respond to a different agent. Younger patients with shorter duration of disease, high inflammatory markers (ESR and CRP), and fewer fixed mechanical problems respond best, but this does not mean that other patients will not respond. Despite the effectiveness of the TNF antagonists in treating AS, there is still some progression of X-ray changes.

The chief risk associated with TNF antagonists is infections. These include reactivation of tuberculosis and diminished resistance to common infectious organisms. There is also a slightly increased risk of certain tumors and autoimmune phenomena (see also tumor necrosis factor antagonists). As this is a relatively new treatment, only being licensed by the FDA for treatment of AS in 2004, the long-term effects remain unknown. The other caution in their use is their considerable cost. Infliximab is given as intermittent infusions that can be spaced out to one every two or three months in good responders. Allergic reactions can occur at the time of infusion, and it needs to be given in a hospital or clinic setting. Etanercept is given as a once or twice weekly injection, and adalimumab is injected fortnightly. Both of these are usually self-administered by the patient. The TNF antagonists have been used in rheumatoid arthritis in conjunction with methotrexate or another DMARD, ostensibly to prevent patients developing antibodies that might neutralize the TNF antagonist (as they are proteins that the immune system may recognize as foreign) but also providing additional anti-inflammatory treatment. In AS, where these DMARDs are considerably less effective, there is limited evidence that TNF antagonists can be used as sole agents without loss of effect due to neutralizing antibodies.

If the hip joint is severely damaged, total joint replacement can dramatically improve a patient's quality of life. This is a common operation in AS. However, many patients are young at the time of surgery and are likely to need a second operation years later to replace the artificial hip when it wears out. Patients with AS who undergo hip replacement surgery have a greater chance of developing heterotopic ossification, a condition where new bone grows around and into the new joint, thus restricting its motion. To prevent heterotopic ossification, many orthopedic surgeons treat the hip with a low dose of radiotherapy before surgery. Surgery is also occasionally used to correct a severe spinal deformity when the patient is bent so far forward that forward vision is impossible. The majority of patients with AS can lead an active life and continue to work. Indeed, some patients with mild disease who have had back pain but never sought medical advice for it are diagnosed only when a routine X-ray late in life shows the typical findings of AS. Patients with AS have a 10 times greater risk of spinal fracture than the general population. Most of these are sustained in simple falls, an unusual cause in those without AS. Patients with early onset of disease, peripheral joint and especially hip involvement, high ESR, or a poor response to NSAIDs have a poorer outcome. Smoking also worsens the prognosis. AS does not, however, significantly reduce longevity.

Risk Factors and Preventive Measures

The major risk factors are genetic. HLA-B27 plays a major role as discussed above, but other genes including those involved in CYTOKINE production clearly play a role. Although 98 percent of AS patients of European extraction will have HLA-B27, only a minority of the general population with HLA-B27 will ever develop AS. It is therefore not a useful test to screen people for risk of developing the disease. If an individual has HLA-B27 and a first-degree relative with AS, then the risk is much higher, but again a positive test does not mean that the disease is inevitable. There are no preventive measures.

anticardiolipin antibody syndrome See ANTIPHOSPHOLIPID ANTIBODY SYNDROME.

antineutrophil cytoplasmic antibody (ANCA) See Appendix II.

antinuclear antibody (ANA)   See Appendix II.

antiphospholipid antibody syndrome   This is also known as anticardiolipin antibody syndrome or lupus anticoagulant syndrome. This syndrome is characterized by an increased risk of venous or arterial blood clots (thrombosis), recurrent mid- to late-pregnancy loss, and thrombocytopenia in individuals who have antibodies to phospholipids. The antiphospholipid antibody syndrome may be primary, when it occurs alone, or secondary, when it is found in association with another autoimmune disease. SYSTEMIC LUPUS ERYTHEMATOSUS (SLE) is the most common cause of secondary antiphospholipid antibody syndrome, but less common causes are RHEUMATOID ARTHRITIS, SCLERODERMA, and SJÖGREN'S SYNDROME.

Antiphospholipid antibodies were first recognized as causing a false-positive test result in early blood tests for syphilis. These antibodies do not always result in complications. When complications such as thrombosis do occur in patients who have the antibodies, they are diagnosed with antiphospholipid antibody syndrome. Approximately 3 percent of healthy people have antiphospholipid antibodies, but many never develop the antiphospholipid antibody syndrome. Treatment with some drugs, for example chlorpromazine, quinidine, and hydralazine, can induce antiphospholipid antibodies. These drug-induced antiphospholipid antibodies, and those found in association with HIV infection, are seldom associated with thrombosis.

The term lupus anticoagulant was coined when it was recognized that some patients with SLE had antibodies that acted as anticoagulants in the laboratory by prolonging tests of blood clotting such as the Russell viper venom time or activated partial thromboplastin time. However, the term lupus anticoagulant turned out to be a misnomer. The anticoagulant effects occur only in the test tube. These patients in fact have an increased risk of blood clots, rather than excessive bleeding that would be expected if the antibody acted as an anticoagulant. It was also a misnomer because many people who had a positive lupus anticoagulant test did not have lupus. The antiphospholipid antibody syndrome and the lupus anticoagulant syndrome are now known to be related, and some patients who have an antiphospholipid antibody also have a positive lupus anticoagulant test. However, the overlap is not complete, and sometimes one test is positive and the other negative. Both tests are associated with an increased risk of thrombosis. In addition to antiphospholipid antibodies, it is now known that other antibodies, for example beta$_2$-glycoprotein antibodies, play an important role in the development of the syndrome.

It is not clear how antiphospholipid antibodies that decrease blood clotting in laboratory tests increase clotting in people. Several theories have been proposed. Normal endothelium (the thin layer of cells lining the inside of blood vessels) has complex protective mechanisms to prevent thrombosis (i.e., has an anticoagulant effect). Many of the antibodies found in this syndrome in fact bind to beta$_2$-glycoprotein I and prothrombin. Beta$_2$-glycoprotein I and prothrombin are proteins that bind to phospholipids on cell walls in the process of thrombus formation. One popular theory of how the antiphospholipid syndrome occurs is that the antibodies interfere with these mechanisms and thereby allow thrombosis to occur. The underlying trigger that results in the formation of antiphospholipid antibodies is not known. Indeed, the presence of the antiphospholipid syndrome simply seems to tip the body's normal balance between thrombosis and anticoagulation in favor of thrombosis. A further prothrombotic event can then more easily lead to thrombosis. Such events include smoking, pregnancy, estrogen use (either in a contraceptive pill or hormone replacement therapy), malignancy, nephrotic syndrome, hospitalization, long-haul flights, or atherosclerotic vascular disease.

Symptoms and Diagnostic Path
Most individuals with antiphospholipid antibodies do not have symptoms unless a complication occurs. A thin, lacy, red-purple rash, livedo reticularis, is common but does not cause symptoms. Patients with associated diseases such as SLE will have the usual symptoms of that disease.

Pregnancy loss   A common complication is repeated miscarriage, often occurring in the second half of pregnancy. Up to 50 percent of women with high levels of IgG antiphospholipid antibodies will have some pregnancy loss. Lower levels and IgM or IgA antibodies are associated with a lower rate of complications. Overall, the antiphospholipid syndrome is not a common cause of pregnancy loss. Pregnancies that do not end in miscarriage have a greater chance of delivering prematurely, thereby placing the immature infant at risk. In pregnancies that carry on to term, fetal growth is often poor because the placenta does not function well and the supply of nutrients to the unborn baby is inadequate.

Thrombosis The antiphospholipid antibody syndrome is often diagnosed when someone spontaneously develops blood clots in his or her arteries or veins. Deep vein thrombosis (DVT) most often occurs in the veins of the legs but can occur anywhere. This can be dangerous if the clot breaks off and lodges in the blood vessels of the lungs (pulmonary embolus) since this is sometimes fatal. Arterial thrombosis reduces blood supply to the organ affected and can result in stroke, myocardial infarction (heart attack), or gangrene of a limb. As with other complications, the antiphospholipid syndrome is not a common cause of these vascular problems. It should be suspected when thromboses occur in young patients, nonsmokers, or in unusual sites.

Other complications These include leg ulcers, heart valve irregularities known as vegetations, and nervous system complications such as stroke. Thrombocytopenia is common but is usually mild and seldom leads to complications such as bleeding. Catastrophic antiphospholipid antibody syndrome is rare but often fatal. It was given this name because in addition to clots occluding the blood supply to limbs, several organs such the lungs, kidneys, and brain are affected.

The diagnosis of antiphospholipid antibody syndrome is difficult and requires a high index of suspicion. Recurrent thromboses, thrombosis in a person for no apparent reason, or recurrent mid trimester abortions usually trigger diagnostic testing. The tests performed should include tests for both anticardiolipin antibodies and lupus anticoagulant (see Appendix II). Because the antiphospholipid syndrome is so common in patients with SLE, lupus patients are often screened to assess their risk of thrombosis. Internationally agreed criteria for diagnosing the antiphospholipid antibody syndrome are known as the Sapporo criteria. These include one or more venous or arterial thrombosis or adverse pregnancy outcome as discussed above, plus a clearly positive test for one of the antibodies or lupus anticoagulant. The blood tests should be repeatable after at least 12 weeks to exclude transiently positive tests associated with an acute event but not causative. Antiphospholipid antibodies can cross-react with the antibodies detected by some blood tests for syphilis, resulting in a false-positive test for that disease.

Treatment Options and Outlook

Patients with primary antiphospholipid syndrome who have not yet had a complication such as a thrombosis are at low risk of thrombosis, and there is no safe medication that will significantly lessen their risk. It is vital for these individuals to avoid other predisposing factors for thrombosis such as smoking and the contraceptive pill. However, those patients with another connective tissue disease such as SLE with positive antiphospholipid antibodies but no thrombosis are at higher risk and are often prescribed low-dose aspirin. They may also benefit from HYDROXYCHLOROQUINE for which there is reasonable evidence although no randomized CLINICAL TRIAL has been done. Patients who have already had a thrombosis are at much higher risk of having recurrent events. Overall, there is an 11 percent recurrence per year, and so prophylactic treatment to prevent this is desirable. The anticoagulant warfarin is the most commonly used medication. This was previously used at high dose, but recent trials have shown that usual dose warfarin is as effective and may be safer, the commonest side effect being bleeding. The dose of warfarin is judged by how long it prolongs a patient's clotting time in a laboratory test. Most patients who have thromboses while taking warfarin do so when the level of this test drops too low. However some patients may thrombose despite good levels and require higher doses of warfarin. In this situation, low-dose aspirin is sometimes added to the usual dose of warfarin, but there is no good evidence that this is effective, at least for venous thrombosis. When there have been serious or recurrent thromboses, prophylactic treatment is recommended for life unless the risks of the treatment become greater than those of the disease.

As with any significant thrombosis, heparin is usually used as the initial anticoagulant. It works differently and much quicker than warfarin but needs to be given by injection. The older "unfractionated" heparin requires laboratory testing to ensure it is at the correct dose, but it has the advantage of being able to be reversed by protamine if there is bleeding. The low molecular weight heparins can be given as under-the-skin injections without monitoring blood tests in many situations. Patients can therefore administer these once or twice a day at home or while traveling. They are particularly useful to cover periods of increased risk such as around surgery or during long-haul flights. Clopidogrel is a newer drug that inhibits platelet stickiness and is therefore useful in preventing arterial clots, as is aspirin. As yet, there is no good evidence concerning its use in antiphospholipid syndrome. The catastrophic antiphospholipid antibody syndrome is often fatal despite all available treatment. The treatments used in this condition include the anticoagulants discussed above, usually in combination, CORTICOSTEROIDS, PLASMAPHARESIS to remove some of the antibodies, and intravenous immunoglobulin.

As warfarin is potentially harmful to a fetus, especially in early pregnancy, low molecular weight heparins are used to treat pregnant patients. This is especially important as pregnancy itself can induce thromboses and the antiphospholipid syndrome has frequent deleterious effects on the fetus. Good results are obtained with self-injection at home often combined with low-dose aspirin. All the heparins can cause OSTEOPOROSIS with prolonged use. Some prophylactic treatment before pregnancy as well as very adequate calcium intake during and after pregnancy is advisable. Although high-dose corticosteroids have been used in pregnancy with some effect, the adverse effects outweigh the benefits.

Risk Factors and Preventive Measures

There are no known risk factors or measures to prevent the development of the antiphospholipid syndrome. Prevention of complications is discussed above.

arthritis Inflammation of joints that results in pain, heat, swelling, and loss of function. Arthritis is not one condition but has many causes, and it affects more than 40 million people in the United States. Arthritis in its many forms causes considerable suffering to the affected individual and is costly for both the individual and society. Direct medical costs for patients with RHEUMATOID ARTHRITIS averaged $8,500 per year in the late 1990s. Half of this was in hospital costs, 26 percent in medication costs, and 8 percent for physician visits. Not only do people with arthritis have these direct costs, but they may also suffer loss of earnings or require modification of their home or workplace. These are known as indirect costs and average out at roughly two and a half times the direct costs.

Approximately 5 percent of people of working age in the United States have some form of arthritis. About 25 percent of workers with rheumatoid arthritis take early retirement because of their disease, as do 14 percent of those with osteoarthritis. This contrasts with 3 percent of those without arthritis taking early retirement because of ill health. Although it is difficult to measure scientifically, several studies now show that effective treatment reduces these costs as well as improves the quality of life.

Treatment of different types of arthritis varies, and classification aids the selection of rational therapy. Arthritis-related conditions can be classified into the following categories:

1. *Degenerative arthritis* (OSTEOARTHRITIS, OA). This is by far the commonest form of arthritis in the world and affects many animal species as well as man. It can be seen as a disease of the cartilage that lines our joints and allows bones to move smoothly, gradually leading to wear and tear (degeneration) of the cartilage. Initially, the characteristics of the synovial fluid between the two layers of cartilage change, allowing abrasion of the outer layer, loss of water content, and then fissuring, and finally progressive loss of cartilage depth. All this reduces the shock- and friction-absorbing functions of cartilage leading to bone changes as well. When the joint no longer functions normally, the joint capsule, tendons, and ligaments and the muscles acting

on that joint may become stressed or weakened, and it is largely these structures that give rise to pain.

There are a number of different types of OA and some important underlying diseases that can give rise to it. A common type known as generalized nodal OA causes the characteristic bony enlargement of the finger joints and carries an increased risk of OA affecting the hips and knees. This type has a strong genetic component, often being passed down in the female line, sometimes skipping a generation. There are other rare genetic types due to a known defect in type II collagen that is an important constituent of cartilage. Overall, however, the major risk factor for OA is being overweight. Some occupations are risk factors for OA in particular joints, e.g., farmers are at increased risk of getting hip OA. Diseases such as HEMOCHROMATOSIS and Wilson's disease can cause metabolic problems in the cartilage and should always be considered when people develop OA at a young age or when there is a strong family history of OA. Injury to a joint (including surgery) or the adjacent bones can lead to OA. Even poor alignment due to postural problems can over a long period of time cause OA of the stressed joints.

Treatment in the early stages consists largely of pain relief and exercises to maintain as normal function as possible. Later on anti-inflammatory medication such as NSAIDs or JOINT INJECTION may be necessary. At this stage, aids, orthotics, and finding different ways of doing things that stress the joints less may be helpful. When the joint fails, surgery can be done to either fuse the joint or replace it with an artificial one. (See also ARTHRODESIS; JOINT REPLACEMENT.)

2. *Arthritis caused by crystal deposition.* When substances such as uric acid reach high enough concentrations in the blood, they form crystals and deposit out in the tissues. This may have no consequences at all. However, under the right circumstances, these crystals can cause intense inflammation or varying degrees of chronic or intermittent inflammation between these extremes. So people who develop GOUT have usually had high uric acid levels for many years with crystal deposition occurring in many tis-

sues, including within the joints. An event such as trauma, change in temperature, change in acid base balance, or sudden intake of purines (the precursors of uric acid) causes the crystals to break free in the joint, and this excites the acute inflammatory response that is called gout. Initially, this will settle even without treatment but over a number of years will become more frequent, last longer, be more difficult to treat, and eventually there will no longer be disease-free periods between attacks. Initially the big toe and ankles are most frequently affected but, if untreated, gout can spread to involve most joints and especially those with previous damage.

Once crystals form, they facilitate the deposition of more crystals and can build up into firm lumps of uric acid that can cause pressure problems, including eroding through skin, and damage bone and joints. When they form in the kidney, there is probably low-grade inflammation, but this is silent (i.e., not felt by the patient). However, over many years, they can cause kidney damage and are a surprisingly frequent finding in end-stage kidney disease in autopsy studies. Treatment involves three distinct aims. Firstly, NSAIDs are usually used to treat the acute attacks although CORTICOSTEROIDS are sometimes required, either orally or injected. If attacks are frequent it may be necessary to use NSAIDs, COLCHICINE, or corticosteroids to prevent recurrent attacks. Thirdly, effectively lowering uric acid levels and keeping them low will largely prevent acute attacks and other adverse health outcomes. This can be achieved through a combination of lifestyle measures such as weight loss, dietary modification, alcohol reduction, alteration of medications, and the use of uric acid–lowering medication. These drugs either slow uric acid production (ALLOPURINOL) or increase its excretion (PROBENECID).

CALCIUM PYROPHOSPHATE DIHYDRATE DEPOSITION DISEASE (CPPD) similarly causes a range of diseases from acute arthritis very similar to gout (pseudogout) to a low-grade grumbling arthritis more like rheumatoid arthritis. Wrists and knees are the most frequently affected joints.

The hallmark of CPPD is chondrocalcinosis, which is a line of calcium pyrophosphate within a joint seen on an X-ray. However, this can exist without causing any problems and not everyone with CPPD will have chondrocalcinosis. The calcium pyrophosphate crystal is difficult to identify in the routine laboratory, and diagnosis is probably frequently missed because of this. Two broad groups of people get CPPD although it is by no means limited to these groups. The first are people with some abnormality in the way their bodies handle calcium. They usually get CPPD at a young age. The other, larger group are older people with established OA. Treatment at one end of the spectrum is similar to that of acute gout and at the other rheumatoid arthritis treatments are occasionally used. (See also MILWAUKEE SHOULDER.)

3. *Rheumatoid arthritis* (RA). The commonest of the chronic inflammatory arthritides, rheumatoid arthritis affects about 1 percent of the population, usually starting between the ages of 40 and 60 years. The cause is not known. It causes pain, swelling, and ultimately damage to many joints. Typically the small joints of the hands, toes, and wrists are affected, but in time major joints such as knees, hips, and shoulders will also become involved. Even joints such as the temporomandibular (jaw) and voice box can be affected. Tissues other than joints can be affected including skin, lungs, heart, and bowel, but this is much less common with the improvement in treatment over the past 20 years. Treatment is aimed at relieving pain, preventing damage, maintaining joint function, and preserving muscle strength and functional capacity. This can be a very complex process and involve altering the patient's situation and use of aids as well as medications including painkillers, NSAIDs, corticosteroids, DISEASE MODIFYING ANTIRHEUMATIC DRUGS, PHYSICAL THERAPY, and surgery. (See RHEUMATOID ARTHRITIS, SYNOVECTOMY, and JOINT REPLACEMENT). Patients with RA develop atherosclerotic complications at a younger age, and consequently efforts to prevent these have become especially important now that patients are living longer and more active lives.

4. *Seronegative arthritis.* This group of inflammatory arthritides was grouped under the term *seronegative* arthritis to distinguish them from rheumatoid arthritis (presumed to be rheumatoid factor positive). As only 70 percent of patients with rheumatoid arthritis are *seropositive* for rheumatoid factor, this is not a very useful term, but the name has stuck. They do however share several characteristics and in practice are easily distinguished from rheumatoid arthritis except for the rheumatoid form of psoriatic arthritis. They all have a strong association with the HLA-B27 gene although for psoriatic arthritis this is only for the spondylitic form. This association is strongest for ANKYLOSING SPONDYLITIS. They tend to affect young adults between the ages of 20 and 40 years, but a number of teenagers are also affected. Spondylitis or inflammation of the spine and large sacroiliac joints at the base of the spine is the hallmark of ankylosing spondylitis and is found to a varying degree in the other conditions. Inflammatory arthritis and tendinitis affecting the legs in a nonsymmetrical manner are other characteristic findings. Manifestations can vary considerably between patients, and studies have shown that primary care doctors have difficulty diagnosing these conditions. PSORIATIC ARTHRITIS can be particularly confusing as there are five distinct subtypes.

   Severity varies considerably, and some patients do very well with intermittent use of NSAIDs, while others have crippling and until recently almost untreatable disease. In the last 10 years, the TNF antagonists have been found to be remarkably effective in severely affected patients. Despite REACTIVE ARTHRITIS being initiated by infection, antibiotic therapy has not been found to be effective with the possible exception of treating *Chlamydia*. (See also INFLAMMATORY BOWEL DISEASE.)

5. *Connective tissue disorders.* These disorders are characterized by inflammatory disease that typically affects a number of different organs and evidence of a high level of autoimmunity. This is when an individual's immune system escapes its normal control mechanisms and attacks parts of the individual's own body. This can be demonstrated in a number of ways, but in practice

the usual way is to look for well-known self-reactive autoantibodies (e.g., see Appendix II for ANTINUCLEAR ANTIBODY). Different autoantibodies are useful in the early diagnosis of these diseases, and some give additional information about the risk of complications. Women are affected more frequently than men. There are two age groups when these disorders present most commonly, first in the 20–40 year group and then in those over 60 years. Skin and joints are frequently involved in all these conditions but in addition muscle, brain, nerves, heart, lungs, kidneys, and blood may all be involved although not in the same person. The different disorders have been separated out because they have distinguishable clinical courses and outcomes, and this allows more effective study of the optimum treatment in different situations. Typically, treatment will depend on the particular manifestation that a patient has. (See also SCLERODERMA; SJÖGREN'S SYNDROME; and SYSTEMIC LUPUS ERYTHEMATOSUS.)

6. *Infective arthritis.* When bacteria get into joints, they can invoke an intense inflammatory reaction that will cause irreversible damage to the joint quite quickly if not appropriately treated. Recognizing that the arthritis is infective is therefore very important. The organism can get into the joint via the bloodstream, because of soft tissue infection close by or because of trauma (including surgery) to the joint. Patients with rheumatoid arthritis are at high risk of infective arthritis both because they are often mildly immunocompromised and because their joints have much increased blood flow. All immunosuppressed patients are also at higher risk. Treatment usually consists of a combination of washing the joint out repeatedly and appropriate antibiotics.

7. *Arthritis caused by metabolic and systemic diseases.* A disparate group of diseases can cause arthritis by causing abnormalities in cartilage (ACROMEGALY, HEMOCHROMATOSIS), bone (PAGET'S DISEASE, SICKLE-CELL DISEASE), or by causing inflammation in joints (HEMOPHILIA). For most of these, early recognition of the primary disorder and its effective treatment will limit the severity of the arthritis.

Symptoms and Diagnostic Path

A diagnosis of a particular type of arthritis is usually made mainly on the symptoms and physical findings. Laboratory tests and X-rays are sometimes helpful but are seldom absolutely diagnostic (see Appendix II). Examination of synovial fluid (see JOINT ASPIRATION) is important in the diagnosis of arthritis caused by infections and crystal deposition, for example gout. For a few rheumatic problems, for example VASCULITIS, a biopsy of tissue, often skin or a superficial nerve, can be diagnostic.

The following clinical features of arthritis aid the diagnosis.

1. Whether it is inflammatory or noninflammatory
2. Whether its onset is acute or chronic
3. The number of joints involved and their distribution
4. The characteristics of the individual that predispose him or her to arthritis
5. The involvement of organs other than the joints

Inflammatory and noninflammatory arthritis Inflammatory arthritis (RA, seronegative arthritis, crystal-induced arthritis, infective arthritis) causes pain, often worse in the morning, swelling, warmth, redness, pain on movement, and several hours of stiffness after arising. Noninflammatory arthritis (degenerative arthritis) causes pain, often worse at night, and stiffness usually lasting only a few minutes after a joint has been in one position for a while. Soft tissue swelling, warmth, and redness are usually absent.

Acute and chronic arthritis Acute onset of severe symptoms occurring overnight is typical of crystal-induced and infective arthritis. Most other types of arthritis have a more gradual onset, and degenerative arthritis typically becomes slowly more noticeable over years.

The number and distribution of affected joints Arthritis can affect many joints (polyarticular), a few joints (pauciarticular or oligoarticular), or one joint (monarticular). The distribution of affected joints can be symmetrical, typically involving the same joints on both sides of the body, or asymmetrical, affecting scattered joints.

Individual characteristics Different types of arthritis are more likely to affect people with certain characteristics at particular stages of their life. For example, gout most commonly affects middle-aged men who are overweight and drink alcohol and elderly women who are on treatment for high blood pressure or heart failure. Connective tissue diseases like systemic lupus erythematosus (SLE) largely affect young women, and rheumatoid arthritis usually starts between the ages of 40 and 60 years.

Organ involvement Connective tissue diseases typically affect organs other than the joints, especially the skin, blood, nervous system, kidneys, heart, lungs, and muscle. The organs involved may give clues to which type of arthritis it is. For example, the skin changes in a patient with scleroderma point to that diagnosis. Other diseases such as acromegaly will usually be diagnosed because of the other organs involved before the arthritis becomes a problem. The characteristics of various types of arthritis are summarized in the following table. There is, however, considerable overlap, and clinical features are only clues and are not diagnostic.

**CLINICAL FEATURES OF
DIFFERENT TYPES OF ARTHRITIS**

Arthritis	Inflammatory	Acute	Symmetrical	Polyarticular
Osteoarthritis	-	-	-	±
Crystal-induced	+	+	-	-
Rheumatoid arthritis	+	-	+	+
Seronegative	+	±	-	±
Connective tissue disorders	±	±	±	±
Infective	+	+	-	-
Metabolic/ systemic	±	+	-	-

Treatment Options and Outlook

The aims of treatment are

1. Relief of pain and suffering
2. Maintenance and restoration of function
3. Prevention of disease progression

The treatment of the various types of arthritis depends on the diagnosis, the severity of disease, the individual patient's response to different therapies, and a person's needs. Treatment may involve a combination of physical therapy and exercises, lifestyle alterations, medications, and surgery. The treatment of specific types of arthritis is described under their individual entries but is summarized in the table on page 19.

The prognosis of arthritis differs according to the diagnosis, severity of disease, and treatment and is discussed under individual entries. People with certain forms of arthritis also develop related health problems such as lung, heart, and kidney disease more frequently than average. Paying careful attention to these will also improve the patient's quality of life.

arthrocentesis   See JOINT ASPIRATION in Appendix II.

arthrodesis   A procedure in which a damaged joint that cannot be replaced is surgically fused. The remains of the joint are removed and the ends of the two bones fixed in place by screws or by a rod running through the bones until they have united. The advantages of arthrodesis are that it gives stability and excellent pain relief to severely damaged joints. However, a disadvantage is that all movement is lost. The procedure is most useful for joints that are causing severe pain and where stability is more important than movement such as the distal interphalangeal joints and the proximal interphalangeal joint of the index finger. Before proceeding with arthrodesis, the future implications need to be considered with regard to the individual patient's functional needs, the demands that will be put on the joint, and the state of the surrounding joints. For example, arthrodesis of one disorganized wrist can improve grip strength considerably. However, if both wrists were fused, personal hygiene would become very difficult. Although arthrodesis of the ankle leads to significant gait problems, it is still sometimes done for crippling pain because JOINT REPLACEMENT surgery at the ankle remains problematic.

COMMON TYPES OF ARTHRITIS AND THEIR TREATMENT

Type of Arthritis	Diagnosis	Goals of Treatment	Commonly Used Drugs*
Inflammatory Arthritis	Rheumatoid arthritis (RA)	Decrease pain, maintain/ improve function, RA remission if possible; if remission is not possible, the goal is to control RA.	One or more of methotrexate, sulfasalazine, hydroxychloroquine, leflunomide, cyclosporine azathioprine, gold, TNF antagonist, ± prednisone, ± an NSAID.
	Gout	Control the pain of acute gout attacks, control the problem by decreasing uric acid levels in the blood and so prevent future gout.	NSAIDs or colchicine to control acute attacks; allopurinol or uricosurics to decrease the uric acid in the blood.
	Pseudogout (CPPD)	Control the pain of acute pseudogout attacks, prevent attacks if possible.	NSAIDs, sometimes corticosteroids or colchicine.
	Psoriatic arthritis, reactive arthritis, arthritis of inflammatory bowel disease	Decrease pain, maintain/improve function, remission if possible; if remission is not possible, the goal is to control disease activity.	An NSAID ± one or more of methotrexate, sulfasalazine, hydroxychloroquine, gold, cyclosporine, TNF antagonist.
	Ankylosing spondylitis	Decrease pain, maintain/improve function, and prevent deformity.	An NSAID, sometimes with methotrexate, sulfasalazine, or TNF antagonist if the problem is detected early.
Degenerative joint disease	Osteoarthritis (OA)	Decrease pain, maintain/improve function.	Acetaminophen; NSAID.
Connective tissue or autoimmune diseases	Systemic lupus erythematosus (SLE)	Prevent organ damage, improve symptoms, control disease activity.	Prednisone + one or more of hydroxychloroquine, azathioprine, cyclophosphamide, methotrexate.
	Scleroderma	Prevent organ damage, improve symptoms, maintain joint mobility.	Blood pressure treatment, antireflux treatment to improve swallowing, treatment of Raynaud's.
	Dermatomyositis and polymyositis	Restore and maintain muscle strength, remission if possible; if not possible, control disease activity.	Prednisone ± one or more of azathioprine, cyclophosphamide, methotrexate, cyclosporine.
Vasculitis	Temporal arteritis	Prevent organ damage (blindness), remission if possible; if not possible, control disease activity.	Prednisone, often alone, but sometimes with azathioprine or methotrexate.
	Wegener's granulomatosus and polyarteritis nodosa	Prevent organ damage, improve symptoms, remission if possible; if not possible, control disease activity.	Prednisone + cyclophosphamide, or sometimes methotrexate, leflunomide, or azathioprine.
Fibromyalgia	Fibromyalgia	Decrease pain, maintain/improve function.	Aerobic exercise, antidepressants, muscle relaxers, sometimes NSAIDs.
Tendinitis/bursitis	Tendinitis/bursitis	Wait for it to get better, decrease pain, maintain/improve function.	Rest, sometimes NSAIDs, sometimes corticosteroid injections.
Osteoporosis	Osteoporosis	Prevent bone loss and prevent fractures.	Adequate calcium and vitamin D plus one of the following: Estrogens, SERMs, bisphosphonates, calcitonin.

*Medicines are only part of the treatment of arthritis problems. For many problems, exercise, physical therapy, or surgery can be very important.

arthroplasty   See JOINT REPLACEMENT.

arthroscopy and arthroscopic surgery   In its simplest form this involves direct visualization of the structures inside a joint through a tube. Modern arthroscopes have improved sources of light, and the image is magnified and transmitted to a video screen via a fiberoptic cable. Instruments can be inserted through separate entry points around a joint, improving surgery by a technique known as triangulation. Arthroscopy is used both to obtain a clear view of anatomical abnormalities that may be the cause of a patient's symptoms and to perform surgery to correct the abnormalities. As recently as the 1960s the value of arthroscopy was still being debated in the United States. However, with improvements in instrumentation and video technology as well as the diagnostic and therapeutic techniques, it has evolved into a widely used and valuable procedure. Although arthroscopic diagnosis has been partially displaced by MRI over the last decade, the role of arthroscopic surgery is continually expanding. Advantages include precise diagnosis, very small skin and joint capsule incisions, relatively brief disability and rapid rehabilitation, as well as a better cosmetic outcome than open surgery. Many arthroscopic procedures can be performed under regional anesthesia, and most patients are discharged home on the same day. The risk of infection is lower than with open surgery.

The knee is a large accessible joint with complex internal organization subject to large stresses that frequently lead to structural abnormalities. It is thus the ideal joint for this type of procedure. The first arthroscopy was performed on the knee using a modified cystoscope (used for looking into the bladder) in Japan in 1931. Lesions in the knee that are amenable to arthroscopic surgery include meniscal injury or degeneration (see MENISCAL TEARS), ligament injury, OSTEOCHONDRITIS DISSECANS, LOOSE BODIES, PATELLOFEMORAL DISORDERS, synovial diseases, OSTEOARTHRITIS, and fractures of the surface of the tibia.

Although most arthroscopic surgery has been done on the knee, several other joints are also suitable. In the shoulder, tears of the glenoid labrum (the rim of supporting cartilage around the shoulder joint—see SHOULDER PAIN), capsule, biceps tendon, or rotator cuff may be identified and repaired. Loose bodies can be removed and synovial or joint surface abnormalities repaired. Arthroscopic surgery is particularly useful in the subacromial space just above the shoulder joint where the rotator cuff tendons can be repaired and the undersurface of the acromion and acromioclavicular joint can be smoothed without disrupting the overlying muscles.

Arthroscopy is frequently used at the elbow to remove loose bodies and osteophytes. The cause of chronic wrist pain can be very difficult to determine, and special arthroscopes have been developed to assist with this. In the ankle, arthroscopy is helpful in diagnosing difficult ankle problems as well as treating synovial impingement, loose bodies, osteophytes, and irregularities caused by healed hairline fractures. Although arthroscopy has been less frequently employed at the hip, the potential benefits from avoiding open surgical exposure of this deep joint suggest that it will continue to have a role despite the disadvantages of limited maneuverability and a small joint space.

assistive devices   These include any device that improves the functional capacity of someone with a disability brought about by a rheumatic disease. Disability in this context means the lack of ability to perform an activity in the manner or within the range considered normal for a human being. In the assessment of the impact of rheumatic diseases, these abilities or activities of daily living are often grouped into functional classes or domains. Some of the important domains are listed below, together with examples of relevant assistive devices.

• *Locomotion* Many types of cane, crutch, or walker may be used to unload a damaged or painful joint. Manual or electric wheelchairs may be used to cover distances that would otherwise be impossible.

• *Transport* Spinner knobs on steering wheels may enable someone with severe arthritis in the hands to drive. Hand controls for the brakes and the accelerator may do the same for those with severely affected legs.

- *Personal Hygiene* Many aids, including handheld shower nozzles, grab rails to aid entry to the bath or shower, long-handled combs, electric toothbrushes, glove-shaped washcloths with soap pockets, and toothpaste squeezers, can make life easier for those with painful joints or loss of range of movement.
- *Dressing* Velcro closures for shoes and clothing as well as modified clothing.
- *Feeding* Large-handled utensils, a rocker knife that is used with a rocking rather than chopping or cutting motion, jar openers, and many nonslip items.
- *Communication* Rubber-tipped devices for typing, voice-activated tape recorders, and auto-dial telephones.
- *Housework* Wheeled carts, long-handled reachers, see-through pots, electric can openers and food processors.

atrial myxoma A rare, benign heart tumor that most often occurs in the left atrium. The diagnosis is often difficult because the symptoms of atrial myxoma can mimic other illnesses, including rheumatological conditions such as VASCULITIS. Symptoms include:

1. Systemic symptoms such as fever, weight loss, myalgia, and arthralgia.
2. Embolic symptoms that result from small fragments of the tumor, or small blood clots from the tumor surface, breaking off into the circulation and finally blocking blood vessels in other organs. These tumor emboli may cause stroke, blood in the urine, and a skin rash.

Blood tests may show nonspecific abnormalities such as anemia and a raised ESR compatible with inflammation. The myxoma can be detected by echocardiography (ultrasound scan of the heart). Treatment by surgical removal is usually curative and recurrence is unusual.

autoimmunity See IMMUNE RESPONSE.

avascular necrosis (AVN; also known as osteonecrosis and aseptic necrosis) Death of an area of bone marrow and bone resulting in loss of normal architecture. Avascular necrosis is not a specific disease but is the end result of any condition that decreases the circulation to an area of bone to the extent that the bone dies. AVN can occur in almost any bone but does so more commonly at the ends of long bones. Thus it often affects bone that contributes to the normal architecture of the hip, shoulder, or knee joints. AVN is relatively common and is the underlying cause of arthritis in approximately 10 percent of people undergoing joint replacement.

The cause of AVN is not well understood. However, a feature common to most theories is that the blood supply to an area of bone is inadequate, resulting in bone infarcts. Interruption of blood supply to bone can result from:

1. Mechanical factors, for example a fracture or dislocation that damages a blood vessel
2. Blockage of a blood vessel by clot (thrombosis or embolus), fat (fat embolus), or nitrogen bubbles (rapid decompression in divers)
3. Damage to a blood vessel, either directly, for example by VASCULITIS, or indirectly by neighboring inflammation causing swelling and pressure

Sometimes AVN occurs without any recognized underlying predisposing factor and is termed idiopathic, but often it occurs in the presence of recognized risk factors. These include trauma, alcohol abuse, corticosteroid therapy, SYSTEMIC LUPUS ERYTHEMATOSUS (SLE), SICKLE-CELL DISEASE, vasculitis, and rapid decompression in deep-sea divers.

Symptoms and Diagnostic Path
Pain in the affected bone is common. The severity of the pain varies from a mild dull ache in chronic forms of AVN to incapacitating pain during acute infarction of bone. If the bone infarct is large, this area can weaken and partially collapse over months or years. If this occurs in bone that forms part of a joint, a relatively small alteration in structure can alter the biomechanics of the joint substantially and lead to severe degenerative arthritis. The symptoms during the late stages of AVN are

those of severe OSTEOARTHRITIS, specifically pain that increases when the joint is used.

The symptoms and clinical findings of AVN are not specific. X-ray changes occur relatively late, and several months must pass before areas of increased bone density are visible. In the early stages of AVN, magnetic resonance imaging or a radionuclide bone scan (see Appendix II) show characteristic features before X-ray changes occur and are useful for diagnosis. AVN is often bilateral. Both hips should therefore be scanned even if only one side is painful.

Treatment Options and Outlook

If AVN affects a weight-bearing bone, then avoidance of weight bearing by using crutches in the acute phase protects against loss of normal architecture. If AVN affecting the hip joint is diagnosed before the bone has collapsed, some orthopedic surgeons recommend a surgical approach known as core decompression. The surgery involves drilling into the head of the femur and removing a narrow core of bone and bone marrow. Research has shown that the pressure in the bone marrow of a joint affected by AVN is high. This increased pressure is thought to compromise the blood supply to the affected area of bone. Removing a core of tissue reduces the pressure and may improve the blood supply to the area of bone undergoing AVN. The efficacy of core decompression surgery to treat AVN of the hip has not been evaluated in rigorous controlled studies. Late in the evolution of AVN, joint replacement surgery may be needed if the normal architecture of a joint such as the hip is destroyed and function is lost or pain is severe.

Risk Factors and Preventive Measures

The two most common risk factors identifiable in patients suffering AVN are corticosteroid therapy and alcohol use, both usually in large doses. However, AVN has been described with both short- and low-dose courses of CORTICOSTEROIDS, and these should never be regarded as trivial. Other well-recognized risk factors include SLE, especially when associated with the ANTIPHOSPHOLIPID ANTIBODY SYNDROME or high-dose corticosteroid use, sickle-

cell disease, vasculitis, and rapid decompression in deep-sea and SCUBA divers. There are well-established maximum dive times at various depths as well as surfacing speeds, adherence to which would prevent most cases of decompression sickness and its complications. Corticosteroids should always be used at the lowest possible dose for as short a period as possible to prevent side effects. Because AVN is a relatively rare side effect this approach is usually adopted primarily for other reasons rather than to prevent AVN. Most patients who develop AVN because of corticosteroid therapy have had prolonged treatment with relatively high doses for life-threatening illnesses, and it is unlikely that the majority of corticosteroid-associated cases of AVN could be prevented. Alcohol should similarly be used in moderation for many other reasons apart from preventing AVN. As AVN is a rare complication of the antiphospholipid antibody syndrome, itself a fairly rare disease, it is not known whether effective anticoagulation prevents it in this situation.

AVN   See AVASCULAR NECROSIS.

Ayurvedic medicine   A complementary, holistic approach to health based on ancient Hindu texts. It is traced back to the sages of ancient India. These rishis are believed to have discovered the principles of Ayurveda during deep meditation. These principles were codified in the Vedas (knowledge) that form the religious texts of Hinduism. The Atharva-Veda is the source of Ayurveda. The basis of Ayurveda is understanding a person's dosha. There are three doshas or types that can be initially viewed as being similar to the common body types: ectomorph (light and slim), endomorph (heavy and big boned), and mesomorph (muscular and medium build). On top of these physical characteristics are layered information about learning styles, emotional tendencies, and spiritual inclinations. The three doshas are termed Vata, Pitta, and Kapha. One is usually dominant and one secondary.

These not only describe people but also determine what foods they should eat and what lifestyles are appropriate for them. According to this model, arthritis is thought to result from weakened digestion, poor diet, and disturbed equilibrium. Treatment of arthritis is not standardized. Individualized therapy can include steam baths, enemas, massage, bloodletting, herbs, exercises, yoga, fasting, and avoiding alcohol, meat, and certain vegetables. Ayurvedic approaches to medicine have not been adequately evaluated in well-designed studies.

B

back pain A surgeon in the United States can operate on someone in the Middle East with a remote-controlled device. Scientists can build specific proteins to block complex molecules secreted by white blood cells in the body or to deliver drugs to a specific subset of cells in the body. Researchers can even predict the later development of certain cancers at the time individuals are born. However, we have no answer to the rising epidemic of simple low-back pain. This does not mean that back pain is new. There is a written description of sciatica dating back to 1500 B.C. and back pain appears to have been a common problem in medical writings from the 1800s. In particular, the disability associated with back pain is on the increase rather than back pain itself. Studies in Scandinavian countries over the last 40 years show no increase in the rate of occurrence of back pain over that time. There is no evidence to suggest that the pathology or nature of the problem is changing. However, the percentage of Swedish workers taking time off work because of back pain increased from 1 percent in 1970 to 8 percent in 1992, and the average number of days they took off increased from 20 to 39 per year. Why, when people do less physical work and the treatment possibilities are so much greater, should disability increase? The answers may be as much sociocultural as medical. Between 1991–93, the Swedish government progressively reduced sickness benefits (although they remain generous), and total sick leave for back pain fell from 28 million days in 1987 to 19.2 million days in 1995. Studies in less developed countries like Oman and Nepal show that back pain is extremely common, but very few people are disabled because of it. Hardly anyone in these countries takes to their bed or stays off work because of back pain.

Population surveys show that around 60 percent of adults have experienced low-back pain at some time, a figure confirmed in several developed countries. In the 45- to 59-year-old age group, this rises to about 70 percent. Many of these people will have had short-lived back pain not requiring any treatment. A third of the population has had back pain lasting more than a day in the previous 12 months. About 6 percent have chronic disabling back pain. This can be compared with the 1 percent that has the most common chronic inflammatory arthritis, RHEUMATOID ARTHRITIS. In the United States, back pain is the commonest cause of activity limitation in people under 45 years of age. There is no significant difference in the numbers of men and women reporting pain.

In any given year, 30 percent of adults who have never experienced back pain will do so. For those who have had back pain previously, the figure is just over 40 percent. In a 12-month study 10 percent of men and 7 percent of women between the ages of 20–59 years had time off work because of back pain. Back pain is conventionally divided into acute or chronic by virtue of persisting for less than or more than three months, respectively. This is because the three-month cutoff separates patients with quite different characteristics and underlying problems. A third group of patients (recurrent) have had back pain for less than three months but have also experienced previous attacks.

Much back pain is attributed to the abnormalities of the intervertebral disc, and sometimes the disc is indeed the culprit. In the adult, the top and bottom of each vertebral body is covered by a thin sheet of CARTILAGE (as found in joints), the outer rim of which is calcified (that is, bony). Attached to this outer rim are concentric layers of tough fibrous tissue (the annulus fibrosis) that spiral round at an angle of 70 degrees to the vertebral body to attach to the next vertebral body. Each successive layer is at right angles to the previous one, thereby increasing the ability to withstand torsion. Contained within these layers is a gelatinous substance called the nucleus pulposus. This allows for free movement as well as providing a shock-absorbing ability. Important changes occur as we age. The nucleus pulposus loses water, becoming smaller and stiffer. Cracks and tears start to develop in layers of the annulus fibrosis after the age of about 30 years. This occurs particularly in the inner two-thirds that has no blood supply. These changes may lead to significant weaknesses and possibly bulging of the annulus fibrosis. The forces on the erect spine are always tending to squeeze the nucleus out of its contained space. Generally, it is most likely to be forced either upward or downward into the adjacent vertebral body or outward through the retaining annulus fibrosis. It is likely that this actually occurs only with a sudden increase in force. Apart from pain, such disc-bulging or protrusion can lead to several spinal problems. Spinal movement will be reduced in the affected segments. Some forward tilting of the spine occurs due to loss of height of the disc. Bony protrusions or osteophytes develop around and abnormal stresses are placed on the posterior spinal or facet joints that may then develop OSTEOARTHRITIS.

However, it is important to see back pain not as a disease entity but as a symptom that can arise from many different diseases or abnormalities. Approximately 90 percent of back pain patients have mechanical back pain. This is defined as pain from overuse of a normal structure or from trauma to or deformity of an anatomic structure (including the disc). The exact source and nature of this pain may be extremely difficult to pinpoint, and specific diagnoses vary between practitioners with different special interests. Some diagnostic labels that are applied to people in this group include disc derangement or disruption, annular tear, spondylosis, degenerative disc disease, disc syndrome, lumbar disc disease, back sprain or strain, facet joint syndrome, spinal osteoarthritis, and sacroiliac injury. While these are all potentially valid diagnoses it is just not possible to be sure of the precise cause of the pain in many people. A common clinical finding among these patients is pelvic or shoulder malalignment together with spinal scoliosis (curvature) and often segmental dysfunction. Segmental dysfunction refers to the situation where one vertebra is held slightly out of alignment to its neighbor by muscle spasm. These abnormalities may result from poor posture, minor or significant injuries, mechanical problems elsewhere in the musculoskeletal system, any cause of a limp, muscle weakness or imbalance, and mechanical abnormalities within the spine. These malalignments are not permanent abnormalities and are what chiropractors and OSTEOPATHS try to correct.

A small proportion of patients with mechanical back pain will have nerve root impingement, usually known as sciatica. This can be due to direct pressure from disc material as the nerve leaves the spinal cord, a gradual narrowing of the canal through which the nerve exits the spine, interference with the nerve's blood supply, or simply swelling and inflammation close to the nerve.

The remaining 10 percent of patients with back pain have an underlying systemic disease, and there are many such possible causes. Inflammatory back pain is typified by ANKYLOSING SPONDYLITIS, but REACTIVE ARTHRITIS, psoriatic arthritis, and SARCOIDOSIS can all cause spinal inflammation (see PSORIASIS AND PSORIATIC ARTHRITIS). Infective spondylitis can be caused by any of the organisms causing INFECTIVE ARTHRITIS. It should be considered particularly in intravenous drug users (where staphylococcal species and gram-negative bacteria such as *Pseudomonas aeruginosa* are common) as well as those with lowered immunity due to cancer, HIV infection, or other causes of chronic ill health. BRUCELLOSIS frequently involves the spine or sacroiliac joints, and 50 percent of bone or joint TUBERCULOSIS is in the spine.

Tumors may arise in the spine (lymphoma, sarcoma, giant cell tumor, osteoid osteoma, hemangioma, chordoma) or metastasize there from a primary cancer elsewhere (lung, breast, prostate, ovary, colon, and myeloma particularly). Bone disease such as PAGET'S DISEASE, OSTEOMALACIA, and OSTEOPOROSIS can frequently cause back pain. Problems outside the spine may occasionally first present as back pain. Such conditions affecting internal organs include abdominal aortic aneurysm, kidney infection, pancreatitis, and colon cancer. Herpes zoster (shingles) may give rise to severe pain of uncertain cause for two or three days before the characteristic rash appears.

There are also well-described associations with back pain. While these might not physically cause the pain, the association is such that effective therapy will necessarily have to address them. These include obesity and smoking. Patients consulting their doctor for back pain are also more likely to have consulted for stress or mental disorders. Depression is thought to be a consequence of back pain more often than a precedent.

Degenerative changes are very much less frequent in children, and other causes of back pain need to be considered. As with adults, much of the back pain in children is nonspecific in that it is difficult to make a precise anatomical diagnosis. Posture is important and backpacks should not weigh more than 20 percent of the child's weight. Psychosocial factors are more common in children with back pain than in their peers. Spondylolysis is a defect in the posterior part of a vertebra as the bone arches around the spinal cord. This can sometimes lead to one vertebra slipping forward relative to its neighbor (known as spondylolisthesis). While this can be seen in adults with degenerative spinal disease it is more frequently a relevant finding in children. It can be congenital (the child is born with it) or acquired as a type of STRESS FRACTURE. Technetium bone scans will show if it has recently occurred and therefore is more likely to be painful. Children may have scoliosis (spinal curvature) due to congenital spinal anomalies or muscle imbalance. Scheurmann's kyphosis is a condition of unknown cause in which the spine angulates forward and pain usually develops gradually after exercise. Disc disease can occur in children but is rare compared to adults, and there is often a family history of disc disease in these children. Discitis is a poorly understood condition affecting very young children and widely believed to be infectious in most cases, although most patients recover without antibiotics. The resultant disc narrowing may cause some disability in later life but this is seldom severe. Children may also develop SPONDYLOAR-THROPATHIES, tumors, and infections.

Symptoms and Diagnostic Path

Almost all patients with a back problem complain of pain. Disability or restriction of activities is the most important association with back pain. Pain and disability are not the same, and there is no close correlation between them. There is also no close correlation between pain or disability and pathology of disease. Of note is that this means the severity of pain does not provide any information on the actual diagnosis. Some people with serious spinal pathology will have little disability while others with minimal pathology are seriously disabled. Many people with low-back pain will have pain elsewhere. This is most commonly in the neck but may be widespread. It is important to note that pain radiating into the leg does not necessarily indicate nerve root entrapment. The sacroiliac joint and associated structures frequently refer pain into the upper leg. Pain with numbness or tingling that radiates down the leg to the foot usually does indicate nerve root irritation, though.

Confusion has arisen because of the difficulty in making a precise anatomic diagnosis in many (some say up to 85 percent) patients with back pain as well as the controversy surrounding various diagnoses. The anatomic diagnosis means identifying which structure the pain is coming from or in which the primary problem lies. Everyone presenting with significant or persistent back pain should have a detailed history taken followed by a thorough examination by a practitioner skilled in this area. The management of back pain is improved if, at this stage, a differentiation or triage into one of three groups is made. These are

- Simple low-back pain
- Nerve root pain
- Serious spinal pathology

Simple Low-Back Pain usually develops in patients aged 20–55 years. The pain may be in the lower back, buttock region, or thighs. It is mechanical in that it varies with time and physical activity, and apart from the pain, the patient is well.

Nerve Root Pain generally radiates to the ankle or foot. Frequently this unilateral leg pain is worse than the back pain. There is numbness or paresthesia in the same area and signs of nerve irritation such as reduced straight-leg raising that reproduces the pain. There may be loss of power, loss of sensation, or altered reflexes in the area supplied by one nerve root.

Serious Spinal Pathology includes the inflammatory conditions, infections, tumors, metabolic bone disease, and other rare diseases mentioned above. Less than 5 percent of back pain is due to these. There is an increasing trend to use so-called red flags to identify these. This requires the clinician to run through a validated list of signs and symptoms that signal the possibility of serious pathology. Red flags include:

- Presentation younger than 20 years or older than 55 years
- Significant trauma such as a motor vehicle accident
- Constant, nonmechanical pain
- Thoracic back pain
- Previous history of cancer
- Steroid use
- Drug abuse or HIV infection
- Systemical unwellness, including weight loss or fever
- Widespread neurological abnormalities (more than one nerve root)
- Deformity of the spine
- Bone destruction or collapse on X-Ray
- A raised ESR

Within the grouping simple low-back pain are of course many different syndromes and a large number of structures that may be giving rise to pain. However, most patients with simple back pain and no red flags do not need any diagnostic tests. Symptom-relieving treatment may be given in the expectation of an early recovery. Many patients with nerve root pain will also recover spontaneously and special investigations will not be required. All patients with positive red flags should have further investigations done immediately. In addition, those in the first two groups who do not improve significantly within six weeks should

have further investigations. These may include appropriate blood tests looking for an underlying systemic condition and imaging. Blood tests may include those indicating inflammation such as ESR, tests for calcium and markers of bone turnover, as well as tests looking for various forms of cancer such as prostate specific antigen. These will be dictated by each individual's circumstances. Plain X-rays show bony lesions well but may take some time to become abnormal. Technetium bone scans on the other hand are very sensitive in showing abnormalities early on but do not give very specific information. They are particularly useful if metastatic cancer (cancer that has spread) is suspected, although one particular cancer (multiple myeloma) may not be demonstrated in this way.

Magnetic resonance imaging (MRI) scans are the investigation of choice for demonstrating nerve root impingement and many other conditions such as tumor or infection. Apart from expense, the chief drawback of MRI scans is the frequent finding of abnormalities in normal people. As MRI scans became widespread in the early 1990s, it was found that 40 percent of adults with no back pain at the time had abnormalities on MRI of their lower spine. It has therefore become important for radiologists reporting these scans to specify the degree of the abnormality along internationally agreed guidelines. In particular, it must be recognized that degenerative changes in the discs are a normal aging process. The MRI abnormalities should also be in keeping with the clinician's expectations before they are accepted as the cause of the patient's problem. CT scans may also be useful, although they show the soft tissues less well. There is very little place for traditional myelograms (injection of dye into the fluid space around the spinal cord), although they are very occasionally combined with CT scanning to assist in the planning of surgery. An electromyogram (EMG) may be helpful in a few instances where nerve lesions are atypical or difficult to interpret.

Treatment Options and Outlook

The treatment of back pain clearly depends on the diagnosis, and this discussion will be limited to mechanical back pain. Many of the other causes will be discussed elsewhere in this book. As indicated above, the vast majority of people with acute back pain will recover spontaneously within a few days. Studies have shown that continuing with normal activities (excluding heavy lifting) actually leads to a better outcome in acute back pain than either specifically designed back exercises or bed rest for a few days. Indeed, it has become apparent over the last 20 years that bed rest for more than a day or two leads to a much worse outcome. This is of course a dramatic change from an earlier era when rest was considered an important treatment for back pain.

Acute back pain   For those people whose acute back pain lasts more than a few days or in whom the pain is very severe, treatment may be necessary. This group should first have serious disease excluded as above and be reassured about this. Aggravating or initiating factors should be looked for, and ways of avoiding or modifying these discussed. An explanation of the pain and possible causes is extremely important in enabling people to continue their normal activities while still having pain. Pain relief is often necessary, and either pain killers or NSAIDs are helpful. Manipulation may help reduce the pain more rapidly and improve mobility. Physical therapy as well as appropriate exercises may be prescribed or a referral made to an appropriate therapist to initiate these. The expected outcome should be discussed since many people have an overly negative view of back pain. Most patients seeking care for back pain (which is not everybody with back pain) will improve considerably over the first four weeks, but only 30 percent will actually be painfree. After four weeks, about a third will continue to have moderate pain and 25 percent will have marked limitation of activity. At 12 months, 70 percent will have had some recurrent back symptoms and 30 percent will have had intermittent or persistent pain of moderate intensity. About 15 percent will still have significant activity limitation at this stage.

Chronic back pain   The treatment of chronic back pain is much more difficult and complex. Psychosocial factors assume greater importance here. Treatment modalities include manual therapies such as massage and manipulation, soft tissue injections, medication, exercise programs, corsets and braces, back schools, COGNITIVE BEHAVIORAL THERAPY, and work hardening (specific training to get fit for work activities). Most modern treatment programs for disabling chronic back pain would include cognitive behavioral therapy and exercise as substantial elements. Factors such as job dissatisfaction, relationship problems, and drug dependency that strongly impact on disability and illness behavior should be addressed. Work activities and the individual's fitness to undertake this must be assessed. Work-hardening programs analyze the individual's physical requirements at work and design a training program specifically to prepare them for this. Posture, both at work and during daily activities, frequently needs correction. Manipulation is less helpful than in acute back pain. Corsets and braces are generally best avoided but may provide some pain relief early in the course of treatment when used in conjunction with an exercise program. Analgesics, NSAIDs, and muscle relaxants are often used with effect.

Evidence-based treatment   Because back pain is such a huge health care problem, the U.S. Agency for Health Care Policy and Research spent over two years and $1 million evaluating the scientific evidence for the effectiveness of the various treatments for back pain in the early 1990s. This has since been updated by both Dutch and British researchers, and the results are very briefly summarized here.

- Good evidence indicates that continuing ordinary activities leads to as good or better symptom relief and less disability than more traditional approaches including specific exercises and short-term rest. Graded reactivation over days or weeks with behavioral management makes no difference initially but leads to less long-term disability.

- Manipulation results in a quicker reduction in pain and better mobility in the first six weeks of back pain, but evidence for its value in chronic pain is inconclusive. When properly carried out, the risks of manipulation are very low. McKenzie exercises (extension or flexion exercises) probably provide some benefit in acute back pain. However, it has not been shown that other back-specific exercise programs are helpful in acute back pain. On the other hand, strong evidence indicates that exercise therapy is beneficial in chronic back pain.

- Local therapies such as ice, heat, short-wave diathermy, massage, and ultrasound may provide some short-term relief, but they do not alter the outcome. Traction is probably not effective for either simple low-back pain or sciatica. There is no evidence that transcutaneous electrical nerve stimulation or TENS is effective for either acute or chronic low-back pain.

- The use of orthotic shoe insoles in appropriate patients is probably helpful, but correction of leg length differences of less than 2 cm is not. There is no evidence for the use of lumbar supports or corsets. Biofeedback is probably not effective in chronic low-back pain.

- The evidence for soft tissue injections is equivocal. Evidence is contradictory regarding the use of acupuncture in chronic back pain. Reasonable evidence is available to support the use of epidural steroid injections in both chronic low-back pain and specifically in sciatica. Facet joint injections have not been shown to be effective.

- Back schools vary considerably in content, but there is some evidence that this form of therapy is more effective than other types of conservative treatment. There is also reasonable evidence in favor of behavior therapy.

- ACETAMINOPHEN, NSAIDs, and acetaminophen-opioid combinations are all effective in acute and chronic back pain, but no one is better than the others. There is strong evidence that muscle relaxants are effective in acute low-back pain and possibly in chronic, but they have significant side effects.

- There is good evidence that narcotics and benzodiazepines for more than two weeks, COLCHICINE, systemic CORTICOSTEROIDS, bed rest with traction, manipulation under anesthesia, and the use of plaster jackets are **bad** for the patient.

Surgery Patients with definite nerve root impingement in whom sciatica is severe, is disabling, and does not improve within four weeks or gets progressively worse will probably benefit from nerve root decompression. Over 90 percent of this group of patients with radiological imaging confirming the clinical findings will have improvement in leg pain after surgery. However, many will continue to suffer intermittent or persistent back pain. Back pain that does not travel into the leg does not usually respond to surgery. Reliable surgical procedures include complete laminectomy (removal of the bony sidewall of the spinal canal), fenestration (enlargement of the nerve root exit canal by removal of some bone), and microdiscectomy (similar to fenestration but minimizing tissue destruction by use of microscope). In all these procedures, as much of the offending disc material as possible is removed. Indirect methods of removing the disc such as chemonucleolysis (injection of an enzyme to dissolve the inner disc) or percutaneous discectomy (removal of inner disc material by insertion of the instrument into the side of the disc) are less successful, although they have all had periods of popularity.

SPINAL STENOSIS, which usually results from multiple factors including soft tissue and bony enlargement and results in a very gradual encroachment on the spinal canal and nerve roots, will usually require complete laminectomy with or without spinal fusion. The cauda equina syndrome characterized by loss of or altered sensation in the saddle area, bladder or bowel disturbance, and often gait disturbance requires emergency surgical decompression.

Risk Factors and Preventive Measures

There are many different causes of back pain, and a number of these are discussed under their own headings, e.g., ankylosing spondylitis and osteoporosis. The common form of mechanical back pain is discussed in this section. Surprisingly perhaps, it is very difficult to show a consistent relationship between heavy physical work and back pain. A recent review of all the literature on this subject found no association with physically demanding leisure activities and conflicting findings as regards activities such as do-it-yourself home repair, gardening, nursing tasks, heavy physical work, or working with the body in a bent or twisted position. This does not mean that back pain does not occur in these situations, just that these activities do not put people at greater risk of back pain than a myriad of other less physically demanding activities. Being overweight and smoking are well recognized risk factors for back pain that are theoretically preventable.

There is strong evidence that a number of different exercise regimens reduce the severity and activity interference from low back pain, but only weak evidence for exercise as a primary preventive measure in adults, i.e., preventing back pain in people who either have not had it or have not had it for a while. In particular, a recent review of studies looking at targeted training programs for people starting work involving moving patients, shifting luggage, or postal workers showed no benefit from these prework training interventions. An intriguing study in children showed that high levels of physical activity (of any kind) predicted a lower prevalence of back pain three years later. There is some evidence that a multidisciplinary approach to patients with workplace-related back pain reduces future back pain (i.e., secondary prevention). Attention to workplace ergonomics frequently shows some benefit in short-term studies. There is strong evidence that orthotic insoles do not prevent back pain. While the studies are not of very high quality, there is reasonable evidence that low back supports do not prevent back pain.

bacterial arthritis   See INFECTIVE ARTHRITIS.

Baker's cyst (popliteal cyst)   A pouch of synovium extending behind the knee that is in communication with the joint. It causes a cystic swelling deep in the tissue behind the knee and can extend into the calf.

Any condition that causes arthritis of the knee, but most often RHEUMATOID ARTHRITIS or OSTEOARTHRITIS, can cause a Baker's cyst. The cyst is thought to form when there is a one-way connection between the knee joint and a pouch of synovium that has tracked behind the knee. When fluid develops in a joint, very high pressures develop under loading. These pressures pump the fluid backward into the lower-pressure cyst. The connection closes as this pressure is removed (when the foot is lifted) and therefore functions as a one-way valve. Any

condition that increases the production of synovial fluid in the knee, such as arthritis, will cause fluid to accumulate in the knee and track into the cyst, making it bigger. In children, Baker's cysts can occur rarely without any underlying arthritis of the knee. These cysts are thought to occur because of variations in anatomy present at birth.

Symptoms and Diagnostic Path
A Baker's cyst accumulates gradually and, if it is small, may cause no symptoms apart from a feeling of fullness behind the knee. Some patients may feel it as a tightness behind the knee and, if very tense, complain of having a golf ball-like swelling there. If the cyst enlarges, it can cause pain and a feeling of fullness behind the knee and in the calf. If it ruptures, synovial fluid tracks down into the muscles of the calf and causes a painful swollen calf—a clinical picture that is very similar to that seen when a clot develops in one of the deep veins in the leg (DVT or deep vein thrombosis).

Diagnostic tests are usually performed only for unexplained pain behind the knee or if a ruptured cyst is suspected. An ultrasound or magnetic resonance imaging (MRI) examination will show the cystic swelling behind the knee and fluid tracking down the calf. If a deep vein thrombosis is suspected, an ultrasound is the appropriate investigation and will usually provide the correct diagnosis.

Treatment Options and Outlook
Good control of the underlying knee arthritis will decrease the production of synovial fluid and thus decrease pressure in the cyst. Treatment with NSAIDs or injection of the knee with CORTICOSTEROIDS often controls knee inflammation and reduces the swelling in a Baker's cyst. Emptying the cysts by drawing the contents out through a needle (aspiration) or removing the cyst surgically is seldom required unless conservative approaches have failed. Surgical treatments may include arthroscopic (see ARTHROSCOPY AND ARTHROSCOPIC SURGERY) repair of underlying mechanical problems in the knee, such as MENISCAL TEARS, or rarely removal of the synovial lining of the knee (SYNOVECTOMY). Recently, resistant or recurrent cysts have been injected with a sclerosing agent

that causes them to fibrose or scar up so that they can't fill up again. While this has been successful in reported cases, in the absence of trials we do not know how often it is successful or how frequent complications are. Most cysts respond to an injection of intra-articular corticosteroid, and although they can recur, surgery is seldom needed.

bee venom (apitherapy) An alternative therapy that uses bee venom to treat medical conditions, most often forms of arthritis and multiple sclerosis. The treatment usually involves allowing bees, often two or three, to sting the patient. The number of bees used, the sites of the body they are encouraged to sting, and the frequency of treatment varies. Bee venom is also sold as tablets, ointments, and injections. In animal models of arthritis, several studies have shown that bee venom decreases inflammation. However, its use in humans is largely based on anecdotes and is not supported by good clinical trials. Side effects are those resulting from bee stings and include pain and swelling at the site of the stings and, rarely, more serious generalized allergic reactions. A newer variation that is growing in popularity is bee venom acupuncture. Here the venom is injected at acupoints aiming to combine the proposed immunological benefits of the venom therapy with those of classical ACUPUNCTURE. While several studies suggest positive results in patients with musculoskeletal pain, the numbers studied are too few to draw any definite conclusions. Interestingly, in a study of all 180 beekeepers in one area of Spain, more than 50 percent had suffered from hand arthritis and 19 percent had a chronic arthropathy thought to be due to their ongoing occupational exposure to bee stings.

Behçet's disease An inflammatory illness of unknown cause that causes recurrent oral and genital ulcers, eye inflammation, arthritis, rash, and gut and nervous system complications. Hippocrates may have been first to describe Behçet's disease, but it is named after a Turkish physician, Hulusi Behçet, who is credited with the first modern description of the illness in 1937. There is a large variation in the frequency of Behçet's disease in different countries. The disease is common in countries along the ancient Silk Route such as Turkey (approximately 100 cases per 100,000 population), Japan, Korea, China, and Iran (approximately 15 cases per 100,000). However, it is uncommon in the United Kingdom and United States (less than 1 case per 100,000).

The cause of Behçet's disease is not known but is thought to involve both genetic and environmental factors. A genetic predisposition is suggested by the observation that an inherited tissue type, HLA-B51, is strongly associated with Behçet's disease in Asian countries. However, there is not a striking association between HLA-B51 and Behçet's disease in Western countries. Many possible infectious causes such as herpes simplex and parvovirus have been investigated, but no infectious agent or environmental factor has been shown to be the cause of Behçet's disease.

Symptoms and Diagnostic Path

The illness typically occurs in young adults in their 30s or 40s, and the pattern of disease is most often one of intermittent attacks separated by periods of good health. The classical symptoms are oral and genital ulcers with inflammation of the eyes, but many other organs can be affected.

- *Mouth and Genital Ulcers* Recurrent, painful oral ulcers that heal without scarring are often the first symptom. The mouth ulcers are most often on the tongue or the mucosal lining of the mouth on the inside of the cheeks and lips. They take about two weeks to heal. Recurrent, painful, deep genital ulcers that heal with scarring can affect the penis or scrotum in men or the vulva or vagina in women.

- *Eye Inflammation* This usually affects deep tissues of the eye such as the uvea and causes redness of the eye, pain, and blurred vision (see EYE PROBLEMS). If the retina is involved, sudden, painless loss of vision can occur.

- *Skin Rash* Rashes are common and can take many forms, ranging from small, acnelike pustules to larger painful red nodules, known as ERYTHEMA NODOSUM, that occur most often on the front of the shin.

- *Arthritis* About half of patients have arthritis that usually involves only one or a few joints, typically large joints such as knees, wrists, or ankles.

- *Gut Problems* Inflammation of the small blood vessels that supply the gut can cause pain, bleeding, ulcers, and perforation of the wall of the small or large bowel.

- *Nervous System Complications* Inflammation of the brain (encephalitis) or the thin tissue that lines it (meningitis) can cause headache, stroke, seizures, and loss of memory.

- *Vasculitis* Inflammation of large and small blood vessels (VASCULITIS) is common and is the underlying cause of many of the clinical manifestations of Behçet's disease. Inflammation of superficial veins that lie just under the skin can cause them to clot and form painful cords that can be felt (superficial thrombophlebitis). Inflammation of larger, deep veins increases the risk of deep vein thrombosis. Inflammation of arteries can lead to formation of aneurysms or to narrowing and blockage of an artery. If the blood flow to an organ is not adequate to supply oxygen and nutrients to the organ, then gangrene and death of tissue will occur.

There is no specific test for Behçet's disease, and the diagnosis is based on the combination of symptoms and disease manifestations. Diagnostic criteria, such as those set by the International Study Group for Behçet's disease in 1990, define criteria that groups of experts have generally agreed are needed to make the diagnosis. According to these criteria, recurrent mouth ulcers must be present with at least another two of the following symptoms: recurrent genital ulcers, eye inflammation, a rash that is typical of Behçet's disease, or a positive pathergy test. The pathergy test is positive when pustules form around areas of minor skin trauma, for example at sites where the skin has been punctured with a needle to draw a blood sample. A test for pathergy is done by pricking the skin on the forearm with a sterile needle and seeing if a pustule forms at the puncture site. These diagnostic criteria have been established mainly for research protocols to make sure that research studies of patients with Behçet's disease are all discussing the same disease. The diagnostic criteria are not always helpful for an individual patient and do not have the same accuracy in different populations. For example, a positive pathergy test is common in Asian and Turkish patients but is less common in American patients.

Treatment Options and Outlook

The treatment of Behçet's disease depends on the organs involved and the severity of disease. If the gut, nervous system, or eyes are involved, the illness is treated aggressively with CORTICOSTEROIDS, usually prednisone, often combined with other drugs. COLCHICINE and topical corticosteroids may also be helpful for oral and genital ulcers and eye inflammation. If these drugs do not control Behçet's disease, then immunosuppressants such as CHLORAMBUCIL, AZATHIOPRINE, METHOTREXATE, CYCLOPHOSPHAMIDE, and CYCLOSPORINE are added. There are good studies showing that azathioprine is effective and that cyclosporine is effective in resistant eye disease, but there are few studies comparing different treatments. THALIDOMIDE is moderately effective for decreasing the frequency of attacks of oral and genital ulcers but has many side effects and is absolutely contraindicated if there is any chance of the patient becoming pregnant. Alpha interferon and the TNF antagonists are being increasingly used in severe disease that is resistant to other conventional agents. Some remarkable successes have been reported, but there are no randomized controlled trials yet to determine the place of these BIOLOGICALS. If venous or arterial thrombosis occur, then anticoagulation, first with heparin and then with warfarin, is used.

Behçet's disease often has periods when the disease is inactive, interspersed with periods when it flares. Complications include blindness, perforation of bowel wall, deep vein thrombosis, rupture of an aneurysm, and neurological damage, but death due to Behçet's is unusual.

Risk Factors and Preventive Measures

Apart from the association with HLA-B51 in Asian countries, there are no known risk factors or preventive measures for Behçet's disease.

biceps tendon rupture See SHOULDER PAIN.

biologicals (biologic agents) Broadly defined as therapeutic agents that have been manufactured using molecular biology techniques. Those used in the treatment of the rheumatic diseases can be divided into three groups: agents interfering with the actions of CYTOKINES; agents interfering with the activation of T lymphocytes (see "cellular immunity" under IMMUNE RESPONSE), and agents causing a depletion of B lymphocytes (see "humeral immunity" under immune response). These agents are different types of molecules and their names have a suffix that indicates this. Soluble receptor antagonists are shortened forms of human proteins that float freely in the blood until they find the specific target to attach to. Their suffix is -cept. ETANERCEPT is an example that binds to TNF in the blood, preventing it from attaching to a cell and having an effect on that cell's function. Monoclonal antibodies are immunoglobulins (see "humeral immunity" under immune response) that can bind to their target in the blood or on the surface of cells. Their suffix is -mab. ADALIMUMAB is a humanized antibody directed against TNF. Its components are identical to that of naturally occurring human antibodies. INFLIXIMAB, also directed against TNF, on the other hand has part human and part mouse protein and therefore has the -ximab suffix. ANAKINRA is a protein that attaches to a cell receptor that recognizes interleukin-1 (see cytokines) and in so doing prevents interleukin-1 from attaching and stimulating the cell. TOCILIZUMAB is a monoclonal antibody that binds to and inactivates interleukin-6 (see cytokines). ABATACEPT is a circulating protein that, in attaching to T lymphocytes, interferes with their activation by other signals. RITUXIMAB is an antibody that attaches to B lymphocytes and causes their death, leading to low B cell levels that can persist for many months.

bisphosphonates A class of drugs that concentrates in bone and decreases resorption (the removal of calcium from bone into the bloodstream). Bisphosphonates are used to treat OSTEOPOROSIS and PAGET'S DISEASE. They include ALENDRONATE (trade name: Fosamax), RISEDRONATE (trade name: Actonel), IBANDRONATE, and ETIDRONATE (trade name: Didronel).

blood tests See Appendix II.

bone marrow transplantation An aggressive therapy undergoing evaluation for a range of autoimmune disorders. Bone marrow transplantation (BMT) involves high-dose immunosuppressive treatment followed by bone marrow replacement. BMT was developed as a treatment for several types of cancer. Virtually all types of chemotherapy for cancer suppress the bone marrow, which makes red and white blood cells and platelets. The theory behind BMT was that much higher doses of anticancer drugs could be used to eradicate cancer throughout the body, including the bone marrow, if physicians did not have to avoid suppressing the bone marrow. Isolated reports that autoimmune disease improved in patients who received a bone marrow transplant for cancer and studies in animal models showing benefits from BMT, have led to widespread interest in it as a potential treatment for autoimmune disease.

Autologous and allogeneic transplants There are two major types of BMT—autologous and allogeneic. In autologous transplantation, patients receive their own marrow or stem cells. In allogeneic transplantation, they receive the bone marrow from a donor closely matched for tissue type (see HLA). The complications and mortality are much lower with autologous transplantation because rejection is not a problem. Virtually all the transplants performed for autoimmune disease have been autologous stem cell transplants.

Autologous stem cell transplants A stem cell transplant involves three phases.

1. The patient receives CYCLOPHOSPHAMIDE and granulocyte colony stimulating factor (G-CSF) to mobilize stem cells from the bone marrow. The cells are harvested by drawing the patient's blood out of a vein, separating the stem cells, and returning the blood to the patient. The stem cells are stored for later use.

2. High doses of chemotherapy that are toxic to the bone marrow are administered. This is sometimes called the conditioning regimen. There are several different conditioning regimens, but most are based on high-dose cyclophosphamide. The treatment causes severe bone marrow suppression, and white blood cell and platelet counts decrease dramatically.

3. The stem cells are injected back into the patient through a vein and repopulate the bone marrow. The stem cells take about two weeks to establish themselves and differentiate into cells that produce white blood cells and platelets. During these two weeks, the patient has almost no white blood cell and platelets, and the risk of infection and bleeding is high. Patients who receive their own stem cells do not need immunosuppression because they will not reject their own cells.

As a Treatment for Autoimmune Disease

A review in 2008 found 26 reports of 854 patients who had received BMT for autoimmune disease. The mortality rate varied from 1 percent with the less intense regimens to 13 percent with the most intense, which included total body irradiation as well as immunosuppressive medication. There are no controlled CLINICAL TRIALS, so knowing how this treatment compares with more standard ones is difficult. The effectiveness of BMT may have been underestimated because patients who received a bone marrow transplant were usually selected because they had not responded to standard treatments.

BMT has been tried in patients with RHEUMATOID ARTHRITIS (RA), SYSTEMIC LUPUS ERYTHEMATOSUS (SLE), SCLERODERMA, and JUVENILE IDIOPATHIC ARTHRITIS. Responses to treatment have been variable, and physicians are not yet certain what the exact response rate will be for each disease. Approximately a third of patients have an impressive clinical response, an other third a moderate response, and the final third no response. The treatment does not cure autoimmune disease. Even patients who respond very well initially often relapse after months or sometimes a few years. Many centers are performing research to define which patients are likely to respond to BMT.

There have also been reports of patients with SLE responding to high doses of cyclophosphamide without stem cell transplantation.

BMT is expensive and can have severe side effects. The risk of death varies from center to center. However, it is approximately 1–2 percent for patients with RA but much higher, approximately 10 percent, for those SLE and scleroderma. The long-term complications of the treatment may include an increased risk of cancer. Overwhelming infection is the most serious complication. BMT is an experimental treatment that is usually limited to research studies and should be performed only at centers that are experienced with this technique.

bone scan   See RADIONUCLIDE BONE SCAN in Appendix II.

brucellosis   An infectious disease, uncommon in the United States, that is a rare cause of arthritis. Brucellosis in humans is caused by a bacterial infection acquired from animals: *Brucella abortus* (cattle), *Brucella suis* (pigs), *Brucella melitensis* (goats), and *Brucella canis* (dogs). Humans usually acquire the infection through eating or drinking unpasteurized dairy produce from infected animals. Workers in close contact with infected animals, for example slaughterhouse workers, can get infected by handling infected animals or carcasses.

Symptoms and Diagnostic Path

The systemic symptoms of brucellosis dominate. The condition often presents as a fever of unknown cause with sweating, loss of weight, arthralgia (joint pains), myalgia (muscle pain), and headache. The arthritis can affect one or a few large joints such as the hip or knee but can also involve the vertebrae and sacroiliac joints (joining the lower spine to the pelvis).

The combination of a history of exposure to infected animals or a diet that includes unpasteurized dairy produce, prominent systemic symptoms and culturing the organism from the blood of a patient, or a positive blood test for antibodies against brucella are the basis for diagnosis.

Treatment Options and Outlook

A prolonged course of combination antibiotic therapy, most often a tetracycline such as doxycycline and another antibiotic such as rifampin or streptomycin, effectively eradicates the infection.

Risk Factors and Preventive Measures

Drinking infected, unpasteurized milk and working in abattoirs or on farms with infected animals are the major risk factors. Thorough testing and vaccination of cattle herds prevents most brucella infections. Drinking only pasteurized milk is safe even if there is residual infection in the source herds.

Buerger's disease (thromboangiitis obliterans) First reported by von Winiwarter in 1879 and then fully described by Leo Buerger in 1908, Buerger's disease in an illness that usually affects young or middle-aged men who smoke heavily. In this illness, smoking causes spasming and narrowing of the arteries of the hands, legs, and feet, sometimes resulting in gangrene. Because there is no specific diagnostic test, researchers do not always agree on the diagnosis and so the true frequency of Buerger's disease is controversial. It is common in the Middle and Far East but is not common in the United States, where it affects about one in 10,000 people.

Although tobacco plays a key part in causing Buerger's disease, why some smokers get it and others do not is not clear. Some experts have reported that Buerger's disease can occur in people who never smoked or used other types of tobacco, but this is exceptional. In all smokers, the endothelium, a thin layer of cells that lines blood vessels, is damaged by smoking so that the blood vessels do not dilate well and cannot increase the blood supply to tissue when it is needed. It is possible that this damage to blood vessels caused by smoking is exaggerated in those smokers who develop Buerger's disease.

Symptoms and Diagnostic Path

Buerger's disease usually affects men in their 40s. The first symptom is often pain in an arm or leg during exercise (claudication). This symptom occurs because tissues need more oxygen, and therefore more blood, during exercise. In Buerger's disease, the arteries are narrow and the blood supply is inadequate to meet the increased need. If the disease gets worse, the pain can be present during rest as well as during exercise and can lead to gangrene. Buerger's disease can also cause inflammation of superficial veins that lie just under the skin so that they clot and form painful cords that can be felt (superficial thrombophlebitis).

No test provides a certain diagnosis of Buerger's disease. In a patient with poor blood supply to a digit or limb, the diagnostic possibilities usually include several conditions: Atherosclerosis, VASCULITIS, CHOLESTEROL EMBOLI SYNDROME, and Buerger's disease. The patient's symptoms and angiogram (X-rays of arteries) can help to separate these conditions. The angiogram in Buerger's disease, in contrast with what is found in atherosclerosis, does not usually show narrowing of large arteries. Typically in Buerger's disease, small- and medium-sized arteries, for example those around the wrist or ankle, have some areas that are blocked and others that are not. These angiogram findings are not specific and are similar to those found in SCLERODERMA, SYSTEMIC LUPUS ERYTHEMATOSUS, and RHEUMATOID ARTHRITIS with vasculitis. To help make the diagnosis of Buerger's disease, diagnostic criteria composed of combinations of several clinical findings have been proposed. Most classification criteria include the following requirements: male less than 50 years old, current or recent tobacco use, and unexplained poor blood supply to an arm or leg. These composite clinical criteria are useful for research studies to ensure patients with a similar disease are studied but are not always helpful in deciding whether an individual patient has Buerger's disease.

Treatment Options and Outlook

The only treatment that can reverse Buerger's disease and avoid amputation is to stop smoking. Smoking even a few cigarettes a day or chewing tobacco can keep the disease active. Drugs that dilate the arteries can help avoid amputation in a critical phase when a limb is almost gangrenous, but these vasodilator drugs do not affect the long-term outcome. Surgery to bypass blood vessels that are blocked is not usually an option because the disease affects many blood vessels and usually affects medium-sized vessels that are not easily treated with bypass surgery.

Ulcers and gangrene can develop at the tips of the fingers, toes, hands, or feet because of poor blood supply. Often more than one limb is affected at the same time. If the blood supply to a tissue is not adequate to supply the oxygen and nutrients needed, then the affected finger, toe, leg, or arm can develop gangrene. These often need to be amputated to prevent infection setting in and spreading from the dead tissue into the bloodstream and throughout the body. Buerger's disease will progress unless the patient quits using tobacco.

Risk Factors and Preventive Measures

Smoking is the major and only known risk factor for Buerger's disease. Not smoking would almost completely prevent it from occurring.

bursitis Bursas are formed where there is significant movement between tissues. They consist of a fibrous envelope lined with fat cells and synovial cells that secrete a thin film of collagen-rich fluid. This allows the tissues on either side of the bursa to move freely with minimal friction. Bursas between deep tissues are formed before birth, but many bursas just under the skin are formed after birth in response to the friction at those areas. These areas include over the elbow, heel, around the big toe, and in certain areas over the spine. Deep bursas exist at most sites where tendons run over bone or cross a joint. Specific bursae that are commonly involved in disease processes are mentioned in the appropriate sections.

Superficial bursas in particular are subject to direct trauma, and bleeding can cause significant pain and inflammation. Some scarring and loss of the synovial cells may result. Any disease that causes synovitis (inflammation of the lining membrane of joints) can cause bursal inflammation. RHEUMATOID ARTHRITIS and GOUT are common causes. Bursitis can result from frequent minor trauma, and infection can occur, especially in the superficial bursae. (See also SOFT TISSUE ARTHRITIS–RELATED PROBLEMS.)

calcium pyrophosphate dihydrate deposition disease (CPPD, pseudogout) A degenerative arthritis associated with the presence of calcium pyrophosphate crystals in the synovial fluid and joint structures. Two broad groups of people develop the disease. The first includes people older than 60 years of age who have had osteoarthritis for some time. In this group, women are affected at least twice as often as men. Second, people with an underlying metabolic disorder may develop CPPD at a much younger age.

The cause of CPPD is not known, but it occurs in association with other conditions, most often OSTEOARTHRITIS (OA) and less often hypothyroidism, HEMOCHROMATOSIS, and conditions that alter normal calcium control. It has been argued that the CPP crystals merely coexist with osteoarthritis and do not actually do any harm. However, many studies now show that people with crystals have a worse outcome than those without. Also, there are families who develop chondrocalcinosis before any arthritis is apparent, suggesting that crystal deposition precedes arthritis. Animal studies have also shown that injection of CPPD crystals into a joint can cause arthritis. Calcium crystals have been shown to stimulate the release of inflammatory CYTOKINES and enzymes that degrade cartilage in models of inflammation. There are therefore a number of potential mechanisms for these crystals either to cause or to worsen arthritis.

Some patients have rare familial or inherited forms of CPPD. In many of these, including Americans of European origin, the genetic abnormality has been linked to chromosome 5. Another large group in New England, however, shows linkage to chromosome 8, and this is therefore unlikely to be due to a single abnormality. The genetic abnormality that leads to CPPD remains unknown.

Symptoms and Diagnostic Path

The symptoms of CPPD usually fall into one of two patterns. The first involves background symptoms caused by chronic degenerative arthritis. The second involves attacks of acute arthritis that punctuate the chronic low-grade arthritis. During attacks of pseudogout, the affected joints become red, hot, swollen, and very painful—symptoms very similar to those of an attack of gout. (The chronic degenerative form of CPPD is indistinguishable from OA. It often affects the same joints that develop OA, such as the knees and hips. However, it can also affect joints that seldom develop OA, such as the wrists and metacharpophalangeal [MCP] joints of the second and third fingers.) These attacks, often in a wrist, knee, or ankle, can develop overnight and usually settle over a few days or weeks, although they can recur. Just as happens with gout, acute attacks of pseudogout can be brought on by other unrelated medical illnesses, such as pneumonia, or surgery. Some patients with CPPD have symptoms resembling RHEUMATOID ARTHRITIS. This pseudorheumatoid form may be very difficult to distinguish from rheumatoid arthritis. Often the presence of chondrocalcinosis or an abnormality of calcium control suggests the diagnosis.

The diagnosis of CPPD is often made clinically based on the symptoms, but X-ray findings can be helpful. Many of the X-ray findings of CPPD are similar to those of OA and include narrowing of the joint and formation of bone spurs. The new bone formation around joints that usually occurs with OA (osteophytes) is more florid in CPPD. Another clue to the diagnosis of CPPD is that fibrous cartilage in joints such as the knees and wrists often calcifies (chondrocalcinosis) and can be seen on the X-ray. The joints involved are also not quite typical of OA (see Symptoms). No blood test is available to help make the diagnosis. The most specific test is when rhomboid-shaped calcium pyrophosphate crystals are seen in the synovial fluid when it is examined under polarized-light microscopy. However, joint fluid is not always examined under polarized light and the crystals may therefore be missed. Also, very small crystals may be too small to see under a light microscope and other techniques are too expensive to be used other than for research purposes.

Treatment Options and Outlook

Treatment of chronic CPPD is difficult. Management is similar to that of OA and includes weight loss to take the load off weight-bearing joints, exercise to strengthen muscles around joints, and analgesics such as acetaminophen or NSAIDs to decrease pain. In an acute attack of pseudogout, it is often helpful for a physician to drain a little of the synovial fluid through a needle so that it can be cultured to make sure the acute inflammation is not caused by an infection in the joint. The synovial fluid can also be examined under a polarizing microscope to see if calcium pyrophosphate crystals are present. NSAIDs are helpful in reducing pain and swelling. Occasionally a short course of CORTI-COSTEROIDS by mouth or an intra-articular injection of a corticosteroid are needed to control the attack. Based on clinical experience rather than evidence from clinical studies, COLCHICINE is sometimes used to prevent recurrent attacks of pseudogout in patients who have had frequent attacks. Patients with chronic CPPD may have arthritis similar to severe OA, but a few progress to develop chronic inflammation more like rheumatoid arthritis. In these patients, METHOTREXATE appears useful in uncontrolled studies.

Acute attacks of pseudogout can be incapacitating but usually settle, either spontaneously or with treatment, over a few weeks and do not cause permanent joint damage. The outcomes of chronic CPPD are similar to those of OA and vary among patients. Some have mild intermittent or chronic arthritis symptoms that can be easily controlled with painkillers such as acetaminophen or NSAIDs. Others have a more severe arthritis that sometimes requires joint replacement surgery.

Risk Factors and Preventive Measures

The familial forms of CPPD are rare but important in that further understanding of their mechanisms may shed light on the causation of the commoner forms. Having established OA and metabolic abnormalities in the handling of calcium are predisposing factors, but only very few of these patients will get CPPD, and so it is not possible to study whether different ways of treating these conditions will alter the incidence of CPPD. Currently there are no known preventive measures.

carpal tunnel syndrome This is the most common entrapment neuropathy. An entrapment neuropathy occurs when there is damage or just impaired function of nerves where they pass through a confining tunnel or are close to the skin and are therefore susceptible to pressure. At the wrist the median nerve passes through the carpal tunnel. This is formed by an arch of four wrist or carpal bones, the ends of which are joined by strong fascia or connective tissue (flexor retinaculum) in the manner of a strung bow. Also passing through this tunnel are nine tendons from muscles that predominantly close the hand, each covered by a tenosynovial sheath.

The many causes of carpal tunnel syndrome (CTS) may be divided into inflammatory, noninflammatory, and idiopathic. This last term is used when there is no apparent cause. Inflammatory causes include all types of inflammatory ARTHRITIS, particularly RHEUMATOID ARTHRITIS and psoriatic arthritis (see PSORIASIS AND PSORIATIC ARTHRITIS). Rheumatoid arthritis is one of the most common causes of CTS, causing 12 percent of cases in one large study. The connective tissue diseases such as SYSTEMIC LUPUS ERYTHEMATOSUS and SCLERO-DERMA are less frequent causes, and GOUT and CAL-CIUM PYROPHOSPHATE DIHYDRATE DEPOSITION DISEASE (CPPD) are rare. Other rare inflammatory causes include gonococcal tenosynovitis, PIGMENTED VIL-LONODULAR SYNOVITIS, EOSINOPHILIC FASCIITIS, LYME DISEASE, and infections including TUBERCULOSIS. Repetitive wrist movements may cause CTS as a form of occupational overuse syndrome, although the frequency of this is debated.

Noninflammatory causes include metabolic disorders such as hypothyroidism, diabetes, AMYLOIDO-

SIS, and ACROMEGALY. Others include hemodialysis for kidney failure, lipomas, or ganglions on the tendons passing through the carpal tunnel, pregnancy, fractures, or contusions close to the carpal tunnel. OSTEOARTHRITIS is a surprisingly common association. Women develop idiopathic CTS more frequently than men.

Symptoms and Diagnostic Path

Typically the person is woken at night by a burning or bursting pain in the hand that is relieved by shaking it or getting up and moving about. Clumsiness such as dropping cups and plates is common, and the hand is often felt to be weak even in the absence of detectable changes in the affected muscles. The pain is usually intermittent and worse at night but may be persistent when severe. Classically, it is felt in the three and a half fingers on the thumb side of the hand because this is the area supplied by the median nerve. Often, people feel that the whole hand or at least the ends of all the fingers are affected. Sometimes there is also an aching discomfort in the forearm. Activities that involve alternating wrist movements or holding the wrist in a flexed position (turned to the palmar side) usually make the symptoms worse or bring them on.

CTS is usually diagnosed on the basis of a typical history with one or more confirmatory signs on examination. These include reduced feeling in the radial (thumb-sided) three and a half fingers, a loss of bulk in the bunch of muscles at the base of the thumb (severe cases only), swelling over the palmar aspect of the wrist (especially with inflammatory causes), and positive Tinel's or Phalen's signs. Tinel's sign is positive if tapping over the carpal tunnel sends tingling or painful feelings into the affected fingers. Phalen's is positive if holding the wrist completely flexed for a minute causes the individual's usual symptoms to come on.

In mild or atypical cases it is best to obtain electrodiagnostic confirmation before embarking on invasive treatment. This is a test that uses low-voltage electric current to measure how well and how fast the median nerve conducts. This is compared with the opposite hand and with conduction in other forearm nerves such as the ulnar. Slowing of sensory transmission (that is, from fingers to elbow) occurs before motor (movement) pathways are affected. The operator needs to be experienced since there is variation between individuals and the results require interpretation. The test is not pleasant for the patient but remains the gold standard. Plain X-rays are sometimes done but seldom give useful information. MRI scans may show distortion of the nerve and swelling of the tendon sheaths in inflammatory conditions. Except in extreme cases, however, they do not give any information about how the nerve is functioning. If both hands are affected or the problem is recurrent or there are other features of a systemic disorder, blood and other tests should be done to look for the causes discussed above.

Treatment Options and Outlook

This is conservative or surgical. Mild or intermittent symptoms may respond to splinting alone. A lightweight forearm *resting* splint that holds the wrist in a neutral position is worn at night and for variable periods during the day. A diuretic is sometimes helpful in idiopathic cases when symptoms are worse just before menstruation. NSAIDs are not very effective but may help when the cause is inflammatory. A one-month course of prednisone has recently been shown to be an effective treatment. Highly effective with inflammatory causes is a CORTICOSTEROID injection into the carpal tunnel. When given by an experienced operator, this is a very safe procedure, although there is a small risk of nerve or tendon damage. Control of inflammation by systemically given medication is essential when the underlying cause is an inflammatory arthritis such as rheumatoid arthritis. Often a steroid injection with splinting is used to give temporary relief while medication changes are made to gain control of the inflammation. Newer treatments such as ultrasound and laser neurolysis are still being tested.

Consideration must be given to precipitating activities, either occupational or recreational, and changes made where possible. Temporarily stopping activities such as meat cutting or plucking chickens is usually necessary to allow resolution of the problem. Typing style may need to be altered. Many people can minimize the everyday stresses to the carpal tunnel once they are made aware of what these are. Wearing a *working* splint with a rigid bar to maintain a relatively fixed wrist position is a good way to become more aware of wrist position during activities.

Surgical release of the flexor retinaculum is a very effective treatment of CTS. It is indicated when the response to conservative treatment is in adequate, when symptoms are recurrent or when progressive nerve or muscle damage exists. Occasionally the inflammatory synovial lining of tendons has to be stripped off in rheumatoid arthritis. Biopsy is indicated when inflammatory tissue is found during surgery since this is often how rare causes such as tuberculosis, fungal infections, or amyloidosis are first diagnosed. The surgery is not difficult and can be done under local anaesthetic.

Risk Factors and Preventive Measures

The wide range of conditions that may be complicated by carpal tunnel syndrome is discussed above. These include most inflammatory arthropathies, hypothyroidism, diabetes, acromegaly, amyloidosis, rarely infections, pregnancy, and dialysis for kidney failure. Aggressive treatment of inflammation will prevent many but not all arthritis-associated cases. Recognition and treatment of hypothyroidism and acromegaly will prevent the associated carpal tunnel syndrome, but those cases associated with these other conditions are not strictly preventable.

In work-related carpal tunnel syndrome, regular wrist flexion, especially beyond 45 degrees and extension beyond 30 degrees, as well as repeated forceful flexion are the major risk factors along with psychosocial factors such as job satisfaction. Repetitive wrist movement in itself does not seem to be a risk factor. The American Conference of Governmental Industrial Hygienists has issued guidelines on work-related hand activity/peak force action limit and threshold limit values that certainly predict increased upper limb pain syndromes including carpal tunnel syndrome. It is not yet known whether adhering to these guidelines will reduce the incidence of these pain syndromes.

cartilage   Specialized connective tissue formed by cells called chondrocytes that synthesize a matrix comprised of collagen and proteoglycans. Cartilage

covers the bony ends of most moving joints and has two main functions. It provides a low-friction gliding surface that enables joints to move smoothly, and it also acts as a shock absorber. As humans age, cartilage retains less water and becomes less pliable and resilient so that small tears develop in the surface that is usually smooth. The aging cartilage is also less effective as a shock absorber. These degenerative changes in cartilage are thought to play an important part in the development of OSTEOARTHRITIS.

celiac disease   An allergic condition affecting the small bowel and leading to malabsorption. The cause of this disease, sensitivity to wheat gluten, was discovered by a Dutch pediatrician who, during World War II, noted that his patients got better when bread became unavailable and unusual noncereal foods were substituted. After the war, bread became available again and his patients deteriorated again. He then performed controlled studies to show that exposure to wheat caused the disease. Using older diagnostic methods, celiac disease was thought to affect about one in 1,200 people in the United Kingdom, rising to one in 300 in parts of Ireland. However, screening programs using modern blood tests have shown that the incidence is much higher. In a large study in the United States using a test for anti-endomysial antibodies, the incidence varied from one in 133 not at risk people to one in 22 of first-degree relatives of patients with known celiac disease. Women are affected more often than men, and the main effect is reduced absorption of important dietary elements.

Well over 90 percent of people in western Europe with celiac disease have the HLA-B8, DR3, DQ2 genetic haplotype (see HLA), although other haplotypes are also common around the Mediterranean. There is often a history of a Celtic ancestor and 10–20 percent of first-degree relatives are affected. All this indicates a strong genetic predisposition to the disease, although the exact abnormality inherited is not yet known. The genetic haplotype above is associated with a number of autoimmune diseases. Celiac disease patients become sensitive to the gluten in wheat. This damages the lining cells of their small intestine, reducing the absorbing capacity. The cause of the arthritis sometimes associated with gluten sensitivity is unknown. Possibly the damaged gut allows antigenic material that would normally be kept in the gut to cross into the body where it sets up an immune reaction (see ENTEROPATHIC ARTHRITIS).

Symptoms and Diagnostic Path

Some patients have diarrhea, loss of weight, poor growth (in children), and anemia, but often the presentation is less obvious. Only 50 percent of patients have diarrhea. Children may be diagnosed when investigated for short stature, infants for vomiting and weight loss, and women when they become severely anemic during pregnancy. Some patients are diagnosed when a physician does a number of screening tests for nonspecific symptoms such as fatigue, depression, or borderline iron deficiency. Diagnosis of these "subclinical" cases is still important as they have an increased risk of nutritional deficiencies, OSTEOMALACIA, low birth weight babies, and possibly malignancy. The risk of the latter is thought to be lower than those with the full-blown disease. Associated autoimmune diseases may lead to the diagnosis. These include thyroid disease, DIABETES, and arthritis. The arthritis is quite variable, but most often the spine, hips, knees, and shoulders are affected. Elbows, wrists, and ankles are affected less frequently. The arthritis is fairly symmetrical and inflammatory with swelling and early morning stiffness but does not often cause damage visible on X-ray. Studies show that people with diagnosed celiac disease are at moderately increased risk of gastrointestinal tumors, particularly lymphomas. It is not yet clear how much successful treatment can reduce this risk although it seems likely that it does. Interestingly, breast cancer seems to occur less frequently in celiac patients than the general population.

The diagnosis should be suspected in arthritis patients who have symptoms of bowel disease, are unusually anemic, or have a low serum calcium concentration. Tests for iron, calcium, folate, and vitamin B_{12} often show low blood levels. The amount of fat passed in the stools is increased, and this can be measured. The diagnosis has recently become much easier with the development of of tests for antiendomysial and tissue transglutamin-

ase antibodies in the blood. These tests are both very sensitive, identifying 85 to 98 percent of people with celiac disease, and specific, being incorrectly positive in less than 5 percent of cases. They are not 100 percent, however, and if negative in someone with otherwise typical symptoms it may be necessary to use the older diagnostic methods. Antibodies to gluten can also be measured but are less often positive. Before these antibody tests were available, it was necessary to biopsy the gut wall, show that the typical changes were present, and then rebiopsy after three months of a gluten-free diet to show that it had recovered. This is still done where the diagnosis is not clear. There is nothing diagnostic about the arthritis other than its coexistence with celiac disease.

Treatment Options and Outlook

Adopting a diet free of gluten not only restores bowel function to normal but also causes resolution of the arthritis. This form of diet should be taken on with the help of a dietician so that the patient can become aware of the many products that contain gluten and learn how to substitute gluten free alternatives. One generally unsuspected source of gluten is many vitamin pills, and so the product label should be carefully read.

Risk Factors and Preventive Measures

An allergy to the gluten in wheat is the cause of celiac disease and avoiding all gluten will prevent the disease. Most supermarkets and delicatessens now carry a range of gluten-free products that are clearly labeled, and eating a gluten-free diet is not nearly as difficult as it was even 10 years ago. However, many patients will find it useful initially to consult with a dietician about the changes they will need to make in their diet when they are diagnosed as having celiac disease.

central nervous system vasculitis A rare form of VASCULITIS (inflammation of blood vessels) affecting the central nervous system, most often the brain. Central nervous system (CNS) vasculitis is classified as primary or secondary. Several illnesses mimic the symptoms and complications of CNS vasculitis. Primary CNS vasculitis affects only the CNS and is also called primary angiitis of the nervous system, isolated angiitis of the nervous system, and granulomatous angiitis of the nervous system. In secondary CNS vasculitis, vasculitis affecting many organs (systemic vasculitis) also affects the CNS.

The cause of primary CNS vasculitis is not known. However, viral illnesses and drugs that suppress the immune system are thought to play a role in some patients.

Secondary CNS vasculitis may be associated with the following conditions:

- *Infections*   (a) Viral infections caused by herpes viruses, cytomegalovirus, human immunodeficiency virus (HIV), varicella virus that causes chickenpox or shingles, and many other viruses (b) Other infections such as syphilis, Lyme disease, tuberculosis, and many other bacterial and fungal infections
- *Systemic vasculitis*   Most types of systemic vasculitis such as WEGENER'S GRANULOMATOSIS, POLYARTERITIS NODOSA, BEHÇET'S DISEASE, and CHURG-STRAUSS SYNDROME can affect the CNS.
- *Other rheumatic diseases*   Several other rheumatic conditions, for example systemic lupus erythematosus and SJÖGREN'S SYNDROME, can sometimes cause CNS vasculitis.
- *Lymphoma*   CNS vasculitis can occur with Hodgkin's and non-Hodgkin's lymphoma, types of cancers that affect the lymph nodes, bone marrow, and other organs such as the spleen.

Conditions that can mimic CNS vasculitis include

- *Lymphoma*   A rare type of lymphoma that occurs inside blood vessels called intravascular lymphoma (also known as malignant angioendotheliomatosis) can mimic CNS vasculitis. A brain biopsy is often needed to differentiate between the two.
- *Drugs*   Many drugs, usually ones that constrict blood vessels, have rarely been associated with nervous system complications such as stroke. These vasoconstricting drugs can also cause abnormal angiograms in that the blood vessels in the brain show irregular areas and spasm that

look identical to the angiograms of patients with CNS vasculitis. Drugs that have caused stroke and abnormal angiograms include cocaine, amphetamines, heroin, and cold remedies, particularly those containing phenylpropanolamine, a drug that was removed from the market by the FDA in 2000 because it increased the chances of having a stroke. Vasoconstrictors do not seem to cause a true CNS vasculitis. However, they can cause clinical findings, for example stroke and an abnormal angiogram, that mimic those of CNS vasculitis.

- *Strokes*   Any condition that causes many small strokes, for example atherosclerosis or blood clots showered off an abnormal heart valve, can be difficult to differentiate from CNS vasculitis.

Symptoms and Diagnostic Path

The first symptom of primary CNS vasculitis is usually a gradual and progressive, diffuse decrease in brain function over many months. This often shows as memory loss, a change in personality, and a decrease in intellectual ability. Headaches occur in just over 50 percent of patients. Symptoms that usually indicate that there is a problem in a localized area of the brain, for example a stroke, occur in 10–20 percent of patients at presentation but in up to 40 percent throughout the illness. A careful examination (as well as MRI scanning) sometimes shows that two or more different areas of the brain are affected, and this is very useful in suggesting vasculitis as the cause of the stroke. Seizures occur at some stage in a quarter of patients. Rarely, vasculitis can affect the spinal cord and result in paralysis of the legs or arms. Secondary CNS vasculitis can cause symptoms identical to those of primary CNS vasculitis. Making a definite diagnosis of primary CNS vasculitis can sometimes be very difficult. Systemic symptoms such as fever, sweats, loss of weight, anemia, and an elevated ESR are absent or mild in patients with primary CNS vasculitis, and if prominent, they usually indicate a secondary cause.

No diagnostic test is always positive in CNS vasculitis or is able to discriminate between primary CNS vasculitis and diseases that mimic it. The diagnosis is based on information from several sources, including the clinical findings, analysis of cerebrospinal fluid (see LUMBAR PUNCTURE in Appendix II), imaging tests such as MRI or angiogram, and sometimes a brain biopsy.

Cerebrospinal fluid (CSF), obtained by lumbar puncture, is abnormal in 80–90 percent of patients with primary CNS vasculitis. It often shows a small increase in the number of white blood cells and protein concentration, findings that usually indicate inflammation or infection in or around the brain. Examining CSF is useful to exclude an infection because in CNS vasculitis all the bacterial and fungal cultures and tests for viruses in the CSF are negative.

The most common MRI findings, many small infarcts deep in the tissue of the brain, are not specific for CNS vasculitis. However, if the MRI and CSF examinations are completely normal, it is helpful because that combination virtually excludes the diagnosis of CNS vasculitis. The MRI provides images of the brain tissue, but an angiogram is often done because it provides images of the arteries in the brain. The angiogram can be normal. However, it is abnormal in more than 60 percent of patients with CNS vasculitis and shows irregular arteries with patchy areas of narrowing and dilation. These angiogram abnormalities are not specific for primary CNS vasculitis but can occur with conditions that mimic it or cause secondary CNS vasculitis.

Because there are no specific CSF and X-ray findings that make the diagnosis of CNS vasculitis, a biopsy of the brain and meninges (the thin layer that lines the brain) is sometimes needed to rule out infections or lymphoma. The biopsy, which samples only a minute area of brain, is also not a perfect test and can be negative in about 25 percent of patients who eventually turn out to have CNS vasculitis.

Treatment Options and Outlook

Because CNS vasculitis is so rare, no clinical trials have compared responses to different treatments. Treatment is with high doses of CORTICOSTEROIDS, often combined with an immunosuppressive drug such as CYCLOPHOSPHAMIDE, and usually continues for at least six to 12 months after the illness has gone into remission.

If CNS vasculitis is not treated, it slowly progresses and causes memory loss, dementia, stroke, and death. Drug treatment usually arrests the process and often improves some neurological symptoms, although some symptoms can be permanent. High doses of corticosteroids and other drugs that suppress the immune system often cause side effects, for example an increased chance of developing a serious infection. Treatment requires careful monitoring.

Risk Factors and Preventive Measures

The many causes of secondary CNS vasculitis are discussed above. These include infections, systemic vasculitis, other rheumatic diseases, and lymphoma. CNS vasculitis is a very rare complication of these conditions and cannot realistically be said to be preventable.

Charcot's joint   See NEUROPATHIC ARTHRITIS.

chemokines   Movement of white blood cells (leukocytes) into tissues and into areas where there is inflammation is controlled by a subgroup of CYTOKINES called chemokines. The synthesis and release of chemokines is stimulated by interleukin-1 (IL-1) and tumor necrosis factor (TNF), cytokines that act to promote inflammation. More than 40 chemokines have been discovered and classified into several families. Chemokines are classified based on their structure. The two largest families are named CC and CXC. The CC family has two cysteine amino acids (designated C) that are always next to each other, and the CXC family has the two cysteines separated by other amino acids (designated X). The nomenclature of chemokines can be confusing because when they were discovered, different researchers often gave the same chemokine different names. Chemokines are often referred to, and are better known, by their abbreviated older names that describe function rather than their newer, official names. For example, the official name of IL-8 (interleukin-8) is CXCL8, MCP (monocyte chemoattractant protein) is CCL2, and RANTES (regulated upon activation normal T cell expressed and secreted) is CCL5.

Chemokines exert their effects by binding to specific chemokine receptors that are found on target cells. The receptors (R) for the CC chemokines are named CCR1, CCR2, and so on, and those for the CXC chemokine family are CXCR1, CXCR2, and so on. Different tissues have different chemokine receptors, and this explains why the same chemokine can have different effects in different parts of the body. There are some inherited variations in the structure of chemokine receptors that affect how well they work. For example, it was discovered that people with a particular genetic variant of the chemokine receptor CCR5 are relatively resistant to HIV infection. This is because the virus enters cells by binding to receptors for this chemokine, but people with the variant CCR5 receptor are less likely to be infected by HIV because their receptors do not bind HIV well.

Chemokines modify several processes that regulate inflammation and growth of cells and tumors. To fight infection in a particular part of the body, cells must move out of the bloodstream and concentrate around the infection so that the inflammatory response can be focused where it is needed. The number and type of white blood cells that are attracted to the area of inflammation is regulated by chemokines. For example, in patients with pneumonia caused by bacteria, the infected tissues of the lungs are infiltrated by many neutrophils, a process that is partly regulated by IL-8, a chemokine that acts as a powerful attractant for neutrophils. Other chemokines, for example MIP (macrophage inflammatory protein) and eotaxin, regulate the movement of macrophages and eosinophils into tissues. Apart from regulating inflammation, chemokines also affect the growth of cancers. Two factors that determine how big and how fast a tumor grows are the ability of its cells to divide rapidly and the speed at which the tumor can make new blood vessels (angiogenesis) and thus provide itself with more nutrition as it grows larger. Some chemokines, for example platelet factor 4, reduce angiogenesis and tumor growth but others, for example IL-8, do the opposite.

The role that chemokines play in regulating inflammation and cell growth in autoimmune disease, infections, and cancer is an area of active research that is likely to produce drugs that will treat these diseases by stimulating or inhibiting specific chemokines.

chiropractic medicine   About a third of the visits patients make to alternative health practitioners are to chiropractors, making this the largest alternative medicine profession in the United States. Chiropractic is a profession that specializes in the manipulation of bones, joints, and muscles to treat medical disorders. Chiropractic has moved from being part of alternative medicine to become mainstream with practitioners licensed in all 50 states. Many health care insurance companies now reimburse for visits to chiropractors, just as they do for visits to mainstream physicians.

Chiropractic was founded in Davenport, Iowa, in 1895 by Daniel David (D. D.) Palmer, a grocery store owner who cured deafness in a man by manipulating his spine. The theory underlying chiropractic was that pressure on nerves irritated them and caused illness that could be corrected by manipulation to relieve the pressure. Palmer developed a school with its name derived from the Greek words *cheir* (hand) and *praxis* (use). His son, B. J. Palmer, developed and popularized the practice further. As it developed, chiropractic attracted practitioners with many different philosophies. Some have believed that all illness is the result of spinal irritation and can be cured by manipulation, but others have restricted their interest to problems affecting muscles and joints. Some chiropractors restrict their treatment to manipulation, but others have incorporated other alternative treatments such as herbal remedies. More recently chiropractic has evolved into a practice that mostly restricts itself to using manipulation to treat problems of muscles and joints.

Osteopathy (see OSTEOPATH), which like chiropractic was based on the concept that manipulation of bones and soft tissues could alleviate symptoms and was also originally thought to be useful for treating most types of illness, has evolved differently. Over the years many osteopaths have increasingly incorporated traditional medicine into their practice. Now many patients treated by osteopaths do not receive manipulation but are treated with medications identical to those prescribed by traditional physicians.

Chiropractic manipulation involves several different techniques. One of the best known is the *high-velocity thrust,* a sudden, sharp thrust applied to the spine, either directly by the practitioner's hands or indirectly by using another part of the patient's body, for example a leg, as a lever to twist the spine. Other techniques involve the relief of muscle spasm through gentle stretching.

Chiropractic has fought a long battle with orthodox medicine that has included hunger strikes by imprisoned practitioners and prolonged legal battles, but it is now generally accepted as a form of therapy. Strong scientific evidence supporting the efficacy of chiropractic is limited to a few conditions. Many studies have compared chiropractic manipulation with other forms of treatment for back pain. An overall synthesis of the many studies, often with conflicting conclusions and interpretations, is that chiropractic treatment improves low back pain and neck pain in the short term but is not useful for other medical problems such as asthma.

cholesterol emboli syndrome First reported in the autopsy of a Danish sculptor, Thorwaldsen, cholesterol embolism is caused by clumps of cholesterol breaking off from a cholesterol plaque in an artery. They float downstream until they reach small arterioles where they lodge, block the arteriole, and cause small infarcts (areas of tissue death) in the organ. Although thought to be rare, cholesterol emboli have been found in 2–8 percent of autopsies.

Atherosclerosis is the underlying cause of cholesterol embolism. Therefore conditions such as diabetes, high blood cholesterol, smoking, and aging that increase atherosclerosis also increase the chances of developing cholesterol emboli. In addition to conditions that increase atherosclerosis, any event that makes the cholesterol plaque lining the walls of arteries less stable can trigger cholesterol embolism. For example, cholesterol plaques can be disturbed by medical procedures, such as angiography when a needle is placed in an artery or when surgery is performed on an artery. If a person is treated with an anticoagulant such as heparin or warfarin to prevent blood clots forming, this can increase the risk of cholesterol embolism. In some patients with atherosclerosis, cholesterol embolism occurs without anticoagulation or any predisposing event.

Symptoms and Diagnostic Path

Cholesterol embolism can cause systemic symptoms such as fever and affect many different organs, depending on where the showers of cholesterol crystals finally lodge. Organs often affected are the skin, brain, and kidneys.

- *Skin* The commonest skin rash is livedo reticularis, a lacy reddish-purplish rash on the front of the legs. This rash is faint, does not itch, and can be difficult to see. Other common skin rashes are small purple or black spots that resemble VASCULITIS and larger purplish nodules. A whole toe or finger can turn blue because its blood supply is inadequate.

- *Kidneys* Worsening of high blood pressure and a decrease in kidney function, shown as a rising level of CREATININE (see Appendix II), in the blood are common.

- *Central Nervous System* If the emboli deposit in the blood vessels of the eye, they can cause sudden blindness or loss of vision. If a physician examines the retina with an ophthalmoscope, shiny yellow cholesterol plugs are sometimes visible. Plugging of small arteries in the brain can cause a stroke, either permanent or lasting a short time (transient ischemic attacks or TIAs).

Cholesterol embolism can be difficult to diagnose because it mimics vasculitis, and the clinical pattern varies according to which organs are involved. The diagnosis is often missed because it is not considered. Although the damage to organs in cholesterol embolism is caused by blocked arterioles, the pulse in an affected arm or leg is usually normal because the plugs are in small arteries, not the large ones that form the pulse. Blood tests are not very useful and can be misleading. The white blood cell count and ESR are often elevated and misleadingly suggest a diagnosis of infection or vasculitis. A high eosinophil count and low COMPLEMENT level can misleadingly suggest a drug allergy or vasculitis. The most helpful diagnostic test is a biopsy of an involved organ (usually the skin is the most convenient site to biopsy) that shows needle-shaped cholesterol crystals blocking small arterioles.

Treatment Options and Outlook

There is no specific treatment for cholesterol emboli. Usually anticoagulants are avoided because of the concern that they may make the atherosclerotic plaque even more unstable and worsen the illness. There are a few reports in the medical literature of patients responding to treatment with one of the *statin* group of drugs that lowers cholesterol. Because the statins (examples are lovastatin, pravastatin, and simvastatin) are relatively safe and because almost all patients with cholesterol emboli need a drug to lower their cholesterol, many physicians start treatment with a statin.

Ulcers and gangrene can develop at the tips of the fingers, toes, hands, or feet if they do not get enough blood and oxygen. Often more than one digit is affected at the same time. Toes are affected more often than fingers because atherosclerosis is more common in the legs than the arms. If the blood supply to tissue is not enough to supply its needs, then gangrene in a finger, toe, leg, or arm can occur. If this happens, amputation is often needed to prevent infection spreading from the gangrenous tissue into the bloodstream and throughout the body. More often the gangrenous tissue slowly shrivels and falls off. The decrease in kidney function caused by cholesterol embolism often plateaus after a few days or weeks and then slowly improves. However, kidney function may deteriorate to the level where a patient needs dialysis. TIAs resolve quickly, but strokes can be permanent. Another serious complication is infarction of the bowel. This can require surgery to remove the gangrenous part of the bowel.

Cholesterol embolism is serious and reported to be fatal in as many as 80 percent of patients, but this figure likely represents the outcome in patients with the most severe form of the disease. Many patients who have a milder form with just a blue toe or a moderate decrease in their kidney function after an angiogram get completely better.

Risk Factors and Preventive Measures

Atherosclerotic plaques are the risk factor for developing cholesterol emboli. In turn, smoking, high blood pressure, high cholesterol, and being overweight are the main risk factors for developing atherosclerotic plaques. It follows that efforts to reduce these will reduce the chances of developing cholesterol emboli. However, because cholesterol emboli are relatively rare, controlled studies to prove this are not feasible.

chronic fatigue syndrome A condition, of unknown cause, characterized by severe, sometimes disabling fatigue and many other symptoms that affect different organ systems. Many people in the population suffer from fatigue at some time, and approximately 25 percent of patients seen by primary care physicians have fatigue that has lasted longer than a month. However, only about 0.2–2.6 percent of people meet the criteria used to define the chronic fatigue syndrome.

The cause of chronic fatigue syndrome is not known and is controversial. Some experts believe that a physical cause exists but has not yet been identified. Others believe that chronic fatigue syndrome does not exist as a separate entity but consists of many physical symptoms that are the result of psychological stress, a process known as somatization. An argument against the theory that chronic fatigue syndrome is the result of a particular personality that responds to stress by developing physical symptoms is the fact that chronic fatigue syndrome often starts suddenly in people who, up until then, have been in relatively good physical and psychological health. However, in spite of intensive research, no clear cause of chronic fatigue syndrome has been found.

Viral infection was first thought to be the cause of chronic fatigue syndrome because many patients have a low-grade fever, sore throat, and enlarged lymph nodes. Epstein-Barr virus, the cause of infectious mononucleosis, was suspected, but studies did not support this suggestion. Several other viruses have been investigated, but none has been found to be consistently associated with the chronic fatigue syndrome.

Many studies have found that psychological distress and psychiatric problems are more common in patients with chronic fatigue syndrome than in the general population. However, clearly separating cause and effect has not been possible. In other words, is psychological distress more common in people with chronic fatigue syndrome because they are feeling sick, or are the psychological symptoms the cause of chronic fatigue syndrome?

An interesting study found that many patients with chronic fatigue syndrome developed low blood pressure and became dizzy when they were placed on a tilt table—a test performed to evaluate why people become dizzy or faint. During a tilt test, people are placed on a table that supports them so that they do not move or use their muscles. Then the table is tilted so that they are standing upright but supported by the table, not their muscles. This test allows blood to pool in the veins and is used to test the body's ability to react to changes in posture. In the initial studies, people with chronic fatigue syndrome could not tolerate the tilt test. However, several later studies, some of which compared people with chronic fatigue syndrome with people who were also out of shape but otherwise healthy, did not confirm the suggestion that altered responses to changes in posture were the cause of chronic fatigue syndrome. A small number of people have a condition known as orthostatic intolerance—symptoms of a very fast heart rate and dizziness after they have been standing for a while. Many of these people also have symptoms similar to those of chronic fatigue syndrome. Most likely chronic fatigue syndrome has several causes and orthostatic intolerance is just one.

Chronic fatigue syndrome often overlaps with the symptoms of several other conditions that cause chronic pain or fatigue and whose cause is not understood. For example, many patients with fibromyalgia have chronic fatigue and vice versa. It is not clear if fibromyalgia and chronic fatigue syndrome are variations of the same condition that have an overlapping spectrum of symptoms or if they are separate problems that sometimes cause similar symptoms.

Symptoms and Diagnostic Path

Chronic fatigue, often worse after a physical activity at an intensity that was previously no problem and that is not caused by another medical problem, is the most common symptom. The onset of fatigue may be sudden and can sometimes be dated from a viral infection. Many other symptoms can occur, including dizziness, poor concentration, unrefreshing sleep, poor memory, tender lymph nodes, muscle and joint pain, headaches, lack of energy, and low-grade fever. Many of these symptoms

overlap with fibromyalgia, and some patients fulfill the diagnostic criteria for both conditions.

No laboratory tests are available to help make the diagnosis. Laboratory tests are helpful because they are usually normal. If they are abnormal, these results may be a clue to some other diagnosis. The diagnosis is made only after other medical causes of chronic fatigue such as anemia, thyroid problems, cancer, hepatitis, autoimmune diseases, and SLEEP APNEA have been excluded. The Centers for Disease Control (CDC) criteria are widely used to define patients with chronic fatigue syndrome for research studies. This definition has the following requirements:

1. Other medical, psychiatric, and substance abuse problems must have been excluded.
2. The unexplained fatigue must be something new (it cannot have been lifelong), is not helped by rest, is not explained by hobbies or activities, and has a big effect on the person's ability to lead a normal life.
3. Unexplained chronic fatigue must be accompanied by at least four of the following symptoms to meet the CDC definition of chronic fatigue syndrome:

   • Poor memory or concentration to the extent that it affects the person's personal activities
   • Sore throat
   • Tender lymph nodes in the neck or armpit
   • Muscle or joint pain without joint swelling or redness
   • Headaches that have a different character from previous headaches
   • Unrefreshing sleep
   • Poor energy level for more than 24 hours after exercising

The fatigue and other symptoms must have been present for at least six months or have recurred over that time.

Treatment Options and Outlook

Many of the studies that have examined treatments for chronic fatigue syndrome have included only a small number of patients, perhaps one of the reasons that the results have not always been reproducible. The strongest evidence supports two therapies, COGNITIVE BEHAVIORAL THERAPY and EXERCISE. In clinical trials, cognitive behavioral therapy was usually administered by experts for several months, usually as six to 16 sessions each lasting 30–60 minutes, and improved symptoms in more than half the patients. The usefulness of aerobic exercise and flexibility training in chronic fatigue syndrome have been studied, usually involving sessions that built up to 20–30 minutes at least three times a week. Aerobic exercise was more effective than flexibility training, and about half the patients improved. Bed rest has not been beneficial and may be harmful. No drug therapy has been consistently helpful.

Several antidepressants have been studied but the results have been inconsistent, although some symptoms, for example poor sleep, have often improved. One promising study suggested that some patients with chronic fatigue syndrome had an alteration of their blood pressure reflexes when they stood up and that treating them with fludrocortisone, a drug that makes the kidneys absorb salt and water and increases the volume of the blood, improved symptoms. A later, more rigorous placebo-controlled study did not confirm these findings. Corticosteroids, such as prednisone, have generally not been effective. Although some trials have found a modest benefit with hydrocortisone, the results have been conflicting.

Chronic fatigue syndrome does not increase the risk of death and it does not cause structural damage to muscles or joints. However, it can have a major effect on quality of life, earning capacity, and activity levels. The outcome of chronic fatigue syndrome has not been clearly defined because most studies have been performed in groups of patients who have been treated by specialists and are likely to have been the most severely affected people. Generally, between 20 and 50 percent of people have some improvement of their symptoms, but only 6 percent reach their previous level of activity and well-being. The personality and beliefs of the patient seem to affect the outcome. A positive outlook and the belief that symptoms can be overcome are associated with a better outcome. (See also FIBROMYALGIA.)

Risk Factors and Preventive Measures

The cause of chronic fatigue syndrome is unknown, and there are no known preventive measures.

Churg-Strauss syndrome   A rare type of vasculitis described by Churg and Strauss in 1951 that is probably a variant of WEGENER'S GRANULOMATOSIS and causes asthma, eosinophilia, and vasculitis.

The cause of Churg-Strauss syndrome is not known but it seems to be associated with allergy. Most patients have a history of preceding nasal allergy. Eosinophils, which are prominent in Churg-Strauss syndrome, are also often elevated in people with allergic asthma and nasal or skin allergy. Immunoglobulin E (IgE), which is also often elevated in patients with allergic conditions, is usually raised in Churg-Strauss syndrome. How allergy proceeds to vasculitis is unclear.

A few patients have developed Churg-Strauss syndrome after starting treatment with a class of drugs called leukotriene receptor antagonists. This includes zafirlukast (trade name: Accolate) and montelukast (trade name: Singulair). Several explanations have been put forward to explain why Churg-Strauss syndrome seems to occur more often in people taking these drugs. One possibility is that the patients with asthma who developed Churg-Strauss had it all along, but it was not diagnosed because the symptoms were suppressed by cortico steroids. Then, when they started treatment with a leukotriene receptor antagonist and were able to decrease or stop their corticosteroids, the symptoms of Churg-Strauss that were previously suppressed became obvious. However, a number of patients not on corticosteroids have developed Churg-Strauss syndrome after starting a leukotriene receptor antagonist. Another possibility, therefore, is that this class of drugs may rarely cause the Churg-Strauss syndrome in a few people through mechanisms that are not clear.

Symptoms and Diagnostic Path

Many patients have allergic symptoms such as asthma or rhinitis (runny nose) for months or years before the diagnosis. It is not clear if these symptoms are caused by Churg-Strauss that has not been diagnosed or if, at some point, Churg-

Strauss develops on top of the allergic symptoms. Eosinophilia does not cause symptoms, but in a patient with vasculitis or unexplained illness, it is often the first clue to the diagnosis. Symptoms can vary a lot and depend on the organs involved.

- *Lung* Asthma, resulting in wheezing and shortness of breath, is usually episodic but can be severe and present much of the time. Vasculitis can affect the lungs causing infiltrates and shortness of breath that resemble pneumonia. Rarely vasculitis can cause bleeding into the lung tissue.

- *Nervous System* Typically vasculitis involves peripheral nerves affecting both sensation and the ability to move. For example, if a nerve to the foot is affected, the patient may lose or have altered feeling in part of the foot and may not be able to pull it up so that it drags while walking, a symptom called foot drop. The nerves affected are usually in different parts of the body, and this symptom complex is called mononeuritis multiplex. The brain and nerves to muscles of the face and eyes are seldom affected.

- *Kidney* The kidneys can be affected, but this is less common than in Wegener's granulomatosis. Kidney involvement causes blood and protein in the urine but does not usually cause symptoms unless the kidneys fail.

- *Others* All types of serious vasculitis can affect virtually any organ. The skin is often affected, and rashes are common. Vasculitis typically causes purple spots that are raised and can be felt (palpable purpura), but almost any type of rash can occur. Muscle pain is common, arthritis rare, and these relate to the activity of the vasculitis. Nasal and sinus problems are common as is abdominal pain and diarrhea. Inflammation of the outer lining of the heart (pericarditis), heart failure, and myocardial infarction are well-recognized complications. Vasculitis affecting the blood vessels to the bowels is uncommon but can cause bleeding, infarction, and perforation.

The diagnosis is clinical and based on three features that are key to the diagnosis: asthma, eosinophilia, and vasculitis. The differential diagnosis usually includes asthma, Wegener's granulomatosis, and other causes of vasculitis such as POLYARTERITIS NODOSA. Asthma is a common disorder, and many patients with asthma also have a mild eosinophilia. Churg-Strauss is differentiated from asthma by the presence of vasculitis and a more pronounced eosinophilia, often more than 1500 cells/mm³. Similarly, marked eosinophilia is uncommon in Wegener's granulomatosis and other types of vasculitis. There are unusual types of pneumonia such as eosinophilic pneumonia that can cause eosinophilia and respiratory symptoms, but vasculitis does not occur.

Laboratory tests provide useful information but are seldom diagnostic. Eosinophilia is often the first clue to the diagnosis but is not specific. Eosinophilia can be caused by several conditions including asthma, allergies, reactions to drugs, parasitic infection, cancer, and vasculitis. If the kidneys are affected, the creatinine level in the blood may be elevated and blood, protein, and white blood cells are likely to be present in the urine. Nonspecific tests that go up with infection and inflammation such as the ESR and C-reactive protein are likely to be elevated. The antineutrophil cytoplasmic antibody (ANCA) blood test (see Appendix II) is elevated in about 70 percent of patients and is more likely to be a P-ANCA than the C-ANCA that is more typical of Wegener's granulomatosis. A negative ANCA test does not exclude the diagnosis of Churg-Strauss. A chest X-ray may show infiltrates. These can be of different shapes and sizes and can change rapidly.

A biopsy of affected tissue, often lung, typically shows eosinophils destroying the walls of medium-sized arteries (vasculitis), eosinophils in deep tissues, and formation of clusters of inflammatory cells around a center, called granulomas.

Treatment Options and Outlook

The treatment is as for any severe vasculitis and usually consists of a combination of corticosteroids and an immunosuppressant such as CYCLOPHOSPHAMIDE. Because Churg-Strauss syndrome is uncommon, there is very little guidance on its treatment from controlled studies (see CLINICAL TRIAL). From the information available, however, many patients apparently do well on corticosteroids alone and drugs like cyclophosphamide should be used only for more severe disease, for example when there is involvement of heart or kidneys. AZATHIOPRINE and intravenous immunoglobulin have also been used with corticosteroids in resistant cases and have fewer long-term adverse effects than cyclophosphamide. Interferon alpha has been used with corticosteroids in a few patients resistant to cyclophosphamide with success, but its place in the treatment of Churg-Strauss syndrome is not yet clear. About 80 percent of patients survive five years or more after diagnosis, but there is a wide range of disease severity that affects the prognosis. Kidney involvement and vasculitis affecting the heart or bowels indicate more severe disease and a potentially worse outcome.

Risk Factors and Preventive Measures

Although the setting in which Churg-Strauss syndrome occurs is well recognized, the actual cause is not known. About 70 percent of Churg-Strauss patients have allergic rhinitis, asthma, and often polyps in their noses. This atopic disposition is however quite common, and Churg-Strauss is rare, indicating there must be other factors involved. There is no known preventive measure.

clinical trial An experiment performed on humans to determine the safety and efficacy of a treatment. The clinical trial is a relatively recent and important scientific advance that has allowed scientists to measure and compare responses to a treatment objectively. Before clinical trials became the standard method for evaluating new treatments, these were introduced into clinical practice empirically, using a trial and error approach, and were then propagated among practitioners based on word of mouth and anecdotal experience. This situation is similar to the approach currently used to evaluate many herbal and other nontraditional therapies that are not classified as drugs and therefore do not require proof of efficacy and safety before they are marketed.

Unscientific, anecdotal approaches to the evaluation of new therapies led to the introduction of many ineffective or toxic drugs. The controlled clinical trial with its unbiased design and objective measurements revolutionized modern medicine. Anecdotal evidence is based on the responses of one or a few patients and is a seriously flawed method for evaluating a treatment. Anecdotal evidence is similar to testimonials from customers—there is a bias to report only the positive responses. A second major problem with the anecdotal approach to evaluating a treatment is that there is a natural tendency for people taking a new treatment to feel better, even if the treatment is an ineffective dummy called a placebo. This positive response to a new treatment, whatever it is, is called a placebo response. Clinical trial design has evolved to overcome these problems. There are several different types of clinical trials.

Uncontrolled, placebo-control, and active-control trials If a new treatment is studied alone, with no comparison group, it is called an *uncontrolled* study. Uncontrolled studies are difficult to interpret because telling if any response is due to a true drug effect or to the placebo response is impossible. Uncontrolled studies, although they can provide useful preliminary information, are not strong evidence in favor of a new treatment, even if the results of the trial are positive.

To decide if a treatment is effective, it is best to compare it with another treatment, and this is called a *controlled* trial. Controlled studies usually compare the new treatment against an inactive substance, like a dummy sugar pill, called a *placebo control*, or else against some treatment that is known to be effective, called an *active control*. Comparing the results of the new treatment with the results of the control treatment makes it much easier to determine if the new treatment is effective.

A placebo-controlled study is generally more efficient in finding out whether a new treatment is effective, but for ethical reasons this design is not always appropriate. Most medical ethicists agree that it is not ethical to treat a patient in a clinical trial with a placebo if an effective treatment is available for that particular condition and if treatment with placebo could result in irreversible, preventable problems for a patient. For example, it is generally considered ethical to evaluate a new drug for pain caused by osteoarthritis against placebo, provided patients have access to adequate pain control if their treatment fails. However, if active rheumatoid arthritis (RA) is not adequately treated for several months it can result in irreversible joint erosions.

Therefore, determining how to perform ethical, placebo-controlled studies in RA is more difficult.

Randomized trials If the researchers in charge of a study could choose to allocate patients to either the treatment or the control groups, there could be a tendency for them to allocate those with the worst problems into one or another of the groups. Then, because the patients in one group were sicker, that group could have a worse outcome, even if their treatment was effective. To prevent this happening, everyone enrolled into a study should have an equal chance of being allocated to receive the new treatment or the control treatment—this is called a randomized study. Patients can be randomized into groups in different ways. One is a simple flip of a coin, but generally a computer generates random numbers.

Open-label trials In an open-label study design, both the individuals in the study and the research staff know which treatment a patient is receiving. This is a scientifically weak design because, even if the study is randomized and controlled, the open-label design allows the enthusiasm of patients and researchers for any new treatment to bias their collection and interpretation of information. Most new arthritis treatments that have been evaluated in exploratory, open-label studies were initially thought to be effective, but many were later found to be ineffective when more rigorous double-blind clinical trials were performed.

Double-blind trials The opposite of an open-label study is a double-blind study. With this design neither the people in the study nor the researchers performing the study know who has been allocated to treatment or control. This means that neither the expectations of patients nor those of researchers can influence the interpretation of the results. To keep a study double-blind is not always easy. For example, the placebo and active drug have to be identical in appearance and taste. A randomized double-blind, placebo-controlled study is the most scientifically rigorous design to evaluate a new treatment but is not always ethical or practical. For example, a placebo-controlled study is not appropriate for evaluating a new treatment for a cancer that already has an effective treatment, and performing a double-blind study to compare a surgical treatment with a drug is very difficult.

Limitations of clinical trials Although clinical trials have been a major scientific advance, they have some limitations.

- Most clinical trials are performed by drug companies and usually compare a new drug with a placebo. Most physicians and patients would be much more interested in how the new drug performs compared with the best-available treatment. Once the new drug is marketed, unless it appears to be better than the standard treatment, there is often no incentive for a drug company to sponsor a study to compare it with standard treatments.

- Most clinical trials study highly selected patients. Typically patients in clinical trials are relatively healthy and are not taking many other medicines. For example, patients with liver or kidney disease, recurrent infections, or recent hospitalizations are excluded from most trials. This means that when a new drug is approved by the FDA and marketed, many types of patients not studied in clinical trials will take the drug.

- Most clinical trials last for only a few months. Knowing the long-term effects of different drugs is more important because many types of arthritis are chronic. Clinical trials cannot provide this information, and it is obtained from observational studies that record the responses of groups of patients followed over many years. Such studies have their own problems because patients are not randomized to a particular drug. Therefore differences in outcome could be due to differences in disease rather than differences in response to drugs.

- Clinical trials determine the average response in a group of patients but do not predict what the response of an individual will be. Thus, although the average response to drug A may be better than drug B in a clinical trial, an individual patient may respond better to drug B.

Cogan's syndrome A very rare type of VASCULITIS described by Cogan in 1945 that affects the eyes, ears, and other organs.

The cause of Cogan's syndrome is not known. An association with smallpox vaccination and upper respiratory tract infections has been reported, but this could be coincidental and no infective cause has been identified. Cogan's syndrome affects younger people, often in their 20s. Recently, researchers identified antibodies against sensory cells of the inner ear in patients with Cogan's syndrome, suggesting that it is an autoimmune illness.

Symptoms and Diagnostic Path
The usual onset is with eye or ear symptoms. Vasculitis can affect the inner ear and cause sudden deafness, dizziness with a sensation of spinning (vertigo), and unsteadiness or poor balance. The eye symptoms are a red, watery eye that feels scratchy and is sensitive to light. The commonest type of eye inflammation is known as interstitial keratitis. This can be diagnosed by an ophthalmologist using a slit-lamp microscope to examine the eye. In addition to eye and ear symptoms, Cogan's syndrome often causes systemic symptoms such as fever and weight loss. Vasculitis can also affect the aorta and cause leaking of the aortic valve or an aneurysm.

There is no diagnostic test for Cogan's syndrome. The diagnosis is made entirely on the clinical manifestations.

Treatment Options and Outlook
Because of its rarity there are no good studies that define the best treatment for Cogan's syndrome. It is usually treated as a systemic vasculitis with high doses of CORTICOSTEROIDS often combined with an immunosuppressant such as METHOTREXATE, CYCLOPHOSPHAMIDE, or CYCLOSPORINE. Vertigo usually improves but deafness (40 percent of patients), blindness (8 percent), and leaking aortic valve (14 percent) can be permanent.

Risk Factors and Preventive Measures
The cause of Cogan's syndrome is unknown, and there are no known preventive measures.

cognitive behavioral therapy A type of therapy most often used to treat chronic pain such as that resulting from FIBROMYALGIA or BACK PAIN or fatigue from CHRONIC FATIGUE SYNDROME. Cognitive behavioral therapy is used with other medical therapy and is not a replacement. It is based on the concept that beliefs about an illness and the strategies people use to cope with illness and other stresses at home or work can affect the outcomes of an illness.

Cognitive behavioral therapy helps patients understand the techniques they are using to cope with illness and substitutes positive coping skills for negative ones. The therapy starts with the patient describing the effect that various symptoms have on activities such as work and hobbies and on attitudes and feelings, for example anxiety, depression, and helplessness. This helps people recognize that what they do is affected by how they feel and think and vice versa. The basis of cognitive behavioral therapy is that by learning positive ways of coping and avoiding negative ones, someone can take an active part in controlling symptoms and improve their quality of life. Therapy focuses on practical strategies to deal with negative attitudes and behavior and to improve physical activity and psychological health. Therapists are usually psychologists or other health professionals with training in cognitive behavioral therapy. A directory of trained professionals is available from the Association for the Advancement of Behavioral Therapy http://www.aabt.org/ (see Appendix III).

Cognitive behavioral therapy techniques Therapists teach several coping techniques. After the patient has mastered and applied them, the program usually also involves a plan to maintain these skills.

Relaxation The technique taught most often involves tensing and relaxing different muscles while resting quietly and focusing the mind on feelings and thoughts of relaxation. After mastering relaxation at rest, the patient learns how to identify muscles that are sources of tension and to relax them during daily activities such as driving, sitting, or standing.

Pleasant imagery Placing pleasant and positive images in the mind's eye helps relaxation and focuses thoughts away from unpleasant sensations such as pain. The patient chooses an image that is peaceful and pleasant, for example a beautiful mountain, and then uses all the senses, smelling the mountain air and feeling the breeze, to make the image more real. The patient chooses images that have personal significance, and the therapist works with the patient to make the image as real as possible.

Alternating rest and activity Many patients overexert themselves on one activity and then have difficulty completing other tasks. Cognitive behavioral therapy teaches patients to break activities down into manageable pieces and plan their days around alternating periods of rest and activity.

Removing negative thoughts Therapists teach patients to identify negative thoughts and feelings and to substitute positive ones. For example, "I am feeling terrible and will never get better" can be replaced with "I have had bad times like this before and I can work through it."

These skills are taught and reinforced by the therapist using several techniques. One technique, cognitive rehearsal, consists of patients imagining situations and their responses. The therapist and patient rehearse healthy responses so that when a similar situation arises in real life, the patient is prepared for it. Role-playing is a similar technique. Therapists also ask patients to keep a journal and then use it as a tool to identify unhealthy attitudes so that these can be redirected.

Results of cognitive behavioral therapy Clinical trials have studied the effect of cognitive behavioral therapy in RA, rheumatoid arthritis, osteoarthritis, back pain, and fibromyalgia. In most studies, therapy was added to other medical treatment and improved outcomes such as pain, depression, anxiety, and quality of life.

complement More than 100 years ago scientists noticed that the cell walls of some bacteria ruptured after they had been exposed to an antibody and placed in fresh serum. As science advanced it was discovered that complement was responsible for this. The activity of complement is the end result of a cascade of interactions between a group of proteins in the blood that forms the complement pathway. The complement cascade has several functions. Two of the most important are defense against bacteria and mopping up antigen/antibody complexes that could otherwise be harmful. There are two main complement pathways, the classical pathway and the alternative pathway. Both work through a series of proteins called *components* that are numbered C1, C2, and so on. The classical pathway is usually activated by a reaction between an antibody and an antigen, but the alternative pathway can be activated without antibody. The two pathways proceed by activating different components initially, then both activate C3. The final steps from then on are identical and result in the formation of a group of proteins, called the membrane attack complex, that can damage foreign cells like bacteria.

There are several inherited abnormalities of the complement cascade that can cause illness. Deficiencies of the early components of the cascade, for example C1, C2, and C4, increase the risk of developing an illness similar to systemic lupus erythematosus (SLE). Complete complement deficiencies are rare. The commonest is C2 deficiency, but only about 1 in 10,000 people have a complete deficiency of it. Half of these develop an illness that resembles SLE, usually with prominent skin problems. Unlike typical SLE, people with C2 deficiency often develop an illness with a negative ANA blood test (see ANTINUCLEAR ANTIBODY in Appendix II). Partial deficiency of C4 is very commonly associated with an SLE-like disease as are deficiencies of the C1 components. About a third of people with C3 deficiency get an SLE-like disease, but they also get many infectious problems. Why a complement deficiency should cause SLE is not clear. However, because complement has the important function of clearing the body of immune complexes, a deficiency in the complement cascade would likely allow immune complexes to accumulate. This would increase the chances of developing an autoimmune disease such as SLE. Deficiencies of the later components of the complement cascade, for example C5, C6, C8, and C9 increase the risk of developing bacterial infections, particularly those caused by *Neisseria meningitidis*, a cause of bacterial meningitis.

Another hereditary abnormality of the complement pathway results in increased rather than decreased activity. Some forms of hereditary angioedema are caused by a deficiency of the enzyme inhibitor that inhibits C1 in the early part of the complement cascade.

COX-2–selective drugs See CYCLOOXYGENASE and NONSTEROIDAL ANTI-INFLAMMATORY DRUGS.

CPPD See CALCIUM PYROPHOSPHATE DIHYDRATE DEPOSITION DISEASE.

CREST syndrome See SCLERODERMA.

Crohn's disease See ENTEROPATHIC ARTHRITIS.

cryoglobulinemia The group of diseases termed cryoglobulinemia all share the laboratory finding of having cryoglobulins on blood testing. When blood plasma is cooled to less than 37°C, one or more immunoglobulin type precipitates out but redissolves on warming. These immunoglobulins are termed cryoglobulins. Immunoglobulins (antibodies) are classified into five major types according to their properties: IgA, IgG, IgM, IgD, and IgE. Within each class of immunoglobulin, particular antibodies may be produced by one B lymphocyte and its progeny (monoclonal) or many lymphocytes and their progeny (polyclonal). The normal response to an infection would always be polyclonal.

Cryoglobulinemia is classified into three subgroups. In type I, there is one monoclonal immunoglobulin, usually IgM. In type II, there are both polyclonal IgG and monoclonal IgM. Type III includes both polyclonal IgG and polyclonal IgM.

Type I cryoglobulinemia is usually caused by Waldenstrom's macroglobulinemia, lymphoma, or multiple myeloma. In these diseases white blood cells called plasma cells have become autonomous, multiplied greatly, and produced excessive amounts of immunoglobulins. In Waldenstrom's macroglobulinemia this is of IgM type, and in multiple myeloma it may be IgG, IgM, or IgA. These immunoglobulins or antibodies have no useful activity in the body. As their concentration in the blood increases, they have a natural tendency to precipitate in the colder parts of the body such as the hands, nose, and feet.

Type II and III cryoglobulinemia, together referred to as mixed cryoglobulinemia, have large amounts of IgG antibodies together with either monoclonal or polyclonal IgM that is directed against part of the IgG molecule. This type of IgM antibody is called rheumatoid factor (see Appendix II). When the IgM attaches to IgG molecules to form large complexes, they become liable to precipitate. These may be associated with chronic infection caused by HEPATITIS B, HEPATITIS C, lymphoma, chronic lymphocytic leukemia, myeloma, and autoimmune diseases such as RHEUMATOID ARTHRITIS, SJÖGREN'S SYNDROME, SCLERODERMA, and SYSTEMIC LUPUS ERYTHEMATOSUS. In a few patients there is no apparent cause, and this is termed *essential* mixed cryoglobulinemia.

In 1989 the hepatitis C virus (HCV) was discovered, and soon it was possible to do blood tests to look for HCV infection. As these blood tests improved, it became clear that HCV was the cause of 80–90 percent of mixed cryoglobulinemia. These patients would previously have been said to have essential mixed cryoglobulinemia.

Whatever the cause, the end result is that cryoglobulins form complexes and precipitate out when the blood temperature drops below 37°C. This is usually just below the skin, especially in the hands, ears, nose, and lower legs. It may form a gel, precipitate, or actual crystals, depending on how much abnormal protein there is and how cold the blood becomes. As a gel it may just cause sludging and poor blood flow. When it precipitates onto the inner lining cells of the blood vessel (endothelium), an inflammatory reaction occurs with damage to the blood vessel (VASCULITIS).

Symptoms and Diagnostic Path

RAYNAUD'S PHENOMENON is common, as are joint pains and mild fever. The typical event that often leads to the diagnosis is leukocytoclastic vasculitis following exposure to cold. This can lead to small purple-black lesions on the lower legs (purpura), larger black crusting lesions that may develop into ulcers, or even dry gangrene of fingers or toes. Occasionally there is inflammation of the filtering part of the kidneys (glomerulonephritis). In type I cryoglobulinemia the protein level can become so high that the hyperviscosity syndrome develops.

This is when the blood is so thick that it does not flow through small blood vessels very well. Hyperviscosity syndrome may cause breathlessness, a fainting feeling, headaches, difficulty in concentrating, and aching in the legs. In addition there may be symptoms of the associated disease. In HCV infection there is usually some inflammation of the liver, but generally this is less severe than in hepatitis B.

There are two aspects to the diagnostic process, first the diagnosis of cryoglobulinemia and, second, the search for an underlying cause. Cryoglobulinemia may be diagnosed when an at-risk individual, for example someone known to have HCV infection or Waldenstrom's macroglobulinemia, complains of typical symptoms and the appropriate investigations are done. On the other hand, someone may, for example, present with purple-black lesions on the legs and have the appropriate investigations done when the biopsy shows leukocytoclastic vasculitis. Blood should be taken in prewarmed syringes and given directly to the laboratory to test for cryoglobulins. The immunoglobulins involved can then be typed and shown to be either monoclonal or polyclonal. The plasma viscosity is measured by seeing how fast the plasma can pass through a very fine tube.

If there is a single monoclonal cryoglobulin, then Waldenstrom's macroglobulinemia or multiple myeloma is likely. Patients with Waldenstrom's macroglobulinemia will have an IgM monoclonal immunoglobulin; may have an enlarged liver, spleen, and lymph nodes; and their bone marrow biopsy will show abnormal collections of lymphocytes and plasma cells. Multiple myeloma patients are less likely to have enlarged livers and spleens but often have bone pain and X-rays show very typical *punched-out* lesions in the bone or a general thinning of bone. The bone marrow biopsy will show an excessive number of plasma cells.

The diagnosis of the autoimmune conditions listed under "Cause" is discussed in the relevant sections of this book. Hepatitis B infection is associated with a small number of cases of cryoglobulinemia. The blood tests reliably show infection and differentiate between past exposure with immunity and current active infection. Blood tests for HCV have proven more difficult. Currently, a second generation ELISA (enzyme-linked immunosorbent assay) is usually done as a screening test and confirmed by a RIBA (recombinant-based immunoblot assay) test. Most doctors would then go on to request an HCV RNA test before starting treatment. This confirms the actual presence of the virus in the blood being tested rather than just the body's reaction to the virus, which the first two tests look at. Because the HCV is present in the blood in very low numbers, it was difficult to find before modern molecular biology techniques became available.

Treatment Options and Outlook

Because cryoglobulinemia is an unusual manifestation of a number of diverse diseases, the treatment may need to be directed at reducing the cryoglobulins as well as treating the underlying disease. In the noninfectious cases treating the underlying condition is usually all that is required. However, in emergencies it is sometimes necessary to deplete the cryoglobulins rapidly. PLASMAPHERESIS is a technique using automated blood cell separators in which 50 percent of the protein in blood can be removed in a couple of hours. This has a temporary effect only. Immunosuppressive treatment with CYCLOPHOSPHAMIDE or high-dose CORTICOSTEROIDS effectively shut down the production of the abnormal immunoglobulins although their effect will take a week or more to become evident.

When the hepatitis B or C viruses are the underlying cause, there is concern that immunosuppressive treatment may worsen the infection. Since the treatment for these infections stimulates the immune system (and may occasionally provoke autoimmune disorders), there is likewise concern that this treatment may worsen the cryoglobulinemia and/or the vasculitis. The best way to approach this dilemma is not known at present. With mild or incomplete cryoglobulinemia, it is probably best to commence antiviral therapy if the patient wishes to have this. If a mild vasculitis is present, it may be best to cover the antiviral treatment with a moderate dose of corticosteroid. If there is limb-threatening vasculitis or renal involvement, this should be adequately settled with immunosuppressive treatment before starting antiviral medication. Hepatitis

B is treated with alpha interferon, an immunostimulatory CYTOKINE. Only about 35 percent of patients will respond to this, and there are considerable side effects. Hepatitis C is treated by a combination of alpha interferon and ribavirin, again with only moderate success. In this difficult situation treatment needs to be tailored to each individual with particular regard to his or her wishes.

Risk Factors and Preventive Measures

The varying causes of cryoglobulinemia are discussed above. The most common, and only potentially preventable, cause is chronic viral hepatitis. See hepatitis C for discussion of routes of infection and therefore possible preventive measures.

crystal-induced arthritis   See GOUT and CALCIUM PYROPHOSPHATE DIHYDRATE DEPOSITION DISEASE.

cyclooxygenase (COX)   There are two COX enzymes, COX-1 and the more recently discovered COX-2, that increase the formation of prostaglandins and thromboxane from a precursor, arachidonic acid. Prostaglandins are a family of chemicals that have many effects on tissues, including some that increase inflammation. An important effect of thromboxane is that it causes platelets to become sticky, clump together, and form blood clots.

COX-1 is found in many different tissues, but COX-2 is usually found only in tissues that have become inflamed. Older NSAIDs, such as aspirin, ibuprofen, naproxen, and many others, inhibit both COX-1 and COX-2 enzymes. Decreasing the amount of prostaglandins made by COX-2 in inflamed tissues is anti-inflammatory and is useful for treating the symptoms of arthritis. Older NSAIDs inhibit COX-2 but also inhibit COX-1 and thus decrease the amount of thromboxane made by platelets. Decreasing thromboxane and making platelets less sticky can be helpful for preventing heart attacks, strokes, and illnesses caused by blood clots, but it can also increase the risk of bleeding. Aspirin is a unique NSAID because it has very long-lasting effects on the platelet COX-1 enzyme, and this is why aspirin is used to prevent heart attacks and strokes. COX-1, in addition to being found on

platelets, is also found in the stomach where the prostaglandins it makes protect against ulcers. The result is that older NSAIDs that block COX-1 and COX-2 are more likely to cause peptic ulcers as a side effect. To overcome this increased risk of peptic ulcer, scientists developed drugs that blocked COX-2 and did not have much effect on COX-1. These drugs are sometimes called COX-2 selective NSAIDs (see CELECOXIB, ETORICOXIB and LUMIRACOXIB).

COX-2 selective drugs are no more effective in decreasing pain and inflammation than nonselective NSAIDs but cause GI side effects less often. Other common side effects of NSAIDs such as hypertension and decreased kidney function do occur with COX-2 selective drugs, perhaps because some COX-2 is present in normal kidneys. COX-2 selective drugs have no effect on COX-1 and therefore do not decrease platelet stickiness and cannot be used to prevent heart attacks.

In fact, a number of studies hinted at an increased risk of cardiovascular events with the COX-2 selective drugs in the early years of their use. In 2004, a large study using rofecoxib to try to prevent large bowel polyps was stopped because people receiving the active drug (see CLINICAL TRIAL) had significantly more heart attacks and strokes than those taking a placebo. Subsequent meta-analysis or grouping together of all the previous studies also showed an increase in the incidence of heart attacks, and rofecoxib was withdrawn from the market. The remaining COX-2 selective drugs have been very carefully studied for their cardiovascular safety. Although judged safe enough for continued use they probably all carry some increased risk which appears to be dose dependent. That is, the risk is higher with higher doses. Currently they should only be used in patients at risk of cardiac events or stroke if the reasons for use are compelling and all precautions possible have been taken to prevent such an event. The commonest such precaution would be to co-prescribe aspirin, but this may then obviate the gastrointestinal benefit of COX-2 selective inhibition.

cystic fibrosis   The most common lethal genetic disorder in western Caucasian populations, cystic fibrosis is the result of an abnormality in the gene for the CFTR or cystic fibrosis transmembrane regulator and affects about 1 in every 3,000 births in Caucasian Americans and 1 in every 15,000 births in African Americans. Cystic fibrosis affects many different glands, including those lining the walls of the intestines, lungs, and sinuses.

Symptoms and Diagnostic Path

Symptoms of the disease often start in childhood. A common symptom is poor absorption of food because the intestinal glands that are important for digesting food are not functional. Repeated attacks of pneumonia are common because the glands in the layer lining the passages of the lungs are not able to stop the normal lung secretions from plugging up the airways and causing infections.

Treatment Options and Outlook

Antibiotics and other medical advances have improved the prognosis and, perhaps because more patients with cystic fibrosis are surviving into their thirties, arthritis-related problems are now recognized more often.

Risk Factors and Preventive Measures

Possession of an abnormal cystic fibrosis transmembrane regulator gene is the risk factor for cystic fibrosis. However, only a minority of cystic fibrosis patients get arthritis and the reason for this is poorly understood. There is therefore no action or treatment modality that is known to prevent these few cystic fibrosis patients from getting arthritis. Hypertrophic pulmonary osteoarthropathy develops because of the chronic suppurative lung infections and the better the control of infection the less likely this will be to occur. This also applies to amyloidosis. Calcium and vitamin D deficiency should be anticipated and tested for with supplements being given when necessary.

Cystic Fibrosis Arthritis A few patients with cystic fibrosis have developed a type of arthritis that seems to be specifically associated with the illness. This arthritis comes in acute attacks lasting days or weeks, can affect one or several joints, and is often accompanied by a skin rash, usually ERYTHEMA NODOSUM. Tests for rheumatoid factor and antinuclear antibodies (see Appendix II) and X-

rays are usually negative. The cause is not known, but because patients with cystic fibrosis suffer from recurrent infections, several investigators have searched for an infectious cause. Infection could cause arthritis either directly or indirectly. According to one theory, infection could trigger an autoimmune response and cause arthritis because the molecular structure of parts of some infectious organisms is similar to that of parts of the human genome. Researchers have not consistently found particular infections to be associated with arthritis in cystic fibrosis. Another possibility is that genetic variability in people with cystic fibrosis may explain why only some get arthritis. Thus, the actual genetic variant of cystic fibrosis a person has, as well as his or her individual immune response genes, may be important. So far there is little information to support this suggestion. A plausible explanation is that because patients with cystic fibrosis have poor pancreatic function and therefore do not absorb food well, they are more likely to develop ENTEROPATHIC ARTHRITIS, a condition that causes a similar type of arthritis. Information about responses to different treatments is limited. NSAIDs can improve symptoms, and some studies show that they may also help the respiratory problems. If possible, immunosuppressive drugs are avoided because patients with cystic fibrosis are already predisposed to developing infections.

Hypertrophic pulmonary osteoarthropathy Any chronic lung problem, including cystic fibrosis that causes clubbing (swelling of the tips of the fingers), can cause HYPERTROPHIC PULMONARY OSTEOARTHROPATHY. The treatment of this condition is based on decreasing the underlying infections, usually with rotating courses of antibiotics.

Osteoporosis Patients with cystic fibrosis often have a low absorption of vitamin D and calcium, two essential requirements for healthy bones. Also, because of chronic illness they are often not very active and therefore have a greater chance of developing OSTEOPOROSIS. The treatment of osteoporosis in patients with cystic fibrosis is similar to that of other patients with osteoporosis, but particular attention is needed to ensure that enough vitamin D and calcium is absorbed.

Vasculitis A few patients with cystic fibrosis have developed VASCULITIS affecting the skin, internal organs, or both. No other cause was found, and therefore cystic fibrosis is thought perhaps to increase the risk of vasculitis.

Amyloidosis Patients with chronic infection or inflammation have an increased chance of developing secondary AMYLOIDOSIS, and a few cases have occurred in patients with cystic fibrosis.

cytokines Small molecules that act as messengers between cells, particularly cells that regulate the immune response. Cytokines are important for local communication between cells, in contrast to hormones, which circulate in the bloodstream and exert their effects on distant organs or tissues. Low levels of some cytokines can be detected in the circulating blood of healthy people, but they exert their main action over the very short distances between cells in the same locality. The first local messenger proteins discovered in 1969 were produced by lymphocytes and so were called lymphokines. The name cytokine soon replaced the name lymphokine because other types of white blood cell also produced these messengers. Cytokines are produced mainly by white blood cells that have been activated. The cytokine is then released into the space between cells. If it comes into contact with its specific receptor on neighboring cells, it binds to the receptor and activates responses in the target cell. These may either increase or decrease inflammation and growth. More than 150 cytokines are currently known. However, the information made available by the human genome project will allow scientists to identify many new molecules that have a cytokine-like structure and then to work forward and discover their biological function. Many cytokines share functions so that often several cytokines can cause the same effects on target cells. Cytokines can be divided according to whether their main effect is to increase or decrease inflammation.

Cytokines That Increase Inflammation

Tumor necrosis factor alpha (TNF-α) Tumor necrosis factor got its name from the observation that if scientists produced inflammation in animals that had experimental tumors, then the animals produced a substance, later called TNF, that could cause necrosis (death) of part of the tumors. TNF-α is produced mainly by monocytes and macrophages but can be produced by activated B and T cells and fibroblasts. It stimulates cells to produce other cytokines that increase inflammation such as interleukin-1 and interleukin-6. If TNF is injected into animals, it causes fever, loss of weight, and shock. TNF-α seems to be particularly important in rheumatoid arthritis because mice that have been genetically engineered to make too much TNF-α develop an illness similar to rheumatoid arthritis (RA). In humans, TNF-α is found in the synovial fluid of patients with RA, and blocking TNF-α with an antibody, or mopping it up with a decoy protein, is an effective treatment for RA (see ADALIMUMAB, ETANERCEPT, INFLIXIMAB). TNF binds to two receptors called p55 and p75. Some of these receptors are bound to cells, but others are not and are called soluble receptors. The soluble receptors can act as a sump to mop up TNF and stop it from reaching receptors bound to cells and activating them.

Interleukin-1 (IL-1) IL-1 is produced mainly by monocytes and macrophages but can be produced by endothelial cells that line blood vessels and by activated B and T cells. A lot of evidence suggests that IL-1 is important in RA. When IL-1 was injected into the knee joints of rabbits, it caused damage. In animal models of arthritis, blocking IL-1 with antibodies decreased the amount of joint damage. In humans, IL-1 is present in the synovial fluid of patients with RA.

IL-1 acts through two types of IL-1 receptors. Type I receptors are linked to cells so that the cells respond if this receptor is activated, but type II receptors are not linked to a signalling system and act as decoy receptors. Another mechanism used by the body to control IL-1 activity is to produce a protein that acts as an antagonist. This protein is called IL-1 receptor antagonist (IL-1ra) and binds to the same receptor site that IL-1 binds to but does not activate the cell. If IL-1ra has bound to the site where IL-1 would otherwise bind, the binding site is blocked and IL-1 cannot bind and activate the cell. This naturally occurring antagonist of IL-1 turned out to be therapeutically useful because it was manufactured and has been developed as a drug that is an effective treatment for RA (see ANAKINRA).

Interleukin-6 (IL-6) IL-6 is produced by monocytes, macrophages, activated T cells, and synovial fibroblasts that line joints and promotes inflammation. It is important in the bone damage that occurs in joints of people with rheumatoid arthritis. Recently, an antibody to IL-6 has been developed (TOCILIZUMAB) for use in inflammatory arthritis.

Interleukin-12 (IL-12) IL-12 is another proinflammatory cytokine that is found in rheumatoid joint lining. However in animal models, targeting this cytokine has not produced consistent improvement in arthritis.

Interleukin-15 (IL-15) IL-15 has a broad range of effects regulating immune and inflammatory cells. An antibody directed against this cytokine was effective in treating arthritis in mice and is in early trials in humans.

Interleukin-17 (IL-17) IL-17 is a family of proteins found in increased levels in joint fluid in rheumatoid arthritis and is under active study.

Interleukin-18 (IL-18) IL-18 appears to act at a very early stage of the formation of pro-inflammatory cytokines and an IL-18 binding antibody is being investigated for efficacy in rheumatoid arthritis.

Cytokines that Decrease Inflammation

Interleukin-10 (IL-10) IL-10 is produced by monocytes, macrophages, and B and T cells. IL-10 acts on cells to stop them from producing IL-1 and TNF-α, cytokines that increase inflammation. IL-10 has been used to treat rheumatoid arthritis, psoriasis, and inflammatory bowel disease but without useful effect so far. Rheumatoid synovium already produces significant amounts of IL-10, presumably as a feedback mechanism limiting inflammation, and it may be that adding more is not going to have much benefit.

Interleukin-4 (IL-4) IL-4 is produced by T cells and acts on them so that they produce less IL-1 and TNF-α.

Transforming growth factor-beta (TGF-beta) TGF-beta suppresses T cells in rheumatoid joint fluid. However, like IL-10, it is already there in good quantities. It may also contribute to the growth of the rheumatoid joint ling (pannus) that contributes to joint destruction.

Interleukin-11 (IL-11) IL-11 reduces production of IL-1 and TNF-alpha, which should be advantageous in rheumatoid arthritis. However, in one small study it was of no benefit.

de Quervain's tenosynovitis Inflammation of the sheath of tissue that lines the tendons of two muscles that pull the thumb away from the other fingers and up away from the palm (abductor pollicis longus and extensor pollicis brevis). This usually occurs as a result of repetitive wrist and thumb movement at work, home, or during recreational activities. Women aged 30 to 50 years are most commonly affected. De Quervain's tenosynovitis may also occur in RHEUMATOID ARTHRITIS, psoriatic arthritis (see PSORIASIS AND PSORIATIC ARTHRITIS), other forms of inflammatory arthritis, following trauma or during pregnancy, and just after delivery.

Symptoms and Diagnostic Path

The maximal inflammation is usually just above the level of the wrist, and the tendon appears hot, swollen, red, and tender. Moving the thumb or wrist is painful. The tendons may be heard to creak as they pass through the tight, inflamed tenosynovial tissue. Finkelstein's test is positive. This involves placing the thumb across the palm, closing the fingers over it, and then turning the wrist away from the thumb side. This reproduces the patient's pain.

Treatment Options and Outlook

Stopping the causative action and splinting is important in treatment. Lightweight splints that hold the thumb slightly up and out while allowing full movement of the fingers and the end joint of the thumb are used. ICE and NSAIDs can relieve pain. Careful injection of CORTICOSTEROIDS along the tendon sheath gives an excellent result in about 70 percent of patients and may be repeated if symptoms do not resolve or recur. If it has not resolved in six months, surgery can be performed to release the tendons from the fibrous pulley that holds them down at the wrist (extensor retinaculum) and remove some of the inflamed tenosynovium.

dermatomyositis and polymyositis Dermatomyositis is an autoimmune disease causing muscle inflammation and weakness together with a number of skin rashes. A very closely related disease, polymyositis, causes muscle inflammation and weakness but no rash. Both conditions will be discussed in this section. There is an association with malignancy in some adults with dermatomyositis and polymyositis. They are rare conditions, each affecting one in 100,000 people at any given time. Women are affected twice as often as men, and African Americans three times as often as Caucasians.

In these diseases the immune system behaves as if there is something in the muscle, skin, and other organs that it needs to attack and destroy. Lymphocytes and other immune cells travel to these organs, leave the bloodstream, and cause inflammation. There are differences between the two conditions. Immune cells, particularly lymphocytes, directly attack muscle cells in polymyositis. In dermatomyositis they seem to cause most of the damage by attacking the blood vessels that supply the muscle fibers. In both the attack damages the muscle and other cells, causing them first to malfunction and then ultimately to die. The reason for this immune attack remains unknown, although certain people seem more prone to it than others.

In 1953 a pair of twins both developed dermatomyositis within a year of each other. Since then a number of families have been found in which more than one person has developed dermatomyositis or polymyositis. In addition other autoimmune diseases have been found in the families of patients with myositis more often than expected. These findings could mean that either hereditary factors or something in the environment shared by these family members influenced the development of the disease. To date no environmental factors have been found to be important. A number of genetic variations (alleles) have been found that predispose people to developing dermatomyositis and polymyositis as well as autoimmune diseases in general. The associations, however, are fairly weak. Likely more than one allele is important in any one person. Also, these genetic factors only predispose people to getting the disease, they do not cause it.

In addition to occurring on its own, polymyositis can occur as a complication of other autoimmune diseases such as SYSTEMIC LUPUS ERYTHEMATOSUS (SLE) and SCLERODERMA and, rarely, as a side effect of treatment with PENICILLAMINE. It is also a common manifestation of the OVERLAP SYNDROME. Hydroxyurea, a drug used to treat certain blood conditions, can occasionally cause dermatomyositis-like skin problems.

Symptoms and Diagnostic Path

Most adults first see their doctor with painless weakness of upper arm, shoulder, buttock, and thigh muscles coming on over three to six months. Children and younger adults may have a more rapid onset and often have fever and fatigue as well. A few people also have muscle aches. This pattern of muscle involvement causes difficulty doing things above shoulder height, such as brushing hair, as well as lower limb activities like running or climbing stairs. The muscles involved in speech or swallowing are affected 10–20 percent of the time, leading to hoarseness, abnormal voice, difficulty swallowing, or food and fluids going up into the back of the nose. There is some tenderness of the muscles in 50 percent of people.

Skin problems may start well before the muscle involvement in dermatomyositis. Occasionally the disease is confined to the skin with no obvious muscle involvement, although sophisticated testing may still show some muscle abnormalities. This condition is called amyopathic dermatomyositis and may constitute up to 10–20 percent of dermato-

myositis patients. The skin lesions are typically flat and purple red and are found on the upper eyelids, cheeks, nose, neck, upper chest and back (shawl area), elbows, knees, and knuckles. A number of other areas are less frequently involved. Quite a lot of swelling may occur early on, and later the lesions become thinner and lose their color. The skin of the hands may become thickened, dry, and cracked, a condition known as *mechanic's hands.* Gottron's papules are typical raised lesions found overlying the outside of the finger joints and are found only in this condition. The small blood vessels in the nail fold become larger and fewer in number so that they can be seen with the naked eye. There is sometimes bleeding in this area. Skin ulcers may occur, and occasionally troublesome itching or sensitivity to the sun is found.

Many patients get joint pain or arthritis early on, but this is seldom severe. Calcification or bone formation under the skin or in the soft tissues especially around muscles can be a serious problem. This usually affects children who have had dermatomyositis for some time and is rare in adults. It particularly occurs at sites of trauma and may cause ulceration of the overlying skin. RAYNAUD'S PHENOMENON is common, especially in dermatomyositis and the overlap syndrome.

Shortness of breath in someone with polymyositis or dermatomyositis may be a symptom of a serious problem, signaling heart, lung, or respiratory muscle involvement. Both the diaphragm and the muscles between the ribs may be affected by the inflammation. This needs vigorous treatment and possibly hospitalization until it can be shown that muscle strength is improving. About 30 percent of patients get inflammation of the gas-exchanging parts of the lung (alveolitis). This starts with a cough and breathlessness when exercising and may progress very rapidly. Patients with weak swallowing muscles or abnormal function of the esophagus are prone to getting chest infections because food or liquids go down the trachea into the lungs.

Mild heart involvement is probably quite common, but it is usually diagnosed only when severe. Abnormalities of heart rhythm are the commonest problem and can be life threatening. Heart failure may occur because of inflammation of the heart muscle or as a complication of severe lung disease.

Adults with dermatomyositis develop an unusual number of malignancies both in the four years before diagnosis and subsequently. The time of greatest risk is the first five years after diagnosis of dermatomyositis. Many different types of malignancy occur, but ovarian cancer is particularly common. The risk of those with *amyopathic dermatomyositis* is the same as those with muscle involvement. Children with dermatomyositis are not at an increased risk of cancer. Although adults with polymyositis do seem to have a slightly higher-than-usual risk, it is not as great as for those with dermatomyositis.

The diagnosis must first be suspected because of the clinical findings and then confirmed by special tests, ideally including a positive muscle biopsy. Special investigations may be required to identify involvement of other organs. The finding of certain autoantibodies may give further information on the type of disease. Depending on the patient's risk profile and treatment, further tests may need to be done to look for cancer or to monitor the safety of the medications.

Confirming the diagnosis   The first step in diagnosis is usually to confirm muscle damage. Enzymes leak from damaged muscle cells and may be measured in the blood. These include creatine kinase (also called creatine phosphokinase), aldolase, and lactate dehydrogenase. Their levels are useful in judging the response to treatment. Creatine kinase is the most useful of these and is raised in over 95 percent of patients. Myoglobin is another protein released into the blood from damaged muscle and can be useful in following progress, although it is less often used. An electromyogram is useful in confirming muscle disease (as opposed to nerve problems) and for showing which muscles are involved. This involves inserting a very fine needle into a muscle and measuring the electrical activity, both spontaneous and on attempted contraction of the muscle. Typical findings of muscle irritability and low-amplitude disordered impulses are found in 90 percent of patients early on but less frequently later on in severely affected muscles.

Trying to obtain confirmation of the diagnosis with a muscle biopsy is important in all patients. In these biopsies, lymphocytes and other chronic inflammatory cells will be seen to be invading muscle cells that will be in varying states of damage or death. Not all the typical findings are seen in all biopsies, and up to 20 percent are normal in definite cases. This is because the disease affects muscle in a patchy manner. Even if an affected patch is biopsied, the changes may still be developing so that it does not look typical. For this reason fairly large biopsies should be taken from muscles with active inflammation. Identifying the best muscle to biopsy may not be easy since weak muscles are not necessarily inflamed. The electromyogram has been used for this purpose, although it may cause muscle changes itself. MRI scanning is more useful, being painless, not causing any muscle changes, and giving information about whole groups of muscles rather than just a small segment of a muscle. The MRI needs to be done carefully since previous damage or simply disuse changes can look very like inflammation on the scan. Special *fat suppression* T2 weighted images need to be taken to avoid this problem. The skin changes of dermatomyositis are usually sufficiently characteristic not to require biopsy. However if there is doubt, biopsy will differentiate them from other autoimmune diseases.

Other organ involvement   Spirometry measures the mechanical ability to move air in and out of the lungs and should be done early on and at subsequent intervals to monitor progress. High-resolution CT scans are excellent at showing inflammation and scarring of the lungs that do not show up on plain X-rays until moderately advanced. Occasionally, a bronchoscope is passed into the main airways and washings taken to count the number of inflammatory cells, or a radioisotope scan (gallium scan) can be done. Both these procedures give information on how much inflammation is going on in the lungs. However with increasing experience using CT scans, they are seldom required.

An electrocardiogram (ECG or EKG), ultrasound scan of the heart, and continuous monitoring of the heart rhythm for a period of time will be used to evaluate the heart if the individual suffers from breathlessness or palpitations and sometimes as a screening investigation. Although the heart is muscle, it does contain slightly different enzymes that can be measured to see if it is affected. These include troponin I, troponin T, and the MB fraction of creatine kinase. Barium X-ray studies are used to identify problems in the gut, including swallowing difficulties.

Autoantibodies A number of patients have positive blood tests for autoantibodies that are also found in patients with other diseases. These include anti-U1-RNP (also found in MIXED CONNECTIVE TISSUE DISEASE), anti-PM-Scl (also found in scleroderma), anti-Ro (found in SJÖGREN'S SYNDROME, SLE, and others), and other nonspecific autoantibodies. These are sometimes called *myositis-associated* antibodies.

Other autoantibodies are found only in patients with inflammatory myositis, so-called myositis specific antibodies. It has been hoped that these antibodies would enable patients to be subdivided into groups with very similar symptoms and complications. In this way it would be possible, by knowing what specific autoantibody a patient had at the outset, to anticipate what complications the individual might develop and even his or her response to treatment. For example, patients with antisynthetase antibodies often have Raynaud's phenomenon, fever, mechanic's hands, more severe arthritis, and inflammatory lung disease. They have an average response to treatment. Antisynthetase antibodies are the commonest autoantibodies found and, of the six known at present, anti-Jo-1 is the most frequent. A second group has antibodies to signal recognition particle (anti-SRP). They have a rapid onset of disease, the heart is often affected, and there is a poorer response to treatment. A third group has anti-Mi-2 antibodies. They frequently have a severe dermatomyositis rash and include children with this condition. They respond well to treatment. How useful these autoantibodies will prove to be in predicting the course of the disease is not yet clear.

Associated malignancy All adults with dermatomyositis should be screened for malignancy at the time of diagnosis. The tests done will vary from person to person but would likely include a chest X-ray, ultrasound scan of the abdomen and pelvis, examination of the stool for blood, and blood tests to look for markers of malignancy, especially ovarian cancer (a CA-125 blood test). Other tests will be done if there are suggestive symptoms or particular risk factors such as a family history of breast or bowel cancer. Although the risk is less in polymyositis, it is still reasonable to screen for the commonest associated malignancies (lung and ovarian cancer) and follow up any suspicious symptoms. A relapse after successful treatment is a warning sign that a malignancy might have developed, and the appropriate tests should be repeated. Screening tests are not necessary in children.

Treatment Options and Outlook

Because polymyositis and dermatomyositis are rare disorders, information about their treatment is based on a relatively small number of patients and very few controlled trials (see CLINICAL TRIAL.) Corticosteroids are the mainstay of therapy in these diseases. This is usually given orally as PREDNISONE, but in severe disease and particularly in children it may initially be given intravenously as methylprednisolone. It has recently been shown that in some patients lower doses of prednisone (30 mg per day or less as a starting dose) result in as good an outcome as the higher doses traditionally used but with much fewer corticosteroid side effects. These side effects are related to both the dose taken and the length of time the drug is used. Management of the side effects becomes one of the major problems with ongoing treatment. To enhance the effectiveness of corticosteroids and allow lower doses to be used, most polymyositis and dermatomyositis patients need an additional medication to suppress the immune system. AZATHIOPRINE or METHOTREXATE is usually used for this purpose, and both are effective.

Patients with dermatomyositis should avoid sunlight or use adequate sun protection as this can worsen the rash. Because of the relatively large doses of corticosteroids used, most patients should receive protective medication against OSTEOPOROSIS. Severely immunosuppressed people are at risk of getting a serious lung infection with *pneumocystis jiroveci,* and if the risk is high, it is better to try to prevent this by taking long-term antibiotics, cotrimoxazole.

When the disease cannot be controlled with these medications or is initially controlled but then returns, it is termed *refractory.* Treatment of refractory disease is difficult. A combination of azathioprine and methotrexate has been shown to be effective, as has INTRAVENOUS IMMUNOGLOBULIN.

The powerful immunosuppressive drugs TACROLIMUS and CYCLOSPORINE have both been shown to be effective in small numbers of patients. Although cyclosporine might theoretically be expected to be more effective in polymyositis than dermatomyositis, this does not seem to be the case in practice. Fludarabine, a drug used to treat certain forms of leukemia, has been used with moderate success.

Alveolitis or inflammation of the gas-exchanging part of the lung is a very serious complication of polymyositis and dermatomyositis and needs to be treated vigorously before there is too much scarring in the lungs since this is not treatable. CYCLOPHOSPHAMIDE, cyclosporine, and tacrolimus have all proven reasonably effective in this situation. The skin lesions of dermatomyositis can be resistant to treatment with corticosteroids, and HYDROXYCHLOROQUINE is very effective in treating them. As well as improving the muscle inflammation, intravenous immunoglobulin is effective in healing the skin lesions and may be used if hydroxychloroquine does not work.

As the muscle inflammation settles (usually indicated by the creatine kinase returning toward normal), it is very important for the patient to begin a gentle stretching routine and progress to a graduated exercise program. This is because inflammation heals by fibrosis or scarring. This shortens muscles that will also have lost a proportion of their muscle cells. Although muscle cells can enlarge with training and exert a greater force, no new muscle cells will develop. The timing of stretching and exercising is important and should be started in consultation with the patient's treating physician.

Polymyositis and dermatomyositis are very serious illnesses. Before corticosteroids were discovered 50 percent of patients died from their disease. With modern treatment, nearly 90 percent of patients can be expected to be alive five years after the onset of the disease, excluding those with a malignancy. There are differences in outcome between the subgroups of disease. The outcome is best for those whose myositis is associated with another autoimmune disease (85 percent alive at five years), second best for dermatomyositis (80 percent), and worst for cancer-associated myositis (55 percent). As mentioned, particular autoantibodies give some information on response to treatment and outcome. Patients with anti-Mi-2 or anti-PM-Scl have a 95 percent chance of being alive at five years, those with antisynthetase antibodies a 65 percent chance, and those with anti-SRP, a 30 percent chance.

One-third of long-term survivors will have enough weakness to interfere with their daily activities, and a few will be left with lung or heart problems. Between 20 and 40 percent will have significant ongoing problems as a result of the side effects of the corticosteroids. There is concern that the powerful immunosuppressive medications may lead to later development of malignancy, and they may also cause bone marrow damage.

Risk Factors and Preventive Measures

Although there are undoubtably genetic influences on the development of polymyositis and dermatomyositis, the known gene associations are weak and do not comprise a significant risk. Penicillamine is the best-known risk factor for polymyositis, but this is a very rare adverse effect, and penicillamine is very seldom used these days. There are no known preventive measures.

DEXA (dual-energy X-ray absorptiometry) See Appendix II.

diabetes mellitus An illness caused by decreased production of insulin or by decreased responsiveness of tissues to it. Insulin, produced by the pancreas, lowers blood glucose levels, and diabetes is characterized by high blood sugar levels. Type I diabetes, also called insulin-dependent diabetes or juvenile-onset diabetes, affects younger people who need insulin injections to control it. Type II diabetes, also called noninsulin-dependent diabetes or maturity-onset diabetes, usually affects middle-aged, overweight people and can often be controlled by a special diet and tablets to lower the blood sugar. Well-known complications of diabetes include blindness caused by damage to blood vessels of the retina, kidney failure caused by damage to the glomeruli that filter urine, and an increased chance of developing infections.

Muscle, Joint, and Soft Tissue Complications of Diabetes

Diabetes is also associated with less well-known complications that can affect muscles, joints, and soft tissues.

Peripheral vascular disease Diabetes accelerates hardening of the arteries (atherosclerosis). The vessels that supply the legs can become so narrowed that they do not carry enough blood. If this happens it can cause pain when the person walks or exercises. This type of pain is called intermittent claudication because the symptoms are intermittent and get better with rest but recur after exercise. Intermittent claudication is caused by a blood vessel problem and is not a type of arthritis. Because it causes pain in the legs while walking, patients can be incorrectly diagnosed and treated for arthritis.

Hand contractures Patients who have had diabetes for many years can develop fibrous tissue in the tendons of their fingers so that they cannot straighten them completely. This is called diabetic cheirarthropathy or diabetic contracture. It causes clumsiness and tightness of the fingers, and other than good control of the blood sugar, there is no effective treatment for it. Diabetes increases the chances of developing DUPUYTREN'S CONTRACTURE and can also cause tight skin on the fingers. An increase in the fibrous tissue of the finger tendons can cause them to catch and then suddenly release when an affected finger is flexed, called TRIGGER FINGER.

Shoulder tendinitis Patients with diabetes have an increased chance of developing shoulder tendinitis that causes pain in the shoulder when lifting the arm and can lead to a frozen shoulder.

Neuropathic arthritis Diabetes can damage the nerves in the feet and legs so that the person cannot feel exactly where his or her ankles and feet are, and the individual walks awkwardly. The person does not feel that the ankle or foot joints are being damaged (see NEUROPATHIC ARTHRITIS).

Diabetic nerve and muscle damage Damage to nerves of the hands and feet (peripheral neuropathy) can cause numbness, tingling, and pain in the *glove and stocking* areas. It can also affect muscles so that they shrink (atrophy) and become weak.

Other conditions DIFFUSE IDIOPATHIC SKELETAL HYPEROSTOSIS (DISH), CARPAL TUNNEL SYNDROME, and infections of bone (OSTEOMYELITIS) and joints (INFECTIVE ARTHRITIS) are more common in patients with diabetes.

dialysis A process used to filter waste products and toxins out of blood and replace the function of the kidneys. There are two common types of dialysis, hemodialysis and peritoneal dialysis. With hemodialysis blood is removed from a patient, filtered through a membrane in a machine, and then returned. Peritoneal dialysis removes waste products from the bloodstream by running clear fluid into a space in the abdomen called the peritoneal cavity and then later removing the fluid after waste products have passed into it. Patients who have been on dialysis for a long time have a greater chance of developing some arthritis problems.

One of the commonest rheumatic problems is pain in the bones caused by increased activity of the parathyroid glands. This is called secondary hyperparathyroidism and is a natural response to the low calcium and high phosphate levels found in the blood of patients with poor kidney function. Secondary hyperparathyroidism is treated with a low-phosphate diet and drugs such as calcium salts that lower the concentrations of phosphate by binding it in the gut and preventing it from being absorbed into the body.

Patients who have been on hemodialysis for a long time have an increased chance of developing arthritis caused by the accumulation of a protein, $beta_2$-microglobulin, that is not removed from the bloodstream by hemodialysis. This substance, a type of AMYLOID, can collect in the carpal tunnel, causing CARPAL TUNNEL SYNDROME, and in the synovial cavity causing arthritis. The diagnosis of this type of arthritis is usually suspected when a patient who has been on hemodialysis for many years develops arthritis, most often affecting the shoulders, wrists, hips, and small joints of the hands. The X-rays show cysts that have occurred because small pieces of bone have been eroded. Some experts believe that the accumulation of $beta_2$-microglobulin by itself is not the entire cause and that secondary hyperparathyroidism, bone problems resulting from aluminum accumulation and deposits of hydroxyapatite crystals, may also contribute. There is no specific treatment for this type of arthritis. However, it can be improved if a patient who has been on dialysis receives a renal transplant and can discontinue dialysis.

The kidneys excrete uric acid in the urine so that poor kidney function causes uric acid levels in the blood to rise and increases that chance that crystals will accumulate in the joints and cause an attack of acute GOUT.

diet Many people believe that diet affects their arthritis or that dietary supplements or vitamins improve their symptoms. A lot has been published about the effects of diet on arthritis. Other than the fact that uric acid levels are elevated in people who drink large amounts of alcohol or eat a lot of red meat or organ meats (see GOUT), the results have not been consistent. Many of the studies have been uncontrolled and open label (see CLINICAL TRIAL), and their results may therefore be biased toward showing a positive effect.

Several studies have shown that total fasting improves the symptoms of rheumatoid arthritis (RA) in some patients, but the effects are temporary. A recent controlled study in overweight people with OSTEOARTHRITIS showed that weight loss through reducing the calories in their diet not only reduced pain and increased physical ability but also lowered levels of inflammatory CYTOKINES. Because it was possible that food allergy aggravated arthritis, researchers have studied the effects of elemental and exclusion diets. Elemental diets contain minerals and amino acids rather than complex proteins and have resulted in a modest improvement in symptoms in some patients but are impractical long term. Exclusion diets eliminate certain food types and have identified a few patients whose arthritis is consistently worsened by a certain food type, for example milk products. These patients appear to benefit by avoiding certain food types, but overall, exclusion diets have not been successful in patients with arthritis.

Several studies have found that a vegan or vegetarian diet resulted in a modest improvement in RA, but the scientific evidence is not strong enough to recommend this as a useful component of routine treatment. Many dietary supplements such as yeast, cider vinegar, honey, copper, zinc, magnesium, garlic, ginger, alfalfa, and shark cartilage have been used to treat arthritis without adequate evidence available to support or refute claims for their efficacy. Oxidative stress resulting in increased production of free radicals appears to be increased in many types of arthritis. Antioxidant vitamins, particularly vitamin E and vitamin C, have therefore been suggested as treatments for arthritis. In some studies, high doses of vitamin E improved the symptoms of RA. Vitamin C did not appear to improve symptoms of RA or osteoarthritis (OA) but was associated with a slower progression of OA in one study.

Some unsaturated fatty acids, particularly those found in fatty fish such as cod and in some plants such as evening primrose oil, decrease the production of inflammatory prostaglandins. Many studies have examined the effects of fish oil and evening primrose oil in arthritis, and some have found modest benefits in RA.

Overall, there are not enough high-quality studies of the effects of dietary supplements in arthritis to be certain of their effects. Most experts recommend a healthy balanced diet without any specific exclusions or supplements for patients with arthritis. If patients do become aware of a foodstuff that appears to make their arthritis worse, it is best to consult a dietician to design an exclusion diet to test whether their impression is really true. The dietician can then advise them on healthy eating with the exclusion of an implicated food. Processed food today is so complex it can be very difficult for the individual to do this.

diffuse idiopathic skeletal hyperostosis (DISH)
Also known as Forestier's disease, DISH is a condition in which there is exuberant bone growth at characteristic sites. It is very common, being found in approximately 10 percent of people over the age of 65 years. It is found twice as often in men as in women and becomes increasingly common with age. DISH is found in all parts of the world. Typical changes of DISH have been found in the spines of dinosaur skeletons, Egyptian mummies, and other ancient skeletons.

Although there are well-known associations, the precise cause is not known. The condition starts at entheses. This is where ligaments, tendons, or joint capsules attach to bone. There is initially a thickening in this area followed by a gradual transformation of the ligament or tendon to bone with increased blood flow to the area. An association with obesity has been recognized for many years, and later a strong association with noninsulin-dependent diabetes (see DIABETES) was shown. Both these conditions have high levels of insulin together with resistance to its action in many tissues. Since insulin acts as a growth factor to many tissues, there is interest in whether this could be one of the factors driving the excessive bone growth.

Symptoms and Diagnostic Path

The powerful ligaments joining the spinal vertebrae are most commonly affected, and in advanced disease, bony bridges can link four to five vertebrae, dramatically reducing spinal flexibility. It is likely that the mechanical disturbance of movement can give rise to intermittent spinal pain, but the process of DISH itself is rarely painful. Most patients have no symptoms, and DISH is discovered only incidentally when an X-ray is taken for some other reason. Spinal DISH may very occasionally cause difficulty swallowing when the bony protuberances press on the esophagus. It can also cause narrowing of the spinal canal and pressure on either the spinal cord or the nerve roots as they exit the spine.

Outside of the spine DISH can cause HEEL SPURS, extra bony growth at the tips of the fingers, thickening of tubular bones, and an increased tendency to form bone in the area of scarring after surgery. Heel spurs in particular can be painful, but again it is probably the disturbance they cause to surrounding tissues that is painful rather than the DISH process.

An X-ray of the spine showing at least four adjacent vertebrae joined by newly formed bone is essential for the diagnosis. Other conditions that can cause similar appearances should be excluded. These are particularly ANKYLOSING SPONDYLITIS and degenerative disc disease (see BACK PAIN). The X-ray changes in DISH are usually quite distinctive, with the extra bone growth appearing to flow from vertebrae to vertebrae like candle wax, affect mainly the right side of the spine and lacking severe changes in the disc or any damage to the vertebral body.

Treatment Options and Outlook

Most people with DISH do not have symptoms and do not need any treatment. Those with spinal stiffness need to understand what the problem is and use occasional painkillers as needed. A very few may need surgical removal of a spur or decompression of the spine or nerve root. Injection of a small amount of CORTICOSTEROIDS around a painful heel spur may be very helpful. Those who are overweight should lose weight and exercise more, but it has not been shown that this will beneficially affect the DISH. More importantly, in these patients the diagnosis of DISH may prove the trigger for them and their physician to recognize that they have the *metabolic syndrome*. These patients often have high insulin levels, insulin resistance, obesity, hypertension, gout, and high lipid levels as well as a high risk of coronary artery disease.

Risk Factors and Preventive Measures

The cause of DISH is unknown, and there are no known preventive measures. The recognition of the metabolic syndrome, however, and institution of effective treatment may prevent subsequent cardiovascular complications.

disease-modifying antirheumatic drugs (DMARDs)
A name that has evolved to mean drugs that alter the course of rheumatoid arthritis by preventing joint damage (see RHEUMATOID ARTHRITIS). DMARDs (pronounced "dee-mards") do not belong to a single class of drug and can be classified as follows.

Anticancer drugs Although these drugs are also used to treat cancer, much lower doses are used to alter the immune response in rheumatic problems. Side effects are much milder and less common than with cancer chemotherapy. Established DMARDs are

METHOTREXATE (trade name: Rheumatrex)
AZATHIOPRINE (trade name: Imuran)

Antirejection drugs These can be used to prevent organ rejection in people who receive an organ transplant. However, because they suppress the immune system, they are also useful for some arthritis-related problems. Established DMARDs are

LEFLUNOMIDE (trade name: Arava)
CYCLOSPORINE (trade names: Sandimmune, Neoral)

Biologicals These are used to treat RA. They are antibodies or cytokines that are similar or identical, to those the body makes and can manipulate the immune response. Established DMARDs are

ETANERCEPT (trade name: Enbrel)
REMICADE (trade name: Infliximab)
ADALIMUMAB (trade name: Humira)
ANAKINRA (trade name: Kineret)
RITUXIMAB (trade names: Rituxan, MabThera)

Other DMARDs Several DMARDs have different mechanisms of action that are not thought to alter the immune response and do not fit neatly into a category. This category includes the following drugs:

AURANOFIN (trade name: Ridaura) oral gold pills
Aurothioglucose (trade name: Solganal) intramuscular gold injection
HYDROXYCHLOROQUINE (trade name: Plaquenil) an antimalarial
CHLOROQUINE (trade name: Aralen) an antimalarial
MINOCYCLINE (trade name: Minocin) an antibiotic
PENICILLAMINE (trade name: Cuprimine) a drug that binds metals like copper and lead
SULFASALAZINE (trade name: Azulfidine) a combination of a sulfa antibiotic and a salicylate

DISH See DIFFUSE IDIOPATHIC SKELETAL HYPEROSTOSIS.

DMARDs See DISEASE-MODIFYING ANTIRHEUMATIC DRUGS.

drug-induced lupus This diagnosis is made if someone with no symptoms of SYSTEMIC LUPUS ERYTHEMATOSUS (SLE) before taking a drug develops clinical SLE while taking a drug and this resolves on stopping the drug. The criteria for diagnosing SLE as well as a detailed description of the clinical manifestations and investigation will be discussed under SLE. This section will discuss how drug-induced lupus differs from idiopathic SLE, the drugs involved, some possible mechanisms, and treatment of this condition.

The antihypertensive drug hydralazine was first recognized to induce SLE 50 years ago. Since then there have been many reports of drugs inducing lupus and even more of drugs inducing the characteristic autoantibodies. It can be very difficult to be sure that the drug did cause the disease in an individual case. Only two drugs, hydralazine and procainamide, have been scientifically proven to induce lupus. With many others the reports of an association are frequent enough to make a reasonable assumption that there is a real association. However, when there are only one or two reports of lupus occurring after use of a drug that has been available for some years, then it is likely to have happened by chance. Rare occurrences with new drugs are always viewed with more suspicion. The table on page 69 includes all drugs in use today, by category of use, that have more than a couple of reports of possibly inducing lupus. The risk associated with their use is approximate for most of them. The risk of developing lupus after taking procainamide for one year is 20 percent and that for hydralazine is 8 percent, although this varies with the dose. The risk for all the other drugs in the table is very much less than 1 percent.

Many of these drugs can cause a positive ANTINUCLEAR ANTIBODY (ANA) test without causing any clinical manifestations of lupus, and this is thought to be harmless. Drug-induced lupus usually develops only after the drug has been taken for months or years, unlike drug-induced flares (see Symptoms). Evaluating some of these associations can be very difficult. This is especially true when the suspected drug is being used to treat arthritis. For example, someone with rheumatoid arthritis taking penicillamine who gets a worsening of pain and swelling could have a flare of their arthritis or be developing penicillamine-induced SLE. While penicillamine is no longer used much, minocycline use has increased, and the anti-TNF drugs are becoming very widely used.

As will be seen from the table, these drugs are very different compounds acting on a wide range of

POSSIBLE LUPUS-INDUCING DRUGS LISTED BY CATEGORY OF USE

Agent	Risk	Agent	Risk
Antiarrhythmics		**Anticonvulsants**	
procainamide	high	carbamazepine	low
quinidine	moderate	phenytoin	very low
disopyramide	very low	ethosuximide	very low
propafenone	very low	primidone	very low
Antihypertensives		**Antithyroid drugs**	
hydralazine	high	propylthiouracil	low
methyldopa	low		
captopril	low	**Antirheumatic drugs**	
acebutalol	low	penicillamine	low
enalapril	very low	sulfasalazine	low
clonidine	very low	phenylbutazone	very low
atenolol	very low	minocycline	low
labetalol	very low	anti-TNF drugs	very low
pindolol	very low		
minoxidil	very low	**Diuretics**	
prazocin	very low	chlorthalidone	very low
		hydrochlorothiazide	very low
Antipsychotics			
chlorpromazine	low	**Miscellaneous**	
perphenazine	very low	statins (cholesterol-lowering drugs)	very low
phenelzine	very low	levodopa	very low
chlorprothixene	very low	aminoglutethimide	very low
lithium carbonate	very low	alpha-interferon	very low
		timolol eye drops	very low
Antibiotics			
isoniazid	low		
minocycline	low		
nitrofurantoin	very low		

tissues in the body. There seems no obvious reason why they should all induce a particular immunological disease. One important finding is that many drugs with the ability to induce lupus undergo breakdown within a class of white cells called neutrophils. This breakdown is through the formation of oxygen radicals and results in a form of the drug (metabolite) that has a high capacity for reacting with other tissues. Because this takes place in white cells (rather than the liver where most drugs are broken down), it suggests a way in which these metabolites may be concentrated in the lymph nodes where they could act on the immune cells that pass through there. Traditional research has looked at ways in which these drugs could stimulate the immune system to attack the individual's own tissues. Recent research, however, suggests that these drugs may interfere with the immune system's ability to recognize what is self and what is not. There is much that remains unknown, however.

Symptoms and Diagnostic Path
Drug-induced lupus differs from idiopathic SLE mainly in that the kidneys and central nervous

system are very seldom affected. The commonest manifestations are arthritis, inflammation of the lining membranes of the heart or lungs (serositis), fever, and feeling generally unwell. The patient will usually have been taking the medication for many months or even years. Several drug-induced autoimmune diseases that can sometimes also be a manifestation of SLE can occur in isolation in the absence of other drug-induced lupus problems. These include autoimmune hemolytic anemia, thrombocytopenia, and skin rashes. Autoimmune hemolytic anemia is the destruction of the person's own red blood cells by their immune system. Likewise immune thrombocytopenia is the destruction of the small blood cells involved in clotting called platelets. Drugs that are known to cause these two problems include penicillin, methyldopa, quinidine, levodopa, chlorpromazine, nomifensine, and alpha-interferon. The antifungal drugs griseofulvin and terbinafine may induce chronic lupus skin rashes. The anti-TNF drugs are unusual in sometimes causing kidney disease, which is very uncommon in other drug-induced SLE.

Another group of drugs is able to cause flares of lupus. This is a completely different situation than that discussed above but is mentioned here because it frequently causes confusion. These patients already have SLE, although it may be very well controlled. It is also different in that the flare typically occurs within a week or two of taking the drug and does not necessarily improve on stopping it. Most frequently the flare is in the form of a rash. These reactions are better seen as drug allergies rather than disease induction. SLE patients have long been known to be particularly prone to drug allergies. Antibiotics are commonly involved in these reactions, including sulfonamides, penicillins, cephalosporins, erythromycin, and ciprofloxacin.

Patients with drug-induced lupus often do not fulfill the criteria used to classify disease as SLE. The diagnosis needs to be suspected in someone taking one of the drugs listed in the table for at least one month but usually longer. Some drugs tend to induce particular problems, for example procainamide often induces serositis, quinidine and minocycline induce arthritis, and minocycline often causes hepatitis.

Most patients will have a positive ANA test, but this may be found in the absence of any disease and may have been present before the drug was started. A specific type of ANA test, the anti-(H2A-H2B-DNA) antihistone autoantibody is often found in drug-induced lupus and very seldom in other situations apart from true SLE and SCLERODERMA. However, this test is not routinely available. Many patients with minocycline-induced lupus or VASCULITIS do not have a positive ANA test but may have a positive ANTINEUTROPHIL CYTOPLASMIC ANTIBODY test. A positive anti-DNA test is very unusual except when the disease is caused by an anti-TNF drug.

Although it may seem difficult to be sure of the diagnosis, the almost invariable improvement within weeks of stopping the drug is very useful.

Treatment Options and Outlook

Once the diagnosis has been made or strongly suspected, the treatment is to stop the drug. Alternative means of managing the condition being treated should obviously be made. A short course of CORTICOSTEROIDS is occasionally required for severe problems, but usually they can be managed with simpler medications such as NSAIDs or painkillers until symptoms settle.

Risk Factors and Preventive Measures

The causative drug is by definition the risk factor here. However, only hydralazine, procainamide, and quinidine cause lupus frequently enough to be avoided in order to prevent the syndrome. It would be unusual to find a situation where there was not a more modern drug that would adequately replace one of these three. By virtue of its frequent use, the antibiotic minocycline causes a number of cases of drug-induced lupus, but these are seldom severe. The other listed medications should all be used appropriately with the possibility of drug-induced lupus in mind so that it is recognized early on the rare occasion that it develops.

drug-induced rheumatic disease   In addition to DRUG-INDUCED LUPUS, there are several other musculoskeletal side effects of drugs.

Arthralgia, Arthritis, and Tendinitis

Quinolones A class of antibiotics, fluoroquinolones, more commonly known as quinolones, can rarely cause musculoskeletal side effects. Examples of quinolone antibiotics are ciprofloxacin, levofloxacin, and norfloxacin. Arthralgia and myalgia occur in less than 1 percent of patients treated with this class of antibiotics. More severe adverse effects such as arthritis, tendinitis, and rupture of a tendon are much less common. In animal studies, quinolones are harmful to cartilage, particularly in growing bones. Therefore quinolones are contraindicated in children and adolescents and pregnant women. Reversible arthritis, most often affecting the knees, has occurred most often in patients who received treatment with a quinolone for several months to suppress chronic or recurrent infection. Tendinitis, resulting in pain in the involved tendon, affects approximately 20 per 100,000 patients treated with a quinolone. The ACHILLES TENDON is affected most often, but others such as the quadriceps (in the area of the knee) or ROTATOR CUFF (in the area of the shoulder) can be involved. Rupture of a tendon is rare, but the risk is higher with prolonged quinolone treatment and in people who have other risk factors that weaken tendons such as being older than 65 years or treatment with corticosteroids.

Vaccines Just as RUBELLA (German measles) can cause arthralgia and rarely arthritis, so too can the vaccine used to prevent it. Arthralgia and arthritis after rubella vaccination are more common in adults than children but usually resolve without treatment. Chronic arthritis is rare.

There have been a few reports of inflammatory arthritis similar to rheumatoid arthritis (RA) developing after vaccination for hepatitis B. One theory is that the vaccine acts as a trigger for RA in people who are already genetically predisposed. Another is that the association is coincidental. RA is a common illness and the onset of RA symptoms and the administration of a vaccine will occasionally occur at the same time coincidentally.

A vaccine called BCG (bacillus Calmette-Guérin) is used to prevent tuberculosis in many countries. More recently it has been used to treat bladder cancer by placing it into the bladder to stimulate the immune response. Arthralgia (0.5–5 percent) and arthritis (less than 1 percent) can develop in patients treated for cancer using this vaccine. The arthritis is often asymmetrical and affects large joints such as the knee. This pattern resembles that of Reiter's syndrome, and other features typical of that condition such as conjunctivitis and urethritis can occur. These clinical features and the fact that people who are HLA-B27 positive have a greater chance of developing arthritis after treatment with BCG vaccine suggest that this type of arthritis may be a variant of Reiter's syndrome. However, BCG may also initiate a RHEUMATOID ARTHRITIS–like disease.

Corticosteroids Inflammatory arthritis often responds dramatically to treatment with corticosteroids. However, if therapy is suddenly discontinued or if doses are decreased rapidly, patients may develop a flare of their original symptoms or an ill-defined syndrome of arthralgia and fatigue that improves when corticosteroid treatment is resumed or the dosage increased. Both oral and locally injected corticosteroids have been associated with tendon rupture, most frequently the Achilles tendon, but also others.

Cytokines Several CYTOKINES that are used to treat illness can themselves rarely cause arthritis, often associated with a positive blood test for autoantibodies such as ANTINUCLEAR ANTIBODY and RHEUMATOID FACTOR. Interferon-α, used to treat hepatitis B and C, and interleukin-2, used to treat some malignancies, can rarely cause inflammatory arthritis affecting small joints.

Statins These drugs are now very widely used to prevent heart attack and stroke, and their association with muscle pain and inflammation (see MYOSITIS below) has been known for some time. Although much less common, they are now being associated with tendinitis and sometimes tendon rupture. This starts suddenly and usually in the first year of taking the statin but can occur at any time. All the statins appear to be involved. The Achilles tendon is involved in half the cases, and the drugs frequently affect tendons on both sides of the body. Although it is a rare complication, it is becoming more important because of the widespread use of statins.

Gout and Hyperuricemia

Several drugs increase the concentration of uric acid in the blood (hyperuricemia) and therefore increase the risk of GOUT. Diuretics, such as furosemide, bumetanide, and thiazides, which are used to increase the amount of sodium and water excreted by patients with high blood pressure or fluid retention due to problems such as heart failure, often increase the concentration of uric acid in the blood. Other drugs that do this are CYCLOSPORINE, an immunosuppressant, and pyrazinamide and ethambutol, two drugs used to treat tuberculosis.

Osteoporosis

A common cause of OSTEOPOROSIS is treatment with high doses of corticosteroids. Osteoporosis associated with corticosteroid therapy is more severe if high doses are administered for a long time but can occur even with low doses, such as 5–7.5 mg of prednisone a day. Corticosteroids cause osteoporosis in several ways: They increase the loss of calcium from the body, reduce calcium absorption from the gut, and also decrease the activity of cells called osteoblasts that form new bone. Individual patients treated with corticosteroids vary in their susceptibility to osteoporosis. Many patients treated with a low daily dose of prednisone, for example 5 mg or less, will not develop osteoporosis, while others do. The reasons for these variations in individual susceptibility are not known. However, there are differences in the way the drug is absorbed and broken down and in the glucocorticoid receptors through which it acts. However, virtually every patient treated with high doses, say more than 20 mg of prednisone a day for more than a few weeks, will lose a significant amount of bone. The risk of osteoporosis caused by corticosteroids can be decreased but not eliminated by taking calcium and vitamin D supplements. Osteoporosis in patients taking corticosteroids is most often treated with a BISPHOSPHONATE or, if the patient cannot take any of the drugs in this group, with other drugs used to treat patients who have osteoporosis not associated with corticosteroid treatment.

Prolonged treatment with heparin, an anticoagulant used to prevent blood clots from forming, can cause osteoporosis. Heparin has to be administered by injection, so few people receive it for more than a week or two. However, because it does not cross the placenta and therefore does not affect blood clotting in the developing baby,

heparin is the anticoagulant most often used during pregnancy. If someone is pregnant and needs to be anticoagulated, then heparin given by subcutaneous injection is often administered during and immediately after pregnancy. These patients have an increased risk of developing osteoporosis. This usually resolves slowly when heparin treatment is stopped.

Osteomalacia

Several drugs such as rifampin, phenobarbitone, and phenytoin stimulate the activity of liver enzymes that inactivate vitamin D. This impairs the body's ability to calcify new bone and can cause OSTEOMALACIA.

Osteonecrosis

Corticosteroids increase the risk of osteonecrosis (see AVASCULAR NECROSIS).

Vasculitis

Several drugs or classes of drug such as penicillins, sulfonamides, cephalosporins, thiazides, phenytoin, and captopril can cause vasculitis that most often affects small blood vessels in the skin and causes a rash that typically consists of purple spots. If a skin biopsy is done, it shows white blood cells invading the walls of blood vessels (leukocytoclastic vasculitis). Propylthiouracil, a drug used to treat hyperthyroidism, can rarely cause vasculitis associated with a positive antineutrophil cytoplasmic antibody blood test (see Appendix II). Vasculitis associated with propylthiouracil treatment has been complicated by glomerulonephritis and occasionally features of WEGENER'S GRANULOMATOSIS. More recently, fluoxetine and paroxetine, antidepressants of the selective serotonin reuptake inhibitor (SSRI) class, have been associated with drug-induced vasculitis. This adverse effect is rare but important, because these drugs are widely used and taken for long periods of time. Drug-induced vasculitis usually resolves when the offending drug is stopped.

Myositis and Myopathy

Drugs can cause inflammation or degeneration of muscle, resulting in weakness, pain, and sometimes elevated blood levels of muscle enzymes such as creatine kinase. A class of drugs used to lower cholesterol known as the *statins* or HMG coenzyme reductase inhibitors, for example lovastatin and simvastatin, occasionally causes myositis. Myalgia occurs in approximately 2 percent of patients treated with a statin, but less than five in 1,000 develop significant myositis with symptoms and levels of muscle enzymes elevated 10 times or more above the normal range. Rarely, muscle inflammation is so severe that death of large amounts of muscle occurs, a condition known as RHABDOMYOLYSIS. The risk of developing muscle inflammation was higher with cerivastatin than other statins, and the drug was withdrawn from the market in 2001. The chances of developing myositis on a statin drug are higher in the first few months of treatment and are greater in patients taking combinations of different drugs to lower their cholesterol. Myositis with a statin is more common in patients who are also taking drugs, for example ketoconazole, an antifungal drug, or cyclosporine, an immunosuppressant, that slow the breakdown or elimination of many statins.

Colchicine, a drug used to prevent and treat attacks of gout, can damage nerves and muscles. This is a rare side effect even in people who have taken an overdose of colchicine or taken it for many years. The first symptoms are usually weakness of the thigh, shoulder, and ankle muscles. Levels of muscle enzymes are usually increased. Muscle weakness is often accompanied by evidence of nerve damage such as loss of sensation in the feet and absent ankle reflexes. Muscle symptoms resolve soon after colchicine treatment is stopped, but neurological symptoms recover more slowly.

Hydroxychloroquine and chloroquine, antimalarial drugs that are also used to treat systemic lupus erythematosus and RA, can rarely cause muscle disease, but this is not usually associated with much inflammation. The commonest symptom is weakness affecting proximal muscles such as the thigh and shoulder, without elevation of muscle enzymes. Even less common is inflammation of the muscles of the heart, cardiomyopathy, which if severe can cause heart failure.

High doses of corticosteroids cause atrophy and weakness of muscles, particularly those around the hip and shoulder, which is therefore called a proximal myopathy. It causes symptoms such as difficulty standing from a seated position or lifting objects above the head. The myopathy caused by corticosteroids is gradual, not associated with pain or elevated muscle enzymes, and more likely to occur in patients who receive moderate or high doses for a long time. Low doses of corticosteroids, for example less than 10 mg a day, seldom cause muscle problems. Corticosteroids are used to treat inflammatory muscle disease such as polymyositis and dermatomyositis, conditions that cause muscle weakness. It is therefore sometimes difficult to know if increased weakness is caused by the disease or the treatment. If there are no clinical or laboratory signs of disease reactivation, such as an increase in creatine kinase, a muscle enzyme that increases in inflammatory muscle diseases but not in corticosteroid myopathy, then the drug rather than the disease is likely to be responsible.

Alcohol can cause acute and chronic muscle problems. Acute myopathy usually occurs in alcoholics after a heavy binge. It causes symptoms of muscle pain, weakness, and elevated enzyme levels. Most muscles are involved, enzyme levels are often very high, and rhabdomyolysis can occur. Usually, unless rhabdomyolysis leads to kidney failure, recovery is complete. Alcohol can also cause muscle atrophy and a chronic, painless proximal myopathy. The onset of symptoms is gradual, and muscle enzymes are normal or elevated only a little. The cause of alcoholic myopathy is not known, but direct toxic effects of alcohol on the muscle combined with the effects of poor nutrition may contribute. Also, many alcoholics have diarrhea or vomiting and thus lose potassium and magnesium. This can increase the severity of muscle symptoms. Patients with chronic alcoholic myopathy are more likely to have alcohol-induced heart muscle disease (cardiomyopathy), a condition that can lead to heart failure and death. Stopping alcohol can lead to improvement in muscle symptoms, but this occurs gradually over many months.

Penicillamine, a drug occasionally still used to treat RA and scleroderma, can cause inflammatory myositis that can be difficult to differentiate from DERMATOMYOSITIS AND POLYMYOSITIS. The risk of developing myositis does not seem to be related to the dose or duration of treatment. Affected patients most often complain of proximal muscle weakness, but features thought to be typical of autoimmune disease such as a rash and difficulty swallowing can occur. Elevated muscle enzymes and symptoms rapidly revert to normal when the drug is stopped.

Cocaine, one of the commonest causes of disease induced by an illegal drug, can cause muscle problems ranging from small, asymptomatic increases in muscle enzymes to rhabdomyolysis with dramatic increases. Cocaine can cause muscle damage in several ways. Not only is it a powerful vasoconstrictor that decreases blood supply to organs such as muscle, but it also increases the tissue concentrations of epinephrine and norepinephrine, fight or flight stress hormones, that can damage muscle. Muscle disease can be the main symptom of cocaine use, but more often it is part of a clinical presentation that can include agitation, coma, confusion, seizures, and chest pain.

Risk Factors and Preventive Measures

The causative drug is by definition the risk factor in these conditions. Medications should always be prescribed only when their expected benefits exceed their potential for serious adverse effects. Many of the conditions discussed above are not predictable and therefore preventable. Corticosteroid use is an exception. Corticosteroids produce a multitude of actions in the body, and most people will experience unwanted effects if they take a sufficient dose for long enough. This is different from most other drugs in which the occurrence of an adverse effect is an idiosyncratic event. Corticosteroids should therefore always be used at as low a dose for as short a time period as possible to minimize effects such as osteoporosis and tendon rupture. Anti-osteoporotic medication should also be used if corticosteroids are going to be used long term (conventionally more than six to nine months).

Osteomalacia (vitamin D deficiency affecting bones) should be anticipated and tested for in long-term users of the antiepileptic drugs phenytoin, carbamazepine, and phenobarbitone, and vitamin D supplements should be used as appropriate. Some adverse events occur because of the interaction between two or more drugs. For example, the myositis associated with statins is more likely to

occur if they are combined with another drug that occasionally causes muscle problems (fibrates) or a drug that affects its metabolism (cyclosporine). These combinations should be avoided if possible and carefully monitored if not possible. The large number of medications available today makes it impossible to remember all possible interactions, but it is important for doctors to know the drugs that often cause interactions and look them up when prescribing new medications. There are a number of online resources that make this process fairly easy. Recognizing drug-induced rheumatic conditions when they occur can be difficult in patients with multiple diseases taking multiple medications but is important as this will lead to early and more effective treatment.

drug metabolism After a drug has entered the body, it can be processed in several ways. Some drugs, for example penicillin antibiotics, are absorbed and then eliminated unchanged by the kidneys. Others, for example codeine, are absorbed as poorly active pro-drugs that are biotransformed by the liver to a more active metabolite, in the case of codeine into morphine. The liver, in addition to activating pro-drugs, biotransforms drugs into metabolites that are less active or toxic than the parent drug. These chemical reactions are classified into Phase I and II reactions and are carried out by enzymes. Many Phase I reactions are mediated by enzymes belonging to a group called the cytochrome P450 (CYP) superfamily. This is classified into families such as CYP1, 2, and 3 and further divided into subfamilies such as CYP1A, 2D, and 3A. Many drugs are metabolized by more than one CYP enzyme, but some depend on a single pathway. Drugs eliminated by a single metabolic pathway are particularly likely to cause side effects if they are administered with another drug that blocks that pathway. For example, CYCLOSPORINE, an immunosuppressant, is metabolized mainly by CYP3A4. If a drug that inhibits this enzyme, for example the antifungal drug ketoconazole, is taken at the same time, the metabolism of cyclosporine will be inhibited and blood levels will increase. Although the liver is considered the primary site of drug biotransformation, Phase I enzymes are also found in other sites and can affect drug levels. For example, CYP3A is found on the surface of the lining cells of the small intestine and acts locally on drugs as they are absorbed. Drug interactions can also occur here. Grapefruit juice, for example, is a strong inhibitor of CYP3A in the gut but not the liver. Several studies have shown that the absorption of drugs that are metabolized by CYP3A, such as cyclosporine and statin cholesterol-lowering drugs, is increased when they are taken with grapefruit juice.

Phase II reactions make drugs more water soluble and therefore easier to excrete in the urine. This is achieved by adding a water-soluble molecule such as acetate (acetylation), sulfate (sulfation), or glucuronide (glucuronidation) to the drug.

There are several genetic variants of drug-metabolizing enzymes that affect how active they are. For example, approximately 5–10 percent of most Caucasian populations have a variant of CYP2D6 that is either inactive or poorly functional. This means that these people poorly metabolize drugs that are substrates for this enzyme. For example, the activation of codeine to the active morphine metabolite is carried out by CYP2D6. Therefore people with an enzyme that functions poorly do not activate codeine well and do not receive the analgesic benefits of codeine when they take it. The older antidepressants such as amitriptyline and nortriptyline are also metabolized by CYP2D6, but in this case they are inactivated. Therefore people with the inactive enzyme have higher blood levels of these antidepressants and are more likely to have side effects if they are given standard doses of the drugs. The ability to predict how an individual will respond to a drug based on his or her genetic makeup, termed PHARMACOGENETICS, is an area of intense medical research.

drug transport Drugs can cross biological membranes is several ways. One of the commonest is simple diffusion. This process is affected by the size of the molecules and whether they are water or lipid soluble. Drugs that cross membranes well tend to be smaller and lipid soluble. Recently several active pathways that pump drugs across cell membranes have been identified. These drug transport pathways are usually specific for a small number of drugs and are termed uptake or efflux transporters, depending on whether they pump drugs into or out of the cell. The best-known transporter is P-glycoprotein (PgP), the product of the multidrug resistance gene. This efflux transporter was intensively studied when it was discovered that some tumors are resistant to chemotherapy drugs because they are able to make this transporter and protect themselves by pumping drug out of their cells. Scientists then discovered that PgP is found not only in some tumors but also in many normal cells, for example those lining the intestine, liver, and the blood vessels that act as a barrier between the brain and the circulation (the blood-brain barrier). Also, in addition to chemotherapy drugs, several other drugs such as CYCLOSPORINE, digoxin, erythromycin, and protease inhibitors are PgP substrates. This means that absorption of these drugs can be affected by the amount and activity of PgP. Some drugs such as the protease inhibitors that are used to treat HIV infection do not cross the blood-brain barrier well. Some scientists believe that the reason HIV infection cannot be cured is because the virus hides from drugs in sanctuary sites such as the brain. Using drugs that inhibit PgP to allow protease inhibitors to penetrate the brain better is an interesting research area that may improve HIV therapy.

Dupuytren's contracture A fibrosing disease leading to clawing of one or more fingers. The soft-tissue layer just beneath the skin in the palm of the hand has many fibroblasts. These are cells that form the fascia or connective tissue here and throughout the body. In Dupuytren's contracture, the fibroblasts multiply and produce fibrosis in the palm of the hand that first causes nodules and then, as the fibrosis contracts, starts to dimple and tether the overlying skin and later to draw the finger into a fixed curved position. It is fairly common as people age, is found mainly in Caucasians, and affects men five times as often as women.

Although the cause of Dupuytren's contracture is not known, there are associations. There is a clear association with heavy manual work or work with vibrating machinery. It is more common in association with epilepsy, DIABETES MELLITUS, excessive alcohol consumption, chronic lung disease, REFLEX

SYMPATHETIC DYSTROPHY, and probably smoking. In some families it appears to be inherited. A few patients also have fibrosing problems in other parts of the body, and this form is inherited.

Symptoms and Diagnostic Path

The dimpling and tethering of the skin on the palm of the hand causes few problems. With progressive disease the fingers become bent at the metacarpophalangeals (MCPs) with an inability to straighten them. The fourth finger is usually affected first, then the fifth, and less commonly the third and second. The fingers may become drawn back right into the palm when they not only become useless themselves but also interfere with the grasping of objects by the other fingers. This process usually takes many years and may stabilize at any stage without further progression. Occasionally there may be fairly rapid progression. Although it may start on one side, both hands are usually affected. Pain seldom occurs.

Treatment Options and Outlook

In the early stages warmth, moisturizing creams and stretching are appropriate. The use of protective gloves for manual work is recommended. When there is pain or rapid progression, injections of CORTICOSTEROIDS into the affected area may be helpful. If the deformity interferes significantly with daily activities, either just the affected fascia or the whole of the fascia on the palm of the hand can be removed surgically. Sometimes a skin graft is used. Unfortunately, recurrences may still happen.

Risk Factors and Preventive Measures

Repetitive trauma, especially if associated with heavy manual work, use of vibrating machinery, and factors that could affect oxygenation of subcu-taneous tissues such as smoking, diabetes, chronic lung disease, and reflex sympathetic dystrophy, is a risk factor for Dupuytren's contracture. It is not clear whether these physical trauma and metabolic (oxygenation) factors are additive or whether many different factors can lead to the development of Dupuytren's as a common final pathway. People with poor posture or malalignment for other reasons such as severe arthritis seem particularly prone to developing Dupuytren's. Malalignment causes widespread myofascial tightening, which may thereby accentuate the trauma to the myofascium of the hand. This has not been studied in a controlled manner.

The use of protective gloves when using machinery, spades, axes, or other equipment makes sense, but there are no adequate studies to say it is effective. Likewise it is not known whether excellent control of diabetes and chronic lung disease or indeed stopping smoking has a protective effect, although it seems reasonable to assume so. Once Dupuytren's has started, regular stretching is most important to prevent progression. Ideally, this should be part of a generalized stretching program. The specific hand stretch is best done by placing the thumb of the non-Dupuytren's hand in the palm of the Dupuytren hand on the wrist side of the contracture and the next two fingers toward the end of the finger affected by the contracture and trying to push thumb and fingers farther apart. Stretches should be held until some give is felt in the contracture, repeated for each affected finger and done twice daily. During painful flares, injecting a small amount of corticosteroid just under the skin where the contracture is painful can settle it down quicker and should be accompanied by stretching.

endocarditis   See INFECTIVE ENDOCARDITIS.

enteropathic arthritis   Inflammatory arthritis associated with bowel disease, most often Crohn's disease and ulcerative colitis (see INFLAMMATORY BOWEL DISEASE). The gut harbors many bacteria and other microorganisms but is also rich in lymphatic tissue that protects the body against invasion. Enteropathic arthritis is thought to occur when infection or inflammation of the bowel allows organisms that would not usually enter the body to do so. Certain bacteria, or even parts of their cell walls, can trigger arthritis in susceptible individuals. Several conditions may cause enteropathic arthritis. These include infectious diarrhea (see REACTIVE ARTHRITIS), inflammatory bowel disease, and bowel surgery that creates a loop of bowel with a dead end that allows overgrowth of bacteria (see INTESTINAL BYPASS ARTHRITIS, WHIPPLE'S DISEASE, and CELIAC DISEASE). The type of bowel surgery creating a loop of bowel used to be done to help people who were extremely overweight lose weight. Because of frequent GI side effects, it has been replaced by other surgical procedures, including stapling of the stomach, that cause fewer problems.

eosinophilia myalgia syndrome   This is a rare illness, similar to scleroderma that usually occurred in people who used the health food supplement, L-tryptophan. There was an outbreak of the disease in the United States in the late summer of 1989, and additional cases were also reported from Europe. The initial group of patients was identified in New Mexico in 1989. Case-control studies suggested that the outbreak was associated with the use of L-tryptophan. This product, an essential amino acid, was marketed over the counter as a health food supplement for 20 years for the treatment of insomnia and depression, although the scientific evidence supporting its efficacy was limited. Approximately 1,500 patients, including 26 who died, were reported to the Centers for Disease Control (CDC) in the 1989–90 outbreak, but it is estimated that between 5,000 and 10,000 people were affected. The disease almost disappeared after L-tryptophan was removed from the market.

The outbreak was traced to L-tryptophan and most often to L-tryptophan manufactured by a single company, suggesting that a contaminant was responsible, but the exact cause is not known. Many people who used L-tryptophan from the same batch that caused disease were not affected, suggesting that the risk to individuals exposed to the same toxic chemical varied. Occasional cases have been reported after L-tryptophan was removed from the market and are thought to be caused by unidentified chemicals that result in the same syndrome. In support of this theory is that a clinical syndrome similar to eosinophilia myalgia syndrome was seen during an outbreak of an illness called *toxic oil syndrome* that occurred in Spain in the 1980s in people exposed to contaminated rapeseed oil. An alternative theory to explain the few cases of eosinophilia myalgia syndrome that still occur is that some people metabolize the naturally occurring L-tryptophan abnormally and actually produce a toxic chemical themselves.

Symptoms and Diagnostic Path
The symptoms of eosinophilia myalgia syndrome can affect almost any organ system. Typically the

most characteristic early symptom is severe and sometimes disabling muscle pain (myalgia). The muscles are tender and later in the illness can become weak. Fatigue, arthralgia (joint pain), fever, cough, edema (swelling), poor memory and concentration, and shortness of breath are common. Most patients have a rash that can be itchy and urticarial initially (wheals) but that later becomes SCLERODERMA-like and can cause contractures. Neuropathy affecting the nerves to the hands and feet can cause numbness and the sensation of pins and needles in the glove and stocking areas. The brain can be affected, resulting in impairment of memory and thinking.

Blood tests show a marked eosinophilia in all patients. Other blood tests are often abnormal, but the findings are not specific. The white blood cell count and ESR can be elevated and liver function tests are abnormal in approximately 50 percent of patients. Despite severe muscle pain, muscle enzymes such as creatine kinase (CK) are usually normal. A biopsy of skin and muscle is abnormal and shows fibrosis and inflammation, findings that can be similar to those seen in EOSINOPHILIC FASCIITIS. The CDC criteria for classification as eosinophilia myalgia syndrome are

- An eosinophil count more than 1,000 cells/mm³
- Generalized myalgia severe enough to affect the patient's ability to perform daily activities
- Absence of an infection or malignancy that could account for the first two criteria

Treatment Options and Outlook

CORTICOSTEROIDS are used to treat the acute illness and the rash. Eosinophilia and swelling usually respond rapidly. Fibrosis in the lungs, thickening of the skin, and neurological damage do not improve with therapy. A range of immunosuppressive therapies has been tried, with little evidence of success.

In some patients the illness has a short duration with complete resolution of symptoms, but approximately 40 percent of patients have chronic symptoms. The central nervous system symptoms of poor memory and concentration are most likely to persist or worsen. Approximately 2–6 percent of affected patients have died, most often from progressive neurological complications.

Risk Factors and Preventive Measures

Eosinophilic myalgia syndrome has become very rare over the past decade, presumably as a result of more attention to the manufacture of L-tryptophan, although as discussed above the exact cause has not been determined. Taking L-tryptophan supplements is unnecessary, although eosinophilic myalgia syndrome is now so rare it need not be avoided for this specific reason.

eosinophilic fasciitis A rare SCLERODERMA-like illness that causes inflammation and thickening of the fascia and is associated with eosinophilia. First described by Dr. L. E. Shulman in 1974, more than 200 cases have now been reported in the medical literature. Eosinophilic fasciitis has occurred in people of all ages but is more common in adults.

The cause is unknown. However, because a similar illness called toxic oil syndrome occurred in people exposed to contaminated rapeseed oil and because isolated cases have been associated with exposure to organic chemicals and solvents such as trichloroethylene, an unidentified environmental toxin is thought to be responsible. In patients presenting with eosinophilic fasciitis, a history of recent strenuous physical exertion is common, but the significance of this observation is not known. A syndrome that has some similar features, EOSINOPHILIA MYALGIA SYNDROME, was recognized after eosinophilic fasciitis. Some authorities believe that some of the early cases of eosinophilic fasciitis were in fact a late stage of eosinophilia myalgia syndrome.

Symptoms and Diagnostic Path

Pain and swelling in the deep tissues below the skin are the first symptoms. Over weeks or months the tissue becomes thick and immobile, and dimpling of the skin can result in a characteristic orange peel appearance. The arms and legs are affected most often, but occasionally, the face and trunk can be involved. The thickening of deep connective tissue reduces the mobility of muscles, tendons, and joints, resulting in contractures. Systemic symptoms include low-grade fever and loss of weight.

The clinical findings and the presence of eosinophilia are clues to diagnosis, but a biopsy of skin and deeper tissues is usually needed. Other than eosinophilia, which is not always present, blood tests are not useful, and tests such as rheumatoid factor and antinuclear antibody are usually normal.

Treatment Options and Outlook

CORTICOSTEROIDS usually control the disease. Occasionally immunosuppressive drugs are added if the response to corticosteroids alone is inadequate. Contractures can limit the mobility of joints. Internal organs are not usually involved, and the prognosis is good in most patients.

Risk Factors and Preventive Measures

The cause remains unknown, and there are no effective preventive measures.

eosinophilic myositis A rare inflammatory muscle disease associated with an increased number of eosinophils in the blood (eosinophilia) or muscle. Up to 1993, only 31 cases had been described in the medical literature. No specific cause has been identified, but some cases have been associated with an allergic response to a drug.

Symptoms and Diagnostic Path

Muscle inflammation can affect several muscle groups diffusely or, less often, can cause focal, nodular lesions. The average age of onset in a review of published cases was 43 years but ranged from 14 to 70 years. Men were affected twice as often as women. Most patients had eosinophilia and increased muscle enzymes such as creatine kinase. The most common symptoms were muscle pain, cramping, and swelling. Weakness was uncommon. Reported associations include arthritis, nerve damage, and blood abnormalities, especially malignant conditions of the blood-forming cells.

Treatment Options and Outlook

Treatment with CORTICOSTEROIDS improved symptoms in most patients and the overall prognosis was good. HYDROXYCHLOROQUINE seems nearly as effective as corticosteroids in an uncontrolled case series and may have fewer long-term adverse effects.

epicondylitis (tennis elbow, golfer's elbow) The bony prominences on the inner and outer side of the elbow are known as the epicondyles. They are the lower part of the humerus (upper arm bone) and form the attachment of muscles that move the wrist. Muscles that move the hand away from the palm (as in a backhand stroke in tennis) attach to the outer or lateral epicondyle. Those that move the hand in the palmar direction (as in a forehand stroke) attach to the inner or medial epicondyle. When these attachments become injured, the condition is called epicondylitis. In common usage they are often called tennis (outer epicondyle) or golfer's (inner epicondyle) elbow, although less than 5 percent of lateral epicondylitis is found in tennis players and an even smaller percentage of medial epicondylitis in golfers.

Lateral epicondylitis is quite common, with between 1 and 3 percent of the population having it at some stage. Although most patients are not tennis players, nearly 50 percent of tennis players will suffer from it at some time. It is most frequent between the ages of 40 and 60 years. Many patients are manual workers, while in others there is no obvious cause. Medial epicondylitis or golfer's elbow is a very similar condition on the opposite epicondyle but is not common.

Small tears develop where the muscle joins the tendon close to the epicondyle. With repeated tears and scarring, chronic or ongoing inflammation develops, and the individual feels a persistent ache with more severe pain on use of the involved muscles. The grip will often weaken. In lateral epicondylitis, there will be marked tenderness over the bony prominence on the outside of the elbow or close to it and the pain will be most severe on extending the wrist up (as in a backhand stroke). Stretching these muscles (tuck the thumb into the palm of the hand, flex the wrist down, and then slowly straighten the elbow) may also produce some pain but is important in rehabilitation after treatment. The opposite movement of the wrist will bring out the pain of medial epicondylitis that is usually less severe and spread over a wider area.

Symptoms and Diagnostic Path

The chief symptom is pain felt in the upper forearm. The pain is made much worse by use of the hand and forearm, particularly with gripping or repetitive movements. Most patients will complain of some weakness of the grip as well. The pain is not confined to the same, usually quite small, area that the tenderness is but will be around the affected epicondyle.

The diagnosis is made based on the history and examination, but an X-ray may be done to exclude OSTEOARTHRITIS of the elbow joint. When the condition does not respond to usual therapy, other causes should be considered, particularly arthritis of the elbow joint, inflammation of the ligament that holds the head of the radius (forearm bone) in place, and nerve entrapments. Compression of the posterior interosseus nerve (a branch of the radial nerve) as it passes backward just below the elbow may be particularly difficult to diagnose while giving rise to complaints very similar to the far more common tennis elbow. Electrical stimulation studies can be helpful in diagnosing nerve entrapments.

Treatment Options and Outlook

Many treatments have been and are still used for epicondylitis. The three most frequently used are

- Rest with some immobilization
- Ultrasound
- Local corticosteroid injection

Although corticosteroids have been injected on the assumption that inflammation is causing the problem, studies show that the inflammatory component is usually quite minor. A number of alternative injection techniques have been tried therefore, and a controlled study showed no difference between injecting corticosteroid, local anesthetic, or saline (salty water) as long as a "peppering" technique was used. Rest of the involved muscles certainly helps healing, but it needs to be for at least six weeks. Since it is bad for joints and muscles to be completely immobilized for this length of time, a variety of movable elbow splints have been developed. It is also possible to use a wrist splint that prevents the wrist from flexing toward the palm and thereby stretching the muscles in lateral epicondylitis. Ultrasound is effective but takes longer and is more expensive than a corticosteroid injection. It has a lower relapse rate, however. Usually a combination of either ultrasound or injection plus rest (or at the very least avoidance of aggravating activities) is used. Strapping of the forearm muscles an inch or two below the elbow reduces the tension on the injured muscle/tendon junction and can be helpful in allowing patients to recommence activities. At this stage gentle stretching should also be undertaken. Similar treatment is used for medial epicondylitis.

Despite such a combined approach to lateral epicondylitis and an excellent initial response rate, about a third of patients will have had a recurrence of their symptoms by six months. Often conservative treatment is repeated with stricter immobilization. However, with repeated relapses and if the diagnosis is certain, surgery may be considered. Many surgical procedures have been done over the years, depending on what the surgeon considered the essential problem to be. However, the most common and least invasive is simply to cut the tendons close to their attachment to the epicondyle. They will heal by fibrosis or scarring, and the effect will be to lengthen them. This approach is successful in nearly 90 percent of cases.

Risk Factors and Preventive Measures

Many different activities, not necessarily very strenuous, can give rise to the forearm pain grouped together as tennis elbow and, less frequently, golfer's elbow. Many but not all sufferers are unable to stabilize their shoulders properly during activity. It seems likely therefore that the forearm muscles are either being overused or used from a position of mechanical disadvantage due to shoulder dysfunction and therefore sustain the minor tears that lead to these conditions. A good level of general fitness and regular forearm stretches as described above will prevent some cases, but few people do these until after they have developed symptoms. Some people such as dentists develop lateral epicondylitis because they have to hold their arm still for sustained periods of time despite this requiring less than 20 percent of their muscle strength. Use of forearm rests may be helpful here and regular breaks for powerful contraction and stretch of the forearm muscles is important.

erythema nodosum An inflammatory skin rash that causes red, painful nodules in the deep tissues under the skin, most often on the shin. It occurs at all ages and in both genders but affects young women more often.

The exact mechanism is not known, but it is thought to result from an immune reaction to an underlying infection or drug. Several conditions are associated with erythema nodosum. These include streptococcal upper respiratory tract infections, SARCOIDOSIS; INFLAMMATORY BOWEL DISEASE; BEHÇET'S DISEASE; pregnancy; infections such as TUBERCULOSIS, coccidiomycosis, histoplasmosis, blastomycosis, and leprosy; and reactions to drugs such as penicillins, estrogen, iodine, and sulfonamides. In approximately one-third of patients no underlying cause can be found.

Symptoms and Diagnostic Path

The first symptom is the development of painful, shiny, red raised lumps on the shin. The lesions are often 1 inch or more in diameter and can occur in other parts of the body such as the thighs or arms. Over four to eight weeks the nodules change color and resemble a bruise slowly turning from red to blue and then to brown. The nodules do not usually ulcerate. Systemic symptoms such as fever, fatigue, and arthralgia (joint pain) are common. Less often there is mild arthritis, most often affecting the knees. The symptoms can be severe and limit walking and other day-to-day activities.

In patients with erythema nodosum associated with sarcoidosis, there may be arthritis of the ankles and enlarged lymph nodes on chest X-ray. This combination of findings is called Löfgren's syndrome.

The diagnosis is usually made clinically from the typical rash. Occasionally if the rash is not typical, a skin biopsy is done. This shows inflammation around the blood vessels in deep subcutaneous tissues, particularly fat (panniculitis). The white blood cell count and the ESR are often elevated, but laboratory tests are not helpful in making the diagnosis. They are, however, helpful in diagnosing the underlying cause. For example, a throat culture may detect the presence of a streptococcal infection, or a chest X-ray may show signs of sarcoidosis or an infection such as tuberculosis or histoplasmosis.

Treatment Options and Outlook

If there is an underlying associated illness, it should be treated. For example, antibiotic therapy, most often penicillin, is the usual treatment for streptococcal infection. If a drug is the cause, it should be discontinued. Treatment of the symptoms may include analgesics to control pain or NSAIDs to decrease inflammation. Occasionally if symptoms are not responding to these drugs, a CORTICOSTEROID is used. A potential disadvantage of corticosteroid therapy is that because it suppresses the immune response, it can aggravate an unrecognized underlying chronic infection such as tuberculosis.

The course is usually self-limited. Symptoms slowly improve and resolve completely over a few weeks or months, even without any specific treatment. A few patients have a more protracted course and the condition can recur.

Risk Factors and Preventive Measures

Although the inciting events are well known (see above), erythema nodosum is not a common or severe complication of these, and there are no realistic preventive measures.

erythrocyte sedimentation rate (ESR) See Appendix II.

exercise Views on exercise range from those enthusiasts who point to its importance in managing obesity, diabetes, hypertension, and arthritis and suggest that it can prevent cancer to the "when I feel the urge to exercise I quickly lie down till it passes" brigade. For people with musculoskeletal disorders, exercise becomes more difficult and at the same time more important. It is important for pain relief, maintaining independence, recreation and quality of life, recovering from surgery or severe bouts of arthritis, improving sleep, managing body weight, and feeling better. Specific problems require specific exercises, and exercises need to be done correctly. Many people will require the help of a physical therapist or personal trainer to achieve this. Specific exercises that may be required, for example those to restore normal scapulohumeral rhythm in a patient with shoulder pain, are beyond the scope of this book. This section will first address some general principles of rehabilitation exercises and then aspects of exercise in general as they apply to people with arthritis.

Rehabilitation Exercise

Rehabilitation is defined as "restoration to a former capacity." In patients with chronic arthritis, restoring or improving functional level may be a more appropriate definition. Rehabilitation may be required in a patient with severe inflammatory arthritis such as RHEUMATOID ARTHRITIS once the inflammation has been controlled, in a patient who has gradually lost functional ability, following an acute injury, and always following surgery. Everybody has different goals and abilities as well as different forms of arthritis at various stages. Rehabilitation programs should be tailored to each individual's needs and abilities. The goals should be realistically achievable and the time frame appropriate. Important aspects of rehabilitation include the following:

- *Muscle Conditioning* When a joint is painful and swollen, the muscles that normally move it weaken rapidly. This is worsened by inactivity, particularly if the muscles are habitually held in a shortened position. So, for example, when an athlete injures a knee or someone with ANKYLOSING SPONDYLITIS develops an inflammatory effusion at the knee, the quadriceps muscles (the large muscles in front of the knee) that extend and stabilize the knee will rapidly decondition. Although this is easily seen as a reduction in size, the weakening is always greater than the size change would suggest. This is because there is an increase in fatty tissue in the muscle with deconditioning. Following resolution of such an

event it is therefore necessary to condition the muscle again.

Muscle conditioning requires overload and activity-specific exercises. The latter is most relevant to athletes and indicates that different types of exercise will produce different conditioning effects. The individual's goals must be known when devising an exercise program. In order to increase muscle strength, power, and endurance, it is necessary to overload it. This means that if a patient with arthritis just wants to be able to walk reasonably well after a knee replacement, walking by itself is not adequate muscle conditioning for the quadriceps muscles that have become small and weak prior to surgery. There are several ways in which overload training is achieved:

(a) Increasing speed of movement, e.g., for quadriceps doing leg extensions (straightening the knee from a sitting position) or climbing stairs faster

(b) Increasing the number of times the exercise is repeated, e.g., more leg extensions or stairs

(c) Exercising more frequently, e.g., from once a day to twice then three times a day

(d) Exercising against resistance, e.g., attaching a weight to the shoe before doing leg extensions

(e) Decreasing the rest time between exercises

(f) Altering the range through which the muscle is exercised

This final method is a very specialized area and should be done only under expert guidance. Usually a muscle is best exercised through its full normal range of movement.

The four components of muscle conditioning that need to be considered in planning rehabilitation exercise are strength, power, endurance, and motor reeducation.

1. Strength is the muscle's ability to exert force. This can improve before any noticeable increase in muscle size. This improvement is thought to be due to the improved blood supply and metabolic efficiency that occur with training. Three main types of exercise are used.

   (a) Isometric exercises are when a muscle is contracted without moving the joint. These can be started before a joint has completely settled down as they cause very little pain and will not cause an inflamed joint to flare. They can prevent a lot of the wasting that occurs with a painful joint and perhaps some of the loss of proprioception (see below). The muscle is usually contracted for six seconds followed by a 20-second rest. Ten to 20 contractions are performed many times a day at increasing intensity with the joint in various positions.

(b) Isotonic exercises involve moving a joint through its range of movement with a constant resistance, e.g., doing a biceps curl holding a dumbbell. These can be concentric (when the muscle shortens) or eccentric (when the muscle lengthens). Eccentric exercise is particularly important in rehabilitation, especially if there has been a tendon or musculotendinous injury. It should be started very gradually, however, since too rapid an increase can damage a deconditioned muscle. The use of free weights is almost always better than using exercise machines. Free weights provide appropriate stress to all the involved tendons and ligaments. They require activation of not only the muscle group being trained but also all the stabilizing and postural muscles and in this way prepares the individual for real-world activity. Exercise machines cut out all postural and supporting muscle action and should be used only to achieve specific, short-term goals.

(c) Isokinetic exercises are when the speed of movement is constant throughout the full range. Because the force that a muscle is capable of exerting is different when the muscle is at different lengths, isokinetic exercises are done against a machine that is capable of varying its resistance in response to the force applied. It is possible to perform more muscle work with this form of exercise than isometric or isotonic exercise, but there is maximal loading at the weakest points of the range of movement. Isokinetic exercise is used mainly for testing rather than for rehabilitation itself.

2. Power is the speed at which muscles can perform work or *explosive strength*. A standing high jump, for example, is a measure of power in the leg muscles. It is important in sports such as sprinting and the jumping and landing of basketball players. Power exercises come later in a rehabilitation program. *Plyometric* exercises such as hopping and bounding are often used before an athlete attempts actual sport-specific maneuvers.

3. Endurance is the ability of muscle to perform repeated contractions. Most marathon runners will have highly developed endurance, although they may have relatively little power compared with a tennis player. Endurance is improved by performing many repetitions of an exercise with relatively little resistance, e.g., walking, jogging, cycling.

4. Motor reeducation is important because muscles do not act in isolation. Rather, the prime mover works with the help of synergistic or supporting muscles on the background of stabilizing muscle action. In addition, human action usually involves a chain of movements (the kinetic chain) rather than one group of muscles moving a joint. For example, a right-handed baseball pitcher's throw (excluding the windup) begins with pressure being exerted onto the ground by the right foot and is then followed by a chain of movements through the body until the right wrist and fingers apply the final acceleration and curve to the ball. Following a significant injury or flare of arthritis it is not uncommon for these chain movements to become relatively *uncoupled* or for stabilizing muscles to become inactivated. This is a frequent cause, for example, of shoulder injuries or tendinitis to fail to settle after what appears to be adequate treatment. Muscle reeducation is required to restore the normal patterns of movement, and this is as important in elderly patients with rheumatoid arthritis as it is in elite athletes. The first step toward muscle reeducation is an analysis of faulty movement patterns by a skilled examiner.

- *Flexibility* The pain of an inflamed arthritic or injured joint causes the person to restrict its movement. The swelling in the joint also reduces the amount of movement possible and there is spasm of the muscles around the joint that cause a variable degree of *splinting*. The joint capsule, ligaments, and other soft tissues can in a short while start to contract so that once the original inflammation has been successfully treated, the joint may be stiff with a limited range of movement and tight muscles and tendons. Joint mobilization is used to free up the joints and stretching to relax the muscles and lengthen tendons. Mobilization should be started as soon as possible before severe restriction develops. There are many mobilization and stretching techniques taught by physical therapists that are appropriate at different stages of rehabilitation.

- *Proprioception* Normally our joints, muscles, and tendons are continuously sending nerve impulses to the spinal cord and brain carrying information about the position of our limbs and joints in space. This is called proprioception. Following injury or surgery these nerve pathways are damaged, leading to poor balance, poor coordination, and reduced sense of joint position. This can lead to reinjury. Proprioceptive training involves retraining these nerve pathways. Following an ankle injury, for example, a patient might start by standing on one leg, progress to standing on an unstable surface such as a wobble board, and then progress to one-leg trampoline jumping.

- *Functional Exercise* Rehabilitation progresses from the conditioning of muscle groups and retraining faulty movement patterns to activities that the individual intends doing for work or recreation. These latter are broadly termed functional exercises. Although basic functional activities such as walking and jogging are started early on in rehabilitation, more advanced activities such as would be required for a soccer player or manual worker to return to sport and work will start only once muscle conditioning, flexibility, and proprioception are progressing well. Initially functional exercises that simulate the individual's desired activity are done in a controlled setting. The intensity is gradually increased with careful monitoring before specific sport or work activities are started. Even then it is advisable to return to previous levels of activity in a graduated fashion.

- *Biomechanical Abnormalities* These may have produced the injury or be the result of either injury or progressive arthritis. They may pres-

ent as muscle tightness or weakness or actual joint abnormalities. Clearly, successful rehabilitation will depend on identifying them and correcting or ameliorating them. This can be achieved by muscle stretching, conditioning, proprioceptive training, taping, and orthotics and shoe modification.

Exercise for Arthritis

One of the major advances in treating musculoskeletal conditions over the past 25 years has been the realization of the dangers of rest, especially bed rest, and the importance of exercise. Much pain and disability suffered by arthritis patients is due to poor posture and muscle function that results from inactivity and muscle imbalance rather than active arthritis itself, although the arthritis may have initiated these problems. Most people with arthritis who take up exercise find it helpful. Benefits that they report include more flexibility, less pain, and improved general health. People find controlling their weight easier if they exercise regularly. They sleep better, have more energy, and find the exercise helps in dealing with stress. In general, exercise should involve some combination of aerobic activities for endurance, stretching or range of movement exercises, and strengthening exercises for muscle conditioning (see Rehabilitation Exercise section above).

For those with severe arthritis, it is advisable to take advice before starting an exercise program. This may be from the patient's doctor, a physical therapist, or both. The Arthritis Foundation in most areas is likely to have appropriate exercise classes or be able to advise on what is available locally. There are also a number of very good self-help exercise books for patients with arthritis. Exercise should be enjoyable, although this will vary among individuals. Many people enjoy exercising to music (in a gym or at home), some like exercising in a group, others alone, some in the morning, and others later in the day. Warming up before vigorous exercise or stretching is important. Gentle exercise is the usual way to warm up, but this can be helped by having a warm environment, using heat rubs, or simply dressing warmly.

Relaxation techniques are a very rewarding way to end an exercise session. Progressive relaxation where each part of the body is first moved (usually contracted) and then relaxed before moving on to the next part is a commonly used technique. There are many others, however, including breathing techniques, imagery, and meditation. Many tapes are available to assist with relaxation. People with muscular pain find this particularly helpful. Walking is the most readily available form of aerobic exercise and can be fun (e.g., with a pet or friend), uplifting (in a beautiful park), educational (listening to a lecture on an iPod), or incorporated into daily life (walk to a friend's house rather than driving). Cycling is also a good aerobic exercise that avoids much of the impact of walking or jogging, especially when using a stationary bike or modern mountain bike.

Two forms of exercise are particularly useful while joints are inflamed or very painful. Exercising in water, especially warm water, can give pain relief as well as useful exercise even when hips, knees, or ankles are too painful to walk any distance on. Not only is the water and the warmth relaxing but it also unloads the weight-bearing joints while providing good resistance to muscle action. The other useful form of exercise is isometric exercises, as discussed above under Rehabilitation Exercise.

Although recreational exercise is generally more fun, activities such as housework and gardening can be turned into therapeutic exercise. It is important to be aware of doing tasks with a good posture and alternating activities frequently. If weeding for example, weed for 10 minutes and then get up and carry the weeds to the compost heap rather than remaining kneeling for 40 minutes. Consider the use of gardening stools, wheelbarrows, high chairs in the kitchen, and ergonomic tools so as not to cause strain. It is clear, however, that the benefit of housework as exercise is less than enjoyable recreational exercise.

eye problems Several rheumatic illnesses can have associated eye problems. All parts of the eye can be involved, but different illnesses are more likely to affect particular parts of the eye.

Conjunctivitis

The conjunctiva is the most superficial layer of the eye. When it is inflamed the superficial blood vessels become dilated and the eye turns red, becomes itchy, and feels painful. Vision is not affected but can be blurred if the eye waters. The most common causes of conjunctivitis are allergy and viral or bacterial infection. Patients with any rheumatic disease that causes sicca syndrome, for example SJÖGREN'S SYNDROME, SYSTEMIC LUPUS ERYTHEMATOSUS, and RHEUMATOID ARTHRITIS, are more likely to develop conjunctivitis. Sicca syndrome causes dry eyes that are easily irritated by minor trauma, and the resulting inflammation causes conjunctivitis. The treatment of conjunctivitis associated with sicca syndrome includes measures to prevent the eye from drying out, for example glasses with side shields, eye drops or lubricant eye ointment to counteract dryness, and antibiotic drops if a bacterial infection is present. Some patients with sicca syndrome get problems because of the mucous layer drying out and forming a crusty material rather than an absolute lack of tears. These patients may be helped by the use of drops that contain acetylcysteine that dissolve mucus.

Episcleritis

The episclera is a layer lining the eye that lies below the conjuctiva and above the sclera. It is superficial. When it is inflamed, the eye becomes red but vision is not affected. Oral or topical NONSTEROIDAL ANTI-INFLAMMATORY DRUGS may relieve symptoms, but often no specific treatment is prescribed and symptoms resolve spontaneously. Rheumatoid arthritis is often associated with episcleritis.

Scleritis

Inflammation of the sclera, the layer below the episclera, causes a red, painful eye. The pain is deep, severe, and aching in character compared with the superficial scratchiness caused by conjunctivitis or episcleritis. A few patients get an associated uveitis. Vision can be affected, and scleritis should be treated by an ophthalmologist. Treatment involves management of the underlying condition and may require CORTICOSTEROIDS and immunosuppressive drugs. Approximately 60 percent of patients with scleritis have no associated systemic disease, 30 percent have rheumatoid arthritis, and the remainder have one of a variety of less common diseases. These include, systemic lupus erythematosus, VASCULITIS (particularly WEGENER'S GRANULOMATOSIS), INFLAM-MATORY BOWEL DISEASE, ANKYLOSING SPONDYLITIS, and RELAPSING POLYCHONDRITIS. In patients with severe rheumatoid arthritis, nodules can occur in the sclera and inflammation can cause the sclera to become thin. If scleral inflammation in rheumatoid arthritis is not controlled, the sclera can become so thin that the globe of the eye perforates and blindness results. This is, fortunately, very rare.

Uveitis

Inflammation of the uveal tract, the tissues lining the inside of the eye, can occur with several rheumatic diseases. Uveitis is usually classified as anterior uveitis affecting the tissues in the front of the eye such as the iris (iritis) or posterior uveitis affecting tissues at the back of the eye such as the retina (retinitis and choroiditis). Approximately 40 percent of people with uveitis have an underlying rheumatic illness.

Anterior uveitis   This often causes a red, painful eye with disturbance of vision and discomfort in bright light (photophobia). Some types of anterior uveitis, particularly the type associated with JUVENILE IDIOPATHIC ARTHRITIS, can be relatively asymptomatic and if not diagnosed and treated can cause gradually progressive, irreversible loss of vision. The diagnosis of uveitis is made by an ophthalmologist using an instrument called a slitlamp microscope that provides a clear and enlarged view of the interior of the eye. Anterior uveitis increases the amount of cells present in the anterior chamber of the eye, and this is visible as a flare on slitlamp examination. Approximately 25 percent of patients with spondyloarthropathies such as Reiter's syndrome or ankylosing spondylitis will develop anterior uveitis at some time during the course of the illness. Typically this uveitis has an acute onset and affects one eye, although if recurrent attacks occur, the other eye can be affected. Anterior uveitis associated with spondyloarthropathies is usually a self-limiting problem and settles over weeks or a few months. Recurrent attacks are common, but the prognosis is good and permanent visual loss is rare. Anterior uveitis usually responds to treatment with local corticosteroids.

Posterior uveitis   The most prominent symptom is often loss of vision. Unless there is associated anterior uveitis, the eye may not be red or painful. It is important to differentiate infectious causes of posterior uveitis such as toxoplasmosis and cytomegalovirus from rheumatic disorders such as BEHÇET'S DISEASE and SARCOIDOSIS. If an infectious cause has been excluded and vision is threatened, posterior uveitis is often treated with systemic corticosteroids and immunosuppressive drugs. In many patients no definite cause for uveitis is found.

Other Eye Disorders

Vasculitis of large- and medium-sized vessels as occurs with TEMPORAL ARTERITIS (giant cell arteritis) can affect the artery supplying the retina and cause sudden, irreversible blindness. Cataracts occur more commonly in patients treated with corticosteroids.

familial Mediterranean fever (FMF) An inherited disorder that causes acute attacks of fever, arthritis, pleurisy, and peritonitis. An illness characterized by paroxysmal peritonitis was first described by T. C. Janeway and H. O. Mosenthal in 1908 and was termed *periodic disease* until the 1950s, when the name familial Mediterranean fever was used to describe the illness. FMF occurs most commonly in populations of Mediterranean origin such as Sephardic Jews, Arabs, Armenians, and Turks. It also occurs sporadically in individuals in other populations.

FMF is the first rheumatic disease for which a clear genetic cause has been found. The gene responsible for FMF was cloned in 1997 and designated *MEFV.* In 1998, Eisenberg and colleagues reported three mutations in this gene that were found in many patients with FMF. Subsequent work has shown that five mutations, designated V762A, M694V, M694I, M680I, and E148Q, account for approximately 75 percent of patients with FMF. These mutations likely derive from single individuals or founders who lived long ago. Other mutations can cause FMF, and so far 29 mutations in the MEFV gene have been described. In American populations in whom FMF is not endemic, not all the mutations responsible for the illness have been identified. The ability to identify the genetic causes of FMF has enabled researchers to study populations in whom the disease is common. In these populations where about one in 500 people are affected, the carrier rate for an abnormal MEFV gene is as high as one in six people. The high frequency of abnormal MEFV genes in healthy people has led to the suggestion that it may impart a biological survival advantage, but this is speculative.

The MEFV gene codes for a single protein named both *pyrin* and *marenostrin* by different research groups. This protein suppresses the inflammatory responses of granulocytes (polymorphonuclear white blood cells). Individuals with FMF produce an abnormal protein that does not efficiently suppress inflammation. It is not clear why some parts of the body such as the pleura and peritoneum are particularly likely to be affected in people with FMF or what triggers acute attacks.

Symptoms and Diagnostic Path
The onset of symptoms occurs before the age of 10 years in 50 percent of patients, and only 5 percent have their first attack after the age of 30 years. Attacks start suddenly and last one to four days. The frequency of attacks varies, but often they occur several months apart. As patients get older the frequency and severity of attacks tend to decline.

Fever occurs with every attack and is often such a prominent symptom that it is not unusual for a patient to have been extensively evaluated for severe recurrent fevers before the diagnosis of FMF is made. Another common symptom is abdominal pain, present in more than 90 percent of patients. The pain has features of peritonitis and can mimic other causes such as appendicitis. Again, it is not unusual for patients to have had emergency surgery performed for suspected peritonitis before the diagnosis of FMF is made. Pleurisy occurs in more than half of patients, but pericarditis is rare, affecting less than 1 percent. Arthritis occurs in most patients and is typically acute and asymmetrical, affecting large joints such as the knee, ankle, and wrist, often at the same time as the acute attack. Arthritis resolves spontaneously and completely. A less common, more chronic arthritis affecting the sacroiliac joints has been described. Other symptoms include myalgia and a red rash that resembles a bacterial infection of the skin, but like the acute attack, these resolve spontaneously.

Common laboratory tests are not helpful for making the diagnosis. During an acute attack, tests that reflect inflammation such as the ESR, CRP, and white blood cell count are often raised (see Appendix II). The symptoms of FMF together with abnormal blood tests are often interpreted by physicians as indicating the presence of a serious infection or surgical problem in the abdomen. The correct diagnosis is often not made until other causes for the symptoms have been excluded. Genetic testing for the common variants of the MEFV gene associated with FMF is now widely available and is helpful in making the diagnosis.

Treatment Options and Outlook

The most effective treatment is COLCHICINE, a drug that prevents white blood cells from leaving the bloodstream to set up inflammation at the affected site. While taking colchicine more than 50 percent of patients have no further attacks, and in the remainder, the attacks are less frequent and severe. Colchicine also decreases the risk of AMYLOIDOSIS and slows progression in patients who develop it.

The most serious complication of FMF is AA amyloidosis. This commonly affects the kidneys and causes protein to leak into the urine and kidney failure. The frequency of amyloidosis varies among different ethnic groups. Preliminary evidence indicates that the different genetic variants associated with FMF impart different risks for developing amyloidosis. The risk of amyloidosis in different populations is also affected by treatment with colchicine. Zemer and colleagues reported their findings in a large series of 1,070 patients in Israel and found that less than 2 percent of patients who took colchicine regularly developed amyloidosis compared with 50 percent who did not.

Risk Factors and Preventive Measures

This is an inherited disorder for which there are no preventive measures. In populations where it is common, genetic counseling is advisable.

Felty's syndrome Patients with RHEUMATOID ARTHRITIS occasionally develop an enlarged spleen and an abnormally low white cell count (leukopenia). This is known as Felty's syndrome. It is quite rare and occurs in less than 1 percent of patients with rheumatoid arthritis. All Felty's syndrome patients are positive for RHEUMATOID FACTOR.

The fact that Felty's syndrome sometimes occurs in members of the same family suggests that there may be genetic factors in its development. This is supported by the very strong association with the HLA-DR4 gene (see GENETIC FACTORS). This association is stronger than with other rheumatoid arthritis patients. There is also an association with a gene that results in less-than-normal amounts of COMPLEMENT factor 4 being produced. Different factors may be more important in different patients with Felty's syndrome, but two main abnormalities are found in all patients to a degree. First, these patients have very high levels of antibodies in the blood that stick both to each other and to the surfaces of white cells. This has three effects on the white cells: They are less effective at attacking invading organisms; they tend to clump on the walls of the blood vessels rather than circulating in the blood as usual; they are removed from the bloodstream and destroyed by the spleen, which enlarges as a result. Second, the bone marrow does not respond to a low white cell count by producing many new cells as it would normally.

Symptoms and Diagnostic Path

The arthritis may not be severe or even active at the time Felty's syndrome develops. It is always an erosive arthritis but in a third of patients is quiescent when Felty's syndrome starts. An enlarged spleen is necessary to make the diagnosis, but this can be difficult to detect early on. If suspected, an ultrasound scan of the abdomen is a good way to show splenic enlargement. The size of the spleen does not predict the severity of the other problems.

Weight loss is common and may be marked. Leg ulcers are frequent and may be very difficult to heal. They are presumed to result from low-grade VASCULITIS or inflammation along the blood vessels of the legs. The most dangerous complication of Felty's syndrome is the frequent infections to which these patients are prone. Infections are mostly with common organisms especially those normally found on human skin, and occur 10 to

20 times more often in Felty's patients than in other rheumatoid arthritis patients. Mild anemia that may be due to more rapid breakdown of red blood cells and a low platelet count are common. Platelets are small blood cells involved in the clotting of blood.

Felty's syndrome is diagnosed when a patient with rheumatoid factor-positive rheumatoid arthritis develops an enlarged spleen and a white cell count of less than 2000 cells/mL of blood. It should be differentiated from a low-grade leukemia of large granular lymphocytes (a small subset of white blood cells), which can give rise to a very similar picture. A quarter of these patients also have rheumatoid arthritis. These large granular lymphocytes have a very typical appearance and, if suspected, can be recognized on examination of a blood sample or a bone marrow biopsy.

Treatment Options and Outlook

The arthritis should be treated along the usual lines for rheumatoid arthritis. Often good control of the rheumatoid inflammation will lead to a rise in the white cell count. Pulse intravenous CYCLOPHOSPHAMIDE is effective in healing ulcers but carries significant risks, especially in blunting the immune response to infection. Growth factors such as granulocyte-macrophage colony-stimulating factor (GM-CSF) can dramatically increase the white cell count and may be useful in managing overwhelming infections but have no role in long-term treatment. Androgenic steroids (similar to testosterone) and drugs like lithium may also increase the white cell count but do not have an established role in treatment.

Splenectomy (surgically removing the spleen) is effective at raising the white cell count in all patients. In a quarter, however, it will drop to low levels again. The anemia and low platelet count also improve as do some leg ulcers. Splenectomy increases the risk of infection with certain types of bacteria. It is possible to vaccinate against some of these before removing the spleen, thereby giving partial protection. Vaccines are available for *Pneumococcus, Haemophilus,* and *Meningococci.* Splenectomy is generally used only in those with severe disease in whom other therapies are ineffective.

People with Felty's syndrome have a shorter life expectancy than others with rheumatoid arthritis. This usually results from infections.

Risk Factors and Preventive Measures

Felty's syndrome develops in a small number of people with rheumatoid arthritis who usually have a strongly positive RHEUMATOID FACTOR (see Appendix II) and possess the HLA-DR4 gene. There are no proven preventive measures.

fibromyalgia A syndrome characterized by widespread musculoskeletal pain, poor sleep, fatigue, and a number of tender points on physical examination. A syndrome is a grouping of symptoms that are characteristic enough to be used to describe a group of patients. It does not imply a disease entity, although some syndromes subsequently become known as diseases as more knowledge accumulates. This point is worth laboring because of the considerable debate still surrounding the term fibromyalgia. The debate is not about whether the pain and suffering are real but rather about what fibromyalgia is and whether it should be separated from other chronic pain syndromes. Surveys show that between 1 and 2 percent of the population in developed countries fit current criteria for fibromyalgia. It is more common in Caucasians, and in women and there is a trend for patients to have slightly higher-than-average social class.

There is no agreement on the cause, and there is unlikely any one specific cause. A proportion of patients describe a traumatic event of some sort before the symptoms first start. These include infections, accidents, emotional trauma, or corticosteroid withdrawal. Women who have been sexually abused as children appear to be prone to developing chronic pain problems in later life including fibromyalgia. Five factors are believed to influence the development of this syndrome.

First, early studies suggested abnormalities in the painful muscles, but more recent controlled studies have shown these to be no different from normal individuals. There are differences in energy utilization and oxygen levels in the affected muscles, but it is not possible to say whether this is a primary (causative) problem or simply the result of muscle deconditioning. More than 80 percent of fibromyalgia patients are deconditioned or unfit by a variety of measurements. Deconditioned muscle is more likely to develop very small areas of trauma that result in pain. Because of this pain the muscle is not used normally, and reflexes in the brain may actually reduce blood circulation in that muscle. Deconditioning therefore worsens, there is more minor trauma to muscle fibers, and the condition escalates. In keeping with this, nervous control of blood flow to the hand has been shown to be abnormal in fibromyalgia patients, and this may be why some patients develop RAYNAUD'S PHENOM-ENON-like symptoms.

Second, although the absence of any recognizable disease might once have led people to think of fibromyalgia as a psychological problem ("it is all in your head"), this is no longer tenable. Indeed, the complex interaction and indivisibility of mind and body mean that very few doctors would find this type of thinking useful, although it may still be encountered in neighbors, workmates, and the like. There are, however, some clear psychological differences when fibromyalgia patients are compared with healthy control groups (see CLINICAL TRIAL for an explanation of controlled studies). Fibromyalgia patients have more psychological symptoms, and a quarter have clinical depression. About 50 percent have had clinical depression at some time in the past, and there is also more depression in their families. There is no personality type, however. Differentiating whether the depression preceded the fibromyalgia or was in part caused by the chronic pain of fibromyalgia is difficult. Nevertheless, it is important that the depression be identified and treated appropriately.

Third, about 80 percent of fibromyalgia patients report that they awake in the morning not feeling refreshed, and many will be aware of several nighttime awakenings. By studying brain waves using an electroencephalogram (EEG), it has been shown that people with painful conditions have many more wakings at night than they are aware of. EEGs show that fibromyalgia patients have frequent interruption of stage 3–4 sleep, which is believed to be the most restorative. Normal individuals who have their stage 3–4 sleep experimentally interrupted fairly soon develop fibromyalgia-like

symptoms. Furthermore, people with other conditions characterized by interrupted sleep patterns, such as those with SLEEP APNEA, frequently develop fibromyalgia. While disturbed sleep is likely important in the development and maintenance of fibromyalgia, the manner in which it acts is unknown and there remain unresolved difficulties in some of the experimental findings.

Fourth, fibromyalgia is a chronic pain syndrome, and there are physicochemical changes that occur in the pain-processing pathways in chronic pain. These changes occur in the nerves that carry signals from skin, muscle, and joints to the spinal cord as well as in areas in the spinal cord where these inputs are processed. In the spinal cord there are nerve networks that allow interaction with messages coming down the spinal cord that can either block or encourage transmission of the peripheral signals upward. It should be remembered that pain is felt only if these signals reach the upper levels of the brain where people become conscious of pain. It is possible for the pain signals from very dramatic injuries to be completely blocked for long periods of time. There are many examples of this in sport and war situations. Initially in chronic pain the constant bombardment of signals coming into the spinal cord produces changes in the ion channels of nerve cells that make it easier for these signals to be transmitted. Later on there are probably permanent changes in these cells. Along with this is the spreading of nerve activity so that a wider area is felt to be painful than was initially the case. These changes are important in understanding the widespread pain and tenderness that can occur with stimuli that would not ordinarily cause pain.

In fibromyalgia, particular interest has focused on high substance P levels in the CSF (fluid surrounding the brain and spinal cord) and low levels of serotonin in the blood. Substance P stimulates nerve endings that initiate pain impulses (i.e., it induces a pain signal) and is also known to play a role in pain transmission in the spinal cord. Serotonin is a substance that is released by nerves in order to stimulate other nerves (a neurotransmitter substance). It also has important effects on blood vessels. The systems in the brain that particularly use serotonin as a transmitter have to do with sleep, mood, and pain experience. Some studies have suggested that levels may be low in fibromyalgia patients as well as in depressed patients.

Fifth, many patients who fulfill the diagnostic criteria for fibromyalgia have segmental spinal dysfunction. Simply put, this means there are areas where two or more vertebrae have a restricted range of movement relative to each other in one or more directions. This can result from many conditions, including a disc prolapse or protrusion, osteoarthritis of the spine, poor posture, obesity, or any injury or condition that results in asymmetrical spinal movement. People with segmental spinal dysfunction frequently develop changes in tissues away from the spine but in the affected segment (the areas supplied by nerves from that level of the spinal cord). The whole body is divided up into these segments according to what level of the spinal cord the nerve supply comes from. If the spinal dysfunction is ongoing, they are at risk of developing a chronic pain syndrome.

Symptoms and Diagnostic Path

Pain described as muscular or around joints is the most frequent complaint. Stiffness often occurs that tends to be worse in the mornings. The pain may vary from day to day and is often made worse by stress, physical activity, poor sleep, and humid weather. Studies have shown that fibromyalgia patients report pain as being similar in severity to those with rheumatoid arthritis (pain is a private, subjective experience; there is no absolute measure) and that the effect on the household's earning capacity is nearly as bad as someone getting rheumatoid arthritis. Patients frequently wake unrefreshed, and fatigue is a significant problem. Sleep is often disturbed even when the patient is unaware of it. This usually takes the form of frequent waking or near waking after which the patient drops off to sleep again. Waking in the early hours of the morning and not being able to get back to sleep again is typical of depression, not fibromyalgia.

Fibromyalgia patients often suffer from other complaints such as frequent headaches, peculiar feelings in different parts of the body (such as tingling or burning in part of the hand), and a feeling of swelling, particularly of the hands (when no swelling can be seen). An increased sensitivity to cold and occasionally Raynaud's phenomenon-like symptoms occur. Dry eyes and mouth, palpitations, dizziness, difficulty in concentrating, and multiple allergies may occur. Anxiety is common. Mood swings and irritability occur. There is an overlap with migraine and irritable bowel syndrome.

Although patients may feel weak, there is no actual loss of muscle strength other than might occur from reduced use. The characteristic findings are numerous tender points mainly around the neck and shoulders but also around the hips and knees together with an absence of signs of other diseases that could cause the same symptoms.

The American College of Rheumatology has issued criteria for the classification of fibromyalgia, and these are widely used as the basis of diagnosis. The patient should have suffered widespread pain for at least three months. Widespread means pain in both left and right side of the body, both above and below the waist, and relating to the spine. In addition, there should be at least 11 out of 18 designated points around the neck, shoulders, hips, and knees that are felt as painful when pressed on with a force of about 4 kg. In practice, not all these criteria need to be met at one time in order for the diagnosis to be made.

Blood tests, X-rays, and scans are all normal in fibromyalgia. Blood tests may be done to exclude other difficult-to-diagnose conditions that can give rise to widespread aching and fatigue. Such illnesses include POLYMYALGIA RHEUMATICA, reduced thyroid function, autoimmune forms of hepatitis, multiple sclerosis, and autoimmune forms of arthritis such as SYSTEMIC LUPUS ERYTHEMATOSUS. It is considered possible to have fibromyalgia and another painful condition such as rheumatoid arthritis (then known as secondary fibromyalgia). As long as this other condition is recognized and treated appropriately, then treatment of fibromyalgia can improve the patient's sense of well-being. The danger lies in diagnosing fibromyalgia and not recognizing the presence of these other conditions (see also the related CHRONIC FATIGUE SYNDROME). Many patients with fibromyalgia will meet diagnostic criteria for chronic fatigue syndrome and vice versa. Some patients with either of these conditions will also meet criteria for irritable bowel syndrome and migraine.

Treatment Options and Outlook

Treatment is aimed at improving the contributing factors discussed above. General commonsense measures include avoiding sitting for long periods, avoiding awkward postures, doing regular stretches, and taking a hot shower in the morning. All these can significantly prevent or relieve the pain and stiffness. Patients should avoid overexertion when they feel well since this is likely to bring on a period of increased pain. More specific treatment should be tailored to the individual patient and might include the following:

- Education about the condition gives the patient some understanding of what may have seemed a strange and frightening condition. It may also allay some of the fears people have such as ending up in a wheelchair or dying young. An understanding of the state of the muscles and musculoskeletal system is necessary before the patient will work through the pain and fatigue to improve matters. Relatives and significant others should also have a reasonable understanding of the condition. This is particularly important because fibromyalgic patients look well and it is counterproductive if they constantly or frequently have to prove that they are suffering. Relatives and workmates should not, however, make a fuss over the patient unnecessarily and should still expect him or her to contribute to family life or the workplace. Education may include information about pacing activities and mini and micro rest techniques at work.

- Supervised general aerobic exercise has been shown not only to improve fitness but also to reduce pain levels and improve the patient's well-being. Unfortunately, unsupervised home exercise programs appear less successful, and many fibromyalgia patients are reluctant to join group exercise classes. The increase in pain after exercise is one reason that patients do not maintain regular exercise programs. They should start exercising slowly, do low-impact exercise, and try to tolerate some increase in pain. Sleep does not appear to be improved by exercise. Specific strengthening exercises and stretches to correct postural problems and spinal dysfunction are important but have not been subjected to controlled study.

- Biofeedback has produced significant improvement in pain, stiffness, and tenderness. Hypnotherapy improved pain, fatigue, and sleep more than physical therapy in one study. Meditation-based relaxation techniques may be helpful especially for the depressive symptoms.

- Good evidence shows that COGNITIVE BEHAVIORAL THERAPY, either alone or as part of a multimodal pain therapy program, is effective in improving fibromyalgic symptoms. In addition, self-management programs emphasizing either coping skills training or exercise provide benefit to some but not all patients.

- Tender points can be injected usually with a small amount of saline or local anesthetic, although dry needling (where nothing is injected) is done as well. This relaxes dysfunctional muscles and is particularly helpful when combined with stretching or manual therapy to correct postural problems. ACUPUNCTURE has not been demonstrated to be effective in fibromyalgia.

- Many medications may be used. Most fibromyalgia patients will have tried various painkillers such as ACETAMINOPHEN and NSAIDs such as DICLOFENAC and IBUPROFEN and possibly even oral CORTICOSTEROIDS without much benefit. There does not appear to be any value in using these medications long-term to manage the condition. However, most patients will find them intermittently useful for headaches or flares of pain. Surveys show that fibromyalgia patients find NSAIDs more helpful than pure analgesics (painkillers).

The most commonly used medications are those to improve the quality of sleep. Low doses of tricyclic antidepressants such as amitriptyline, imipramine, and cyclobenzaprine have consistently shown improvements in sleep, pain, and general well-being in controlled trials. The tricyclics not only promote stage 4 sleep but also act on pain pathways. Not all patients benefit, however, and many do not tolerate these medications even at low doses. Antidepressants of the SSRI class such as FLUOXETINE and PAROXETINE have been shown to reduce pain in fibromyalgia, independent of their effect on depression. Fluoxetine combined with low-dose amitriptyline is more effective than either alone. A newer drug, DULOXETINE, has a similar effect to this combination, and early studies suggest it may be useful although side effects are relatively common. There is little information on the benefit of the newer antidepressants, and the benzodiazepines should be avoided because of their addictive potential.

Ketamine works on the central pain mechanisms believed to be operative in chronic pain syndromes. It has been shown experimentally to relieve muscle pain and referred pain as well as to lower pain sensitivity in fibromyalgia patients. Using ketamine as a regular medication is not possible, but there is a lot of interest in developing a drug with similar actions that could be taken regularly. Two medications primarily developed as anticonvulsants, GABAPENTIN and PREGABALIN, have been shown to improve pain and sleep in fibromyalgia. Carisoprodol is a muscle relaxant with some promise but further studies are required.

Clinical depression should be treated in the usual way if present. Many fibromyalgia patients are reluctant to consider the possibility that they may be depressed. This probably reflects a societal view that mental illness is somehow bad or evidence of weakness of character combined with a rigid separation of mind and body. While neither of these views has any medical validity, they will likely continue to be prevalent in society for some time. Frank discussion between the clinician and patient is the best way to bring these concerns out into the open.

While fibromyalgia is not a life- or limb-threatening condition, it is a long-term problem in many patients. Over two-thirds of patients still have some symptoms 10 years after diagnosis, and 10 to 20 percent receive disability payments at some time because of the fibromyalgia. For many patients, however, the symptoms are controllable and are at a nuisance level rather than being disabling. Men and those who are depressed or single tend to do less well. Those who do best tend to share a number of beliefs in common. The most important of these are a feeling of control over their pain, believing that they are not disabled, and a recognition that their pain is not a sign of damage.

Children, in whom fibromyalgia is less common, seem to do very well, with 75 percent having fully recovered within 12 months in one study.

Risk Factors and Preventive Measures

The factors associated with fibromyalgia are discussed above. Deconditioning or lack of fitness, poor sleep, and segmental spinal dysfunction or postural problems are found in the majority of fibromyalgia patients at diagnosis but are more correctly seen as associated factors rather than risk factors as there is no clear etiological connection, or at least not a widely accepted one. It is difficult to study large numbers of the general population before they develop conditions like fibromyalgia. Relatively defined populations have therefore been studied. None of the industrial studies have shown any effective measures to prevent fibromyalgia. Members of the armed forces suffering from post-traumatic stress disorder have been shown to have a high incidence of developing fibromyalgia. Engaging in regular exercise reduced this significantly. Given the associated factors discussed above, there is some logic to extending this to other groups of people, but this would need to be studied further.

fibrositis   See FIBROMYALGIA.

foot pain   Since the feet bear the body's entire weight, abnormalities and lesions, whether severe or minor, frequently cause pain and disability. For problems affecting the heel area, see HEEL PAIN and ACHILLES TENDON injuries. Many forms of inflammatory arthritis such as RHEUMATOID ARTHRITIS, psoriatic arthritis (see PSORIASIS AND PSORIATIC ARTHRITIS), REACTIVE ARTHRITIS, SARCOIDOSIS, and GOUT affect the ankle and foot, and these are discussed in the relevant sections. There is a considerable difference between adults and children as to the causes of foot pain. This section will discuss foot pain under the following headings:

Musculoskeletal foot pain in children
Musculoskeletal foot pain in the adult
Nerve lesions causing foot pain

Musculoskeletal foot pain in children Foot pain in children usually results from developmental problems.

- Flat feet may be congenital (the child is born like that) or acquired (it develops only after weight bearing is established at around two years of age). Congenital flat feet may be flexible or rigid. Note that infants are naturally flat-footed and only when this is severe is treatment required. Flexible flat feet are treated with exercises and insoles that hold the feet in the correct position until there is sufficient maturity and strength. In severely affected children, hinged casts that can be easily applied and removed are used intermittently to promote soft tissue maturation in an appropriate position. While casts and insoles are useful, they merely provide support. Only exercise will strengthen muscles sufficiently to hold the correct position. Good exercises include walking on tiptoes and picking up marbles and moving them with the toes. The Achilles tendon may need stretching to achieve a good foot position. Acquired flat feet in children are often a manifestation of HYPERMOBILITY SYNDROME. Treatment is similar. Rigid flat feet are more difficult to treat. Here the heel bone (calcaneus) is semifixed in a turned-out position and the talus (the bone at the heart of the ankle that acts as a universal joint) points in and down, almost reversing the normal arch along the inner border of the foot. A series of casts that progressively correct this malposition are used. In severely affected children, though, some surgical correction is often required as well. Fusing of the affected joints (ARTHRODESIS) may be necessary later in life.
- Claw foot or pes cavus is the opposite of flat feet, with an exaggerated arch and sometimes a short foot. It is usually inherited but can also occur in other conditions such as polio, Friedreich's ataxia, and spina bifida. The foot is very stiff and therefore has little shock-absorbing capacity. Athletes and people who do a lot of walking therefore frequently develop pain. Stretching the muscles that pull the toes up and wearing modified shoes helps. It is also possible to lengthen the tissues that support the arch of the foot while removing slices of bone to lower the arch toward normal surgically.

- Metatarsus varus refers to a condition in which the feet turn inward toward each other midway along the length of the foot. This can lead to an awkward gait and tripping. This should be differentiated from an intoeing gait, which may have many causes, and clubfeet. The diagnosis is best made by a foot specialist. Mild degrees of metatarsus varus can sometimes be corrected by wearing the shoes on the opposite feet. More commonly, though, progressive corrective casts are required. Good results are obtained with early treatment.
- Congenital clubfoot or talipes equinovarus occurs in about one in 1,000 births and affects both feet in half the affected infants. The foot is turned in and down and the heel is also turned in (unlike metatarsus varus above). It cannot be brought up to 90° because of a very tight Achilles tendon. Gentle stretching followed by taping or use of a cast is begun early and may correct the milder 30–40 percent. In those that cannot be adequately corrected in this way, surgery is usually performed between three and six months of age.
- Although tarsal coalition may cause a rigid flatfoot, it is usually unsuspected until it causes foot pain in adult life. In tarsal coalition, a bony bar links two of the mid- or hindfoot bones and does not allow any movement at that joint. This loss of movement causes increased stress on the other midfoot joints, which eventually give rise to pain. This commonly begins after some increased stress such as weight gain or sudden increase in the amount of walking or time spent standing. The diagnosis is evident on plain X-ray and in difficult cases can be confirmed by a CT scan. The bony bar can be removed surgically, but pain may continue because of established OSTEOARTHRITIS in the adjacent joints.

Musculoskeletal foot pain in the adult Most musculoskeletal foot pain that is not due to an inflammatory arthritis (see ARTHRITIS for classification) results from abnormal stresses on normal tissues, normal stresses on structurally abnormal tissues, or highly repetitive stresses on normal tissues.

- Acute foot strain may result from a sudden unaccustomed increase in walking or other activity. This could include walking on unusually rough surfaces or in poor footwear. The pain may arise from muscles, ligaments, tendons, joint capsules, or a combination of these. Treatment, if required, is with rest, ice, massage, or NSAIDs. If the activity is repeated before adequate recovery of the tissues, damage may occur and result in chronic (ongoing) foot strain. This not only takes longer for the pain to subside but may lead to permanent alterations in the tissues and, in the long term, osteoarthritis of the joints. An example of chronic foot strain is PLANTAR FASCIITIS.

- Metatarsalgia refers to a condition in which pain is felt under the balls of the feet. It is often described as walking barefoot on pebbles. Normally most of the weight is borne on the ends of the first and fifth metatarsal bones (the bony enlargements just before the toes start). The ends of the second, third, and fourth metatarsals form an arch between these two at toe off and therefore do not normally take as much weight. Toe off is that point in the stride just before the foot leaves the ground when only the metatarsal heads and toes are in contact with the ground. However, if the arch flattens (splaying of the foot), they then take as much weight as the first and fifth but without as good padding as these two. As a result they become painful and develop calluses. There are many reasons for this anterior arch to flatten. The most common is loss of tone in the supporting muscles as people grow older, together with increasing weight. Along with the flattened arch the toes tend to ride up and become curved in shape (cock-up toes). Exercises to strengthen the small muscles of the foot, weight loss, and orthoses to prevent the heel bone from turning out too much and to take the pressure off the ends of the metatarsal bones are all helpful. Surgery is useful in relieving pain but will not restore normal foot biomechanics.

- In hallux valgus the first metatarsal (the longer bone on the inner border of the foot that runs down to the big toe) moves toward the other foot and away from its neighboring metatarsals. As a result the big toe deviates the other way, often pushing the second toe out of position. A bunion then develops at the base of the big toe. The cause of this abnormality has been debated for some time and there is still little agreement on it. Even if high-heeled shoes that constrict the toes are not the cause, they will undoubtedly make a mild hallux valgus worse. Most patients are older women with a broad front part of the foot and a flat arch. Many of these women will remember deviation of the big toe occurring when they were quite young, but generally, they seek treatment only when the condition becomes painful. This is usually when BURSITIS develops over the bunion. If hallux valgus develops before the age of 20 years, it should be treated prophylactically to prevent or delay progression. Appropriate footwear is important, especially flat heels and a broad front end. Corrective insoles for the flat foot are used, and splints that hold the foot in the desired position can be worn at night. In older patients, molding the shoe to accommodate the bunion helps relieve pain. Many surgical procedures are established for hallux valgus that work reasonably well. Two of the commonly used ones are known as Keller's and McBride's procedures. Surgical correction is reasonably successful, although it does not restore normality and many patients continue to have some pain and often some stiffness. It should be done for pain and disability, therefore, not appearances.

- Bunions may develop anywhere there is excessive pressure against a person's shoe. This is commonly on the inside of the big toe associated with splaying of the foot or hallux valgus. They are also common on the outside of the base of the little toe where there is often an underlying bursitis. This is known as a Tailor's bunion from the days when tailors used to sit cross-legged. They can also result from poorly fitting shoes. Shoe modification and bunion pads are helpful. Surgical correction of the underlying bony prominence may be indicated.

- Two small bones called sesamoids are found in the tendons beneath the end of the first metatarsal bone. Inflammation can occur here, termed sesamoiditis. Temporary rest with a shoe insert to relieve pressure is the usual treatment. Occasionally in resistant cases the sesamoid is surgically removed.

- Hallux rigidus refers to stiffness of the joint at the base of the big toe such that it no longer bends enough to allow normal walking. This usually results from osteoarthritis in older individuals but can occur in younger people as a result of trauma or following recurrent attacks of gout. If mild, the wearing of a stiff-soled shoe relieves pain. CORTICOSTEROID injection may give temporary relief. If severe, surgery can be done either to fix the joint in a usable position (see ARTHRODESIS) or to put in a joint replacement.

- Morton's syndrome describes a condition in which the first metatarsal bone is congenitally short. This is different from Morton's neuralgia (see below). Morton's syndrome causes problems around the joint at the base of the second toe because the second metatarsal bone, being longer than the abnormal first, takes an unusual amount of weight and stress during walking and running.

- A march fracture is a STRESS FRACTURE of the second metatarsal bone. This occurs as a result of overuse stress, as for example new army recruits marching on the parade ground. Initial X-rays may be normal and should be repeated two weeks later if the diagnosis is considered likely. Treatment is with initial immobilization and then more gradual conditioning.

Nerve Lesions Causing Foot Pain

- Lesions in the lower spinal cord that irritate or press on the L5 or S1 nerve roots can give rise to pain in the foot. In young people, this is usually due to a lumbar disc prolapse and in older people to osteoarthritic changes in the lower spine (see BACK PAIN). Especially in younger people there may be little or no back pain, and if there is no muscle weakness, the foot pain can be both puzzling and distressing.

- The common peroneal nerve is a branch of the sciatic nerve that winds around the fibula bone just below its head that can be felt as a bony prominence just below the outside of the knee.

Because the nerve is close to the skin here, it can be easily damaged by trauma in this area. This can cause pain over the top of the foot and front of the ankle. However, there is usually clearcut weakness in raising the foot and turning it outward so the diagnosis is relatively easy. In addition, numbness is more common than pain. The nature of the trauma should also point to the diagnosis.

- The superficial peroneal nerve is a branch of the common peroneal. It can become trapped as it comes up through the fascia in front of the ankle and cause a similar unpleasant burning pain on the top of the foot. Because it supplies only relatively small muscles, the weakness is less obvious. The diagnosis can therefore be puzzling. The clue is that the web space of the big toe and the inside of the second toe are not affected since they are supplied by the deep peroneal nerve.

- The deep peroneal nerve (also called the anterior tibial nerve) enters the foot running across the front of the ankle toward the inside. Here it passes underneath a retinaculum known as the cruciate crural ligament, where it can become compressed. This is the equivalent of CARPAL TUNNEL SYNDROME in the hand and is known as the anterior tarsal tunnel syndrome. It causes pain in the web space of the big toe and inner surface of the second toe. Runners, skiers, dancers, and people who repeatedly sprain their ankle are at particular risk.

- The posterior tibial nerve passes down and across the inner surface of the ankle and heel bone and is covered by a ligament. It can become compressed here and cause pain in the sole of the foot.

- The small nerves supplying sensation to the toes, the interdigital nerves, can become stretched by cock-up toes or suffer direct pressure, especially in patients with rheumatoid arthritis. Occasionally these nerves enlarge, and this is known as Morton's neuroma.

- REFLEX SYMPATHETIC DYSTROPHY is a complex disorder that most often affects the foot or hand.

frostbite Damage to peripheral tissues (especially toes, fingers, nose, and ears) caused by prolonged exposure to extreme cold. Frostbite affects the extremities, particularly the hands and feet. If the acute injury is severe, tissue death occurs and digits may need to be amputated. The cold injury can also damage blood vessels and cartilage in joints, resulting in OSTEOARTHRITIS many years later. The problem of frostbite arthritis is a late complication. No treatment will alter the course if applied between the cold injury and the development of arthritis. Other than the usual treatments for osteoarthritis, no specific treatment is available for arthritis caused by frostbite.

ganglion   A small cystic lump found close to joints or tendons. Ganglia occur more often in people with arthritis but also occur in people with healthy joints. Any type of arthritis, injury, or overuse is believed to increase the chances of developing a ganglion.

Symptoms and Diagnostic Path

Ganglia occur most often in the area of the wrist and do not usually cause symptoms. Usually, a patient will report finding a small lump that feels as if it contains fluid in the area of a wrist, ankle, or knee. Some ganglia can become painful if they are bumped or injured. However, most ganglia do not cause symptoms and many patients notice a ganglion because they are concerned about the development of a new lump. Ganglia that have formed recently feel soft and can be compressed like a small balloon that is filled with water, but as they age, they develop a thicker wall of fibrous tissue and feel much more solid.

Treatment Options and Outlook

Some ganglia resolve by themselves or after the application of firm compression. Many ganglia do not cause symptoms and do not require specific treatment. The traditional treatment for a ganglion was to strike it firmly with a heavy book such as the family Bible. As a consequence of this, ganglia have sometimes been called *Bible cysts*. A firm blow will rupture a newly formed ganglion, causing the swelling to disappear when its mucus-like contents escape into the surrounding tissues. However, many ganglia treated in this way recur. An alternative treatment is for a physician to empty the cyst by aspirating its contents through a needle. Again, recurrence is common. An injection of a CORTICO-STEROID into the cyst after aspiration may decrease the chances of recurrence. Ganglia that recur after conservative treatment and cause symptoms may require surgical removal.

Risk Factors and Preventive Measures

Arthritis and repetitive overuse of the tendon in question are risk factors. Apart from ensuring good technique in repetitive manual jobs, there are no known preventive measures.

genetic factors   Most rheumatic problems are thought to have a genetic component. Some conditions such as FAMILIAL MEDITERRANEAN FEVER, HEMOCHROMATOSIS, and HEMOPHILIA are entirely due to a defined mutation in a single gene. For most conditions, though, the genetic component is likely to be smaller and to involve many genes.

The sequencing of the human genetic code (genome) has greatly increased the ability of researchers to identify genetic variability that may be associated with an increased risk of disease. The genetic code of most humans is almost identical, but occasional changes result in the genetic differences known to exist among individuals. Many of these changes are the result of single nucleotide polymorphisms or SNPs (pronounced "snips")—a change in one of the millions of bases that make up the genetic code. Two common approaches have been used to identify genetic variations related to disease. The first is called a *genome-wide scan*. With this technique, investigators have no preconceived idea of which genes are likely to be involved but use markers to screen the entire genome for differences among affected and nonaffected people. The genome wide-scan approach requires a large number of subjects and is more powerful if it is performed using affected and nonaffected members in the same family. The second technique is called a *candidate gene approach*. This strategy examines variability in genes that are thought to play a key role in the cause of a disease. There are many large studies using both of these approaches to identify genetic variants that are important in rheumatic diseases.

A strong association between the HLA-B27 tissue type (see HLA), an inherited factor, and ANKYLOSING SPONDYLITIS (AS) is well-known. Approximately 95 percent of Caucasian patients with AS carry the HLA-B27 gene. However, approximately 10 percent of healthy people also carry this gene and the majority do not develop AS. The implications of these observations are that the HLA-B27 gene increases the risk of developing AS significantly, but other factors that have not been identified are also required before the illness occurs.

Many rheumatic illnesses occur more frequently in some families, but for most, no reproducible genetic causes have been identified. Genetic variation in the collagen gene has been associated with a rare familial type of osteoarthritis, but the genetic factors underlying the common form of osteoarthritis in the general population are not clear. RHEUMATOID ARTHRITIS (RA) has been known to be associated with HLA tissue types (DR4) since the 1970s. The risk of RA is increased fourfold in individuals with HLA-DR4 tissue type (new nomenclature HLA-DRB1 0401, 0402, and so on for the different variants of the 04 tissue type). The strength of the association varies in different populations and has been weaker in African Americans than in Caucasians. In SYSTEMIC LUPUS ERYTHEMATOSUS, several studies have reported associations between SNPs in the gene coding for tumor necrosis factor, but the association has been variable.

Considerable genetic variability occurs among individuals and populations affecting both the metabolism and efficacy of drugs (see PHARMACOGENETICS).

German measles   See RUBELLA.

giant cell arteritis   See TEMPORAL ARTERITIS.

glucocorticoids   See CORTICOSTEROIDS.

golfer's elbow   See EPICONDYLITIS.

Goodpasture's syndrome   This is a rare, life-threatening autoimmune illness that causes lung hemorrhage and kidney failure. Ernest W. Goodpasture (1886–1960) first described the illness in 1919 when he was examining the lungs of patients who had died in the 1918–19 influenza epidemic and noted a new illness that affected the lungs and kidneys of one patient. In 1958, almost 40 years later M. C. Stanton and J. D. Tange attached the name Goodpasture's syndrome to an illness that caused severe lung and kidney disease. In subsequent years scientists discovered that Goodpasture's syndrome was a unique illness caused by antibodies directed against a component of the kidney and lung. In retrospect, the original patient Goodpasture described may have had a systemic vasculitis affecting the lungs and kidneys rather than the autoimmune condition that now bears his name.

Goodpasture's syndrome is rare, affecting about one person per million per year. It affects Caucasians more than other races and men more often than women. It can occur at any age but most often affects people in their 30s.

Goodpasture's syndrome is caused by antibodies against type IV collagen, a component of the cells that line the lungs and the glomeruli of the kidneys. The glomeruli are lined by a thin layer called the basement membrane that is rich in type IV collagen. Because it produces antibodies directed against the basement membrane, Goodpasture's syndrome is sometimes known as antiglomerular basement membrane disease. The underlying cause that turns on the production of autoantibodies is not known. In some patients the disease is preceded by a respiratory tract infection or some other illness that could damage the lungs. Often there is no preceding event, and no specific infectious or toxic cause has been identified.

Symptoms and Diagnostic Path

In most patients, symptoms start suddenly with coughing, often producing blood-stained sputum, and shortness of breath. A chest X-ray shows widespread shadowing. Hemorrhaging into the lungs can cause severe shortness of breath and the coughing up of large amounts of blood. Lung hemorrhage is more common in smokers. Kidney failure can progress rapidly and cause symptoms of nausea, fluid retention, and poor appetite. In most patients both the kidneys and the lungs are affected, but in a few the lungs are spared. Blood tests show an elevated creatinine concentration, indicating poor kidney function, and the urine usually contains protein, blood, and cells.

Several different illnesses, including WEGENER'S GRANULOMATOSIS and SYSTEMIC LUPUS ERYTHEMATOSUS, can cause sudden lung and kidney failure. Goodpasture's syndrome is diagnosed from the clinical picture and a positive blood test for antiglomerular basement membrane antibodies. The test is positive in more than 95 percent of patients with Goodpasture's syndrome. A tissue biopsy, most often from the kidney, is usually obtained to confirm the diagnosis. The biopsy shows inflammation in and around the glomeruli and deposits of antiglomerular basement membrane antibodies.

Treatment Options and Outlook

Patients are often critically ill when the disease is diagnosed and need aggressive therapy not only to suppress the production of antibodies but also to support lung and kidney function. High doses of CORTICOSTEROIDS combined with CYCLOPHOSPHAMIDE are used to suppress the production of antibodies, and PLASMAPHERESIS is used to remove antibodies from the bloodstream. Many patients require DIALYSIS to support kidney function during the acute phase of the illness. If treatment is started early though, kidney function can recover and long-term dialysis be avoided.

Before effective treatment was available, Goodpasture's syndrome was usually fatal. If treatment is started early, before kidney failure is established, more than 90 percent of patients survive. If severe lung hemorrhage is present, oxygen transport from the air to the bloodstream in the lungs is often decreased and a patient may need to be treated in an intensive care unit on a ventilator (a machine that breathes for the patient). With time and immunosuppressive therapy, lung function improves and

the patient can be weaned from the ventilator. If kidney failure has set in before treatment is started, kidney function may not recover and the patient will require permanent dialysis.

Risk Factors and Preventive Measures

There are no known risk factors or preventive measures.

gout   Described by Hippocrates in 500 B.C., gout is one of the oldest forms of arthritis known. The urate crystals that start an attack were discovered more than 400 years ago. One of the medications still used today, COLCHICINE, was isolated from its herbal origins nearly 200 years ago. Once known as the "king of diseases and disease of kings," gout became associated with excessive eating and drinking. Although there is some truth to this, there are many other reasons that people get gout. About eight in every 1,000 people suffer from gout, making it one of the more common forms of arthritis. This translates to 2.1 million people in the United States having gout, with men being affected three times as often as women.

Uric acid is the final breakdown product of purines in humans. Purines are essential for manufacturing DNA and RNA and are therefore present in all animal cells. Humans have higher uric acid levels than most other animals because the animals produce an enzyme called uricase that breaks uric acid down further. Humans actually have the gene for uricase but have inactivated it at some stage during evolution. Uric acid is a powerful antioxidant. It is believed that the uricase gene was inactivated because of the advantages of having a powerful antioxidant. Given the current enthusiasm for taking antioxidants such as vitamin C and vitamin E as well as a host of others marketed as health supplements, it is interesting to look at how much trouble one of our natural inbuilt antioxidants has caused the human race.

Although hyperuricemia (high blood levels of urate) is not the same as gout, it is the major risk factor for gout. Generally speaking, anything that tends to raise the blood urate level is a risk factor for gout. However, not everyone with raised urate levels will get gout. About 95 percent of uric acid in the blood combines with sodium to form molecules of monosodium urate, which is much more soluble than uric acid in both blood and joints. Many people use the terms uric acid and urate interchangeably. Although they have different chemical structures, for everyday purposes, it does not really matter. At levels up to about 0.35 mmol/L (5.8 mg/dL) urate dissolves well in body fluids, and levels are similar in joints and blood most of the time. Above that level it can form a stable supersaturated solution. The higher the concentration, the more likely it is to crystallize out of solution. When it crystallizes out into joints and soft tissues, it may initiate an intense inflammation called gout. The easiest way to view the relationship between blood urate levels and gout is to look at the risk of developing gout in either one year or five years given a certain urate level as in the table below.

In males, there is a significant rise in urate levels at puberty. Although this rise is less marked in women, they have a further rise after menopause. Since most people probably have raised urate levels for 10 to 20 years before getting gout, this may explain the typical age of onset in men in their 30s and 40s and in women in their 60s.

Causes of hyperuricemia Either the formation of too much urate or not getting rid of it quickly enough can lead to a buildup. Two-thirds of a person's urate is eliminated in the urine. In most people there will be a variety of factors operating to cause significant hyperuricemia.

- Enzyme deficiencies can lead to overproduction of uric acid. The best-known one (that of an enzyme abbreviated as HGPRT) is extremely rare and when severe, also results in mental retardation (the Lesch-Nyhan syndrome). Minor abnormalities in this enzyme can cause high uric acid production without mental problems. Many other enzyme abnormalities have recently been discovered, but at present these account for only an extremely small number of people with gout. People developing gout under the age of 20 years are very likely to have an enzyme abnormality predisposing them to hyperuricemia.

- Many Polynesian groups of people have genetically determined hyperuricemia as well as frequent gout. Chinese and Filipino people living traditionally in their own lands have normal urate levels but are prone to hyperuricemia on modern diets or when living in Western countries. This is probably due to an interaction between diet and genetic makeup. Even in Western populations the genetic contribution to the urate level has been calculated as 40 percent.

- Body bulk is the strongest predictor of urate level in the vast majority of people. This is true for straightforward weight measurements as well as for weight corrected for height. This is not just related to dietary intake, because weight loss will actually increase the amount of uric acid passed in the urine.

- Dietary intake of foods high in purines is important (see later under Treatment Options and Outlook). Regular alcohol intake (not necessarily excessive) increases urate levels in a number of ways. It slows down uric acid excretion in the urine as well as speeding up the breakdown of some purines to form urate. In addition, beer contains a large amount of purine itself.

- Many drugs may increase urate levels. The most common are the diuretics (water tablets), especially the thiazides but also furosemide and bumetanide. Low-dose aspirin is now com-

RELATIONSHIP OF GOUT TO BLOOD URATE LEVELS IN MEN		
Blood Urate	Risk of Developing Gout	
	In One Year	In Five Years
< 0.42 mmol/L (7 mg/dL)	<1 per 1,000	5 per 1,000
0.42–0.47 mmol/L (7–7.9 mg/dL)	1 per 1,000	6 per 1,000
0.48–0.53 mmol/L (8–8.9 mg/dL)	4 per 1,000	10 per 1,000
> 0.54 mmol/L (> 9.0 mg/dL)	49 per 1,000	220 per 1,000

monly used for the prevention of heart disease and will slightly increase urate levels (although high doses lower it). Others include most cytotoxic (anticancer) drug regimens, levodopa, and the antituberculous drugs ethambutol and pyrazinamide.

- Diseases such as PSORIASIS in which there is an increased rate of cell turnover also lead to higher urate levels. An extreme degree of this happens when treatment for leukemia and lymphoma is begun.

- Lead exposure can lead to kidney disease and high urate levels.

- Patients who have received an organ transplant, usually a kidney or heart, develop high urate levels, frequently get gout, and have particular problems with its treatment.

Given a high urate level for many years, there are many events that may precipitate an attack of gout. These include any sudden illness, trauma (even minor), surgery, a large intake of alcohol or large purine-containing meal, or starting on one of the drugs listed above. Bleeding from the gut (which may be due to taking NSAIDs to settle the previous attack) seems to be a particularly potent initiator of gout.

Symptoms and Diagnostic Path

Typically the patient awakes in the early hours of the morning with pain in the great toe, less commonly the heel, ankle, or midfoot. This becomes progressively worse and is often excruciating. In severe attacks there may be fever and chills. Most first attacks (90 percent) occur in the great toe. This is probably because of the frequent minor trauma this toe suffers as well as the fact that cold precipitates gout (the urate becomes less soluble) and feet are often the coolest part of the body. Only one joint is affected in 90 percent of first attacks, but as time goes on, more and more joints are likely to be affected during an attack. Somebody having a first attack of gout has a 60 percent chance of having another within one year and a 90 percent chance of having another within five years. Ankles, knees, and hands are commonly affected. Not all attacks are severe and may be put down to sprained ankles or bruised heels because they do not appear to be a typical gout attack.

Even if untreated, most attacks of gout will settle down after 10 to 14 days. Initially there are no abnormalities to see once the attack has settled. However, after years of gout with no treatment to lower the urate levels, it may become chronic; that is, the gaps between attacks become shorter and shorter until it is continuous. When this happens there are always many joints affected and it may occasionally look very like rheumatoid arthritis. By this time damage has occurred to the joints with loss of cartilage and cysts in the bone.

Tophi may also develop in longstanding gout. Tophi are collections of urate crystals that steadily grow larger if the urate level remains high. If close to the skin surface they may periodically break open and discharge chalky, white material (the urate crystals). They may also cause pressure symptoms on nerves and other deeper tissues. The spine, heart, eyes, and voicebox are among the unusual places to be affected by tophi. Tophi seldom develop within 10 years of first developing gout and are becoming much less common with better treatment of hyperuricemia.

Gout may be difficult to diagnose when attacks are not typical. Women develop gout later than men (usually in their 60s), and it more frequently affects more than one joint from the beginning. In older patients, attacks may be less severe but longer lasting, and frequently other forms of arthritis are suspected. Gout has a tendency to develop in damaged joints and may not be suspected if these are joints not commonly affected by gout. Gout in the shoulder and hip joints is particularly difficult to diagnose. Some people with OSTEOARTHRITIS of the hands develop gout there that causes intermittent pain and swelling that should be distinguished from erosive osteoarthritis. In these situations the danger is that the intermittent gout will accelerate the damage to the joint if unrecognized. In severe gout the joint is fiery red and hot, hugely swollen, and exquisitely painful. This is exactly what an acute joint infection looks like. In addition the sufferer is likely to have sweats and chills, and it is not surprising, therefore, that they are frequently treated as infective arthritis initially.

High urate levels can lead to two kinds of kidney disease, and these can occur in patients who have not had gout as well. In the first, uric acid crystals form in the small tubules of the kidney or the ureters that drain urine from the kidney to the bladder and, often together with calcium crystals, form kidney stones. This can lead to intense pain (renal colic) as well as blockage of tubules or ureter. In the second type, uric acid crystals form in the tissues of the kidney and cause inflammation there. These patients may go on to develop kidney failure.

A number of conditions are closely associated with gout and should be addressed or looked for as part of the management plan:

Obesity Nearly 80 percent of people with gout are more than 10 percent overweight, and nearly 60 percent are 30 percent overweight. Not only does this indicate a poor health outcome, but increased weight has a direct effect on raising urate levels.

Diabetes This association may simply be because of the obesity since there is some disagreement about the strength of the association in different studies.

Hyperlipidemia A risk factor for heart disease, this is especially likely to be present in those who drink alcohol. About 80 percent of gout patients have hyperlipidemia.

Hypertension Approximately 30 percent of gout patients are hypertensive, and nearly 30 percent of hypertensives have a high urate level.

Atherosclerosis Patients with gout develop atherosclerotic problems (angina, heart attacks, strokes, and poor circulation to the legs) at a younger age than others. However, the high urate levels and gout do not cause this but probably a combination of the other associated conditions mentioned above do.

Diagnosis It is necessary to take fluid from a joint or material from a tophus and see urate crystals under a polarized-light microscope to diagnose gout definitely. This not always possible, however, and in typical presentations not necessary. When the setting is not typical, however, every effort should be made to find the crystals. In long-standing gout, the X-rays show bony damage that is very typical of gout and useful in the diagnosis.

The blood urate levels are not very useful in making the diagnosis during a sudden attack. First, many people with mildly raised urate levels will never develop gout, and second 40 percent of people with acute gout will have a normal level during the attack. All of this second group will, however, have a raised urate level later on when the attack has settled. Because the diagnosis may still sometimes be difficult, the American College of Rheumatology has developed criteria for the diagnosis that relies on at least three of 12 suggestive symptoms, signs, and investigations being present.

Treatment Options and Outlook

There are several quite different aspects to the treatment of gout:

- Treatment of the sudden painful attack of gout
- Prophylactic or preventive treatment of the gout
- Treatment to lower the urate levels
- Transplant gout
- Management of the associated conditions listed above, which will not be discussed here

The acute attack Rest has been shown to shorten the sudden attack of gout. Cold compresses help relieve pain but do not shorten the attack. COLCHICINE has been used for 200 years and is still an effective drug. The traditional high doses used for acute attacks are, however, not well tolerated mainly because of the severe diarrhea. In lower doses it also does not work as quickly as the NSAIDs and is therefore usually used only when these drugs cannot be used or for prophylaxis (see below). All the traditional NSAIDs work in gout. PHENYLBUTAZONE should not be used because of its severe side effects, especially on the blood-forming parts of the bone marrow. INDOMETHACIN is often preferred by gout patients because it is very powerful. However, it also causes more side effects than the others. IBUPROFEN, DICLOFENAC, NAPROXEN, PIROXICAM, tenoxicam, and SULINDAC have all been used with success. The most important factor in using colchicine or the NSAIDs is to take them as early as possible in the attack. It is usual to start with a high dose and reduce it as the attack comes under control. There is limited experience with the COX-2 inhibitors, but both LUMIRACOXIB and ETORICOXIB have some controlled trial data showing that they are as effective as indomethacin in treating acute attacks.

CORTICOSTEROIDS may be used when colchicine and the NSAIDs are contraindicated. They are most effective if injected directly into the affected joint but can be taken orally as well. On average, an acute attack will get better in seven days. The more joints involved, the longer before improvement.

Prophylactic treatment When there is a large urate load in the body, urate-lowering therapy may take some time to reduce this load sufficiently to prevent gout. The initial period of urate-lowering therapy may also increase the frequency of attacks in a quarter of patients. For these reasons, many patients are given prophylactic or preventive treatment during the initial urate-lowering phase. Low-dose colchicine (one to two tablets a day) is very effective, preventing attacks in 85 percent of such patients. The NSAIDs may also be used. Typically this therapy will be continued for six to 12 months but possibly longer in those with numerous tophi. It is usual to continue this treatment until the patient reaches the target urate level and remains free of attacks for three months at this level.

Urate-lowering treatment In severe or frequent gout or gout with complications, lowering the urate level to less than 0.35 mmol/L (5.8 mg/dL) is essential for good management. If this can be achieved, tophi will resolve and the risk of further attacks will be very small. There are drug and nondrug means to achieve this, and a combination of the two is usually required. Urate-lowering treatment has been shown to be cost-effective if an individual is having more than two attacks of gout a year.

(a) *Nondrug Urate-Lowering Therapy* Weight loss will lower the urate level by 0.05 mmol/L (0.83 mg/dL) for every 10 kg lost. It will also improve blood pressure, diabetes, and hyperlipidemia if present. A low-protein diet will reduce urate levels by 0.06 mmol/L (1mg/dL). A high fluid intake assists urate loss in the urine and prevents kidney stone formation. The urate-lowering effect is small, however. Reducing alcohol intake and giving up beer altogether is very effective at lowering urate levels because of the mechanisms discussed under Cause above. Avoiding foods high in purines should be part of every gout patient's management plan. These are listed below in three groups according to their purine content. The first two groups should be avoided altogether and the third eaten in moderation.

- Very high purines—heart, herring, meat extracts, mussels, yeast
- High purines—anchovies, bacon, liver, mutton, salmon, venison, wild fowl, cod, haddock
- Moderate purines—asparagus, brains, chicken, beef, eel, kidney beans, lentils, lima beans, lobster, mushroom, peas, spinach, oysters, other fish, and meat products

(b) *Drug Therapy* ALLOPURINOL partially blocks the enzyme that forms uric acid from xanthine. This leads to higher levels of xanthines. However, these are more soluble than urate and do not cause the same problems. It is the most effective urate-lowering drug and is commonly used first whether the patient is forming too much urate or not getting rid of it quickly enough. It is important to start at low doses and slowly build up so as not to cause increased attacks of gout during the early stages of treatment (see Prophylactic Treatment above). Allopurinol is also used to treat patients about to start chemotherapy for certain kinds of tumors (especially lymphomas and leukemias) since they can get massive release of uric acid. Unfortunately, somewhere between 5 and 20 percent of patients develop side effects on allopurinol that requires stopping it. Allopurinol also interacts with several other drugs, and patient and doctor need to be aware of these. This can be a particular problem in transplant patients.

If allopurinol is not tolerated, there are a number of drugs that increase the amount of uric acid passed in the urine. These are known as uricosuric drugs. The most effective is benzbromarone, which causes a similar degree of urate lowering to allopurinol. It is also a very useful drug in transplant patients. Although used in Europe for many years, it is not available in the United States. PROBENECID is somewhat less effective, although reasonably well tolerated, with only 2 percent of patients stopping the drug because of side effects. It too has a number of interactions with other drugs (mainly in blocking their excretion by the kidneys), which can lead to serious problems if not taken into account. SULFINPYRAZONE is probably more effective than probenecid, but more people have side effects with it. It also has an anticlotting effect by reducing platelet function. This can be an advantage if someone needs antiplatelet treatment because of heart disease and the low-dose aspirin is being stopped while the urate levels are being lowered. Once urate levels are stable at the required level, low-dose aspirin can usually be restarted without any problems. Sulfinpyrazone and benzbromarone are more effective than probenecid when there is poor kidney function. Febuxostat (Uloric) is a new xanthine oxidase inhibitor.

Transplant gout Cyclosporine is used to prevent rejection in most transplant patients. Unfortunately, it causes high uric acid levels by altering blood flow through the kidneys, and many transplant patients get gout. There are several special problems in this situation. Allopurinol causes much higher-than-usual levels of AZATHIOPRINE, another commonly used transplant drug, and this combination can lead to serious side effects. Colchicine very rarely causes damage to nerves and muscles, but this side effect becomes more frequent if cyclosporine is also being used. In addition, some of the uricosuric drugs may not be effective if kidney function is not adequate. Treatment of transplant gout is best undertaken in consultation with an experienced rheumatologist. Some strategies to overcome these problems include:

- Reducing the dose of azathioprine to about a third and monitoring carefully when starting allopurinol

- Using urate oxidase to break uric acid down; this needs to be given into the veins once a month and is still experimental

- Using MYCOPHENOLATE MOFETIL instead of azathioprine

- Using benzbromarone, which is an excellent urate-lowering drug in this situation

Risk Factors and Preventive Measures

Hyperuricemia is the risk factor for gout. This is usually due to a combination of a genetic predisposition and the hyperuricemia risk factors discussed above. Addressing these latter factors is the best preventive measure. Reducing weight to the ideal range is the most effective action to prevent hyperuricemia and therefore the risk of gout. Eating only moderate amounts of high purine foods (see above) is also helpful. Doctors should take their patients' other risk factors into account when prescribing drugs that may increase uric acid and monitor levels if appropriate. Proper protective equipment should be used when stripping old paint as this may still contain lead. Appropriate preventive treatment is usually given when treating tumors that can give rise to high uric acid levels.

Gulf War syndrome A collection of symptoms occurring in veterans of the Gulf War. In January and February 1991, a coalition army led by the United States fought a war against Iraq. The war was unusual in that the risk of exposure of soldiers to biological agents was thought to be high and because burning oil wells exposed soldiers to potentially toxic substances. Approximately 700,000 U.S. troops were deployed in the Gulf War. In January 1992, reports appeared of an increased frequency of unexplained, unusual illnesses in soldiers who had returned. The term *Gulf War syndrome* appeared to come into usage more as a result of media attention than scientific definition of a unique constellation of symptoms that constituted a new syndrome. Much research has focused on the question of whether Gulf War syndrome exists as a unique illness. Although the answers are not clear, the weight of scientific evidence does not indicate the existence of a unique syndrome or illness.

The cause of Gulf War syndrome is not known. There are several conflicting opinions that can be divided into three main camps.

First, Gulf War syndrome does not exist as a discrete entity and was created by the media, not medical evidence. The term *syndrome* implies a unique grouping of symptoms, but no such grouping has been found in Gulf War veterans. In most studies of U.S., U.K., and Canadian soldiers, almost every symptom studied occurred more frequently in veterans of the Gulf War than in soldiers who were not deployed. There was no unique pattern to the increased symptoms. Opponents of this position argue that the word syndrome is a semantic definition and that the absence of a defined syndrome does not imply the absence of illness. Renaming the condition *Gulf War illness* would overcome the inability of researchers to define reproducibly a clear syndrome. However, the term illness also requires a definition, something that has been difficult to establish.

Second, Gulf War syndrome is a poorly defined entity that is caused by psychological stress. Similar syndromes have been reported after many wars and variously named shell shock, soldier's heart, and neurasthenia. The level of psychological stress resulting from the Gulf War may not have been as great as in previous wars if one considers the duration and intensity of fighting or the numbers of casualties; however, the type of stress was different. The risk of exposure to biological or chemical weapons was greater and may have resulted in prolonged anxiety and psychological stress, particularly in those people who believed they were exposed to harmful substances.

Third, Gulf War syndrome was caused by exposure to infectious or toxic substances, either alone or in combination. Several candidates have been proposed and studied. There is no reproducible relationship between exposure to depleted uranium, smoke from oil fires, vaccines, insecticides, and chemicals such as pyridostigmine that were used to protect against nerve gas and risk of developing Gulf War illness. However, many studies, particularly those examining the role of multiple vaccinations and exposure to potentially harmful agents, are ongoing. No infectious agent has reproducibly been associated with the illness. Some researchers reported finding an atypical mycoplasma and clinical response to treatment with an

antibiotic, doxycycline, but others found no evidence of infection. Clinical trials with doxycycline are being conducted.

Symptoms and Diagnostic Path

Many symptoms have been reported, but the most common are fatigue, poor memory, myalgia, arthralgia, diarrhea, rash, weakness, and neuropathy. Many of the symptoms overlap with FIBROMYALGIA and CHRONIC FATIGUE SYNDROME, and some patients fulfill diagnostic criteria for these conditions.

No diagnostic laboratory test is helpful. Laboratory tests are usually normal. The diagnosis was usually applied to veterans of the Gulf War who developed symptoms that were not explained by another medical diagnosis.

Treatment Options and Outlook

No specific treatment is available for Gulf War syndrome. Treatment is symptomatic and similar to that prescribed for fibromyalgia. Low doses of antidepressants are used to improve sleep and decrease fatigue. Clinicians often prescribe COGNITIVE BEHAVIORAL THERAPY and EXERCISE. These treatments have been found to be effective in fibromyalgia. A large, randomized study of the efficacy of these interventions in Gulf War syndrome is underway.

Veterans with Gulf War syndrome report more symptoms and a poorer quality of life than those who were not affected. Studies that have examined deaths and hospitalizations in Gulf War veterans and the frequency of birth abnormalities in their children have found an increased risk of death from accidents but no indications of more frequent complications of medical illnesses.

Risk Factors and Preventive Measures

Despite considerable research and all that has been written, the causation of this syndrome remains unclear and apart from the obvious solution of not having wars there is no known preventive measure.

heat A therapy used to alleviate musculoskel-etal symptoms. Physical therapy often involves the application of heat or cold (see ICE) to relieve symptoms and improve function. Patients with inflammatory arthritis often suffer from stiffness and decreased mobility that is particularly severe in the morning after arising and then slowly improves during the day. Many have noticed that these symptoms improve more rapidly if they take a hot bath or shower. It is not known how heat relieves arthritis symptoms, but it increases blood flow in tissues. This could either wash out chemicals that cause inflammation or, alternatively, deliver chemicals that oppose inflammation. Some of the beneficial effects of heat may occur because it changes the pain threshold. Heat and pain messages are transmitted through different nerve fibers, but traffic in one group of nerves could decrease transmission through others. Also, if the sensation of superficial heat is strong, it can distract the brain from processing pain messages from joints. Heat could also act on muscles and connective tissue to make them more flexible. Superficial heat can be applied using hot water, heating pads, or paraffin or wax baths. Heat that reaches the deeper tissues is applied by a physical therapist using ultrasound. Local application of heat causes few side effects unless the temperature is too hot or heat is applied for a long time, in which case burns can result. In most patients the painful sensation caused by excessive heat prevents this from happening. However, patients with nerve damage, such as peripheral neuropathy that decreases their ability to feel heat and pain, may sustain burns by applying excessive heat without being aware of it. Regular application of heat such as hot-water bottles to an area can lead to a mottled reddish brown discoloration of the skin known as erythema ab igne without actually causing a painful burn.

heel pain The heel is the first part of the body to strike the ground while walking and, during slow or moderate speed running, does so with a force several times that of the individual's weight. Given these large forces operating on the heel, it is perhaps surprising that heel pain is not more common. However, sophisticated biomechanical factors are operating to reduce the stress of foot impact on the ground. These include movements of the pelvis, hips, knee, and rotation of the tibia (shinbone) that smooth out the gait. These will not be discussed here. However, if their function is disturbed for any reason, the stresses at the heel and ankle may be greatly increased and therefore more likely to give rise to painful conditions. The heel bone (calcaneus) itself has a special protective pad (see below under Painful Heel Pad), and the foot has a complex mechanism to help absorb the impact (see below under Plantar fasciitis). Needless to say, a painful heel will dramatically affect walking or running. The important causes of heel pain are discussed below.

Plantar fasciitis This is the most common cause of heel pain. People usually complain of pain underneath the foot just in front of the calcaneus (heel bone). The pain often comes on after unaccustomed standing, walking, or athletic activity. It is more common in the overweight and in those with flat feet.

Shortly after the heel strikes the ground in normal walking, the foot goes into pronation to absorb the force of impact. Pronation involves a loosening of the joints of the midfoot so there is more give, the arch of the foot drops and there is a slight turning out of the forefoot while the calcaneus itself tilts over to the inside and dips its nose down. This results in the force of impact and weight bearing being spread through a number of bones, joints, ligaments, and muscles rather than just in a direct line through the heel to the ground. One of the important structures in this mechanism is the plantar fascia. This is a tough, flat, fibrous tissue that spans from the front lower edge of the calcaneus to the base of the toes, supporting the long arch of the foot like an unusually wide bowstring. It also sends further slips along the toes that serve to tighten the plantar fascia when the toes are curled up (as when taking off from that foot). As the foot goes into pronation, the long arch tends to collapse slightly and the plantar fascia is stretched and stressed. This is a normal event. However, if the stresses are suddenly increased by, for example, rapid weight gain or a large increase in the distance walked, microtears can develop in the plantar fascia. This results in small areas of inflammation that can accumulate and cause pain. This commonly affects the middle section of the plantar fascia or its attachment to the calcaneus.

A similar process can occur with normal or minimal stresses if the structures themselves are abnormal. This can occur in patients with inflammatory arthritis such as RHEUMATOID ARTHRITIS who are prone to develop overpronation, or in people who are naturally flat-footed. Patients with SPONDYLOARTHROPATHIES are also prone to develop inflammation at the attachment of the plantar fascia to the calcaneus with relatively little stress.

Typically the pain is felt on walking or prolonged standing and is worse after a rest or first thing in the morning, easing a bit with continued activity. Tenderness can be produced by pressing on the front end of the calcaneus toward the inner border of the sole or toward the middle of the long arch of the foot. Pain will also be felt when the toes are pulled upward since this tightens the plantar fascia. X-ray may show a HEEL SPUR, but this seldom affects treatment.

Relieving the pressure over the attachment of the plantar fascia may improve pain on walking, especially if there is a spur. This is achieved by using a heel pad either with a cutout below the tender area or a softer gel material in this area. However, this does not address the cause. Since pronation is an important factor in most cases, an insole that supports the long arch along the inner border of the foot and acts to limit pronation is often used. This can be combined with a pressure-relieving cutout. Weight loss and appropriate footwear are important for some people. Injection of a local anaesthetic and CORTICOSTEROID around the attachment of the plantar fascia is helpful in settling down the inflammation quickly.

Subcalcaneal bursitis This may cause pain in the same area as plantar fasciitis or heel spurs. It differs from plantar fasciitis in that pulling the toes up does not make the pain worse. BURSITIS or inflammation of the bursa below the calcaneus usually happens in older people following trauma (falls, prolonged walking, or badly fitting shoes).

Painful heel pad The thick elastic pad beneath the calcaneus acts as a shock absorber. This is made up of fatty and elastic tissues separated into numerous cells by tough, fibrous sheets. These may become damaged and sometimes burst, either by severe trauma as when falling from a height or by repetitive minor trauma as occurs in elderly overweight individuals or martial arts practitioners. Treatment is by using a heel pad with or without raising the heel in order to shift weight forward into the foot. An injection of local anaesthetic can relieve pain in severe cases. It is usually a short-lived condition.

Dupuytren's contracture An exactly similar condition to the Dupuytren's contracture seen in the hand may affect the plantar fascia. It may be inherited and is also related to alcohol intake, epilepsy, and diabetes. The nodules are easily felt beneath the skin, and treatment is similar to that of the hand.

Posterior calcaneal bursitis This bursitis affects mainly women who wear high-heeled or narrow-counter shoes or people who play sport in inappropriate footwear. The red swollen bursa may be seen below the skin surface behind the heel. Treatment is to avoid the offending shoe. A triangle can be cut out of the counter of an old shoe to be worn until the bursitis has healed. Aspiration and injection of a small amount of corticosteroid may be used in resistant cases.

Calcaneal apophysitis (Sever's disease) This is a painful condition of the back of the heel usually affecting active boys between the ages of eight and 13 years. In growing children most of the bones of the body have large areas of cartilage that have yet to be converted to bone. This involves a gradual spreading of bone from both the middle of the bone and one or more areas near the ends of the bone, the secondary epiphyses. The cartilaginous area where these two bone centers have not yet joined (the epiphysis) can become injured by the pull of a powerful tendon. In Sever's disease, the epiphysis just below the attachment of the ACHILLES TENDON is involved. It becomes tender, mildly swollen, and causes pain when standing on tiptoes or jumping. Only one side is usually involved, but it may affect both sides.

Radioisotope bone scans will show up the area as hot, and MRI scans can confirm the diagnosis. X-rays will show differences between the two sides later on. However, the diagnosis can be made clinically without these investigations. Treatment is to avoid activities that involve powerful contraction of the calf muscles such as sport and outdoor play. This can be difficult to achieve with young boys, and a slight heel raise is helpful in reducing Achilles strain. If very severe, crutches can be used or an above-knee walking plaster applied for a period. Once the inflammation has settled, recovery is complete.

Subtalar arthritis The talus is an important bone in the ankle that has a joint above with the two lower leg bones, two joints below with the calcaneus or heel bone, and in front with the bones of the midfoot. Arthritis affecting its two joints with the calcaneus causes pain felt deep inside the heel. When severe this can cause disabling pain on walking. It may occur after significant trauma to the ankle and is a complication particularly of RHEUMATOID ARTHRITIS and juvenile arthritis. If the foot is brought up with the toes toward the head, the talus is locked in place and the calcaneus can then be moved from side to side to test this joint. This movement will be painful in subtalar arthritis, and there will usually be tenderness on the outside of the ankle just in front of the prominent bone there, the lateral malleolus. Treatment is with relative rest and NSAIDs. Injection of local anaesthetic and corticosteroid into the joint gives temporary relief. Molded orthotics may help long term. When very severe an ARTHRODESIS will relieve pain but reduce walking ability.

Calcaneal fractures The calcaneus or heel bone is strong and fractures only with considerable force or when an individual's bone is generally weak, as might be found in OSTEOPOROSIS. Fractures usually result from a fall from height onto the feet. Just over half the people suffering this fracture have a good outcome. Surgical fixation of the fracture probably gives slightly better results than conservative management. The outcome tends to be worse if the fracture involves the subtalar joint (see Subtalar Arthritis above). Early range of motion exercises and non-weight-bearing for eight to 12 weeks is important for a good recovery.

Pump bumps These are firm swellings near the attachment of the Achilles tendon. They are bony enlargements on the calcaneus associated with wearing high-heeled shoes or other shoes with a tightly fitting heel counter. They are usually painless unless there is an overlying bursitis.

Achilles bursitis Bursitis can occur between the skin and the Achilles attachment at the heel or between the Achilles and the heel bone. When boots are worn and the bursitis is ongoing, it is known as *winter's heel.*

Rheumatoid nodules These are found on the Achilles tendon one or two inches up from its bony attachment. They are intermittently painful, and treatment is to prevent shoes from rubbing against the nodules either by use of padding or by wearing different shoes.

Black heel Occasionally athletic teenagers or young adults develop a bluish black area underneath the back of the heel. The shearing forces of vigorous running and jumping cause minor bleeding into the skin, giving this appearance. No treatment is necessary.

heel spur A spur is a small bony outgrowth that occurs where a tendon or ligament attaches to a bone. This is commonly as a result of inflammation at that site (termed an enthesis) and may represent a healing phase. The lower front edge of the heel bone or calcaneus is a common site for spurs to form. These usually develop because of plantar fasciitis (see HEEL PAIN). In ANKYLOSING SPONDYLITIS, associated SPONDYLOARTHROPATHIES, and Achilles tendinopathies, a spur may form at the back of the heel pointing up the leg.

Symptoms and Diagnostic Path

The heel spur by itself is seldom painful. When there is pain it is usually due to the associated plantar fasciitis or enthesitis or an unrelated but nearby condition. However, if the biomechanics of the foot alters, with, for example, a lowering of the long arch of the foot, the altered angle of the spur in relation to the foot and plantar fascia may set up inflammation and pain.

Treatment Options and Outlook

Treatment of a spur behind the heel may involve a local CORTICOSTEROID injection to reduce the inflammation and padding or alternative footwear to relieve the pressure until healed. The plantar spurs from the lower calcaneus are subject to greater pressures, and treatment is much the same as for plantar fasciitis. Occasionally these spurs are surgically removed together with release of the plantar fascia when there is a poor response to other treatments.

hemarthrosis Bleeding into a joint that causes pain and swelling. There is often significant inflammation leading to pain, warmth, redness, and tenderness. Depending on the cause, it will usually settle within a few weeks. Aspiration to remove as much blood as possible will speed resolution. In cases that do not resolve adequately, ARTHROSCOPY may be done to wash out the joint thoroughly and possibly remove inflamed synovium. The many causes of hemarthrosis include HEMOPHILIA, hemangioma (a benign tumor of the synovial joint lining), scurvy (vitamin C deficiency), trauma causing fracture or ligament rupture, surgery, leukemia and malignant tumors of the adjacent bone, GOUT and CPPD, anticoagulant therapy, and PIGMENTED VILLONODULAR SYNOVITIS.

hemochromatosis This is usually an inherited disease that leads to excessive buildup of iron in the body and damage to a number of organs. A famous German pathologist, F. D. von Recklinghausen, described the disease in 1889, but it was only in 1927 that Sheldon suggested it was due to an inborn error of metabolism. It was finally proven to be genetically linked in 1975. The nature of the two most common abnormalities leading to hereditary hemochromatosis (HHC) was discovered only as recently as 1996. This discovery by Feder and his coworkers has lead to an explosion of research and knowledge about the disease and huge benefit to carriers of the abnormal gene.

The disease is most common in northwestern Europe and in populations that have migrated from there. Between three and five people in every 1,000 of such a population have the disease. It is therefore one of the most common genetic diseases. Unlike many hereditary diseases, it is relatively simple to treat in the early stages, and therefore early diagnosis is crucial. Occasionally certain unrelated diseases can lead to iron overload, which causes problems similar to the inherited disease.

Iron is both essential for the normal functioning of the human body and a poison in excess. Since iron is all around us, we have developed mechanisms for keeping excess iron out of our bodies. In this sense the gut contents are outside of our bodies. The cells lining our gut are continually being turned over. That is, they are lost into the gut as they get older and replaced by new cells. The new cells start at the bottom of little folds in the gut wall called crypts and move toward the top, where their function is to absorb all the nutrients we need. As they are being formed at the bottom of the crypts, they are programmed as to how much iron to absorb according to the body's iron need at the time. This programming is achieved by altering the amount of a protein known as HFE. The more HFE protein produced, the less iron absorbed. HFE therefore acts to keep iron out of the body.

More than 90 percent of patients with HHC will have two copies of a mutated (changed) gene that codes for the HFE protein (i.e., these genes carry the information each cell needs in order to make the protein). Since people normally inherit one gene from each parent, patients actually have to have two mutated genes to be unable to make the normal protein. The mutations are very minor differences but clearly alter the protein's function quite dramatically. The most common mutation is known in shorthand as C282Y and the other as

H63D. Some people have one copy of C282Y and one of H63D, and a proportion of them can also develop the disease. The abnormal protein allows excessive amounts of iron to enter the bloodstream and become stored throughout the body. An adult man needs to absorb about 1 mg of iron a day and a woman about 1.5 mg to remain healthy. Typically HHC patients absorb two to three times as much iron as other people, i.e., 4 mg a day. After many years the iron load can become enough to interfere with the function of a number of organs.

Because of a property of genes known as incomplete penetrance, not everyone with two C282Y genes will develop the disease. An even smaller percentage of those with two H63D genes or one C282Y plus one H63D gene will do so. A small number of patients with hemochromatosis have neither of these mutations. A number of other mutations in the HFE gene have been found in these patients, as well as mutations in other molecules involved in the control of iron metabolism such as transferrin receptor 2 and hepcidin. However none of these are frequent enough to test for routinely, and there are still patients with a presumed but unknown mutation. One such disorder causes iron overload in children and is known as juvenile hemochromatosis.

A number of other diseases can lead to iron overload without any known genetic tendency to overabsorb iron. Black Africans who drink a traditional beer brewed in nongalvanized iron pots sometimes develop iron overload. This condition, previously known as Bantu siderosis, is especially seen in southern Africa, but a similar condition has been rarely reported in African Americans. Because only a minority of such beer drinkers are affected, it is thought that there is some as yet undiscovered genetic tendency involved as well as the high dietary iron load. Blood contains a lot of iron, and patients requiring regular blood transfusions over a long period of time will develop iron overload as a result. This includes patients with severe thalassemia, complicated sickle-cell anemia (see SICKLE-CELL DISEASE), bone marrow failure, or following aggressive treatment of cancer. The pattern of iron loading in all these patients is different than that in HHC, but the resulting organ damage is much the same.

Symptoms and Diagnostic Path

Many years of iron accumulation are required to cause symptoms, and these usually start between the ages of 40 and 60 years. This varies considerably among patients, however. Women tend to develop problems later than men because they lose modest amounts of iron with regular menstruation. The sudden increase in iron accumulation after menopause probably causes the characteristic development of symptoms in women a few years after menopause. Liver and joint problems are common, together with weakness, tiredness, reduced sexual drive, and skin discoloration. Heart failure, diabetes, and other hormone abnormalities tend to occur later. The disease can be divided into four stages.

- Stage I is when someone is diagnosed as having the genetic predisposition to the disease. He or she is perfectly healthy and may never develop problems related to HHC. However, there will still be concerns related to screening other family members and getting insurance.

- Stage II is when iron stores reach two to five times normal and blood tests begin to show iron overload, although the patient still has no symptoms. These stage II patients need regular blood monitoring, and some will need treatment.

- Stage III is when symptoms due to iron overload start.

- Stage IV is when one or more organs (usually the liver) have developed irreversible damage.

The liver is usually affected first and will be enlarged in most symptomatic patients. Blood tests of liver function may not be abnormal until very late in the disease. Loss of body hair, blotchy redness of the palms, smaller testicles, and increased breast size in men can occur. Cirrhosis (widespread and irreversible scarring of the liver) will develop in the long term. This can lead to bleeding from the esophagus (gullet) due to high pressure in the veins taking blood to the liver. Of patients with cirrhosis, 30 percent will develop cancer of the liver. These complications can be largely avoided by early treatment.

The joint disease is a form of OSTEOARTHRITIS coming on prematurely. It typically affects the second and third metacarpophalangeal joints (and sometimes proximal interphalangeal joints) that are seldom affected in the usual type of osteoarthritis. Wrists, shoulders, hips, knees, and ankles are also affected. Some patients have an unusually destructive form of osteoarthritis. HHC is also one of the possible underlying causes of CPPD during which there may be episodes of quite intense joint inflammation. Unlike many of the other complications of HHC, the joint disease is not much improved by treatment. The osteoarthritis in particular progresses regardless of treatment once it has developed.

Darkening of the skin used to be quite common but is becoming less so with the earlier diagnosis of HHC following the development of genetic testing. DIABETES MELLITUS used to affect 65 percent of patients but again should become increasingly preventable with early diagnosis. Involvement of the heart occurs in 10–15 percent of symptomatic patients and usually causes heart failure. The heart enlarges and abnormal rhythms (which may be life-threatening) are particularly common. Heart failure is more common and develops earlier in the hemochromatosis caused by repeated blood transfusions.

Lower sex hormone production can occur in both sexes. This may cause loss of body hair, lowered sex drive, impotence, loss of menstrual periods, and smaller testicles. Very occasionally there may be dysfunction of the adrenal, thyroid, or parathyroid glands, all of which produce important hormones. Patients with hemochromatosis are also unusually prone to getting certain infections. These include *Vibrio vulnificus, Listeria monocytogenes, Yersinia enterocolitica, Salmonella* sp., *Klebsiella pneumoniae, Escherichia coli,* and *Rhizopus infections.*

The most important step is considering the diagnosis. This is both because the onset of symptoms is usually very slow and subtle and because the various manifestations may be diagnosed as diseases themselves (osteoarthritis, diabetes, cirrhosis of the liver, etc.) without realizing that there is an underlying disease causing these problems. Once suspected, confirming the diagnosis is easy. Iron is carried around the body by a carrier protein called transferrin. The percentage saturation of transfer-

rin can be measured. This rises with rising body iron, and levels over 55 percent in woman and 60 percent in men strongly suggest iron overload. Ferritin is a protein involved in iron storage, and levels rise with iron overload although somewhat later than transferrin saturation. In someone with HHC, the transferrin saturation will typically rise between the ages of 20 and 30 and ferritin will rise between 30 and 40 with symptoms beginning after age 40. This is quite variable, however. Confirming whether someone carries one or both of the C282Y and H63D mutations has now become relatively simple with a blood test. Thus stage I and II HHC can be diagnosed with these three blood tests. Transferrin levels are less reliable in detecting the iron overload due to repeated blood transfusions. Ferritin levels are a reasonable indicator in this situation, but liver biopsy is still the most accurate measurement.

A liver biopsy has been the traditional way to confirm iron overload and is still required to show the degree of damage to the liver. This involves passing a hollow needle into the liver and removing it quickly with a core of liver tissue. There is a very small but measurable chance of bleeding after this, and it is not infrequently uncomfortable or painful. It is therefore done less frequently now that improved blood tests are available. Sophisticated CT and MRI scanners can also measure the amount of iron in the liver, but this capability is not yet widespread.

Further tests may then need to be done to assess the degree of organ damage depending on the stage of the disease. Hormone testing can evaluate the sex hormones, adrenal hormones, and thyroid and parathyroid function. An EKG and echocardiogram (ultrasound scan of the heart) should be done in all symptomatic (grade III) patients, and continuous electrical monitoring of the heart may be indicated by the patient's symptoms. X-rays are useful in evaluating the arthritis and are sometimes diagnostic. Marked involvement of the second and third metacarpophalangeal joints is characteristic. The finding of thin lines of calcification along the cartilage in joints is suggestive of CPPD. MRI scans can also be useful in evaluating the joints.

A number of features of this disease suggest that routine screening would be a good idea:

- HHC is common.
- There are relatively easy tests to determine carrier status (the C282Y and H63D genes) and iron overload (transferrin saturation and ferritin).
- Treatment is cheap, technically easy, and acceptable to most patients.
- Early treatment can prevent considerable disability, suffering, and costly treatment of the complications of HHC.

Despite these arguments, most public health bodies and governments are not recommending screening. Their arguments revolve around the fact that not everyone who has two copies of C282Y develops the disease (although the vast majority do) and the ethical problems relating to prediction of disease. However, everyone agrees that once a patient has been diagnosed, his or her first-degree relatives should be offered screening. This is done by checking for the presence of the C282Y and H63D mutations on a blood test. If present, the transferrin and ferritin should be measured to assess the iron load. In younger stage I patients these should be repeated periodically. If the gene tests are negative, it means that individual has not inherited the same susceptibility to develop HHC as his or her family member. As explained above, there is still a theoretical chance that the individual could develop the disease through some other as yet unknown mutation, but this risk is extremely small.

Treatment Options and Outlook

The treatment is to remove iron from the body until body stores are normal and then maintain this level. Blood contains about 0.5 mg of iron per mL. Removing a unit of blood (the normal amount given during a blood donation) therefore removes 200 to 250 mg of iron. As long as the patient is healthy, it is possible to remove a unit of blood every week or fortnight without any adverse effects. In the presence of heart failure or other chronic disease this may have to be slowed down. Frequent removal of blood (termed venesection or phlebotomy) is continued until the ferritin level is below 100 µg/L. This may take up to two years. Venesection is then continued just often enough to keep the ferritin at this level. This is usually two to four times a year.

Although patients do not have to limit their dietary intake of iron strictly, which they may find unpleasant, they should take some precautions. Vitamin C and iron supplementation should be avoided. Vitamin C promotes iron absorption. Both of these may be found in multivitamins or other health supplements or health drinks. Red meat is a potent source of iron and should be limited. Alcohol should be avoided in those with clinical liver involvement and limited in stage II. Raw shellfish are best avoided since there have been deaths in HHC patients from *Vibrio vulnificus* infections.

Complications of HHC such as diabetes, heart failure, or endocrine deficiencies are treated as they would be in any other patient. See the OSTEOARTHRITIS and CPPD sections for treatment of these forms of arthritis. In the past transfusion services generally did not accept blood for transfusion into other patients if the donor suffered from a chronic illness. Many HHC patients are very healthy, however, and there is nothing wrong with their blood. Increasingly, therefore, transfusion services are accepting HHC blood, and many patients welcome the opportunity to help provide this service.

Obviously, venesection is not an option for patients who require regular transfusions to maintain an adequate red cell level (thalassemia, sickle-cell anemia, etc.). Currently the only alternative for these patients is desferrioxamine. Desferrioxamine is a chelating agent, which means that it binds very tightly to iron and therefore removes fairly large amounts of iron from the body as it is excreted. It is given as an infusion under the skin and can remove 10 to 20 mg of iron per day. If done on a daily basis, this is just less than half the amount removed by weekly venesection.

Roughly a third of untreated HHC patients die of heart failure, a third of liver failure or its complications, and a third from liver cancer. Treatment has been shown to improve the five year survival of these patients from only 33 percent to 89 percent. Since Feder and colleagues' discovery of the two important gene mutations and the development of relatively simple blood tests to aid the diagnosis, many more patients have been diagnosed at a much earlier stage. It is hoped that this will bring their life expectancy very close to that of the normal population. However, further long-term studies of patients being currently diagnosed will be needed to see if this in fact happens.

With successful treatment the liver and spleen get smaller, liver function improves (although any cirrhosis present remains), heart failure resolves, and diabetes improves in about half the patients. Reduced sex hormone production and the arthritis are not affected by treatment. If the disease is treated before cirrhosis develops, there is no increased risk of liver cancer.

Risk Factors and Preventive Measures

Although hemochromatosis is a hereditary disease, the adverse effects are theoretically preventable because they are caused by the iron overload that is the result of the genetic abnormality in the HFE gene. It is relatively easy to remove iron from the body by venesection as long as the diagnosis is made early enough so that there need never be excessive iron buildup. Most people with HHC in the Western world have the C282Y gene with a smaller number having the H63D gene. Not everyone with two copies of these genes will develop HHC, and some without these genes will develop HHC. Thus, it is necessary to show early evidence of iron buildup to be sure of the diagnosis. Theoretically, if everyone was checked for these two genes prior to leaving school, those found to be at risk (homozygous or compound heterozygous) could have iron levels checked at regular intervals and start preventive treatment at the appropriate time, thus preventing a very large majority of the disease consequences of HHC. However, public health authorities around the world have deemed this not cost effective, and screening is limited to contact tracing. This means that when someone is diagnosed with HHC, all their close relatives should be screened for the two common abnormal genes. Those found to be homozygous or compound heterozygote then have regular iron testing.

hemophilia An inherited disorder of the blood-clotting mechanism that increases the risk of bleeding. Hemophilia A, caused by a deficiency of clotting factor VIII, affects about 80 percent of hemophiliacs and is more common and more severe than hemophilia B which is also known as Christmas disease and is caused by deficiency of clotting factor IX.

Hemophilia results from mutations in the genes for factor VIII and IX. These genes lie on the X chromosome, and males, because they carry only one X chromosome, are affected by hemophilia if they have the abnormal chromosome. Women, on the other hand, because they have two X chromosomes, one inherited from each parent, are unlikely to have two abnormal chromosomes and are protected from disease. However, if they have one abnormal X chromosome they are carriers, and their children will have a 50 percent chance of having hemophilia if they are male and a 50 percent chance of being a carrier if they are female. Approximately one-third of patients with hemophilia do not have a history of affected family members, and the disease is then thought to have arisen from a new mutation. Although hemophilia is thought of as being a disorder of blood, one of the problems it causes, bleeding into muscles and joints, can result in acute and chronic musculoskeletal problems.

Symptoms and Diagnostic Path

Patients with a very low level, less than 1 percent of normal, of factor VIII or IX activity are severely affected and often develop symptoms caused by spontaneous bleeding before they are two years old. Patients with less severe hemophilia often have factor levels that are 5 percent or more of normal and may develop symptoms only after surgery or trauma.

The symptoms caused by bleeding depend on the site affected. Bleeding into soft tissue and muscle causes pain and swelling in the area. A large collection of blood (hematoma) can cause damage to nerves and other tissues directly through pressure and indirectly by cutting off the nerves' blood supply. Hematomas slowly resorb but cause damage and scarring to the surrounding tissues and can result in contractures that prevent a limb from straightening. Bleeding into a joint is called HEMARTHROSIS and causes severe pain, swelling, and difficulty moving. Most patients with severe hemophilia suffer spontaneous hemarthrosis in early childhood, usually when they start to walk. In later life, acute hemarthrosis can occur spontaneously or after minor trauma. Acute hemarthrosis usually resolves over two weeks, but recurrent episodes of bleeding into a joint damages it and can cause chronic inflammation resulting in swelling, deformity, pain, and loss of function. How blood damages the joint is not known exactly. Activation of platelets and white blood cells and the release of iron are all thought to play a role in damaging cartilage and stimulating abnormal growth of the synovium or joint lining.

Hemophilia is diagnosed from the family history of a bleeding problem, the clinical features, tests of blood clotting, and levels of factors VIII and IX. By the time musculoskeletal problems occur, the diagnosis of hemophilia is often known.

Treatment Options and Outlook

Patients with hemophilia are usually treated by specialized centers. The basis of treatment is avoiding medications, such as aspirin, and environmental situations such as contact sports, that increase the risk of bleeding and replacing the deficient clotting factors. The focus is on early and intensive home administration of the appropriate clotting factor by patients at the first symptom of a bleed. Factors VIII and IX are available as either a concentrate made from human blood from many donors and treated to inactivate viruses or as a recombinant product made using molecular biology techniques. In the early years of the HIV epidemic many patients with hemophilia were treated with factor concentrates made from blood before it was routinely screened for HIV infection. Many of these patients became infected by HIV and subsequently developed AIDS. Because there is no risk of transmitting viral infections with recombinant clotting factors, they are often preferred. Desmopressin is an agent that increases production of factor VIII by the lining cells of blood vessels. This is most effective in people with mild deficiency and can be used before surgical procedures in hemophilia A. It can be given by injection under the skin, infused into a vein, or taken by an intranasal spray.

The best treatment for hemophilia arthritis is to prevent it by adequate and early replacement of clotting factors. Giving the appropriate clotting factor as early as possible and drugs to control pain treats acute hemarthrosis. In the early stages of hemarthrosis draining the blood by drawing it out of the joint through a needle (arthrocentesis) may decrease the long-term damage to the joint. Short courses of CORTICOSTEROIDS for a few days can help resolve the resulting inflammation quicker, although it is not always necessary. Chronic arthritis can be improved by intensive clotting factor replacement, pain control, and physical therapy to prevent contractures and strengthen muscles. A few patients do not respond to treatment and have recurrent, frequent bleeding into a joint. Tranexamic acid and aminocaproic acid interfere with the normal mechanisms of breakdown of clots and therefore can stabilize clots in patients with bleeding problems. They can be used in hemophilia patients along with clotting factor replacement when there is difficulty controlling bleeding despite adequate replacement. Some of these patients benefit from surgery to remove the inflamed lining of the joint (SYNOVECTOMY). Joint replacement surgery has been performed in patients with end-stage hemophilia arthritis with a severely damaged, painful joint. However, joint replacement surgery is avoided if possible because complications occur more often in patients with hemophilia. Also, most of the patients are young with a long life expectancy and will therefore almost certainly need future surgery to revise the replaced joint.

Risk Factors and Preventive Measures

Hemophilia is a hereditary disease and therefore not preventable. Genetic counseling should be available to those carrying the gene. Early intensive administration of the missing factor at home at the first sign of a bleed is the key to preventing the long-term sequelae. Prophylactic factor replacement should also be given for any surgical procedures.

Henoch-Schönlein purpura (HSP) This is the commonest form of VASCULITIS in children. Although it may affect anyone from six months to 80 years old, the vast majority of patients are aged between two and 10 years. It occurs mostly in the fall and winter months and often follows an infection. In this form of vasculitis, small blood vessels become damaged by inflammation. Skin, bowel, joints, and kidneys are commonly affected.

The cause is not fully understood. IgA antibodies clearly play an important role. Of the five classes of immunoglobulins or antibodies, IgA is most involved with protection against infection and other events at mucosal surfaces, i.e., the inner lining of the nose, throat, lungs, gut, and genital areas. In HSP not only are IgA levels in blood raised, but there is increased formation of chains of IgA molecules and complexes of IgA and other molecules. When these relatively heavy complexes settle out on the walls of small blood vessels, they cause inflammation. The white cells attracted to this area then cause damage to the blood vessel wall, which may result in blood cells leaking out or the blood vessel actually blocking off (thrombosis). On biopsy this appearance is called *leukocytoclastic vasculitis,* but HSP is only one of several causes of this.

It is well known that HSP often follows an infection, usually of the throat or chest. Many organisms have been implicated, including streptococcal bacteria, *Helicobacter pylori,* hepatitis B virus, herpes simplex virus, human parvovirus B19, Coxsackie viruses, and adenovirus (a cause of the common cold). HSP has also followed the use of medications, but there do not seem to be any particular properties of the drugs or infecting organisms that might initiate this abnormal immune response. Rather, there may be subtle abnormalities in the IgA of some people that predisposes them to develop HSP. A lot of research is being conducted in this area at the moment.

Symptoms and Diagnostic Path

HSP cannot be diagnosed without the characteristic skin rash. This comprises small 2–10 mm diameter blue-black spots on the legs and buttocks. These spots are easily felt to be lumpy. They may start as reddish lumps or wheals. About 75 percent of patients get arthritis, usually affecting the ankles or knees, that may start before the rash. A smaller number develop gut problems, usually colicky pain, vomiting, and passing of blood in the stools. A serious complication of gut involvement is intussusception. This is where one section of bowel pushes through the next section so that the first

lies inside the second. This double tube of bowel causes obstruction. If it does not resolve, it can lead to perforation or bursting of the bowel wall. In HSP this usually affects the small bowel.

About 40 percent of patients also get inflammation of the kidneys. This is recognized by finding small amounts of blood and, less often, protein in the urine. Kidney involvement usually starts a couple of weeks after the rash and may last much longer than the other manifestations. A large number of other complications rarely occur, including inflammation of muscle, testes, bladder, eye, heart or pancreas, bleeding in the lungs, seizures, reduced level of consciousness, movement disorders, loss of nerve function, and paralysis. These are fortunately all very rare.

In children, the clinical manifestations are characteristic and the diagnosis can be made without any special tests. The urine should be tested to look for kidney involvement. Adults often have atypical disease and may require more intensive investigations. A throat swab may grow streptococcus. Biopsy of the rash shows the picture of leukocytoclastic vasculitis with destruction of small blood vessel walls by white cells and the remains of broken-up white cells close by. Biopsy of the kidney is done occasionally and shows the presence of IgA and varying degrees of damage to the filtering part of the kidney (glomerulonephritis). Blood levels of IgA are often raised.

Treatment Options and Outlook

In the absence of severe complications, HSP will resolve spontaneously in about four weeks. CORTI-COSTEROIDS are very helpful in treating the arthritis and abdominal pain. Kidney involvement is the one manifestation that may not resolve, and the outlook for most patients depends on how badly their kidneys are affected. Although nearly half of HSP patients continue to have minor abnormalities on urine testing, only 1 percent go on to develop end-stage renal failure. Up to a third of patients may get recurrent attacks, usually within six months. Adults with HSP are more likely to develop serious kidney problems than children. Those with a lot of blood or protein in the urine initially or severe damage on kidney biopsy have the worst outcome. These patients should therefore receive aggressive treatment with large doses of corticosteroids intravenously initially and then in tablet form together with AZATHIOPRINE or CYCLOPHOSPHAMIDE.

Risk Factors and Preventive Measures

Although HSP is well known to follow a number of infections as discussed above, its occurrence is unpredictable and not preventable.

hepatitis See HEPATITIS, AUTOIMMUNE; HEPATITIS, DRUG-INDUCED; HEPATITIS B; and HEPATITIS C.

hepatitis, autoimmune A subset of hepatitis that is thought to be caused by an autoimmune illness. Chronic autoimmune hepatitis can be divided into two subtypes:

1. An illness previously called *lupoid* hepatitis that affects mainly young women and is associated with a positive antinuclear antibody (ANA) test
2. An illness that affects mainly children and is associated with a positive test for antibodies to liver-kidney microsomal antigens (anti-LKM) and not with ANA

The cause is not known. However, it is thought that a genetic predisposition and an environmental trigger act in synergy to trigger and sustain an autoimmune inflammatory process that targets liver cells.

Symptoms and Diagnostic Path

The onset of symptoms varies and can be acute, with an illness similar to acute viral hepatitis, or insidious. Fatigue, nausea, arthralgia, jaundice, and decreased appetite are common. Less common are arthritis, pleurisy, sicca syndrome symptoms, rash, and VASCULITIS.

The diagnosis is based on the clinical presentation, elevated liver enzyme tests, a positive ANA or anti-LKM test, and negative tests for viral hepatitis. A liver biopsy is often performed to assess the severity of the illness and to exclude other causes of hepatitis. In addition to a positive ANA test, which usually has a smooth or homogenous pattern, positive tests for other autoantibodies such as RHEUMATOID FACTOR and smooth-muscle antibodies are common.

High levels of immunoglobulins are usually present.

Treatment Options and Outlook

The severity and course of autoimmune hepatitis is highly variable. If severe and chronic with features that on liver biopsy are called chronic active hepatitis, then treatment with CORTICOSTEROIDS is prescribed because cirrhosis and liver failure may result. Autoimmune hepatitis is one of the few types of liver disease that responds to corticosteroid treatment. Prednisone, initially in high and then in decreasing doses, will induce remission in 80 percent of patients. Some physicians add another immunosuppressant drug such as AZATHIOPRINE or CYCLOSPORINE for patients who do not respond to corticosteroids alone or who require high doses to maintain remission. Studies have shown improvement in both symptoms and liver biopsy samples, and more than 90 percent of treated patients survive longer than 10 years. Prolonged treatment, often for a year or longer, is required. Approximately 50 percent of patients remain in remission or have only mildly active disease for a time after the initial course of therapy is completed. However, most patients relapse within a few years of stopping treatment and require further courses or often indefinite maintenance treatment.

Risk Factors and Preventive Measures

There are no known risk factors or preventive measures for this group of illnesses.

hepatitis, drug-induced The liver is the organ primarily responsible for the metabolism and detoxification of most drugs, so it is not surprising that several drugs can cause liver damage and result in hepatitis. Drugs can cause two major types of liver damage, toxic hepatitis and idiosyncratic hepatitis.

Toxic Hepatitis is liver damage that is predictable and will occur in most people exposed to a certain dose of the toxic chemical or drug. Examples are acetaminophen overdose, carbon tetrachloride, and the *Amanita* species of mushroom. Often toxicity extends beyond the liver and other organs are affected.

Idiosyncratic Hepatitis is unpredictable, does not depend on the dose of drug taken, and occurs in only a few people who have taken a particular drug. Why a few people develop hepatitis after exposure to a drug and others do not is not known. Affected individuals are thought to be more susceptible to liver damage from a particular drug because either they develop an allergic response or they metabolize the drug differently and form toxic by-products that damage liver cells. Idiosyncratic hepatitis can be further subclassified according to whether the primary damage is to the liver cells (hepatitic) or to the system that excretes bile (cholestatic). However, there is often overlap, and many drugs can cause a mixed hepatitic and cholestatic illness. Drugs that have caused a hepatitic pattern of liver damage include halothane, NSAIDs, LEFLUNOMIDE, METHOTREXATE, SULFASALAZINE, and many others. Drugs that have caused cholestatic liver damage include oral contraceptives, erythromycin, anabolic steroids, and chlorpromazine.

Methotrexate and leflunomide, drugs used to treat RHEUMATOID ARTHRITIS, can rarely cause chronic liver damage resulting in scarring or cirrhosis.

Symptoms and Diagnostic Path

Drug-induced hepatitis can result in symptoms and liver enzymes tests that are similar to those of viral hepatitis. Unless severely affected, many patients have no symptoms and hepatitis is suspected only when routine blood tests are performed.

No diagnostic test enables a particular drug to be identified as the cause of hepatitis in an individual patient. The usual clinical approach is to perform blood tests for viral hepatitis and if these are negative and drug-induced hepatitis is suspected to stop the drug that is thought to be responsible. To be sure that a particular drug was the cause of a patient's hepatitis would require that once the hepatitis had resolved, the patient be treated with the drug and develop hepatitis again. This rechallenge test would be very helpful in pinning down a particular drug as the cause of a patient's hepatitis but is seldom performed because there is a risk that reexposure to the drug could induce severe hepatitis.

Treatment Options and Outlook

Most types of drug-induced hepatitis are treated by stopping the offending drug. The outcome depends on how severe the liver injury is. It ranges from rapid reversal of mildly abnormal liver function tests to death from liver failure.

Risk Factors and Preventive Measures

Hepatitis due to predictable drug toxicity such as acetaminophen overdose or carbon tetrachloride is prevented by avoiding exposure although the former is usually intentional and the latter accidental in industrial settings. The use of drugs that cause idiosyncratic hepatitis must be preceded by an assessment of their expected benefit to the patient versus the likelihood of an adverse effect, including hepatitis. For most drugs used in short courses including a number of antibiotics and NSAIDs, the risk is very small in a patient with no other liver problems or risk factors. When drugs are used for prolonged periods however, such as the DMARDs methotrexate and leflunomide in inflammatory arthritis, the risk of getting hepatitis at some stage is considerably greater. It is therefore important to do regular monitoring of liver blood tests. Some rise in these tests is very common, and it is customary to only make changes when they reach two to three times the normal limit. They should be stopped immediately if the tests reach five times the upper limit. Symptoms are of no use in picking up these early changes. Leflunomide particularly is more likely to cause hepatitis if it is taken together with other drugs that affect the liver, and particular caution has to be exercised if this is necessary. Combining methotrexate and alcohol increases the toxicity and should be avoided.

hepatitis B A common viral infection transmitted from person to person by blood or body fluids that results in acute and chronic liver inflammation, cirrhosis, and liver cancer. In the United States, approximately 200,000 cases occur annually. The liver complications of hepatitis B infection are the most frequent and serious ones, but musculoskeletal symptoms can also occur.

Hepatitis B virus is found in blood, semen, and other body fluids, and like HIV, it is transmitted from person to person by blood or body fluids. Hepatitis B virus is more infectious than HIV and is able to survive for longer outside the body. Therefore, transmission of hepatitis B from person to person can occur by sharing toothbrushes. However, sexual contact and sharing of needles are the commonest ways the virus is transmitted. Intravenous drug users who use dirty or shared needles have a very high risk of contracting HIV and hepatitis B and C. Needle exchange programs that provide clean needles have been started in some countries to combat this form of transmission. Transmission of hepatitis B to patients by medical procedures is rare. Blood products are screened for viruses such as hepatitis B, and medical instruments are either disposable or sterilized between patients. Health workers can be infected by accidentally pricking themselves with a needle used on a patient with hepatitis B. If this happens, the chance of getting hepatitis B can be as high as 30 percent and is much higher than the chance of getting HIV infection from a needle stick (less than 1 percent). Outbreaks of hepatitis B have occurred from contaminated equipment in tattoo parlors. Pregnant women who are infected with hepatitis B can transmit the infection to their babies.

Symptoms and Diagnostic Path

Symptoms may not appear until several months after transmission of the virus. Ones such as arthralgia, poor appetite, and fatigue are usually mild and nonspecific, and approximately a third of people have no symptoms. Some patients become visibly jaundiced, with the white parts of their eyes turning yellow and their urine becoming dark. Severe hepatitis resulting in liver failure is rare and occurs in approximately five out of 1,000 infected people. Most patients develop antibodies to the virus and eliminate the acute infection, but approximately 5 percent become chronic carriers and can transmit the infection to others. Carriers are at risk of long-term complications. Some chronic carriers seem to carry the virus without it causing much liver inflammation, but others have chronic hepatitis that can lead to cirrhosis and eventually liver failure. Patients who carry the virus, even those with ongoing liver inflammation, usually have no symptoms unless chronic liver disease develops. This may cause jaundice, swelling of the abdomen due to fluid (ascites), swelling of the legs, and symptoms of liver failure such as confusion and coma.

In addition to nonspecific musculoskeletal symptoms such as fatigue and arthralgia that are common during acute hepatitis B infection, there are two well-recognized rheumatic syndromes, the arthritis-dermatitis syndrome and hepatitis B vasculitis.

Hepatitis B arthritis-dermatitis syndrome After infection has occurred and immediately before hepatitis develops, approximately 20 percent of people develop symmetrical arthralgia affecting many joints, typically the small joints of the hands, and a rash that can be urticarial. The symmetrical involvement of the small joints of the hands can lead to an incorrect diagnosis of rheumatoid arthritis. The joint pain is severe and often out of proportion to the degree of swelling, which is usually minimal or absent. The arthritis-dermatitis symptoms seem to herald the hepatitis. As soon as it develops the musculoskeletal symptoms settle without causing any permanent joint damage. A similar pattern of arthralgia and arthritis resembling rheumatoid arthritis has occurred in a few patients after they were vaccinated against hepatitis B (see DRUG-INDUCED RHEUMATIC DISEASE).

The symptoms of arthritis and rash occur just before, or at the same time, as the first symptoms of hepatitis. Blood tests show elevated liver enzymes with a positive HBsAg test.

Hepatitis B vasculitis Approximately 25 percent of patients presenting with POLYARTERITIS NODOSA have hepatitis B vasculitis. Unlike the hepatitis arthritis-dermatitis syndrome, which occurs just before hepatitis develops, hepatitis B vasculitis can occur at any stage in the course of hepatitis B infection. Polyarteritis nodosa and hepatitis B vasculitis have identical symptoms. The symptoms depend on the organs affected. Fever, loss of weight, rash, abdominal pain, neuropathy, glomerulonephritis, kidney failure, and hypertension are common.

In patients with polyarteritis nodosa or a similar type of systemic vasculitis caused by hepatitis B, the tests for viral infection and replication (HBsAg and HBeAg) are positive. Other diagnostic tests are performed to establish the diagnosis of vasculitis. These include an angiogram of the arteries to the kidneys and bowel that arise from the aorta. The findings on angiogram are identical to those of polyarteritis nodosa and show small aneurysms and irregularity of small and medium-sized arteries. A biopsy of affected tissue, usually muscle, nerve, or skin, shows vasculitis.

Hepatitis B infection   In many patients hepatitis B infection does not cause symptoms and infection is not diagnosed until blood tests, often performed for another reason, suggest that infection has occurred. This usually happens in one of two ways. The first is when an otherwise healthy person donates blood. All donated blood is routinely screened for HIV and hepatitis B and C. People whose blood tests are positive for one of these infections are often advised that they should see their physicians for further tests. The second is when an otherwise healthy person has a routine physical examination and blood tests show elevated levels of alanine and aspartate aminotransferase enzymes (see LFTs in Appendix II). Specific blood tests for markers of hepatitis B and C infection are then performed to make the diagnosis. The hepatitis B surface antigen (HBsAg) test is positive in patients with acute infection but becomes negative in the majority who develop hepatitis B surface antibodies and eliminate the virus. Chronic carriers who do not eliminate the infection remain positive for HbsAg. In those patients in whom the virus is actively multiplying, another marker, hepatitis B e antigen (HBeAg), is also positive. Viral DNA can also be measured in patients in whom the virus is replicating. A liver biopsy is not performed routinely to diagnose hepatitis B infection but can be useful for assessing the activity and severity of chronic disease.

Treatment Options and Outlook

Hepatitis B   A very effective vaccine prevents the disease. In addition to vaccination, other measures are used in developed countries to prevent people from becoming infected. These include testing all blood products for hepatitis B, sterilization of medical instruments, and educational programs to encourage drug users not to share needles. In developing countries hepatitis B is a serious problem, and in some countries as many as 10 percent of the population are chronic carriers. In people who have been exposed by a needle stick, hepatitis B infection can be prevented by rapid injection of immune globulin and hepatitis B vaccination.

Acute hepatitis B infection is usually not treated, and more than 90 percent of people clear the infection without problems. Combination treatment with alpha-interferon and lamivudine has been reasonably successful in treating chronic hepatitis B patients with good liver function. Treatment options have increased considerably in recent years for patients with poor liver function, resistant disease, or other special situations. Adefovir is useful against lamivudine-resistant virus. Entecavir works very quickly and is effective against resistant virus. Telbivudine is a rapid-acting alternative, and tenofovir is a new drug with wide efficacy. The treatment of hepatitis B, especially in those who fail initial therapy, is evolving and has become quite complex. Liver transplantation is reserved for patients with severe cirrhosis and deteriorating liver function. People who develop cirrhosis have an increased risk of developing a type of liver cancer, hepatocellular carcinoma.

Hepatitis B arthritis-dermatitis syndrome   Most patients do not need any specific therapy. The illness is short-lived and settles spontaneously.

Hepatitis B vasculitis   Treating hepatitis B vasculitis is difficult. The standard treatment for serious vasculitis, CORTICOSTEROIDS combined with an immunosuppressant such as CYCLOPHOSPHAMIDE, is often needed to control the vasculitis but has the negative effect of promoting viral replication. The approach usually used is to control the vasculitis and then to start treatment with antiviral drugs. The largest experience with this type of sequential immunosuppressant/antiviral therapy for hepatitis B vasculitis is from a group in France headed by Dr. Luc Guillevin. They report good results, with approximately 80 percent of patients surviving five years.

Risk Factors and Preventive Measures

Exposure to infected body fluids is the route of infection for hepatitis B. This can occur through sexual contact, sharing needles, through accidental injury to health workers, occasionally through sharing toothbrushes, tattoo equipment, and the like, and transplacentally from mother to infant. Needle-exchange programs have helped reduce some new infections, and not sharing other equipment, such as razors, toothbrushes, or the straws used for inhaling recreational drugs, is important. This should be part of school health education programs. Correct use of condoms is essential for sex with anyone other than a long-term partner. Careful screening of blood for transfusion has largely eliminated this as a source. Overall, however, vaccination is the most effective way to reduce the effects of hepatitis B. Since the early 1990s, most developed and many developing nations have introduced universal vaccination, aiming to vaccinate all children by the age of three. Vaccination is compulsory for all health workers in many countries. A recent survey in the United States showed that just over 80 percent of teenagers were vaccinated.

hepatitis C   The cause of an illness previously called non-A, non-B hepatitis was identified in 1989 and the illness renamed hepatitis C. Approximately 170 million people worldwide and 3 million in the United States are chronic carriers of hepatitis C. In the United States, it is the commonest cause of chronic hepatitis and hepatocellular carcinoma.

Hepatitis is caused by an RNA virus belonging to the family of flaviviruses. There are many variants of the hepatitis C virus (HCV) with minor differences in their genetic structure that allow them to be classified into six genotypes. Different genotypes predominate in different parts of the world. In the United States genotypes 1, 2, and 3 are common. The different genotypes vary in their response to therapy, with genotype 1 being the most resistant.

Before 1990 hepatitis C was often transmitted through transfusion of blood or blood products, but routine testing of donors for hepatitis C has virtually eliminated this route of transmission. However, new infections still occur, and as is the case with hepatitis B, sexual contact and sharing of needles are the most common ways the virus is transmitted. Intravenous drug users who use dirty or shared needles have a very high risk of contracting HIV and hepatitis B and C. Transmission

of hepatitis C to patients by medical procedures is now extremely rare. Health workers can be infected by accidentally pricking themselves with a needle used on a patient with hepatitis C. If this happens, the chance of getting hepatitis C is about 3 percent, much lower than the 30 percent risk of getting hepatitis B in this way. A pregnant mother can transmit the virus to her infant but it happens less often than with hepatitis B.

The cause of rheumatic problems associated with hepatitis C is not known. Autoantibodies such as rheumatoid factor and antinuclear antibody (ANA) are often found, but it is not clear if they are directly implicated in the cause of musculoskeletal disease.

Symptoms and Diagnostic Path

Most people infected with hepatitis C do not know that they have been infected because the symptoms of the acute infection are usually trivial. In a few people acute hepatitis develops and they have symptoms of nausea, jaundice, and fatigue. Approximately 20 percent of infected people clear the virus spontaneously and have no further problems, but in the other 80 percent the infection persists. In these people some liver inflammation occurs. The exact risk of severe liver disease in hepatitis C carriers is not known because it can develop 30 or more years later, but about 20 percent of infected people are thought to progress to severe liver disease. If this happens it may cause symptoms of jaundice, swelling of the abdomen due to fluid (ascites), swelling of the legs, and symptoms of liver failure such as confusion and coma. Several conditions that affect organs other than the liver can occur in patients who carry hepatitis C. Because the virus was discovered only in 1989, the range of clinical conditions it may cause or be associated with is still being defined. Hepatitis C is widely accepted as causing two rheumatological conditions, CRYOGLOBULINEMIA and inflammatory polyarthritis, but several other associated problems have been described.

Cryoglobulinemia   Both hepatitis B and C can cause cryoglobulinemia, but hepatitis C is more likely to do so. It is estimated that this develops in between 10 and 60 percent of HCV infected people with large variations between different countries.

Hepatitis C is one of the most common causes of cryoglobulinemia, and in some studies 80 to 90 percent of patients with this condition have had hepatitis C.

Inflammatory polyarthritis Arthralgia is common and is found in about a third of infected patients, but arthritis occurs in only about 4 percent. Some patients develop symmetrical inflammatory polyarthritis that is very similar to rheumatoid arthritis, with symptoms of pain and swelling that affect mainly the small joints of the hands. This type of arthritis is not a feature of acute hepatitis C infection but can occur at any time during the course of the illness. Unlike most types of arthritis associated with viral infections, hepatitis C arthritis persists, often for years. Many patients have symptoms of both cryoglobulinemia and arthritis. Hepatitis C and rheumatoid arthritis are both relatively common illnesses and will therefore occur together in some patients by chance. The arthritis associated with hepatitis C can be very difficult to distinguish clinically from true rheumatoid arthritis. To add to the confusion, many patients with hepatitis C, even those without arthritis, also have a positive blood test for rheumatoid factor. Hepatitis C arthritis differs from classical rheumatoid arthritis because it is less likely to cause joint deformities or erosions and tends to cause more pain than swelling in affected joints.

Other conditions SJÖGREN'S SYNDROME, POLYARTERITIS NODOSA, VASCULITIS, NEUROPATHIC ARTHRITIS, FIBROMYALGIA, and MYOSITIS have occurred in association with hepatitis C infection.

Diagnosis Because most patients who have acute hepatitis C infection or are chronic carriers have no symptoms, the diagnosis is often not made until blood tests, performed for some other reason, raise the possibility. This often happens in one of two ways. The first is when an otherwise healthy person donates blood. All blood is tested for HIV and hepatitis B and C. People whose blood tests are positive for one of these are often advised that they should see their physicians for further tests. The second is when an otherwise healthy person has a routine physical examination and blood tests show elevated levels of alanine and aspartate aminotransferase enzymes suggesting some liver disturbance (see LFTs in Appendix II). Specific blood tests for markers of hepatitis B and C infection are then obtained to make the diagnosis.

The usual blood test performed to screen for hepatitis C infection is an ELISA test that detects antibodies to viral protein. This test can be falsely negative but this is rare, occurring in less than 1 percent of patients. A false negative ELISA is more likely to occur in patients with a poor immune response, for example those who also have HIV infection and patients with cryoglobulinemia. A false positive ELISA test can also occur, and therefore a positive (enzyme-linked immunosorbent assay) ELISA test is followed by a more specific confirmatory test for hepatitis C. This could be a recombinant-based immunoblot assay known as a RIBA test or directly measuring the virus RNA using polymerase chain reaction (PCR). In patients receiving treatment, the PCR test can be used to measure the amount of virus present and therefore monitor the patient's response to treatment. A liver biopsy is often performed to provide information about the activity of the disease and the amount of scarring.

All patients with cryoglobulinemia and polyarteritis nodosa should be tested for hepatitis B and C infection. In patients with other rheumatic conditions, hepatitis C is usually diagnosed when routine blood tests reveal elevated liver enzymes. In patients with rheumatoid arthritis, hepatitis C infection is sometimes discovered when screening blood tests are performed before starting treatment with methotrexate or leflunomide, drugs that can rarely damage the liver.

Treatment Options and Outlook

Hepatitis C infection is treated to reduce the chance of a person developing cirrhosis, liver failure, and hepatocellular carcinoma. All infected patients should be considered for therapy. However, for some the risks associated with treatment may be more than those of continuing low-grade infection. For example, women with normal liver function and little change on liver biopsy have a low risk of developing cirrhosis and may be better off with monitoring of the infection and only having treatment if their condition deteriorates. Also type 2 and 3 hepatitis C virus respond better to treatment than type 1. People who continue to drink alcohol have more rapid development of cirrhosis while those still using intravenous drugs may reinfect themselves. Persistently raised liver enzymes and significant changes on liver biopsy predict a poorer outcome. All this should be considered when deciding whether to treat or not, and each person should be assessed individually.

Treatment for hepatitis C has advanced rapidly, and a combination of a long-acting form of interferon alpha (pegylated interferon) and another antiviral drug (ribavirin) has given the best results so far. Patients treated with this combination for 48 weeks have a 40 percent chance of clearing the viral infection permanently. Preliminary information suggests that treatment decreases the risk of long-term complications of hepatitis C even in patients who relapse or do not clear the infection.

Inflammatory arthritis associated with hepatitis C infection is difficult to treat because many of the drugs that could be used, such as methotrexate and leflunomide, are contraindicated in people with liver disease. There are no large studies to guide therapy but most rheumatologists use NON-STEROIDAL ANTI-INFLAMMATORY DRUGS, low doses of CORTICOSTEROIDS, and DMARDS such as HYDROXY-CHLOROQUINE, SULFASALAZINE, or GOLD. Treatment of hepatitis C infection with antiviral drugs usually improves cryoglobulinemia but is less effective in controlling arthritis.

Risk Factors and Preventive Measures

As the hepatitis C virus was only discovered in 1989, it was possible to become infected by blood or blood products prior to the early 1990s (different countries brought in universal testing of blood products at different times). Since that time the major source of infection has been injecting or inhaling recreational drugs through shared syringes and straws and less frequently sexual contact. As noted above, hepatitis C is significantly less infective than hepatitis B. Health workers may be exposed to infected blood especially those treating trauma victims. Potentially anything that involves exposure to infected blood can lead to infection. As it has not been possible to develop a vaccine yet, prevention relies on avoiding exposure to infected blood. Needle-exchange programs aim to lessen the sharing of needles. Education should be given at schools to avoid poorly controlled tattoo parlors or other unhygienic body piercing, acupuncture, and needlestick injuries, not to share toothbrushes, shaving equipment, or straws used for inhaling drugs, and to use condoms for casual sex.

herpes zoster   Also known as shingles and caused by the *Varicella zoster* virus, this is the cause of the common childhood illness chicken pox. Once the individual is over chicken pox, the virus is able to stay alive but dormant in the dorsal root ganglia. These ganglia are nodes along the large sensory nerves just before they enter the spinal cord. Later in life the virus can become reactivated, causing inflammation of that particular nerve (with severe pain) and a day or two later a rash in the area that the nerve serves. This is known as zoster or shingles and is most likely to occur when the individual's immune system is suppressed. Common reasons for this are older age (over 60 years), malignancy (especially lymphomas and leukemias), and immunosuppressive treatment. Both chicken pox and shingles can be very severe illnesses in those with poor immune function. The many clinical manifestations and treatment of this virus will not be discussed here. As far as rheumatic diseases are concerned, there are two main circumstances in which herpes zoster is important: immunosuppressive therapy and vasculitis.

• *Immunosuppressive Therapy*   Drugs such as CYCLO-PHOSPHAMIDE, AZATHIOPRINE, METHOTREXATE, and CYCLOSPORINE are often used to treat severe VASCULITIS or resistant RHEUMATOID ARTHRITIS and other inflammatory arthritis. Use of these drugs always requires a balance between suppressing the immune system enough to stop the damage it is causing and not suppressing it so much that the patient becomes too susceptible to infections. With the above drugs, zoster or shingles is often the first infection to occur and can serve as a warning that the immune system is oversuppressed. The number of white cells in the blood drops with immunosuppression, and shingles becomes more likely when the lymphocyte count drops below 0.6×10^9 per liter.

- *Vasculitis* Rarely, herpes zoster can cause a VAS-CULITIS. Unlike many other infectious causes of vasculitis, the zoster virus actually invades the lining cells of blood vessels, thereby provoking an immune response that damages the blood vessels.

hip pain The hip is a true ball-and-socket joint with the head of the femur (thigh bone) fitting into a round socket in the large pelvic bone. The joint is crossed by very powerful muscles that work to move the lower limb under the entire body weight or hold the body upright on one grounded leg while the other is in the air. It is also crossed by the nerves and blood vessels of the lower limb. Pain in the hip region may arise from the joint itself, the bones, the tendons, muscles, ligaments, and the bursas in the area or be referred there from elsewhere.

- *Joint Disease* Pain from the hip joint is usually felt in the groin but also characteristically radiates down the front of the thigh to the front of the knee. If it is long-standing, then the gait becomes abnormal, muscles weaken, and pain may be felt in a wider area. All the inflammatory forms of arthritis may affect the hip, especially ANKYLOSING SPONDYLITIS (often early on), REACTIVE ARTHRITIS, psoriatic arthritis (see PSO-RIASIS AND PSORIATIC ARTHRITIS), and RHEUMATOID ARTHRITIS (often quite late). These will usually be diagnosable by occurring in the context of disease elsewhere. OSTEOARTHRITIS frequently affects the hips, and farmers are at increased risk of this. If osteoarthritis of the hip is causing pain, X-rays will confirm its presence. GOUT may occasionally affect the hip joint, especially if there is already some degree of osteoarthritis, but this is an unusual joint to be affected by gout. Pseudogout or CPPD may affect the hip joint. Although rare, INFECTIVE ARTHRITIS such as TUBERCULOSIS can occur here. A fibrosing or scarring process affecting the joint capsule that usually occurs at the shoulder causing a frozen shoulder (see SHOULDER PAIN) can also affect the hip joint occasionally. This is more common in DIABETES.

- *Bone Disease* Regional osteoporosis is an unusual, painful form of OSTEOPOROSIS that quite commonly affects the head of the femur when it does occur. This is often during pregnancy. AVASCULAR NECROSIS often affects the head of the femur. PAGET'S DISEASE commonly affects the head of the femur, the pelvis, or both. Pain can result from the Paget's disease itself or the arthritis that results from the softer bone deforming and losing its congruity. Cancers may occasionally spread to the pelvis or upper femur and cause pain there. In OSTEOMALACIA it is not uncommon to get a specific type of insufficiency fracture called Looser's zones at the upper end of the shaft of the femur. Especially since there is often weakness of the surrounding muscles, osteomalacia can present as hip pain. Fractures of the hip are usually easily diagnosed because of the trauma that causes them, the inability to walk, and the abnormal position of the leg. However, in people with osteoporosis, they can sometimes occur with minimal trauma, and because the bones are not displaced, the individual can continue to walk. In these unusual situations an X-ray is required to make the diagnosis.

- *Soft Tissue Disease* A number of bursas around the hip commonly cause pain. People with inflammatory arthritis such as rheumatoid disease are more likely to get bursitis, but there are many causes. Weakness of the hip-stabilizing muscles leading to an abnormal gait is a common cause. This may develop due to lack of fitness, an increase in weight, or following pain in or injury to the back or a leg. It may also be the result of disease in the hip joint so that bursitis and hip arthritis not infrequently coexist. The most common bursas involved (TROCHANTERIC BURSITIS) are just above and below the greater trochanter. This is the bony point felt at the outermost part of the hip area. It is sometimes confused with the hip joint itself, which is actually several inches deeper than this point.

TENDINITIS may affect any tendon, but three specific tendons are worth mentioning. The tendon of the gluteus medius muscle (one of the large buttock muscles) is frequently stressed by the same conditions that cause bursitis around the greater trochanter, and tendinitis here is often confused with bursitis. It is important to correct the causative abnormality and strengthen the muscle to treat this tendinitis effectively. The other tendon in the hip area that can cause confusion is that of the iliopsoas muscle. The psoas muscle originates from the lower spine and runs through the pelvis, where it joins up with the iliac muscle coming off the inside of the pelvis. They form a common tendon that attaches to the upper femur. Especially in sports enthusiasts with faulty technique, a tendinitis with or without an associated bursitis can develop and cause pain that is felt deep in the groin. A bursitis here is not infrequent in rheumatoid arthritis. Since the pain worsens with movement, it can be thought to be arthritis of the hip joint unless a very careful examination is done. Adductor tendinitis causes pain at the inner upper thigh and is worsened by stretching the adductor muscles that run down the inner thigh. Horse riders are particularly prone to this, as are ballet dancers, martial arts practitioners, and other sportspeople.

- *Referred Pain*   Pain referred from the lower back may be felt at the back or side of the hip area. Pelvic abscesses or those at the back of the abdomen as well as some cases of appendicitis may refer pain to the hip, usually when they irritate the psoas muscle.

HIV   See HUMAN IMMUNODEFICIENCY VIRUS.

HLA   A genetic region that codes for tissue types and is important in determining whether a transplanted organ is accepted or rejected was identified and called the major histocompatibility complex (MHC). The MHC area in humans is on chromosome 6 and is called the HLA (human leukocyte antigen) region; it contains many genes involved in regulating an individual's immune response. The HLA region is divided into three regions called class I, II, and III.

HLA class I antigens include HLA-A, B, and C antigens. One of the best-known genetic markers of a rheumatic disease is the HLA-B27 tissue type, which is strongly associated with ANKYLOSING

SPONDYLITIS. At each location (locus) in the map of human genes are different possibilities (alleles) that can code for proteins that are virtually identical but differ in only a few amino acids. This slight difference can, however, change their function. Advances in molecular biology have led to the ability to subclassify genetic variants. For example, the HLA-B27 tissue type is now divided into subgroups such as HLA-B2701, HLA-B2702, and so on. More exact subclassification allows clearer identification of the genetic component of an illness. If we can obtain information about the differences in risk or severity of illness in people with different genetic variants, it will allow us to understand and predict better what having a particular genetic makeup (genotype) means for an individual.

HLA class II antigens are divided into DR, DQ, and DP antigens that are usually found on B lymphocytes and monocytes, although inflammation can induce their expression on other cells. DR antigens are classified into subgroups that can impart risks for different diseases. For example HLA-DRB1*0401 and *0404 are associated with rheumatoid arthritis in many ethnic groups.

Just as HLA antigens determine whether an organ transplanted from one person to another is likely to be accepted or rejected, so too they affect the immune response to other stimuli and thus alter disease susceptibility. HLA tissue type affects the development of T cells, the antigens they recognize, and the antigen peptides that are processed and presented to the immune system. One theory to explain the association between inherited HLA antigens and disease susceptibility is that part of a foreign molecule, for example a bacterium, could have a similar DNA code to an HLA molecule. Via this molecular mimicry an infection could trigger an immune reaction that targets both the bacterium and self-antigens, in other words, an autoimmune disease.

homeopathy   The name is derived from the Greek *homoios* meaning "like" and *pathos* meaning "suffering." This is taken to mean treating like with like. Practitioners of homeopathy trace their roots back to Theophrastus Bombastus von Hohenheim, otherwise known as Paracelsus, in the 16th century and Samuel Hahnemann in the 18th century. Despite studying medicine, Hahnemann became a translator of texts. While translating a text on treating malaria with quinine (still used), he began experimenting on himself with quinine and believed this caused the symptoms of malaria. He therefore developed his theory that giving a patient a substance that caused symptoms similar to the disease the patient was suffering from would bring about a cure.

Hahnemann then set about testing a wide variety of remedies on himself, his family, and his friends. Since some of these made people feel quite unwell, he started diluting his remedies until the side effects disappeared. At this point the effects disappeared as well. He is then said to have discovered that vigorous shaking of the by now extremely dilute remedy not only restored its effect but made it even more effective. He called this potentisation. Potentisation and treating like with like remain the cornerstones of homeopathy. Another key concept is that there is a vital force that was disturbed by illness. There are now several thousand homeopathic remedies that are used in such dilute preparations that they are extremely unlikely to retain a single molecule of the original substance.

Hahnemann wrote a book explaining why homeopathic treatment was effective for acute illnesses but not chronic ones. Some would argue that this is because many acute illnesses are self-limiting and will get better with or without treatment (e.g., most common viral infections), whereas chronic diseases (e.g., most common forms of arthritis) by definition will not. James Kent was largely responsible for spreading homeopathy in the United States, and Edward Bach promoted it in the first part of the 20th century in London, England. While there is no doubt that some homeopaths are and have been remarkable healers in the broadest possible sense of the word, there is nothing to suggest that homeopathic remedies have any effect.

homocystinuria A rare group of inherited enzyme deficiencies can lead to the accumulation of excessive amounts of the sulfur-containing amino acid homocysteine. Amino acids are the building blocks of proteins. High homocysteine levels interfere

with the way collagen links together. Collagen is important in forming connective tissues, which include tendons, ligaments, support for skin and other structures, as well as being an important constituent in bones and joints. Patients with homocystinuria may therefore develop problems from weakness of these structures.

The ligaments holding the eye lens in place are often affected, and 80 percent of patients develop dislocation of the lens. Half the patients have some reduction in intellectual capacity. OSTEOPOROSIS and HYPERMOBILITY SYNDROME are common. The vascular problems associated with homocystinuria are life-threatening. A quarter of patients die from vascular complications before the age of 30. These complications include blockage of arteries to the heart, kidneys, and brain, causing heart attack, kidney failure, and stroke, respectively.

The condition can be diagnosed by blood and urine tests, and some of the enzyme deficiencies can be identified from pieces of tissue. Successful treatment depends on early diagnosis. Special diets can then be introduced that restrict the amino acid methionine and provide extra cystine. Half of all patients respond partially to supplementation with pyridoxine, a B vitamin.

housewife's knee   See PREPATELLAR BURSITIS.

human immunodeficiency virus (HIV)   A retrovirus that infects T lymphocytes, replicates, damages the immune system, and causes AIDS (acquired immunodeficiency syndrome). In addition to the well-known infective complications of HIV infection, several musculoskeletal problems occur.

HIV is found in many body fluids, but infection is transmitted from person to person by sexual contact, by injection of blood or blood products, or by an infected mother to her child during pregnancy. HIV is not highly infectious and is not spread from person to person by casual contact. The cause of the rheumatic problems associated with HIV infection is not known, but there are several theories. One is that HIV itself triggers a local reaction that damages joints and muscles. In support of this idea, HIV can be found in inflamed joints. However, it is not clear that the presence of virus means that the HIV is causing the arthritis because the virus can be found in most parts of the body. Another theory is that HIV, because it suppresses the immune system, increases the frequency of infections and that some of these cause a REACTIVE ARTHRITIS. A third possibility is that the dysregulation of the immune system that occurs with HIV infection results in autoimmune rheumatic problems.

Symptoms and Diagnostic Path

The diagnosis of HIV infection is usually suspected when a patient develops an infection that would not otherwise occur in a person with a healthy immune system. There are several diagnostic blood tests. The most common one is an ELISA screening test, but a western blot or detecting the virus itself using polymerase chain reaction (PCR) are more specific. If a patient known to have HIV develops arthritis, few specific tests help diagnose its cause. If the clinical picture suggests that a direct infection of the joint may be the cause of the arthritis, then the joint will need to be aspirated and the fluid sent for culture. In patients suspected of having myositis or vasculitis, a biopsy of muscle or skin confirms these diagnoses.

Some patients have symptoms of acute HIV infection within days or weeks after infection. These symptoms are similar to those of many viral illnesses and include a nonspecific rash, fever, sore throat, headache, cough, flulike symptoms, mouth ulcers, diarrhea, enlarged lymph nodes, and arthralgia. The acute illness settles spontaneously over a few weeks and is followed by a period, which may last years, during which patients do not have symptoms. As the immune system becomes more severely affected, patients develop symptoms of AIDS such as loss of weight, diarrhea, enlarged lymph nodes, and opportunistic infections (infections that are not common in healthy people).

Most patients with HIV infection have nonspecific rheumatic symptoms like joint or muscle pain and fatigue over the course of their illness, but a minority also develops more specific musculoskeletal problems. These often occur months or years after the diagnosis of HIV infection but can sometimes be the first symptom leading to the diagnosis. The following musculoskeletal symptoms or syndromes, all of which also occur in patients without HIV infection and are discussed in detail elsewhere, can occur.

- ARTHRITIS and Reiter's syndrome
- PSORIASIS AND PSORIATIC ARTHRITIS
- INFECTIVE ARTHRITIS
- AVASCULAR NECROSIS
- VASCULITIS
- SJÖGREN'S SYNDROME
- SLE and OVERLAP SYNDROME
- MYOSITIS and RHABDOMYOLYSIS
- FIBROMYALGIA
- HYPERTROPHIC PULMONARY OSTEOARTHROPATHY

Arthralgia, arthritis, and Reiter's syndrome Arthralgia is a common nonspecific symptom that can occur in any chronic illness, but some patients with HIV develop attacks of acute severe joint pain without any swelling. These attacks of acute arthralgia often subside spontaneously over a few days. Several types of arthritis may occur. The most common is a type of arthritis that overlaps with reactive arthritis and Reiter's syndrome. Asymmetrical swelling of large joints such as knees and ankles and inflammation of tendons such as the Achilles tendon and of sites where tendons join bone (enthesitis) may occur. These are sometimes accompanied by other symptoms of Reiter's syndrome such as urethritis and conjunctivitis. Experts disagree whether the incidence of this type of arthritis is really increased by HIV infection. Some believe that HIV infection is often a marker for high-risk sexual behavior, and therefore the incidence of Reiter's syndrome would be expected to be higher because of this and not because of the HIV infection. The strongest argument against this point of view comes from studies performed in Africa where Reiter's syndrome and reactive arthritis were uncommon before the HIV epidemic but are now common medical problems, almost always occurring in patients with HIV infection. Reiter's syndrome in patients who do not have HIV infection is usually triggered by a clearly diagnosed infection such as diarrhea caused by salmonella or urethritis caused by chlamydia. However, in

HIV-associated arthritis a specific trigger is seldom identified. HIV-associated arthritis is usually treated with NONSTEROIDAL ANTI-INFLAMMATORY DRUGS to control pain and swelling. In most patients the arthritis settles over a few months, but in some it persists. There are no large scientific clinical trials to provide information how best to treat this type of arthritis. Clinical experience suggests that some patients with persistent arthritis respond to SULFASALAZINE, a drug also used to treat inflammatory bowel disease and rheumatoid arthritis, or to HYDROXYCHLOROQUINE. METHOTREXATE is avoided because some patients have developed Kaposi's sarcoma, a type of cancer that occurs more often in patients with HIV infection. If a single joint is particularly inflamed and bacterial infection of the joint has been excluded, it may respond to an intra-articular corticosteroid injection.

A handful of patients have developed a type of arthritis that is similar to rheumatoid arthritis with symmetrical inflammation of the small joints of the hand. It is not clear if this is just coincidence and rheumatoid arthritis has developed in a person who is also infected with HIV or if this is part of the spectrum of arthritis associated with HIV.

Psoriatic arthritis Severe psoriasis and psoriatic arthritis can occur for the first time after a person is infected with HIV. The rash is often pustular. The arthritis is typical of psoriatic arthritis with asymmetrical involvement of large joints such as the knee or smaller joints of the fingers or toes, causing *sausage digits*. Psoriatic arthritis in patients with HIV infection can be difficult to treat. Methotrexate, a drug that would usually be used to treat severe psoriatic arthritis, is avoided because it increases the risk of infection and may increase the risk of Kaposi's sarcoma. However, in severe cases, low-dose methotrexate as well as AZATHIOPRINE and SULFASALAZINE have been successfully used.

Infective arthritis Joint infections are more common in patients with HIV infection and are most commonly caused by a bacterium, *Staphylococcus areus,* the same organism that is often the cause of infective arthritis in patients without HIV infection. The symptoms and treatment are similar. Patients with HIV infection, because of immunosuppression, can have joint infection caused by unusual organisms, including fungi and mycobacteria. Intravenous drug users with HIV infection are more likely to get infected joints.

Avascular necrosis Some people who are infected with HIV get avascular necrosis (AVN) in bones, and this causes acute pain and eventually weakening of the bone. Scientists do not know how HIV causes AVN.

Vasculitis Most types of vasculitis have occurred in patients with HIV. Whether this is just coincidence or in some way related to the virus is not clear.

Sjögren's syndrome Patients with HIV infection can develop a condition similar to Sjögren's syndrome with enlargement of the salivary glands and symptoms of dry mouth and eyes. Sjögren's syndrome is caused by proliferation of CD4 lymphocytes in salivary glands and other tissues. The syndrome associated with HIV is caused by CD8 lymphocytes and is sometimes called diffuse infiltrative lymphocytosis syndrome (DILS). It can involve the lungs and cause difficulty breathing.

SLE overlap syndrome HIV infection does not cause SLE. In fact, because of the immunosuppression it causes, it may protect against it. Because many of the symptoms of HIV and SLE overlap, the two conditions can be mistaken. For example, fever, loss of weight, arthralgia, arthritis, facial rash, hair loss, glomerulonephritis, leukopenia, thrombocytopenia, seizures, coma, pneumonia, and a positive ANA blood test can occur in both. A false positive ELISA HIV test can occur in patients with SLE, but more specific tests for HIV are negative.

Myositis and rhabdomyolysis HIV is associated with several types of muscle disease. Myalgia (muscle aching) is very common but occurs with many chronic conditions. Severe loss of muscle mass occurs with advanced AIDS and in some countries was called *slim disease*. An illness very similar to DERMATOMYOSITIS AND POLYMYOSITIS with weakness of proximal muscles and elevated muscle enzymes can occur. Some of the drugs used to treat HIV can affect muscles, for example zidovudine (AZT) can cause myositis. Muscles are remarkably resistant to infection, but in patients with HIV infection abscesses can occur in big muscles such as those of the thigh (pyomyositis). Rhabdomyolysis with severe muscle damage, very high levels of muscle enzymes, dark urine caused by a protein called myoglobin (the result of muscle breakdown), and impaired kidney function have occurred in approximately 20 patients with HIV. Sometimes recognized causes of rhabdomyolysis such as prolonged seizures or drug therapy have been present, but in some cases HIV infection has been the only predisposing cause.

Fibromyalgia   Chronic pain, fatigue, and fibromyalgia are symptoms that occur more often in HIV infection and many other chronic illnesses.

Hypertrophic pulmonary osteoarthropathy (HPOA)   Chronic bacterial infection, particularly lung infection, can cause swelling of the ends of the fingers (clubbing) and pain and swelling at the end of long bones close to joints like the knee and wrist. Treatment of the infection improves the rheumatic symptoms.

Treatment Options and Outlook

HIV treatment has been revolutionized by highly active antiretroviral therapy (HAART), and the prognosis for affected patients has improved from almost certain death to a five-year survival rate of more than 90 percent. Treatment is prolonged and usually lifelong. It consists of combinations of drugs from different classes such as nucleoside analogs, protease inhibitors, and reverse transcriptase inhibitors. Measuring the amount of virus in the blood (viral load) can monitor the response to therapy. Many patients respond well to therapy, and the viral load can decrease to an undetectable level. However, treatment does not cure the infection and the viral load rapidly increases if treatment is stopped.

Risk Factors and Preventive Measures

HIV is transmitted by unprotected sex, sharing of needles, and from mother to child, either at birth or during breast-feeding. Careful testing of blood products has virtually eliminated this as a means of infection. Tattoos and body piercing are risk factors but less so than for HEPATITIS B. Although HIV may be found in other secretions such as saliva and tears, these have not been shown to transmit the infection. If the mother is known to be HIV-positive, giving antiretroviral drugs and then doing a cesarean section delivery will reduce the rate of transmission to about 1 percent from about 25 per-

cent for a normal delivery without antiretrovirals. Education at school about modes of transmission and the importance of not sharing needles, straws for inhaling recreational drugs, toothbrushes, shaving equipment, and the correct use of condoms is important. It should be noted that condom use only reduces the infection rate by 85 percent; it does not provide complete protection.

hypermobility syndrome   The occurrence of musculoskeletal symptoms in a hypermobile patient who does not have another recognizable generalized rheumatic disease. The exclusion of another rheumatic disease is important because many of the manifestations of hypermobility can also occur in people who do not have hypermobility, and it is more the number and wide range of problems that typifies this syndrome. Despite hypermobility first being described by Hippocrates more than 2,000 years ago, it is a difficult concept for many people and remains poorly understood and underdiagnosed. Hypermobility is a feature of many inherited disorders of connective tissue such as Marfan's and Ehlers-Danlos syndromes. These are considered to be separate from what is sometimes termed benign hypermobility syndrome.

Unusual looseness of the ligaments can be found, at least in one or two joints, in up to 10 percent of the population. It is particularly common in children and diminishes rapidly during childhood and then more slowly in adulthood. In general, African Americans have a greater range of joint movement than Caucasians, and Asians a greater range than African Americans. People with hypermobility will frequently have been called double-jointed as children and may make career choices as a result of their condition. All contortionists are hypermobile as are many ballet dancers. It should be emphasized that not everyone with hypermobility will develop problems because of it (see definition above).

Patients with the inheritable connective tissue diseases Ehlers-Danlos and Marfan's syndromes have reasonably clear-cut abnormalities in the makeup of their collagen or fibrillin (connective tissues). Very likely hypermobility syndrome has similar as yet undefined causes. Hypermobility syndrome often runs in families, and some differences in the make up of collagen have been shown in these families. The connective tissues form most of the substance of tendons, ligaments, and cartilage as well as supporting structures such as the skin, arteries, and heart valves. It is therefore these organs that show weakness or abnormal function if the connective tissue is slightly abnormal.

Symptoms and Diagnostic Path

The problems experienced by people with hypermobility syndrome can be divided into four groups.

- More traumatic and overuse injuries occur than average. These include partial or complete tendon or ligament tears, especially around the shoulder and ankle, and injury with inflammation at the attachment of ligaments and tendons to bone (enthesitis). Back pain is also common.

- The ligaments are looser than normal, thus joints may become unstable. This can lead to dislocation, either complete or partial (known as subluxation). Commonly affected joints are the shoulder, kneecaps, metacarpophalangeals, and jaw joint. Flat feet may be a manifestation of subluxed joints.

- A chronic arthritis develops. Usually this is OSTEOARTHRITIS, which is likely to develop earlier than average. A few patients also develop a mild inflammatory arthritis (see ARTHRITIS for the difference) that is secondary to the repeated trauma but is probably often misdiagnosed. Many people with hypermobility syndrome suffer from joint and muscle pain with no obvious abnormalities to be found on examination. If the hypermobility is not recognized, these people may be told there is nothing wrong with them and frustration and depression is then understandably common.

- Organs outside the musculoskeletal system may be affected. The skin may be thin and stretchy and develop striae (scarlike lines similar to those that women develop on their abdomens after pregnancy). Prolapse of the mitral valve may occur. This allows blood to leak back from the main pumping chamber in the heart (the left ventricle) to the collecting chamber (left atrium). Individuals with hypermobility syndrome prob-

ably have more abdominal hernias, rectal and vaginal prolapse, stress fractures, and the head of the thighbone pushing through the pelvic bone (protrusio acetabuli). A number of patients have a physical appearance similar to patients with Marfan's syndrome (marfanoid habitus).

Many different sets of criteria for diagnosing hypermobility syndrome are still used, although there have been international efforts to form an agreed method. The commonly used major criteria are a Beighton score (see below) of 4/9 or greater and joint pain in four or more joints for longer than three months. Marfan and Ehlers-Danlos syndromes must be excluded first. Beighton described a series of tests that led to a scoring system for generalized hypermobility. These are positive if the little finger bends back more than 90°, the thumb can be bent back to touch the forearm, the elbows and knees bend backward (hyperextend) excessively (score 1 for each side), and if the hands can be placed flat on the ground with the legs straight (score 1).

If either four out of nine Beighton criteria or pain in four joints are not present, minor criteria can be used to make the diagnosis, but more are needed. These include a Beighton score of less than 4, more than one joint dislocation, skin striae, recurrent tendon and ligament injuries, Marfan-like body build, mitral valve prolapse, and hernias or rectal prolapse.

Treatment Options and Outlook

The first step in managing hypermobility syndrome is actually to make the diagnosis and provide information about it. Many patients have suffered unexplained pain for some time, and understanding their condition can give considerable relief. An assessment of the impact on the patient's life should be made and sensible advice concerning career and recreational choices given. Treatable complications such as tendinitis are identified and treated as they occur. Special caution should be taken before embarking on surgical procedures due to poor tissue healing and the frequently disappointing results from surgery.

Ideally, the patient should be referred to a physical therapist with special experience in hypermobility, although such a person may not always be available. Physical therapy involves teaching the patient to recognize his or her (greater-than-normal) range of movement and do regular stretches through this range. Muscle strengthening, with most exercises done in the middle of the range of movement, and proprioceptive exercises (such as standing on a wobble board) have been shown to reduce pain in patients with hypermobility syndrome. Many patients with generalized hypermobility have flat feet, and appropriate use of orthotics is important. Acute pain is treated with analgesics and NSAIDs, and chronic pain may require use of low doses of antidepressants and/or COGNITIVE BEHAVIORAL THERAPY.

The outcome for individual patients will vary considerably. Some people may be troubled by so-called growing pains as children and then grow out of it as their tissues tighten up with aging. Others with severe hypermobility may experience many of the problems listed above; develop hip, knee, and back problems in early adulthood; and go on to get early osteoarthritis.

Risk Factors and Preventive Measures

Although benign hypermobility syndrome is thought to result from minor genetic changes in collagen, these remain poorly understood. There are no known preventive measures.

hypertrophic pulmonary osteoarthropathy (HPOA)

A condition involving abnormal growth of skin and the outer coating of bone (periosteum) most commonly in the hands and wrists and feet and ankles. There is a rare inherited primary form, but HPOA is more commonly secondary to a tumor or heart or liver disease. The primary form is called pachydermoperiostitis, and there will usually be a family history. It results from a deficiency in an enzyme that breaks down prostaglandin E2 (PGE2), leading to abnormally high levels of PGE2. High PGE2 levels have also been found in some patients with the secondary form.

This can lead to quite rapid onset of pain that usually affects hands, wrists, and ankles but also occasionally the elbows and knees. Typically the area around the nail bed becomes swollen, giving the fingers a drumstick appearance, a finding called clubbing. The pain may be described as deep and burning, and there may be associated sweating in the hands and feet. The affected areas are mildly swollen, warm, and dusky red. A careful examination may show that the swelling extends beyond the joint margins and that the ends of the long bones are exquisitely tender.

HPOA is most frequently caused by lung cancer and may present some months before the cancer becomes apparent. Other tumors in the chest region, both benign and malignant, can cause it as can chronic infections of the lung and heart valves. Occasionally inflammatory conditions affecting the liver or bowel are the cause. The diagnosis is usually made on the characteristic findings on X-Ray of lifting of the outer layer of the affected bones, termed periostitis. The ESR is raised, but if fluid is removed from a joint the appearances are not inflammatory.

Successful treatment of the underlying cause results in prompt improvement in HPOA. Painkillers and NSAIDs are helpful. The outcome depends on whether the underlying cause is treatable.

hypnosis During hypnosis the subject passes into a trance. This is an altered state of consciousness in which the subject's attention is intensely focused while attention to other stimuli is reduced. It is not a deep sleep or unconsciousness. The subject is awake and can respond to the therapist. Perception, memory, behavior, and suggestibility are altered. In therapy the increased suggestibility can be used to influence behavior and feelings. Hypnotherapists claim benefit in chronic pain and chronic fatigue syndrome among many other medical and psychological problems. About 85 percent of the population are hypnotizable. A typical therapeutic hypnosis session will go through six stages:

1. An introduction explaining what hypnosis is and is not and answering the patient's questions and concerns
2. Induction
3. Deepening of the trance using two or three deepening techniques
4. The therapeutic work, which may include ego strengthening, addressing a specific problem,

and suggestions for behaviors following the hypnosis (posthypnotic suggestion)

5. Dehypnotizing
6. Debriefing

Hypnosis should not be performed on people with psychoses, severe depression, or drug abuse, if the subject is opposed to it (for example on religious grounds), or if the problem being addressed is beyond the therapist's competence.

hypophosphatemic rickets An inherited condition in which the kidneys do not reabsorb phosphate normally, resulting in an excessive loss in the urine. This leads to a condition similar to rickets but does not respond to vitamin D (as rickets would). Patients are usually short with poor teeth development and as adults develop OSTEOMALACIA (weak bones). Hypophosphatemic rickets is one of the causes of CPPD and also results in calcification of ligaments and new bone formation around joints. Both calcium and phosphate levels in the blood are low, and urinary phosphate levels are inappropriately high. Treatment is with large amounts of phosphate by mouth together with an activated form of vitamin D.

ice A therapy used to alleviate musculoskeletal symptoms. Physical therapy often involves the application of heat or cold (see HEAT) to relieve symptoms and improve function. The major symptom of arthritis, painful swollen joints, can sometimes be improved by local application of icepacks. Ice can be applied directly, but this is messy. Many patients prefer to use a packet of frozen vegetables to apply the cold for 10 to 20 minutes. Some patients with chronic arthritis find that application of cold makes their symptoms worse. Acute trauma such as sporting injuries to joints, muscles, tendons, and ligaments are treated with rest, ice, compression, and elevation (RICE).

Cold and pain messages are transmitted through different nerve fibers, but traffic in one group of nerves could decrease transmission through others, thus decreasing pain. Also, if the sensation of superficial cold is strong, it can distract the brain from processing pain messages from joints. Cold causes blood vessels to constrict, decreasing blood flow to the inflamed area and thus decreasing swelling and heat.

Provided ice is not applied for too long, it is safe. A few patients develop urticaria after exposure to cold, but this usually resolves without treatment. Ice treatment is avoided in patients with RAYNAUD'S PHENOMENON because it worsens their symptoms.

idiopathic thrombocytopenic purpura See THROMBOCYTOPENIA.

immune response A complex system of related defenses against foreign organisms. Immunity is innate and acquired. The innate immune response can act immediately and does not require previous exposure to an organism or the production of antibodies. Innate immunity is provided by phagocytic cells that engulf and digest invading organisms; as well as a particular type of lymphocyte called the natural killer or NK cell. Acquired immunity is targeted against specific parts of organisms called antigens that the immune system recognizes as being foreign. It has two components, humoral and cellular immunity. The COMPLEMENT system is an important part of the immune response. Complement helps the process of ingestion and destruction of foreign organisms that have been coated with antibody as well as recruiting inflammatory cells to sites of inflammation.

The cause of many rheumatological conditions, for example RA and SLE, is not known. However, because antibodies (rheumatoid factor and antinuclear antibody [ANA], respectively) against normal components of the body occur, they are considered autoimmune diseases. The presence of autoantibodies does not automatically imply the presence of an autoimmune disease, for example low levels of ANA are common in healthy people. Some autoantibodies do not cause damage directly but may do so when they bind to complement and lodge in tissues such as the kidney. Others directed against a patient's cells can damage them. For example antiplatelet antibodies can cause THROMBOCYTOPENIA. Why autoantibodies develop and cause disease in some people is not clear. One theory is that autoreactive T cells that are normally destroyed in the thymus gland escape destruction and trigger an autoimmune response. Another is that the ability of the immune system to tolerate self-antigens is broken down.

Innate immunity Several different types of phagocytic cells are important mediators of innate immunity. Monocytes are a type of white blood cell that circulate in the bloodstream and move into inflamed tissues where they change their structure a little and are called macrophages. These mononuclear cells are important phagocytic cells, but they also serve another important function. They ingest and break up foreign proteins into smaller pieces. These pieces (antigens) are then carried to the surface of the cell where they may be recognized by T cells. Because of this function they are sometimes called antigen-presenting cells. Neutrophils, also called polymorphonuclear leukocytes or polys make up 80 percent of the circulating white blood cell population and are important phagocytic cells that also contain enzymes that are able to kill and digest ingested cells. NK cells are also called large granular lymphocytes and are T cells that are able to phagocytose invading cells. People with a deficiency of NK cells have an increased risk of viral infection.

Humoral immunity B lymphocytes that produce immunoglobulins mediate humoral immunity. These proteins are also called antibodies and are targeted at antigens on invading cells that the body recognizes as foreign. There are five major subtypes of immunoglobulins, IgG, IgA, IgM, IgE, and IgD, that have different properties. For example, IgM is produced rapidly after an antigen is recognized and IgA is produced mainly by lymphocytes in the gut and other mucosal surfaces.

When B cells are exposed to an antigen, they proliferate and differentiate into activated B cells that produce antibodies that bind to the antigen and neutralize it. Some B cells become memory cells so that when they come across the same antigen at a later time, they are able to recognize it rapidly, multiply, and produce antibodies.

Cellular immunity T lymphocytes that produce CYTOKINES and other mediators to inhibit or stimulate other immune cells to carry out the immune response largely mediate cellular immunity. T and B lymphocytes look similar under a microscope, but they can be differentiated by markers on their surface. These markers can be detected by antibodies and cells categorized into subtypes designated CD (cluster of differentiation) types. Most T cells are CD4 (helper cells) or CD8 (cytotoxic/suppressor) cells. The importance of CD4 cells in the body's defense against infec-tion is illustrated by the susceptibility of HIV patients with depleted CD4 cell counts to a range of infections.

immunodeficiency A state in which the body's ability to fight infection is decreased. Immunodeficiency can be primary, caused by genetic abnormalities, or secondary, due to drugs or infections that affect the number or function of white blood cells (see IMMUNE RESPONSE). The major complication of immunodeficiency is increased susceptibility to infection. Patients who are unable to make antibodies efficiently (deficient B lymphocyte or humoral immunity) are particularly susceptible to recurrent bacterial infections. Those with a decreased cellular immunity (deficient T lymphocyte or cell-mediated immunity) have a greater chance of getting viral or fungal infections.

Primary immunodeficiencies are a group of disorders caused by genetic defects that affect the function of the immune system. Many of the primary immunodeficiencies are also associated with an increased risk of developing malignancy and autoimmune disease.

A drug, infection, or radiation usually causes secondary immunodeficiency. This suppresses or damages bone marrow and decreases the number of white blood cells or affects their function. Human immunodeficiency virus (HIV) infection is the most common cause of immunodeficiency worldwide. In countries where HIV infection is less common, the common causes are cancer chemotherapy and immunosuppressive treatment to prevent rejection after organ transplantation. Many serious rheumatic diseases such as VASCULITIS are treated aggressively with drugs such as CORTICOSTEROIDS and CYCLOPHOSPHAMIDE that suppress the immune system and increase the risk of infection. Several other conditions such as diabetes, decreased kidney or liver function, malnutrition, and severe burns also suppress the immune system.

Cause of Primary Immunodeficiencies

These rare inherited illnesses are subdivided into several subgroups classified according to whether their main effect is on antibody production, cellular immunity, or both.

Combined immunodeficiencies Patients have defects that affect both cellular and antibody components of the immune response. Symptoms usually start in the first years of life with serious, recurrent infections. Without treatment these diseases are often fatal in infancy. Several different genetic conditions cause a similar clinical picture. For example, severe combined immunodeficiency (SCID) is caused by mutations in the interleukin-2 receptor, and adenosine deaminase (ADA) deficiency is caused by mutations in the gene coding for the enzyme adenosine deaminase.

Disorders in which antibody deficiency predominates Patients can have defective antibody formation because B lymphocytes either do not develop or do not function normally. Immunoglobulin A (IgA) deficiency is the most common primary immunodeficiency. It affects approximately one in 700 Caucasians and results in absent or very low levels of IgA. The range of symptoms and severity is wide. Some people are completely healthy, and others have recurrent sinus, lung, and gastrointestinal infections. Another disorder is common variable immunodeficiency (CVID), with an estimated incidence of between one in 50,000 and one in 200,000. It affects men and women and is often diagnosed only in early adulthood. The symptoms are recurrent sinus and lung infections, diarrhea, and autoimmune disease. Infections with *Streptococcus pneumoniae* and *Haemophilus influenzae* are frequent, but infections with other organisms occur. In CVID levels of all antibodies are decreased, but because another function of B cells is to signal T cells, T cell responses (cell-mediated immunity) can also be affected. IgA deficiency is increased in the families of people with CVID, and there are families where some members have CVID and others IgA deficiency.

Rheumatic Symptoms and Primary Immunodeficiencies

Autoantibodies occur more often in patients with primary immunodeficiencies than in healthy people, and autoimmune illness can occur. This is most common in CVID, affecting approximately 20 percent of patients. A range of autoimmune disorders can occur, including thyroid disease, hematological disease, polyarthritis resembling RHEUMATOID ARTHRITIS, SYSTEMIC LUPUS ERYTHEMATOSUS, and SJÖGREN'S SYNDROME. The arthritis associated with CVID is usually chronic and affects knees, wrists, ankles, and fingers but unlike rheumatoid arthritis does not cause erosions of bone. In the primary immunodeficiencies there is an increased risk of developing lymphoma.

The treatment for the primary immunodeficiencies associated with severe T cell or enzyme defects is bone marrow transplantation. In patients with defective antibody production immunoglobulin replacement therapy with intravenous immunoglobulin (IVIG) decreases the risk of infections.

inclusion body myositis (IBM) This form of inflammatory muscle disease (compare with DERMATOMYOSITIS AND POLYMYOSITIS) was discovered just over 30 years ago. Since then it has been increasingly recognized and is now the most common muscle disease in people over the age of 50 years. It occurs mostly in older people and is more frequent in men.

The cause is unknown. Biopsy of involved muscle shows characteristic pinkish-colored inclusions and rimmed vacuoles (cavities) under the ordinary microscope. There are also some lymphocytes invading the muscle and wasting of some muscle fibers. The electron microscope shows the inclusions to be filaments just like those found in the brains of people with Alzheimer's disease. Further investigations have shown that they contain beta-amyloid protein as in Alzheimer's. While this does not identify what is causing the disease, it does throw light on the process of muscle damage. It should be stressed that patients with IBM are not more likely to develop Alzheimer's disease.

Symptoms and Diagnostic Path

Weakness in affected muscle groups is the main problem. Unlike other inflammatory muscle disease, the weakness of IBM comes on very slowly. Although, like polymyositis, it affects the muscles around the hips and shoulders, IBM is distinct in also affecting the muscles of the forearms and lower legs. Characteristic problems are weakness in gripping objects and in lifting the toes and feet upward. Weakness and thinning of the quadriceps muscles (large muscle group in front of thigh) is also very characteristic of IBM. Some patients develop signs of nerve damage as well.

There is usually a slow increase in weakness over a period of years. The muscles used for swallowing are often affected later on, and this can cause not only problems with getting adequate nutrition but also recurrent chest infections.

Because of the very gradual onset of weakness, the diagnosis is often delayed. Indeed, deciding when the disease actually started can be very difficult. When the disease is established, the characteristic distribution of the muscles affected should suggest the diagnosis in an older individual. A good muscle biopsy, examined by electron microscopy as well as routine light microscopy, should confirm the diagnosis, showing the changes described under Cause above. The biopsy will also show the extent of scarring and replacement of muscle tissue with fat.

Other tests may give supportive evidence. The enzymes released by damaged muscle can be measured in the blood and are usually only slightly raised. Creatine phosphokinase is the most useful of these. However, these tests are normal in 20 percent of patients. Very high levels, on the other hand, suggest a different diagnosis. Electromyography, involving measurement of electrical activity by putting very fine needles into muscle, may suggest the diagnosis by showing abnormalities not usually found in inflammatory muscle disease as well as evidence of nerve damage. Occasionally the antinuclear antibody test is positive but this is not typical.

Treatment Options and Outlook

The treatment of IBM is difficult. One reason is the very slow progression of the disease so that it can take over a year to be sure that the treatment is working or not. Another is that much of the weakness is degenerative (accelerated aging) in nature and not inflammatory, and only the inflammation can be treated. Early attempts to treat the disease with CORTICOSTEROIDS (effective in other forms of MYOSITIS) were not successful. In many patients the weakness actually seemed to get worse. Corticosteroids are of course recognized to cause muscle weakness as a long-term side effect. In the 1990s

however, it became clear that up to half of patients show some response to immunosuppressive treatment. In IBM response means that the deterioration stops or slows down rather than the patient returning to normal strength.

Because IBM is uncommon and the response to treatment not dramatic, doing good controlled CLINICAL TRIALS is difficult. Therefore, treatment recommendations are necessarily based on inadequate information. Between 30 and 50 percent of IBM patients respond to immunosuppression with AZATHIOPRINE or METHOTREXATE. Trying treatment early on in the course of the disease before too much muscle is damaged is best. Although people with higher muscle enzyme levels (and therefore presumably more inflammation) at the start of treatment have a better response rate, the degree of their physical improvement is not related to the improvement in enzyme levels. Responders should continue with therapy long term. If no response to treatment is seen, it is best withdrawn to prevent possible side effects. A progressive resistance strength-training program is safe and effective. Very few patients have been treated for more than five to 10 years, and it remains to be seen how successful treatment is in prolonging the health and life expectancy of those who respond.

A number of other immunosuppressive agents have been tried in small numbers of patients without notable success. These include CYCLOSPORINE, CYCLOPHOSPHAMIDE, and intravenous immunoglobulin. Most patients require assistance with normal daily activities between five and 10 years after diagnosis. Eventually they become wheelchair dependent or bed bound. Progress is quite variable, however, and some patients remain independent after 20 years.

Risk Factors and Preventive Measures

There are no known risk factors or preventive measures for this condition.

infective arthritis (infectious arthritis) Arthritis caused by a foreign organism infecting a joint. Several viral infections (see VIRAL ARTHRITIS) cause arthritis. Whether this is caused by direct infection of joints or by a reaction to the virus is not clear.

Bacteria are the most frequent cause of infective arthritis, but given the right conditions, virtually any organism can infect a joint. Bacterial arthritis is sometimes called septic arthritis. Infection with the spirochete *Borrelia burgdorferi* can cause arthritis (see LYME DISEASE).

For an organism to infect a joint two things have to happen. First, the organism has to reach the joint. Second, the organism has to multiply in the joint. Usually joints are sterile with no organisms present and have excellent defenses to protect against the few organisms that might settle there. Organisms can reach a joint by (1) direct penetration, for example trauma such as surgery or an intra-articular injection; (2) traveling in the bloodstream to the joint from another infected site, for example pneumonia, meningitis, and gonorrhea can be complicated by septic arthritis; and (3) spreading from a nearby skin or bone infection into the closest joint. Several conditions increase the chance of a joint getting infected.

- *Immunosuppression* Any condition that decreases the immune response (see IMMUNODEFICIENCY) will increase the risk of infective arthritis. This is because the body's immune defenses and those in the joints are suppressed, and therefore, organisms are more likely to gain access to the joint through the bloodstream and multiply.

- *Trauma* Joint damage from any cause increases the risk of infective arthritis, but injuries or procedures that penetrate the joint are particularly high risk. If something that is contaminated with bacteria penetrates the joint, infection is likely. Penetrating injuries of this type contaminate the joint with a bacterial load that its defenses cannot overcome and occur most often in motor vehicle and other accidents and in warfare. Penetration of the joint by a sterile medical instrument, for example as occurs in JOINT INJECTION or ARTHROSCOPY, is very low risk.

- *Arthritis* Any type of arthritis damages a joint and increases the chances that bacteria circulating in the bloodstream will be able to settle in a joint and infect it. RHEUMATOID ARTHRITIS is the most common risk factor for developing infective arthritis.

- *Artificial Joint* The metal and plastic hardware used to replace a joint does not have natural defenses against infection, and prosthetic joints are more likely to become infected than natural ones.

- *Infection* If someone has an infection in another site, organisms will more likely circulate in the bloodstream, settle in a joint, and cause infection. This can happen with virtually any infection, including pneumonia, urinary tract infection, meningitis, diverticulitis, and INFECTIVE ENDOCARDITIS. Intravenous drug users who inject drugs that are not sterile have low levels of circulating bacteria that need not cause systemic infection but can settle in joints and infect them.

Virtually any organism can infect a joint, but gram-positive bacterial infections occur most frequently. *Staphylococcus aureus* is the most common cause of bacterial arthritis in both natural and prosthetic joints in adults. *Haemophilus influenzae* is a common cause of septic arthritis in children aged one to five years, but the introduction of routine vaccination of children in the United States against this infection has decreased the frequency. Infections with gram-negative bacteria occur more often in the elderly, children, patients who are immunosuppressed, and intravenous drug users. *Neisseria gonorrhoeae*, the organism that causes gonorrhea, is a common cause of septic arthritis in young, sexually active adults. Septic arthritis is usually caused by a single organism but about 10 percent of infections are caused by several organisms. Such polymicrobial infection is more likely after penetrating injury or surgery to a joint and in patients who have polymicrobial infection elsewhere, for example in the abdomen after rupture of a diverticulum.

Mycobacterium tuberculosis, the organism that causes TUBERCULOSIS, is a common cause of infective arthritis in countries with high rates of tuberculosis infection. Arthritis caused by other mycobacteria and by fungi are rare and usually occur only in patients with immunodeficiency. Other types of mycobacteria, called atypical mycobacteria, can also cause arthritis.

Fungal arthritis Several types of fungi can rarely cause arthritis in immunosuppressed patients. These include *Coccidiodes immitis, Histoplasma capsulatum, Blastomyces, Aspergillus, Cryptococcus,* and *Candida.*

Symptoms and Diagnostic Path

Bacterial arthritis Symptoms usually start suddenly and are often severe. In 80–90 percent of patients only one joint is infected. The knee is infected in 50 percent of patients, but hip, wrist, shoulder, and elbow infection are common. Infection of the sternoclavicular joint, where the collarbone joins the breastbone, is more likely in intravenous drug addicts. An infected joint throbs and becomes red, hot, swollen, and very painful. It is difficult for the patient to bend or move the joint at all. There are often systemic symptoms such as fever, but elderly and immunosuppressed patients can have septic arthritis with a normal temperature.

Gonococcal arthritis Gonococcal infection of the genital organs can spread to involve the joints and causes somewhat different symptoms. Usually it infects the joint by spreading through the bloodstream; this is called disseminated gonococcal infection. There is often a rash, which may range from large purple spots to small inconspicuous blisters about the size of the head of a match. Two types of arthritis can occur. The first affects several joints, can migrate from one joint to another, and often occurs with inflammation of tendons (tenosynovitis). The second is much more similar to classical septic arthritis and infects a single joint. Some experts believe these types of arthritis are different stages of one process that first affects many sites and then localizes in one joint. The genital gonorrhea infection usually causes symptoms of urethritis (burning when urinating and a discharge at the end of the penis) in men, but women may carry an infection without knowing it. Disseminated gonococcal infection is more common in women and is more frequent at the time of menstruation.

Tuberculous or fungal arthritis These types of arthritis do not cause acute symptoms but, rather, slow and progressive arthritis with swelling, warmth, and pain in a single joint. Tuberculosis is particularly likely to affect the spine, and then it causes back pain localized to one area.

Diagnosis If a patient develops a rapid onset of pain, redness, and swelling in a joint, there are only a few likely causes. These include infective arthritis, trauma, and arthritis caused by crystals (see GOUT or CALCIUM PYROPHOSPHATE DIHYDRATE DEPOSITION DISEASE). Acute gout can be indistinguishable from septic arthritis. In both conditions a single joint is red, hot, swollen, and acutely tender, and the patient may have fever and an elevated white blood cell count and erythrocyte sedimentation rate. X-rays are often normal and unhelpful in the early stages, the time when making the correct diagnosis is most important. A bone scan will show increased concentration of the radioisotope in the infected joint, but this also occurs with inflammation without infection so it is not helpful in differentiating the two. MRI is helpful to evaluate pain in deep joints such as the hip.

Clues to diagnosis of septic arthritis are a history that the joint has been punctured, infection at another site, a prosthetic joint, and preexisting arthritis. The diagnosis can be difficult in patients with rheumatoid arthritis because in RA a single joint can sometimes become much more painful and swollen than others, without being infected. The most reliable way to make the diagnosis of septic arthritis, and the only way to exclude it, is for a physician to aspirate synovial fluid (see JOINT ASPIRATION in Appendix II) and send it to be examined and cultured. Synovial fluid in septic arthritis is often white or yellow and looks like pus. Many polymorphonuclear white blood cells are present. If the fluid is stained and examined under a microscope, bacteria may be visible in 50 percent of cases. The bacteria may take one to five days to grow in culture, and therefore, antibiotic treatment is usually started before the culture result is available if septic arthritis is strongly suspected. However, culture is still the most accurate way to diagnose septic arthritis and identify the responsible organisms. Joint fluid should also be examined for crystals, because if these are present it suggests that the diagnosis may be gout or pseudogout rather than septic arthritis. However, infection may occasionally coexist with gout.

The diagnosis of gonococcal arthritis is not as straightforward. It may be suspected because of the patient's lifestyle and the presence of a rash. Sometimes the diagnosis is confirmed when the gonococcus is cultured from the blood or synovial fluid. However, in many patients synovial fluid cultures are negative, but the bacterium can be cultured from other sites such as the urethra, cervix, and vagina even though patients may not have symptoms there. The organism can be difficult to culture unless special techniques are used.

The diagnosis of tuberculous or fungal arthritis is usually suspected if there is a destructive arthritis in a single joint that progresses slowly over weeks. The X-rays are often abnormal by the time a patient consults a physician. In spinal tuberculosis there can be destruction of the body of a vertebra, the disc between two vertebrae, and an abscess alongside the spine. Diagnosis requires the culture of the organism, sometimes from synovial fluid but more often from a synovial biopsy.

Treatment Options and Outlook

The principles of treatment are aggressive, appropriate antibiotic therapy and drainage of the infected synovial fluid. Antibiotics are usually given intravenously for the first week or two to ensure that blood levels are high. Once an infection is under control oral antibiotics can be used. The choice of antibiotic ideally depends on the identity of the infecting organism. However, when treatment is started before the results of the joint fluid cultures are back from the laboratory, a choice is made based on the most likely organism in that setting and the appearance of organisms seen under the microscope. The initial antibiotic therapy is usually chosen to cover staphylococcal infection and is often cephazolin for infections that started in the community and vancomycin for infections acquired in a hospital. If a gram-negative infection is suspected, different antibiotics are selected or another antibiotic is added to broaden the spectrum of organisms covered. Once an organism is cultured from the joint fluid, then the antibiotic treatment can be changed to target that organism specifically. Antibiotic treatment often lasts four to six weeks.

Joint fluid can usually be drained by aspirating it through a needle. This may need to be repeated if the fluid reaccumulates. The number of white blood cells in the synovial fluid decreases as the infection responds to treatment. Completely draining a joint using a needle can sometimes be difficult because the fluid is thick and accumulates in pockets. If this happens ARTHROSCOPY is often performed to drain the fluid. Because draining the hip joint through a needle is difficult, surgical drainage is usually performed, either directly or by arthros copy. The outcome of septic arthritis varies a lot depending on the causative organism, how long the infection has been present, and the response to antibiotic therapy. Gonococcal arthritis usually responds rapidly and completely to treatment, while staphylococcal infection responds much more slowly and often causes permanent joint damage. The outcome is worst in patients with other serious medical problems, immunosuppression, and polymicrobial infection.

Prosthetic joints In patients with infected artificial joints the joint often needs to be surgically removed to allow the antibiotics to clear the infection. Prolonged antibiotic therapy, often for many months, is required to clear such an infection. If the infection clears, the surgeon may be able to reoperate and put in a new artificial joint.

Tuberculous or fungal arthritis Tuberculous arthritis requires standard treatment with a combination of drugs used to treat tuberculosis. Fungal arthritis is treated with an antifungal drug that is selected according to the sensitivity of the organism.

Risk Factors and Preventive Measures

As discussed above in more detail, the risk factors for joint infection include immunosuppression, trauma, inflammatory arthritis, an artificial joint, and infection circulating in the bloodstream. For major joint surgery where the joint will be open to the atmosphere for a long time, most modern hospitals have laminar flow air-conditioning in theater with very fine air filters to reduce the risk of infection. There are also well-established antiseptic procedures for the theatre staff. Injections into joints are very safe but should not be done in patients with a bacteremia (active infection with bacteria in bloodstream) or with infected skin nearby. Needle exchange programs and controlled methadone programs for addicts may reduce infection in intravenous drug users.

There are no recognized preventive measures for the many other possible joint infections discussed above.

infective endocarditis This is an infection of the inner lining of the heart, usually involving one of the valves that controls the flow of blood through the heart. Of people who develop infective endocarditis, 75 percent have a previously damaged heart valve. This can be following previous RHEUMATIC FEVER, an aortic valve with two rather than the normal three cusps, a leaking mitral valve (mitral valve prolapse), congenital heart disease, or an artificial heart valve. Others at risk of developing infective endocarditis include intravenous drug users and those with long-standing intravenous lines for various reasons such as intravenous feeding and chemotherapy.

Subacute endocarditis is caused by organisms that are usually not very effective at causing infections. However, if they are physically introduced into the bloodstream and land on an abnormal valve, they may do so. Even in these circumstances infection is rather unusual. The most common such organism is *Streptococcus viridans*, which may enter the bloodstream after dental work or because of infected gums. Instrumentation or surgery on the bowel or genitourinary system may introduce organisms that live in those areas such as *Escherichia coli, faecalis*, and *bovis*. Other bacteria include *Streptococcus pyogenes, Haemophilus parainfluenza, Neisseria, Pseudomonas*, and *Brucella*.

Acute endocarditis is caused by vigorous organisms that cause severe infections and often affect previously normal heart valves. The most common of these is *S. aureus*, which is frequently found on human skin and may be introduced by putting needles in veins or injections.

Culture-negative endocarditis refers to those patients in whom the blood cultures do not grow any organisms. This may be because the patient has been given antibiotics before being investigated (e.g., when another doctor has not suspected the diagnosis of endocarditis) or because the infection is with an unusual organism that does not grow easily. These include chlamydiae, rickettsias, fungi, and *Brucella*.

Symptoms and Diagnostic Path
Acute endocarditis is a dramatic life-threatening illness with fever and rapidly worsening heart failure. Subacute endocarditis comes on more slowly, often with a low-grade fever, loss of appetite, weight loss, feeling generally unwell, and shortness of breath. Joint pain is common as the disease progresses.

The infection causes little collections of cells and debris on the valves (vegetations) that can break off and cause a stroke; gangrene of finger, toe, or even limb; or block other important blood vessels. Anemia and heart failure develop, and small amounts of blood in the urine are common. Changes in the hands such as flat red spots, tender lumps at the ends of fingers, little black splinter-like bleeds under the fingernails, and a curving over of the nails (clubbing) are very characteristic and, once present, lead to the diagnosis.

Arthralgia and back pain are common in infective endocarditis, but arthritis occurs less often. Sometimes this is due to the organisms settling in the joint as well as on the heart valve and causing septic arthritis (see INFECTIVE ARTHRITIS). More often the arthritis is not due to direct infection of joints and the synovial fluid is sterile. Knees and ankles are most often affected.

No diagnostic test is available. The diagnosis must be suspected in any patient with an unexplained fever and a heart murmur and then as much evidence as possible gathered, some of it before treatment is started. At least three separate lots of blood should be taken to try to grow the organism, and this should be done before antibiotics are given. Blood tests show anemia and a raised white cell count. The ESR and C-reactive protein (markers of inflammation) are raised. Special antibody-based tests may detect the presence of unusual infections such as chlamydiae, rickettsias, and *Brucella*. Rheumatoid factor may become positive.

Examination of the urine may show small amounts of blood and protein. The EKG may be abnormal or may just show a rapid heart rate. Echocardiography is a method of scanning the heart using the echoes of sound waves (ultrasound) and may show the vegetations on the valves, leaking valves, or just the preexisting abnormalities. This is usually done by placing a probe on the chest wall. In difficult cases, though, better pictures can be obtained by passing a probe down the esophagus or gullet and scanning the heart from behind.

Treatment Options and Outlook

Once the diagnosis is made, best bet antibiotics are started until organisms are grown from the blood and tested against specific antibiotics to indicate the optimal treatment. Successful treatment should lower the temperature in 10 days and the C-reactive protein within two weeks. Especially in acute endocarditis there may be severe damage to the valve, and emergency surgery may be the only way to save the patient's life. Despite the advances in antibiotics and surgery, nearly one in five patients with infective endocarditis dies. Rapid diagnosis, being able to grow the causative organism, and access to urgent surgery when needed are the most important ways of preventing death.

Following successful treatment, the risk of reinfection should be assessed and reduced. For example, teeth may require removal if they are the source of bacterial infection and preventive antibiotics should be given at the time of minor surgery.

Risk Factors and Preventive Measures

There are no risk factors or prevention for acute infective endocarditis, which is an unpredictable and devastating disease. Subacute infective endocarditis usually develops in people with a previously abnormal heart valve. This can be due to previous rheumatic fever, congenitally abnormal valves, or those that become abnormal because of hypermobility or ANTIPHOSPHOLIPID ANTIBODY SYNDROME. In these cases, the bacteria sometimes enter after a defined procedure. Previously an injection of appropriate antibiotics was given to many people with abnormal heart valves 30 to 60 minutes before they had dental work, gastroenterological or urological endoscopic procedures, or other surgery to prevent bacteria that entered the bloodstream from settling on the heart valve and causing infection. In 2008, the American College of Cardiology and American Heart Association dramatically revised their guidelines to the effect that only patients with the highest risk heart valves should receive antibiotic prophylaxis and then only for dental work that caused some injury to the gum or lining of the mouth. No prophylaxis is required for most gastroenterological or urological procedures. This recommendation has not been universally accepted.

inflammatory bowel disease (IBD)   A term that describes two illnesses, ulcerative colitis and Crohn's disease, both of which cause chronic inflammation of the bowel and sometimes associated arthritis. There are ethnic and geographic differences in frequency. IBD is rare in most developing countries and is more common in developed countries where approximately four out of every 10,000 people have Crohn's disease and eight out of 10,000 have ulcerative colitis.

Despite a great deal of research, the precise cause is not known. There is a genetic predisposition to IBD. Studies in identical twins suggest that this is stronger for Crohn's disease than for ulcerative colitis. If one identical twin has Crohn's disease, the risk that the other will get it is approximately 50 percent. For ulcerative colitis this risk is approximately 10 percent. Genetic studies have linked IBD to a gene on chromosome 16 that codes for a protein called NOD2, but the overall contribution of this gene to the risk of IBD is small and other genetic factors are likely to be involved. The fact that if one identical twin has IBD the other often does not suggests that environmental factors predispose or protect against the disease. One such environmental factor is infection. Infectious causes have been suggested and sought, but no reproducible evidence implicates a particular agent. Studies performed in animal models suggest that the presence of bacteria in the bowel seems to be important. One theory is that ulcerative colitis results when the body's immune system becomes intolerant of the normal bacterial flora in the bowel. Many other environmental factors have been studied. Smoking may protect against ulcerative colitis but increase the risk of Crohn's disease, and NSAIDs and psychological stress have also been proposed as triggers by some researchers.

IBD is often regarded as an autoimmune disease, partly because symptoms outside of the gut such as arthritis occur and because treatment with immunosuppressive drugs is often effective. Also, there is abnormal activation of immune cells with production of inflammatory cytokines; however, this often reverts to normal when the disease is quiescent. The cause of arthritis is not known, but the observation that IBD and several other types of gut problems are associated with arthritis (see ENTEROPATHIC ARTHRITIS) suggest that perhaps bacteria, their cell walls, or toxins they produce leak through the inflamed bowel wall into the circulation and trigger an immune response in joints.

Symptoms and Diagnostic Path

The symptoms of Crohn's disease and ulcerative colitis overlap considerably, but it is usually possible to distinguish them clinically. Crohn's disease can affect any part of the bowel but typically affects the small bowel more severely and causes abdominal pain, diarrhea, and loss of weight. Ulcerative colitis typically affects the colon and rectum more severely and causes diarrhea with blood. Crohn's disease can cause fistulas (narrow channels between the bowel and the skin) around the anus. Both diseases can be associated with fever, ERYTHEMA NODOSUM, and uveitis (see EYE PROBLEMS). Uveitis, usually acute, recurrent, and affecting one eye occurs in 5–10 percent of patients and is more common in patients with the HLA-B27 tissue type (see HLA) and arthritis affecting the spine.

IBD can be associated with arthritis affecting peripheral joints, the spine, and sacroiliac joints (see ANKYLOSING SPONDYLITIS and SPONDYLOARTHROPATHY) in 20–40 percent of patients. The peripheral arthritis tends to affect a few joints (pauciarticular) and is asymmetrical. Large joints such as the knee and ankle are often affected, but the small joints of a digit can become swollen, causing the whole finger or toe to swell (a *sausage digit*). The arthritis can flit from joint to joint, is rarely destructive, and often settles spontaneously over a few months. The sites where tendons join bones are often inflamed (enthesopathy). Bowel symptoms of IBD often occur before arthritis, but rarely joint symptoms can occur first. Flares in arthritis are related to flares in bowel disease more so with ulcerative colitis than with Crohn's disease, but the relationship is not strong.

If the spine is involved, inflammation typically affects the large sacroiliac joints at the base of the spine and the small joints between vertebral bodies

and between ribs and vertebral bodies (spondylitis). This leads to pain and stiffness that is most severe in the mornings and tends to improve with exercise. The lower back and neck are affected more than other parts of the spine. The symptoms are similar to those of ankylosing spondylitis and are discussed in detail in that section.

The diagnosis of inflammatory bowel disease is usually made by a gastroenterologist on the basis of the symptoms and endoscopy or X-ray studies. The specific findings are beyond the rheumatologic focus of this book.

Arthritis associated with IBD is easy to diagnose because the patient is usually already known to have IBD. Blood tests are not particularly helpful. Anemia caused by a combination of chronic disease, blood loss, and poor absorption of iron, folate, and vitamin B_{12} is common. The erythrocyte sedimentation rate (ESR), a nonspecific marker of inflammation, is often elevated (see Appendix II). Approximately 50 percent of patients with IBD and sacroiliac arthritis carry HLA-B27, but this test is not useful for diagnosis. X-rays of affected peripheral joints are usually normal. X-ray changes in the spine and sacroiliac joints are similar to those of ankylosing spondylitis.

Treatment Options and Outlook

Treatment of the gastrointestinal symptoms of Crohn's disease and ulcerative colitis is not discussed in detail here. Briefly, ulcerative colitis is treated with a combination of oral and rectal corticosteroids and aminosalicylates. Aminosalicylates such as mesalamine are drugs related to SULFASALAZINE but that lack the sulfa antibiotic component. If the disease remains difficult to control, AZATHIOPRINE or the closely related drug mercaptopurine is added. Emerging treatments under evaluation include TACROLIMUS, MYCOPHENOLATE MOFETIL, and TUMOR NECROSIS FACTOR ANTAGONISTS (TNF). A similar range of drugs is used to treat Crohn's disease, but rectal enemas are not used because the colon is seldom affected. The TNF inhibitors INFLIXIMAB, ADALIMUMAB, and CERTOLIZUMAB are established treatments in severe Crohn's disease and are particularly helpful in healing fistulas.

The treatment of arthritis associated with IBD is very similar to that of ankylosing spondylitis (see

ANKYLOSING SPONDYLITIS for a detailed description), but there are few controlled clinical trials to guide decisions about treatment. NSAIDs can worsen the gastrointestinal symptoms of IBD in some patients and are used cautiously. Sulfasalazine is a useful treatment for both inflammatory bowel and joint symptoms. Azathioprine, methotrexate, and TNF antagonists are useful treatments for arthritis associated with IBD.

Risk Factors and Preventive Measures

The genetic risk for these conditions remains to be clarified and there are no other definite triggers. Although smoking does seem to protect against ulcerative colitis, it is not recommended as it causes many other poor health outcomes.

intestinal bypass arthritis   Intestinal surgery may be done to assist weight loss in patients who are morbidly obese or to bypass a blockage from a tumor that cannot itself be removed. Up to 25 percent of these patients will develop an arthritis affecting the small joints of the hands, wrists, ankles, and sometimes the knees and neck. The arthritis may start two to nine months after surgery and will last a variable time, from weeks to years. There is often a rash, which can range from small pustules to red blotches. The illness is caused by overgrowth of bacteria in a loop of bowel that is a dead end. Intestinal bypass arthritis has become very rare since this type of operation is seldom done these days. It was initially replaced by surgery that limited the size of the stomach (gastric banding). However, this was only effective for a few years in many patients and in recent years is often combined with a partial bypass operation that does not seem to have the same incidence of adverse effects as the older style operations. Treatment of intestinal bypass arthritis is with NSAIDs and occasionally corticosteroids. Antibiotics can improve symptoms by decreasing the bacterial overgrowth. If symptoms are severe, reversing the bypass will cure the arthritis.

joint aspiration See Appendix II.

joint fusion See ARTHRODESIS.

joint injection A technique for delivering drug directly into inflamed joints. In RHEUMATOID ARTHRITIS, other inflammatory types of arthritis, and OSTEOARTHRITIS, a long-acting, depot corticosteroid can relieve symptoms when injected into a swollen joint. This is called an intra-articular injection— *intra* meaning "in" and *articular* meaning "joint." The advantage of injecting a drug into a joint is that a high concentration can be delivered directly to the site where it is most needed. Most drugs diffuse slowly out of the joint into the bloodstream, but the dose injected into the joint is low. Therefore the risk of systemic side effects from drugs such as corticosteroids are minimized.

Intra-articular injections of corticosteroids start to work within a day or two, and their benefit can last for weeks and sometimes months. Occasionally there is little benefit from the injections. If one or two injections into a joint are not effective, there is not much point trying repeated injections. Steroid injections can weaken tendons and, although there is no definite proof, there is concern that repeated injections into a joint may damage it. Most rheumatologists will try to limit the number of times a particular joint is injected. Tendinitis and bursitis can also be improved by a depot cortico steroid injection into the bursa or around a tendon. In some people the results are dramatic and symptoms resolve rapidly, but in others there is little response. Corticosteroids can be injected into most joints, but the hip is usually not injected because it is a deep joint and difficult to reach.

Apart from corticosteroids, the other group of drugs often injected into joints are the hyaluronans (sodium hyaluronate, trade name: Hyalgan, and hylan GF 20, trade name: Synvisc) that are ap proved for the treatment of knee osteoarthritis. They are administered as a course of three to five injections one week apart.

The usual procedure for a joint injection is that the physician explains the risks and benefits of the procedure, sterilizes the skin with alcohol or iodine, and then injects the drug, keeping the needles and the injection site sterile. Most rheumatologists perform this procedure in their offices and do not drape the injection site with sterile surgical drapes. Some numb the skin with a local anaesthetic before injecting the joint, others numb the injection site by using a spray of ethyl chloride that causes local freezing, and others do not routinely use either numbing procedure because the discomfort from a straightforward joint injection is usually minimal and may be less than the pain caused by injecting local anaesthetic. After a joint has been injected patients are usually asked to rest the joint as much as possible for a day or two and are warned that the joint symptoms may flare immediately after the injection. Joint flares are much more likely to occur after hyaluronan than corticosteroid injections.

Intra-articular injections cause few side effects. Allergy or skin irritation from iodine or adhesive tape can occur. Corticosteroids can cause a small area of skin around the injection site to lose pigment. A few people feel flushed in the face for six to 24 hours after an injection. Serious side effects are rare; the most serious is joint infection. The chance of this happening after a joint injection is low and estimated at about one in 1,000 or less. If a joint becomes infected the symptoms of INFECTIVE ARTHRITIS develop days or weeks after injection. Most physicians warn patients about this possibility and ask them to return immediately if the joint, becomes red, hot, and acutely painful. Intra-articular injections can rarely cause bleeding into a joint but this is extremely rare in a person whose blood clots normally.

joint protection   The principle of joint protection is to reduce the load on a joint or change its use in some way so as to provide a mechanical advantage. This may be important in caring for painful or unstable joints. It is best illustrated by a few examples:

- Using a walking stick in one hand reduces the load on all the joints in the opposite leg.
- A high chair reduces the load through the knees on rising (and the muscular force required to do so).
- Long-levered faucets give a mechanical advantage to the hand turning them.
- Using a wrist splint supports a grip that is weak because of a painful or unstable wrist.
- Long-handled reachers do away with the need to bend to pick clothes up off the floor.
- Buy potatoes that do not need to be peeled (and make other lifestyle changes).

joint replacement   Joint replacement is a salvage procedure for a severely damaged joint. The prime reason for replacing a joint is relief of pain with secondary goals being improving or maintaining function and maintaining personal independence. Joint replacement must be planned within the context of the whole patient and his or her disease. A fit 65-year-old man disabled by advanced OSTEO-ARTHRITIS in one hip poses no problem for this type of surgery. However, patients with RHEUMATOID ARTHRITIS may require surgery at a much younger age, frequently have more than one severely damaged joint at the time of surgery, and may well have other significant conditions such as OSTEOPO-ROSIS or coronary artery disease that make surgery more difficult or dangerous. Factors that may need to be addressed in planning surgery include:

- The demands that the patient is going to put on the joint and his or her expectations following surgery. This includes age, as the expected lifespan of a weight-bearing total joint replacement is about 10 years in a moderately active middle-aged to elderly person. Although the technique and results of repeat joint replacement have improved markedly over the past 10 years, the complication rate does increase slightly with repeat surgery.

- The order in which joints are operated on. It is no good replacing a painful and disordered right knee, for example, if the right foot is too painful to stand on. Similarly, the results of replacing the knuckle joints in rheumatoid arthritis will be poor if that wrist is painful and disordered. Assuming all joints to be equally affected, the order of surgery in the leg is usually foot, hip, knee, and lastly ankle. In the arm the order would usually be wrist first, then hand, elbow, and finally shoulder. Obviously, people seldom have all joints equally affected, but considering the reliance of one joint on another for normal function is important.

- The state of the other limbs. During rehabilitation after a right knee replacement, for example, the left leg must be able to carry the patient's weight. After lower limb surgery the patient often needs to start walking with the help of crutches or a walker, and his or her arms need to be able use these and take some of the weight. If not, this may need to be improved first (for example by local corticosteroid injections into painful joints or use of splints). Lower-limb surgery is usually done before the upper limb.

- Sometimes two or more operations can be performed at the same time. This reduces the time the patient has to spend rehabilitating and is also cost-effective in requiring only one hospitalization. Lower-limb and upper-limb surgery can often be combined, and both hips or both knees may be replaced simultaneously. A hip and knee on the same side, however, could not be replaced together because the rehabilitation required is very different for knees and hips.

- The state of the cervical spine (neck). This is a particular problem in people with rheumatoid arthritis who may develop instability between the upper two cervical vertebrae that can lead to damage to the spinal cord if moved excessively during anesthesia. The cervical spine should always be x-rayed with the head tilted both forward and backward to look for instability before any general anesthetic. If there is evidence of early damage to the spinal cord, the cervical spine would have to be stabilized before any other surgery was contemplated.

- Ongoing medication. NSAIDs and ASPIRIN are usually stopped five to seven days before major surgery to reduce bleeding. DMARDs are also sometimes stopped because of the surgeon's concern about healing. However, this can lead to a flare of arthritis during the rehabilitation phase that can set back the patient considerably and add to the cost of the procedure by prolonging hospitalization. Evidence now suggests that patients with rheumatoid arthritis who continue taking METHOTREXATE throughout surgery and rehabilitation may do better than those who stopped it for a few weeks. LEFLUNOMIDE on the other hand increases the incidence of postoperative infection and should be stopped some weeks before surgery. Some other DMARDs like SULPHASALAZINE have no material effect on surgery, but medication changes are best discussed with the patient's rheumatologist or internist.

- The choice of surgeon. This is one of the most important decisions the patient must make. Undoubtedly, outcomes from joint replacement do differ among different surgeons and among different hospitals. While it is possible in some health systems to find out the rate of infection or unplanned readmissions following surgery in particular hospitals, getting this type of information on individual surgeons is seldom possible. The referring doctor should have a reasonable knowledge of a number of potential surgeons and be able to discuss the patient's choice. The surgeon should clearly explain the proposed surgery, including personal experience with the particular operation, what to expect afterward during both rehabilitation and the long term, the range of possible adverse outcomes, and the surgeon's assessment of the likelihood of

these happening. Obviously, in some HMO and government-funded systems the choice may be limited.

- The most common serious complications of total joint replacement are infection, blood loss, and joint instability. Deep-vein thrombosis and possible pulmonary embolus (clots in the leg that can travel to the lungs, blocking vessels there) should be rare, with modern management with low-molecular-weight heparins (blood-thinning treatment), compression stockings, and early mobilization.

Total or partial joint replacement may be done on a wide range of joints.

Shoulder joint replacement is best when done for severe osteoarthritis. This is because the shoulder is essentially an unstable joint that requires normal muscle and soft tissues to hold it in place. This is usually the case in osteoarthritis. On the other hand, in rheumatoid arthritis the soft tissues have often been damaged by years of inflammation and results of surgery are less predictable. Of prime importance here is that the rotator cuff be intact (see ROTATOR CUFF SYNDROME for a description of the rotator cuff). When the shoulder blade side of the joint is too damaged to accept the prosthesis, providing good pain relief is still possible by just replacing the head of the humerus (upper-arm bone).

In a normal *elbow* joint the bones making up the joint are not constrained. That is, if there were no tendons, ligaments, or capsule holding them together, they would fall apart. Because there is usually considerable damage to these soft tissues by the time joint replacement is considered, the early elbow joint replacements were designed like a gate hinge (i.e., constrained). This means there is none of the usual give in the joint and high forces are transmitted to the cement between the bones and the metal joint prosthesis. This led to early failure of the joint replacement. Where the soft tissues are healthy (for example in posttraumatic osteoarthritis), using a nonconstrained prosthesis is possible. Advances in design have led to the use of semiconstrained prostheses where an axle prevents the joint from falling apart (dislocating) but is not part of the weight-bearing surface and therefore does not create the same forces at the cement interface. Results of total elbow replacement are therefore much improved, and about 90 percent can be expected to function for at least five years. Pain relief is good and function usually improved. Heavy lifting and significant physical work will lead to early wear and the need for repeat surgery or ARTHRODESIS. Patients having this operation most frequently suffer from osteoarthritis, rheumatoid arthritis, JUVENILE IDIO-PATHIC ARTHRITIS, or REACTIVE ARTHRITIS.

Hand and *wrist* surgery needs to be particularly carefully planned with regard to the patient's requirements, what is surgically possible, and what other joints are involved. Ideally an occupational hand therapist will draw up a list with the patient detailing all the hand functions that have been lost or compromised. The patient can then roughly grade these into necessary (e.g., feeding, dressing, personal hygiene), useful (e.g., typing, cooking), and desirable (e.g., hobbies) categories. Cosmetic appearance should never be a reason for surgery. Once the surgeon has assessed the hand, he or she can then discuss with the patient what can be done to improve the functions the patient has identified. Therapy following hand surgery is essential for a good outcome. In general, joint replacement in the hand and wrist can be done only when the subsequent demands on the joint are going to be light. Otherwise arthrodesis is often a better surgical option.

The *small joints of the hand* can be replaced. Joint replacement of the distal interphalangeal joints is seldom a good surgical choice since arthrodesis gives better results. In the proximal interphalangeal joints, soft tissue procedures and arthrodesis are also generally preferred to joint replacement, although this can be done if the soft tissues are healthy and the surrounding joints well preserved. In carefully selected patients joint replacement at the metacarpophalangeal joints can be very beneficial. This is almost always combined with soft tissue procedures to realign, tighten, or release the surrounding tendons and other soft tissues. This is necessary to straighten the joint and get it moving closer to its original plane of motion. A variety of prostheses are used. A full range of movement is not possible, and the amount of movement post-operatively will gradually reduce over a few years.

Failure or loosening of the prosthesis is relatively more frequent here than at other joints. Joint replacement at the wrist is possible but indicated only for a severely damaged joint where movement is required since it is less reliable than fusion. In someone with two severely affected wrists it may be appropriate to fuse the nondominant wrist and replace the dominant wrist.

Total *hip* replacement is now a reliable, commonly performed procedure with excellent outcomes. It has one of the highest benefit-to-cost ratios of all surgical procedures. Pain is almost always improved and function usually improves. Although running should be discouraged, limited recreational activities are possible. A prosthesis can last up to 20 years, but in general, the more active the patient, the shorter the life span of the prosthesis.

Knee movement is complex, and designing prostheses that adequately mimic the original joint has been difficult. Design has improved rapidly, however, and over 90 percent of total knee replacements can be expected to be functioning after 10 years. Redoing the joint replacement increases the risk of complications. Knee joint replacement is particularly likely to cause clotting in the leg veins, and this can occur despite the most diligent precautions. Having strong quadriceps muscles (those in front of the thigh) and being able to straighten the leg are important for good joint function after surgery. Sometimes the surgeon will need to release the tissues behind the knee to get it straight enough. A continuous passive motion (CPM) machine is often used after knee replacement to improve the range of movement.

Ankle joint replacements have proven difficult, and a range of interventions is being explored. These are some way from becoming routine procedures.

juvenile idiopathic arthritis (JIA) This is a group heading for inflammatory arthritis affecting children under the age of 16. Older terms such as juvenile rheumatoid arthritis used in the United States and juvenile chronic arthritis in Europe have been replaced with this internationally agreed term. While the changes in names and classification may seem like nitpicking, the aim is to be able to place children with a similar disease into the same groups to advance knowledge about these diseases and their treatments. The classification categories are:

- Systemic arthritis (Still's Disease)
- Polyarthritis
- Pauciarthritis
- Enthesitis-related arthritis
- Psoriatic arthritis

The first two groups will be subdivided according to age of onset, pattern of joint involvement, and whether they have a positive antinuclear antibody (ANA) test. PSORIATIC ARTHRITIS will be discussed under that heading. The major difference with adult psoriatic arthritis is that more children get the arthritis before the rash, and so patients can be classified into this group without having a rash as long as a first-degree relative has psoriasis.

The frequency with which these diseases occur varies considerably among different populations, with the occurrence generally being higher in Northern Europe and populations that originate from there. For example, 86 per 100,000 Swedish children are affected compared with 31 per 100,000 Puerto Rican children. There are also differences in the types of diseases found in different populations. The pauciarticular type is much more common in populations of Caucasian European origin, and polyarticular disease is more common in African and Indian populations.

The cause of JIA is not known. Infectious and autoimmune causes have been proposed, but research to identify the mechanisms responsible has not been successful. Juvenile spondylitis, or enthesitis-related arthritis, as with spondylitis in adults, is associated with the HLA-B27 tissue type, indicating that there is an underlying genetic predisposition.

Symptoms and Diagnostic Path

The different types of JIA have different symptoms.

- *Pauciarthritis*   About half the patients with JIA have this subtype. It affects fewer than five joints in the first six months of the disease. These are most frequently the knees, ankles, wrists, and elbows. It occurs in girls five times as often as in boys. In many children, the disease is relatively benign and may settle in six to 12 months, although recurrences can occur in up to 20 percent of children. A few children go on to develop arthritis in more joints as time goes on, and in these the disease usually remains active into adulthood. The most serious complication is uveitis, which occurs in 20 to 25 percent of patients (see EYE PROBLEMS). Between 10 and 20 percent of this group of patients have a positive ANA test, and 90 percent of patients developing uveitis will have a positive test. The ANA, and age under six years at disease onset, is therefore useful in identifying children at increased risk of uveitis, but some with a negative test will also develop uveitis. Children often do not complain of eye symptoms until there is significant damage, and so it is important that they undergo regular screening to pick it up early. The greater their risk, the more frequent the screening should be. When only one knee is inflamed, more blood supply goes there and it can grow faster leading to unequal leg length. Uveitis can occur in other types of JIA but less frequently.

- *Polyarthritis*   Arthritis affecting five or more joints in the first six months occurs in about 30 percent of patients with JIA. This group is divided into those with or without a positive rheumatoid factor test. Those with a positive test have an arthritis very similar to adult RHEUMATOID ARTHRITIS. Those with a negative test tend to have more fatigue, low-grade fever, and anemia but a better outcome. The rheumatoid factor-negative disease involves very similar joints to the systemic onset type, knees, wrists, and ankles being most common. Girls are affected four times as often as boys.

- *Systemic Arthritis (Still's Disease)*   About 10 percent of children with JIA have mainly systemic symptoms when their illness starts. It affects equal numbers of boys and girls. Symptoms start suddenly, and a high, spiking fever for several hours every day is classical. Other symptoms can include sore throat, myalgia, arthralgia, loss of weight, fatigue, abdominal pain, enlargement of the spleen and lymph nodes, pericarditis, and rash. The rash is typically a salmon pink, flat patch that does not itch and is evanescent, fading over a few hours. The rash tends to come back with the spells of high fever, often late in the afternoon. If a typical rash is present it is a useful clue to the diagnosis of Still's disease. The symptoms of systemic arthritis can last for weeks and can recur, sometimes years later. In most patients polyarticular arthritis develops a few weeks or months after systemic symptoms.

Still's disease usually occurs in children but can rarely occur in adults and is then called adult-onset Still's disease. The symptoms in adults and children are similar. Still's disease starts for the first time in some adults, but in others a careful history reveals a previous similar, nearly forgotten, episode in childhood.

- *Enthesitis-related arthritis* This group includes children with a number of different forms of arthritis. One group that used to be classified as pauciarthritis may have little arthritis but have frequent enthesopathies (inflammation at the attachment of tendon to bone), often have a positive HLA-B27, and can develop spondylitis. This subgroup, often affecting teenagers, is sometimes called seronegative enthesopathy and arthritis (SEA) syndrome. Some of these children will go on to develop ANKYLOSING SPONDYLITIS, which can also start de novo in childhood. Other pointers to this group of arthritis are a family history of uveitis, SPONDYLOARTHROPATHY, or inflammatory bowel disease. REACTIVE ARTHRITIS and inflammatory bowel disease–associated arthritis can also affect children.

No specific diagnostic test is available. The diagnosis is made on the basis of the clinical findings and excluding other causes of arthritis. Viral infections such as RUBELLA and PARVOVIRUS can cause arthritis in children, but the symptoms do not usually last longer than a few weeks. Leukemia can be mistaken for JIA in children. Acute bone pain can be a symptom of leukemia, and this can be mistaken for arthritis. In children with leukemia pain is usually much greater than joint swelling, and examination of blood or bone marrow usually provides the diagnosis. Arthralgia, but not arthritis, is common in children with HYPERMOBILITY and can mistakenly be diagnosed as JIA. Other types of inflammatory rheumatic diseases such as SYSTEMIC LUPUS ERYTHEMATOSUS and VASCULITIS can occur in children and be mistaken for JIA.

Systemic arthritis and adult-onset Still's disease are particularly difficult to diagnose because high fever, elevated white blood cell count, and other symptoms in a child usually indicate the presence of an infection or a malignancy. The white blood cell count in Still's disease can be high enough to suggest a possible diagnosis of leukemia. The correct diagnosis, particularly in an adult, is usually suspected only after extensive investigations for infection are negative.

In all types of JIA, blood tests for rheumatoid factor are usually negative. About 20 percent of children with polyarthritis have a positive blood test for rheumatoid factor and a greater chance of developing severe chronic arthritis with deformities and erosions. In pauciarthritis many patients have a positive ANA test but do not have other features of systemic lupus erythematosus. Eye complications such as uveitis are more likely to occur in young girls with pauciarthritis and a positive ANA test.

In systemic-onset JIA and adult-onset Still's disease, the white blood cell count and erythrocyte sedimentation rate (ESR), markers of infection, or inflammation, are often elevated. Liver function tests are also often abnormal. An extremely high blood level of ferritin, a protein that increases with inflammation, can be a clue to the diagnosis of Still's disease, but it is not a specific or sensitive test. In all types of JIA, the ESR, although not useful for diagnosis, can be a useful guide to response to treatment in some patients.

X-rays are seldom helpful, because they are often normal in the early stages of JIA. X-rays of the sacroiliac joints are very difficult to interpret even in normal children and are therefore seldom helpful in patients with JIA with symptoms that suggest spondylitis.

Treatment Options and Outlook

As is the case for most types of inflammatory arthritis in adults, JIA is treated with nonsteroidal anti-inflammatory drugs (NSAIDs), corticosteroids, and disease-modifying antirheumatic drugs (DMARDs). In Still's disease the systemic symptoms often respond dramatically to treatment with an NSAID. Traditionally aspirin has been used, but more modern NSAIDs, which do not have a risk of causing Reye's syndrome, are effective. NSAIDs and corticosteroids can control symptoms but do not affect the progression of arthritis. In patients with ongoing joint inflammation, treatment with a DMARD is added. The choice between DMARDs is similar to that in adults (see RHEUMATOID ARTHRITIS). In approximately three-quarters of patients with JIA the illness becomes inactive without causing significant disability.

JIA itself, and the corticosteroids that are often used to treat it, can slow the growth and development of children. Inflammation caused by arthritis can affect the nearby growth plate that determines how fast a bone grows and can lead to asymmetrical bone growth. The jaw is often affected, resulting in an underdeveloped jaw (micrognathia). Hip arthritis in childhood can cause severe joint damage so that eventually hip replacement surgery is needed later in life, even though the disease may have been inactive for many years. Patients with JIA, particularly those with pauciarthritis, should be examined regularly by an ophthalmologist. If uveitis is diagnosed early and treated effectively, loss of vision can be prevented. In addition to medications and physical therapy, children with severe arthritis need psychosocial, educational, and vocational support to help them deal with chronic illness and its consequences.

Risk Factors and Preventive Measures

Like ANKYLOSING SPONDYLITIS in adults, the enthesitis-related arthritis group have a high incidence of HLA-B27. There are no risk factors for the other forms of JIA discussed here. There are no known preventive measures.

juvenile rheumatoid arthritis See JUVENILE IDIOPATHIC ARTHRITIS.

Kawasaki disease Also known as mucocutaneous lymph node syndrome, this is a form of VASCULITIS occurring mostly in young children and having life-threatening complications. It is particularly common in Japan and is named after Dr. Tomisaku Kawasaki, who described the disease as recently as 1967. It occurs worldwide but is more common in developed countries. In the United States, there are about 18 cases per 100,000 population per year, varying from 33 per 100,000 in Asians and Pacific Islanders to nine per 100,000 in Caucasians. Boys are affected more than girls, and nearly 90 percent of affected children are under the age of five years.

Despite a lot of research, the precise cause is not known. It appears to involve an abnormally strong immune reaction to an infection. This immune response causes the damage. The precipitating infection is most likely to affect the throat or lungs and is likely to be any of several infections rather than just one particular organism. The evidence suggests that the affected child's immune system is primed to respond in this way whereas most people will not.

Although many blood vessels are affected in the early stages, the main brunt of the immune attack is borne by the medium-sized arteries, especially those taking blood to the heart, kidneys, and gut. The neutrophil count in the blood is very high, and these cells, as well as lymphocytes, move into the walls of the affected blood vessels where they cause inflammation. This tends to affect scattered patches of the wall rather than the entire blood vessel. After the second week, the intensity of the inflammation starts to subside and the area heals with scarring. There may be clotting in the blood vessels during this stage. By the seventh week most of the inflammation has settled, but the scarred areas of artery wall are weakened and bulge outward. These bulges are called aneurysms and frequently lead to narrowing of the artery itself and may lead to clotting and obstruction of blood flow.

Symptoms and Diagnostic Path

The child becomes ill very suddenly with a high fever that usually lasts one to two weeks but sometimes longer. Reddening and thickening of the conjunctivas (thin outer layer of the eye) starts on the second or third day. Then the lips become dry, red, and cracked and the inside of the mouth very red. The lymph glands in the neck swell and are tender to touch. There may be a reddish rash over the body while the fever is high. A very characteristic finding is the reddening of the palms and soles at about the same time as the mouth. This is followed by peeling of the skin, starting at the fingertips, from about the tenth day.

During the first two weeks there is often inflammation affecting much of the heart. This causes a rapid heart rate, sometimes leaking heart valves, breathlessness, and changes in the heart sounds and EKG. If aneurysms and narrowing of the arteries in the heart develop, the child may develop angina or even a myocardial infarction (heart attack). These aneurysms can occasionally affect arteries to the gut, arms, and legs and cause gangrene there. The brain may be affected, resulting in drowsiness, loss of consciousness, or seizures. Paralysis of limbs and the nerve to the face have occurred.

There is often some protein leak into the urine, and pustules may develop on the elbows and knees. Arthritis affecting many joints develops in 20–30 percent of children with Kawasaki disease.

Kawasaki disease is diagnosed on the basis of clinical findings rather than special tests. The diagnosis requires the presence of fever for five days plus four out of five signs of mucocutaneous inflammation. These include the reddened swollen conjunctivas with no discharge from the eye; the rash; the red, dry, cracked lips and reddened lining of the mouth; the swollen lymph glands; and the characteristic changes in the hands.

In addition, the neutrophil count will be very high in the blood and markers of inflammation such as ESR and C-reactive protein will be raised. Kawasaki disease may be difficult to differentiate from acute infections, and attempts to grow organisms from the child's blood and throat swabs should be made. These will be negative in Kawasaki disease. The fluid surrounding the brain and spinal cord (CSF) will show increased numbers of cells, but again no organisms will grow from it. Echocardiography (ultrasound scanning of the heart) can show the aneurysms on the blood vessels and is done at regular intervals throughout the illness. If present, they should be followed up by echocardiography at one- or two-year intervals. Angiogram (injecting dye into the arteries of the heart and then taking X-rays of the outlined arteries) is done when angina is severe, following a heart attack, or if surgery is thought necessary.

Treatment Options and Outlook

Treatment with intravenous immunoglobulin (IVIG) has dramatically improved the outcome of these children. The immunoglobulin is obtained from the blood of many donors and is treated to destroy all known infections before being used. It has complex effects on the immune system but has been shown to be very useful in treating a number of diseases caused by the immune system, especially various forms of vasculitis. Studies have shown that giving one large dose of immunoglobulin (2 grams per kg body weight) up front when Kawasaki disease is diagnosed is more efficacious at preventing aneurysm formation than the older regimens where the dose was spread out over a few days. This should be given within the first 10 days of the illness. Fairly high doses of aspirin are used until the fever settles and then low doses until all the laboratory tests are back normal, usually within two months.

The use of CORTICOSTEROIDS in Kawasaki disease is controversial. A controlled trial (see CLINICAL

TRIAL) in Japan of oral corticosteroid for two weeks showed that it settled the acute illness quicker and prevented some aneurysms from forming. However, a trial in the United States using one large dose of intravenous corticosteroid showed no effect. At the moment therefore, it is difficult to know whether corticosteroids will prove to be a useful treatment.

The use of immunoglobulin therapy in this manner has brought the incidence of aneurysms in the arteries of the heart down from 25 percent to 4 percent, but it cannot prevent them completely. Echocardiographic monitoring of patients is still required. Those children who develop aneurysms or generally enlarged blood vessels leading to sluggish blood flow are at risk of developing heart attacks, heart failure, or arrhythmias. The larger the aneurysms, the greater the risk. Low-dose aspirin is continued long term in these patients as an antithrombotic agent. They should therefore also get annual influenza vaccinations to protect them from the possibility of Reye's syndrome (a serious illness associated with aspirin use in children with influenza or chicken pox). They are at increased risk of getting angina and heart attacks as adults as well. Cardiac surgery may be necessary in a small number. Very few patients may get a second attack of Kawasaki disease. Children without aneurysm formation remain asymptomatic after at least 20 years of follow-up.

Risk Factors and Preventive Measures

In spite of the general belief that Kawasaki disease is an immune response to an infection, no clear associations with infections have been established, and there are no known preventive measures.

knee pain The knee is not only the largest joint in the body, it is in fact two joints. The larger of the two is the joint between the thighbone (femur) and the larger of the lower leg bones (tibia). The kneecap or patella is a bone within the tendon of the quadriceps muscle (the large muscles in front of the thigh). The patella forms a joint with the femur that shares the same capsule as the joint between the femur and tibia. The latter joint has two half-moon-shaped pieces of cartilage called menisci that both guide the bones as they move and take about 60 percent of the weight going through the knee. In addition, there are a large number of muscles, ligaments, and tendons acting to move or stabilize the knee. Pain may arise from all these structures either singly or in combination. Some causes of knee pain are obvious while others may require expert examination and special investigations to diagnose. Some may arise outside the knee. A well-known source of pain referred to the knee is arthritis of the hip, for example.

Situated as it is in the middle of a weight-bearing limb, the knee is especially susceptible to injury from falling, twisting, direct trauma, long-term overload, and various forms of arthritis. Generally speaking, the causes of knee pain differ in various age groups and they will be discussed accordingly. This does not mean that these conditions occur only in children or adults, just that they are more common in those age groups. Because so many structures can give rise to pain, it may help to think about pain arising within the joint, around the joint, and being referred from elsewhere separately.

Knee Pain in Children

Within the knee joint OSTEOCHONDRITIS DISSECANS can occur in many joints but is most frequently in the knee. A fragment of cartilage and often the underlying bone comes loose and thus causes symptoms. Boys are affected more often than girls.

PATELLOFEMORAL DISORDERS (between the kneecap and thighbone) are common causes of pain in children and adolescents, particularly adolescent girls. The pain is felt in front of the knee, and the other specific conditions listed in this section should be excluded. The pain is often felt during or after sports and may wake the child at night. These girls tend to be more knock-kneed than average, but no dislocation or subluxation can be demonstrated (compare with other patellofemoral disorders). They generally have weak quadriceps (large muscles in front of thigh). Some patients have tight hamstrings (back of thigh muscles), and wearing high-heeled shoes may bring it on. Both of these latter conditions increase the pressure between the kneecap and the thighbone in the patellofemoral

joint. The treatment is a combination of stretching the hamstring and strengthening the quadriceps muscles. Surgery should be avoided.

MENISCAL TEARS are less common in children than adults but may occur because of a discoid (abnormally shaped) meniscus. The reason for this shape is not known. These are either treated conservatively or by limited surgery, usually by ARTHROSCOPY, leaving the outer rim of the meniscus intact. Cysts can also occur in the meniscus and may be felt as a bulge along the joint line.

Bipartite patella refers to a condition where the two bone centers in the patella do not grow together as normal and leave a thin layer of cartilage between them. Because cartilage is weaker than bone, this can fracture following repetitive stress. It heals well with splinting.

During development of the embryo the knee is divided into three sections by shelves of tissue called plicae. These normally disappear but can cause later problems if they persist. The one running down the inner aspect of the joint (medial plica) most frequently causes problems by getting caught in the moving joint and becoming inflamed. This is known as the plica syndrome. It is sometimes diagnosed on clinical examination but often only during arthroscopy done for unexplained knee pain. Treatment is by removal during arthroscopy.

INFECTIVE ARTHRITIS is a relatively more common cause of knee pain in children and adolescents than in adults. It usually complicates a blood-borne infection but may follow a puncture wound. Infection should always be considered in a child with a markedly swollen, painful knee that comes on suddenly since a delay in diagnosis can lead to long-term damage. Occasionally, infection can spread from the bone to involve the joint.

Inflammatory joint disease is relatively less common in children compared with adults. JUVENILE IDIOPATHIC ARTHRITIS of the pauciarticular type is the most common to cause knee arthritis in children.

Around the knee The tendon of the quadriceps muscle includes the kneecap or patella and then continues as the patellar tendon to attach to the larger of the lower leg bones (the tibia) at a little bump in the bone called the tibial tuberosity. At the stage when the tuberosity is still attached to the main bone only by cartilage, it can be excessively strained. The resulting inflammation causes pain, tenderness, and minor swelling. This is known as Osgood-Schlatter's disease. It occurs particularly in active children between the ages of 10 and 14 years. X-rays may show some breaking up of the tuberosity. Treatment is with rest, avoidance of activities such as jumping, and control of weight gain if this is a problem. The condition usually disappears as the cartilage separating the tubercle from the main part of the tibia changes to bone in the midteens. Occasionally a loose fragment of bone remains in the tendon and needs to be surgically removed.

A condition very similar to Osgood-Schlatter's disease can occur where the patellar tendon attaches to the lower end of the patella. This is known as Sinding-Larsen-Johansson syndrome. It is managed in a similar way.

Tumors and OSTEOMYELITIS in the adjoining bone can also cause pain felt in the knee.

Referred pain Pain may be referred to the knee as a result of hip disease. Conditions at the hip that are particular to children include Perthes disease, transient synovitis of the hip, and slipped femoral epiphysis (see HIP PAIN).

Knee Pain in Adults

Within the knee joint Meniscal tears become more common in young adults, often being sustained during sport. They often occur together with a ligament injury, especially a torn anterior cruciate ligament.

OSTEOARTHRITIS can start in early adulthood if there has been significant trauma to the joint, removal of a meniscus, or certain metabolic diseases. Otherwise it is usually a disease of the older adult.

Chondromalacia patellae describes softening of the cartilage at the back of the kneecap where it forms a joint with the thighbone or femur. This gives rise to an aching pain in the front of the knee especially when it is kept bent for long periods, e.g., in the movies, climbing stairs, or cycling. It may result from poor alignment of the patella with the femur so that there is increased shear force on the cartilage during movement or from tight ham-

strings. Treatment is primarily with strengthening the quadriceps and stretching the hamstrings.

Inflammatory types of arthritis such as RHEUMATOID ARTHRITIS, ANKYLOSING SPONDYLITIS, psoriatic arthritis (see PSORIASIS AND PSORIATIC ARTHRITIS), and REACTIVE ARTHRITIS all commonly affect the knee.

The large joint between the femur and tibia is divided into two halves, the medial or inner compartment and the lateral or outer compartment. Between these compartments two ligaments, the anterior and posterior cruciates, wind around each other and provide resistance (and therefore stability) to forward and backward sliding as well as rotation of the knee. The anterior cruciate ligament is one of the most common structures in the knee injured in sport. When an athlete is taking weight on a foot with that knee bent and receives a force pushing the knee inward (either an external force or the individual's own body weight through loss of balance), the anterior cruciate may be torn along with other ligaments such as the medial collateral ligament (see below). It can also be torn alone by a twisting force when the knee is fully straightened. The patient may hear a pop and feel the knee giving way, followed by pain and swelling. A complete tear of the anterior cruciate usually causes the joint to fill up with blood, although it may sometimes leak out of the back of the joint if the capsule is also torn. The patient feels the knee is unstable to twisting movements.

An incompetent anterior cruciate ligament will often lead to meniscal tears and early osteoarthritis. In athletes complete tears should be surgically repaired as soon as possible. People with lesser demands from their knees are usually treated by physiotherapy first to see if they can gain adequate function through appropriate muscle strengthening. A number of surgical techniques try to replace the ligament. These involve using either a whole or part of a tendon from another area, for example cutting a strip of the patellar tendon and sewing it in the place of the anterior cruciate ligament.

Tears of the posterior cruciate are much less common and cause less disability. They usually occur when a powerful force drives the tibia backward on the femur with the knee bent. Surgical repair is not often required, and treatment is by putting the leg in a cast with a slight bend for six weeks followed by intensive physiotherapy.

Synovial chondromatosis is a disease in which cartilage starts to grow within the synovium or lining layer of the joint. Many separate areas of cartilage grow, with enlargement and swelling of the synovium in the early stages. In addition to stimulating the synovium, the cartilage can interfere with the joint by becoming lodged between the moving surfaces. Later on the swelling of the synovium reduces and the areas of cartilage become partly calcified so that they stand out clearly on X-ray. Synovial chondromatosis can affect any joint but the knee is by far the most common. It begins between the ages of 15 and 50 and usually presents as pain in the knee but can also cause locking where the person is unable to straighten the knee because a piece of cartilage has become jammed in the joint. Feeling the cartilage bodies is often possible on examining the joint. Treatment is to remove those cartilage bodies likely to cause problems and a portion of the synovium. This is usually done by arthroscopy and may need to be repeated.

PIGMENTED VILLONODULAR SYNOVITIS affects the knee more frequently than any other joint.

Around the knee BURSITIS is common around the knee and can be puzzling if the location of the bursas is not known. The bursa overlying the kneecap frequently becomes inflamed in people who do a lot of kneeling on hard surfaces. Although known as housemaid's knee, it is more commonly seen in builders, carpet layers, and electricians. People with inflammatory arthritis or gout are also more prone to this condition. The swelling with some redness is very obvious. Often it settles just with avoidance of kneeling. Occasionally needle aspiration is required and may be repeated. The bursa should not be lanced since this may lead to a slowly oozing wound that can allow infection to enter the joint. Occasionally resistant cases require surgical removal of the bursa.

Just below the kneecap is another bursa, and inflammation of this is known as *parson's knee*. The anserine bursa lies over the inner aspect of the tibia just below the joint line. Bursitis here frequently occurs in association with a tendinitis of one of the overlying tendons. Treatment is with rest and NSAIDs.

TENDINITIS may affect any of the many tendons in the knee area, but some of the more common problems will be listed here. In general, patients with an inflammatory arthritis are more likely to develop these. *Jumper's knee* is a tendinitis of the patellar tendon as it attaches to the lower end of the patella. As the name suggests it often affects those involved in running and jumping activities.

Three inner thigh muscles all attach to the inner front portion of the upper tibia just below the knee joint. Their common attachment is known as the pes anserinus, which is another site of tendinitis. This is difficult to separate from inflammation of the medial collateral ligament (medial ligament syndrome) and anserine bursitis (see above).

The iliotibial band is made up of fibrous tissue and forms part of the support mechanism for the knee on its outer aspect. This may become inflamed from repeated rubbing against the lower end of the thighbone, or a bursitis may arise between the two. Long-distance runners are most at risk, particularly if they run on a camber. It is therefore usually known as *runner's knee.*

The knee is particularly susceptible to ligament injuries. In addition to the cruciate ligaments inside the knee, a powerful ligament is on either side of the knee (medial and lateral collateral ligaments) that together with a thickening of the joint capsule function as supporting ligaments. The lateral collateral ligament is a thick, cordlike structure fairly easily felt over the outer aspect of the knee. It is damaged by a force pushing the knee outward with the foot or lower leg relatively fixed. The medial collateral ligament on the other side is broad and not easily felt in healthy people. It is frequently injured at the same time as the anterior cruciate ligament, sometimes with a medial meniscal injury as well. Following injury the patient can sometimes be left with a tender nodule at the upper end of the ligament. X-ray shows some calcification in this area. This is known as Pellegrini-Stieda disease. If it does not settle with rest and NSAIDs a local injection of a low dose of a corticosteroid is helpful.

Popliteal cysts (also called BAKER'S CYSTS) are swellings at the back of the knee. Most of these communicate with the knee joint, some being bursa and others protrusions of the joint capsule itself. They are common in people with rheumatoid arthritis and osteoarthritis. Popliteal cysts can burst and cause pain and swelling down the back of the leg. They are then often mistaken for a thrombosis in the leg veins (DVT). The cysts can be aspirated and injected with corticosteroid but may recur. They can also be surgically removed or drained, but small cysts may not require any treatment.

Referred pain Pain referred to the knee from another part of the body is usually from osteoarthritis of the hip joint.

leukocytoclastic vasculitis   See VASCULITIS.

loose bodies   Sometimes called *joint mice,* these are any objects that move freely within a joint. They may have been part of the joint such as pieces of bone, cartilage, or meniscus that have broken off or objects that have entered the joint such as fragments of bullets. Loose bodies often get coated with cartilage and bone in time and can then be seen on X-ray. Many get drawn into the synovial joint lining and can no longer float about the joint. If they impinge on the joint surfaces, they can cause pain and limitation of movement. The treatment is surgical removal if they are troublesome.

lupus   See SYSTEMIC LUPUS ERYTHEMATOSUS.

lupus anticoagulant   See ANTIPHOSPHOLIPID ANTI-BODY SYNDROME.

Lyme disease   This is a relatively new illness that was first recognized in the mid-1970s by Dr. Alan Steere and his colleagues as the cause of an unusual outbreak of what first appeared to be juvenile arthritis in Lyme, Connecticut. A previously unrecognized spiral-shaped organism belonging to the spirochete family was identified as the cause of Lyme disease by Dr. W. Burgdorfer and colleagues in the 1980s and named after him. Lyme disease is an illness that can affect the heart, skin, nerves, and joints and is caused by a spirochete transmitted to humans by a tick bite. It affects about 15,000 people in the United States annually, making it one of the commonest diseases transmitted to humans by animals. In the United States it occurs mostly in certain geographic areas, the northeastern states (Maine to Maryland), the Midwest (Wisconsin and Minnesota), and the West (California and Oregon). In 1999, more than 90 percent of cases of Lyme disease in the United States occurred in nine states—Connecticut, Rhode Island, New York, Pennsylvania, Delaware, New Jersey, Maryland, Massachusetts, and Wisconsin. Lyme disease also occurs in Europe and has been reported from most parts of the world.

Lyme disease is caused by a spirochete, *Borrelia burgdorferi.* In the United States most infections are caused by *B. burgdorferi,* but in Europe two different species, *B. afzelli* and *B. garinii,* are more common. The spirochete is transmitted from its usual host, most often a small animal such as the white-footed mouse or dusky-footed woodrat, to humans by the bite of a tick of the *Ixodes ricinus* group such as *I. pacificus* and *I. scapularis* (also called *I. dammini*). The white-footed mouse and other hosts harbor the spirochetes without becoming ill, and therefore, an infected animal can serve as a reservoir for infection for an entire summer. A young larval form of the tick feeds on an infected mouse and then harbors the spirochetes until the next year when the tick develops into a more mature nymph form and attaches to another host such as a human and transmits the infection. The ticks are small, approximately the size of a pinhead, and have to remain attached to their host for a long time, 24 hours or more, to transmit infection efficiently. There are color pictures of the ticks that transmit Lyme disease in the *New England Journal of Medicine* 1992; 327:542. The infection rate is as high as 20 percent if a tick harboring the organism is attached for more than 72 hours and as low as 1 percent if it is attached for less than 72 hours. Infection is more common during the seasons when ticks are abundant, usually spring and summer. White-tailed deer, which do not carry the spirochete, are often the preferred host for the species of tick that carries the infection. Thus deer, although not directly responsible for the infection but because they carry the ticks, are an important determinant of how frequently infection occurs in different parts of the country.

Symptoms and Diagnostic Path

One would expect that the first symptom would be a tick bite. But because the ticks are so small, less than half the patients with Lyme disease recall a tick bite. The symptoms of Lyme disease are highly variable, can mimic many other illnesses, and seem to differ in the United States and Europe, perhaps because different species are the predominant cause of infection. Symptoms can be divided according to the stage of infection and the affected organ system.

Skin In about 90 percent of patients in the United States, even in those who cannot remember being bitten by a tick, a typical skin rash called erythema migrans develops about a week after the tick bite. Although it usually develops soon after the bite, it can occur several weeks later. The rash typically develops at the site of the bite, is reddish, is annular (like the rings in the trunk of a tree), and slowly increases in size. The rash, as it slowly expands over several days or weeks, clears in the middle. Similar but smaller secondary skin lesions can occur at sites where there was no tick bite, and these are thought to be caused by spirochetes that have spread through the bloodstream from the site of the initial bite. Erythema migrans fades even without treatment, usually over about a month, but can persist for up to 14 months and can recur. The rash itself does not usually cause much itching or pain but may be warm and may be associated with systemic symptoms such as arthralgia, myalgia, fatigue, and headache. These systemic symptoms are thought to result from the infection spreading through the bloodstream to other parts of the body and are similar to those that occur with a viral infection such as flu.

In Europe, erythema migrans tends to last longer, spread more slowly, and be associated with fewer systemic symptoms. A chronic skin rash called acrodermatitis chronica atrophicans that causes patches of skin to become thin and unhealthy has been described in Europe but seems to be rare in the United States. The organism has been cultured from these skin lesions up to 10 years after the initial infection.

Neurological A few weeks (two to eight on average) after erythema migrans has developed, approximately 15 percent of patients who have not received antibiotic treatment have symptoms indicating that the nervous system has been infected. These include headache, neck stiffness, difficulty thinking, and inflammation of nerves resulting in neuropathy. The nerve that provides movement to the face is often affected, resulting in weakness or paralysis to half the face (Bell's palsy) or if both nerves are affected, to both sides of the face. The neurological symptoms usually resolve even without treatment. However, about 5 percent of patients who are not treated develop chronic neurological damage than can sometimes show up years after the initial infection, even though the patient may have had no symptoms in the intervening years. A wide range of chronic neurological complications has been described, including dementia, peripheral nerve damage leading to shooting pain and numbness in affected areas, damage to the spinal cord causing weakness of the legs (paraplegia), and damage to the nerves that supply the muscles of the eyes and face.

Cardiac Involvement of the heart occurs in 5 percent of patients, usually several weeks or a few months (two to eight weeks on average) after the initial infection and at the same time or soon after neurological symptoms. Lyme disease can affect the heart in several ways. Most often it affects the conducting system that transmits messages about heart rhythm, resulting in the most common symptom—heart block. There are varying degrees of heart block of increasing severity. In first-degree heart block the only abnormality is that the distance between the P wave of the ECG, reflecting electrical messages to the atria, and the QRS complex, reflecting messages to the ventricles, is a little prolonged. Patients have no symptoms and there are no adverse effects on the function of the heart. In second-degree heart block the delay in transmission of messages can lead to skipped beats and symptoms of palpitations. Third-degree heart block is the most severe and reflects a total lack of coordination between the atria and the ventricles. Patients may complain of fainting, dizziness, shortness of breath, and weakness. Heart block can be intermittent and fluctuate in severity. Inflammation of heart muscle (carditis) can occur and, if severe, can decrease the ability of the heart to pump blood and cause symptoms of heart failure such as edema and shortness of breath. Inflammation of the outer lining of the heart, the pericardium, is less common.

Musculoskeletal Arthritis occurs in more than half of infected patients who do not receive antibiotics. Of these patients, 90 percent develop arthritis within a year, usually after about six months, but it has occurred anywhere between four days and two years after infection. The arthritis often affects one joint (monoarthritis) but can migrate from one joint to another. In most patients with Lyme arthritis the knee is affected at some time in their illness, but virtually any joint, including the temporomandibular (jaw) joint, can be involved. Arthritis can cause an affected joint to swell a lot, but there is usually less pain than would be expected for the amount of swelling. Arthritis is often intermittent. After several attacks, though, some patients develop chronic arthritis even after several courses of antibiotic therapy have eradicated the infection. A few patients have developed symmetrical swelling of the small joints of the hands, much like rheumatoid arthritis. It is not clear if this unusual event occurs simply because two common conditions, Lyme disease and rheumatoid arthritis, have developed in the same person or if this is a rare presentation of Lyme arthritis. It is also not clear how the infection causes arthritis. *B. burgdorferi* has seldom been cultured from joint fluid, although it is often possible to detect DNA of the organism using molecular biology techniques. Some patients who have had multiple courses of antibiotics and have no evidence of infection with live spirochetes have recurrent arthritis, suggesting that Lyme arthritis may be a type of REACTIVE ARTHRITIS.

Diagnosis The unequivocal way to diagnose Lyme disease is to culture the organism from an affected tissue. However, this approach is seldom practical and is helpful only early in the disease. The organism is easily cultured from a small biopsy of the erythema migrans rash. If the rash is typical, physicians in an endemic area usually make the diagnosis based on its appearance without a biopsy. Cultures from sites other than the skin in patients who have early disease and develop heart, CNS, or joint complications are seldom positive. The usefulness of molecular biology techniques such as polymerase chain reaction (PCR) to detect *B. burgdorferi* DNA is limited as a diagnostic tool because even though the organisms may have been killed by antibiotic therapy, fragments may remain, causing a positive PCR test. Urine tests to diagnose Lyme disease are unreliable.

Blood tests are useful in people who have been infected for at least a month. In the first two weeks after infection immunoglobulin M (IgM) antibodies to *B. burgdorferi* can be detected in only about 30 percent of patients. After four to six weeks most patients have positive antibody tests for IgG antibodies. If a patient who has been infected for more than four to six weeks has a test that is positive for only IgM and not IgG antibodies, this is likely to be a false-positive result. The initial blood test usually done to detect antibodies to *B. burgdorferi* is an ELISA (enzyme-linked immunosorbent assay) that has not been well standardized across laboratories. Because *B. burgdorferi* shares antigens with other common organisms, false-positive tests are common and have given rise to a condition sometimes called *pseudo–Lyme disease* that is discussed later. For most laboratory tests the upper limit of normal is set at a level that excludes about 2 percent of the healthy population with the highest measurements. The incidence of Lyme disease in states with the highest rates of infection is approximately six new cases per 100,000 population per year (0.006 percent), much lower than the 2 percent cutoff for the laboratory tests. This means that if one performed Lyme antibody tests in the healthy population or in all patients with arthritis, false-positive results would be more than 100 times more common than a true-positive result. A more accurate test to detect antigens that are specific to *B. burgdorferi* is called a Western blot. This test is unlikely to detect antigens from other organisms and is usually performed if the ELISA is positive and Lyme disease is suspected.

There are several problems with blood tests for Lyme disease that have led to confusion. The key problems are as follows:

- Early in the course of infection all blood tests can be negative.
- Some patients who receive antibiotics early in the course of infection do not develop antibodies.
- A false-positive ELISA test for antibodies is very common.
- Tests are poorly standardized, and different laboratories can report different results on the same sample.
- In patients with Lyme disease the test for antibodies can remain positive years after the acute infection. Therefore, even if the infection is eliminated, the blood test can remain positive.

Because of these difficulties, Lyme disease can be overdiagnosed, and any symptoms that develop later can be ascribed incorrectly to *chronic Lyme disease*. The firm diagnosis of Lyme disease is made on the basis of both clinical findings and blood tests to detect antibodies to the organism. The Centers for Disease Control has proposed criteria to be used for surveillance purposes. These are erythema migrans or at least one clinical symptom of Lyme disease affecting the heart, CNS, or joints and also laboratory evidence of infection. A positive ELISA test should be confirmed with a Western blot. This is known as conditional, two-tier testing and is necessary to avoid the problems discussed above. All blood samples testing positive with the ELISA go on to a Western blot looking for both IgM and IgG antibodies to *B. burgdorferi* or just IgG in late disease. It should not be assumed that all laboratories are doing the correct test.

Treatment Options and Outlook
In most patients symptoms of Lyme disease resolve without treatment, but antibiotics speed the process and prevent long-term complications. Several antibiotics are effective against Lyme disease, and the stage of disease often determines which is most appropriate. Most patients with Lyme disease recover completely.

- In patients with early disease and erythema migrans and systemic symptoms, doxycycline for 14–21 days is preferred, except in children and pregnant women in whom amoxicillin is an effective alternative. In patients unable to take these drugs, cefuroxime is the third choice. Studies have shown that these drugs clear the infection in more than 90 percent of people and relapse is rare.
- If patients have CNS or cardiac involvement, intravenous ceftriaxone for two to four weeks is effective. If someone is unable to take ceftriaxone, intravenous penicillin is an alternative.
- Lyme arthritis is treated for 28 days either with one of the oral antibiotic regimens such as doxycycline as used to treat early disease or intravenous ceftriaxone for 14 days. Oral treatment is more convenient, has fewer side effects, and is cheaper, but some patients have developed late CNS symptoms despite having received oral antibiotics for Lyme arthritis. The usual approach is to try a course of oral antibiotics first and, if this fails, to follow with a course of intravenous ceftriaxone. The arthritis can resolve and then recur despite effective treatment that has eliminated the infection. About 10 percent of people with Lyme arthritis, despite repeated courses of antibiotics, go on to develop chronic inflammatory arthritis. This is thought to be a reactive arthritis and not due to persistence of the organism, because a PCR test on the joint fluid or synovial tissue looking for *B. burgdorferi* DNA is usually negative. These patients have been treated with NSAIDs and occasionally SYNOVECTOMY.
- Chronic Lyme disease is a controversial entity. Some patients who have had Lyme disease have chronic symptoms of fatigue and pain similar to FIBROMYALGIA. Repeated courses of antibiotics do not improve symptoms and may be harmful. Several unconventional treatments for this condition, including prolonged courses of high doses of antibiotics, have not been proven to be effective. Also controversial is the entity of pseudo–Lyme disease. This condition describes patients who have chronic pain, fatigue, and disability and have had a positive blood test, usually an ELISA test, for Lyme disease but have

no classical physical findings. Some physicians believe that these patients have fibromyalgia and a false-positive blood test for Lyme disease and have been given an incorrect diagnosis.

- Antibiotics are not the only treatment for Lyme disease. Prevention is important, and the risk of acquiring Lyme disease can be decreased by wearing long trousers and socks that prevent the ticks from attaching, by using insect repellents, and by checking for ticks after returning from the outdoors. Lyme disease can also be prevented in two other ways, preventive treatment after a tick bite and vaccination. The risk of Lyme disease after a bite by the species of tick that transmits the disease is usually less than 1 percent, probably because most ticks do not stay attached long enough to transmit infection very efficiently. A single dose of doxycycline can prevent Lyme disease if it is given within 72 hours of a bite, but preventive antibiotic treatment is seldom used because the infection rate is so low and the species of the offending tick is seldom known.

A vaccine to prevent Lyme disease was developed and appeared to be safe and reasonably effective but was removed from the market in 2002, probably because profits from the limited sales did not cover the risks of litigation from patients who developed arthritis or other symptoms after vaccination. Disadvantages of vaccination were the need for three injections in the first year and booster injections later. Vaccination was recommended only for people with a high risk of infection.

Risk Factors and Preventive Measures

Exposure to *Ixodes* tick bites in endemic areas is necessary for infection with *B. burgdorferi*. Although widespread these areas are predominantly temperate regions of the United States, Europe, and Asia and the highest risk areas in the United States are discussed above. Summer months carry the highest risk. Preventive measures can be taken to protect individuals entering the countryside where the infection is endemic and to modify the environment to make infection less likely. Ticks are most likely to be encountered in wooded areas or tall grass, as well as in stone fences and woodpiles. Being aware of these high-risk places and wearing protective clothing is important. Diethyl-meta-toluamide (DEET) is effective in repelling ticks as well as mosquitos. It is recommended that DEET-containing insect repellents should not be applied underneath clothing and should be washed off thoroughly at least once a day. Checking the entire body and removing any ticks at least once a day is important as the risk of infection is very low if the tick has been attached for 24 hours or less. If a significant tick bite is sustained, the antibiotic doxycycline as a single dose will reduce the likelihood of Lyme disease developing. A vaccine was developed but has been withdrawn because of concerns about adverse effects and low take-up rate. Spraying stone walls, sheds, woodpiles, and other areas likely to harbor ticks with an insecticide to kill them can make a property safer. Establishing deer-feeding stations that apply an insecticide as the deer feeds will reduce the tick carriage rate in the area.

magnetic resonance imaging (MRI) See Appendix II.

magnets In about 1000 B.C., a shepherd, Magnes, found that his sandals were attracted to the ground and that this was due to the metal tacks in them. On digging, he unearthed magnetic oxide of iron, commonly known as lodestone. Later, in the 18th century, scientists discovered how to magnetize ordinary iron, and these magnets became popular both for performing tricks and "healing." Mesmer (of hypnosis fame) used them extensively in achieving miracle cures in the 1770s. In 1938, a Scandinavian doctor reported experiencing pain relief when she applied magnets to painful areas.

Electric fields are always accompanied by a magnetic field, and a pulsed or variable magnetic field induces an electric field (Maxwell's law). Most of the evidence for the biological effect of magnetism is in the use of electromagnetic fields. Researchers in this area have also developed the microwave oven, cellular telephones, and magnetic resonance imaging (MRI). There is good evidence that pulsed electromagnetic fields (PEMFs) stimulate bone growth and are effective for treating nonhealing fractures. The 80 percent success rate is similar to open surgery but less invasive. Approximately 3 percent of long-bone fractures result in nonhealing, and the U.S. Food and Drug Administration approved PEMF stimulators for their treatment in 1979.

Experimental evidence also indicates that PEMF affects cartilage growth although not in the human body. Several short-term placebo-controlled studies (see CLINICAL TRIAL) show that PEMF has some effect in relieving pain in OSTEOARTHRITIS. Treatments are quite time consuming, typically for two hours a day, five days a week for six weeks. Note that experimental work has shown very different effects on cells at different frequencies, and specific frequencies may be required to achieve specific results.

Evidence for the use of the static magnets so widely advertised is less convincing. Several small studies show improvement in a number of chronic painful conditions as well as arthritis in rats. Recent randomized, double-blind, placebo-controlled studies have shown no effect on BACK PAIN or CARPAL TUNNEL SYNDROME but efficacy in osteoarthritis of the knee. Given the ease of studying the use of static magnets it is surprising that there are not more studies reported, and this may indicate the tendency to report only positive studies. Despite the considerable enthusiasm over the past 10 years for the use of many forms of magnetic therapy, the other side of the coin is the debate over possible adverse effects. There has been concern particularly about whether people living near power lines or cellular telephone stations are at increased risk of developing tumors. In 1995, the American Physical Society reviewed all the evidence regarding power lines and issued a statement that they could find no relationship with an increased risk of cancer.

meditation Meditation is defined as any activity that calms the mind and keeps it focused in the present moment. This means that the individual is neither reacting to things that have happened in the past nor making plans for the future. There are many forms of meditation but they can be divided into two basic types.

1. Concentrative meditation involves focusing on the breath, an image, or a sound (mantra) so

that the mind becomes still and aware. Zen meditation is usually begun by counting breaths and progresses from simply being aware of the breath to more advanced techniques. The well-known transcendental meditation involves the use of a unique meaningless sound, the mantra.

2. Mindfulness meditation involves opening the mind to thoughts, feelings, and images and allowing them to float through without reacting to them. This has been described as noting thoughts and feelings in a similar way to which a postal worker might note stamps, without either positive or negative feelings about them.

Successful meditation induces a state of deep relaxation. Studies have shown that this relaxation is associated with a lower heart rate, blood pressure, and breathing rate and with reduced muscle tension and skin conduction. The levels of lactate (from burning energy) and catecholamines and cortisol (stress hormones) go down and the brain waves change. Meditation is part of many mind-body programs and, in some form, is often included in multidisciplinary pain programs. There is good evidence that meditation can reduce pain levels in a number of conditions, including FIBROMYALGIA. In RHEUMATOID ARTHRITIS, several studies have shown significant improvement in pain and distress scores with mindfulness meditation techniques without having any effect on the activity of the disease.

meniscal tears The menisci are two half-moon-shaped structures in the knee that guide the movement of the femoral condyles (lower end of the thigh-bone) against the tibia or lower leg bone (see KNEE PAIN). They are made of a tough fibrocartilage, different from the cartilage lining the bones in the joint. Menisci are joints other than the knee, such as the temporomandibular joint, that can occasionally cause problems, but it is those at the knee that tear. As people age, the cartilage in the menisci develops degenerative changes and stiffens and the meniscal problems are therefore different at different ages.

Children very occasionally have an abnormal disc-shaped meniscus that can catch in the joint and tear. Normal menisci are very unlikely to tear in children. If they are troublesome, the treatment is to trim them back using ARTHROSCOPY, leaving a rim around the joint margin.

Most meniscal tears occur in young adults, usually during sporting activities. The typical injury involves a twisting movement on a weight-bearing knee with the foot relatively fixed. Examples include a basketball player landing unbalanced from a jump or a soccer player turning suddenly on a heavy field. In this sort of injury the meniscus is torn longitudinally so that the inner torn portion may flap into the joint and cause locking, the hallmark of meniscal tears. With a locked joint the individual cannot take his or her weight on that leg and cannot fully straighten it. There is often damage or complete rupture of a ligament at the same time. This is most often the anterior cruciate ligament. With a severe tear there is immediate, severe pain followed by swelling of the knee within a few hours. If the anterior cruciate ligament is also torn, blood will be inside the joint.

Lesser tears or those that do not result in cartilage getting between the moving bones may become chronic. These may cause clicking with intermittent pain and tenderness along the joint line. The diagnosis is made on the history and use of provocation tests to demonstrate that a piece of meniscus interferes with normal joint movement (McMurray's or Apley's grinding test). An MRI scan will confirm the diagnosis and also show the extent of the tear and associated ligament damage, which will help in planning surgery. Arthroscopic surgery is used if treatment is required. The outer third of the meniscus (i.e., closest to the skin) is the only part with a blood supply and therefore the potential to heal. Tears in this portion may therefore heal and are often sewn together. If the tear is through the inner two-thirds, however, the best treatment is to remove the inner torn bit and clean up the remaining edges (a partial meniscectomy).

In older individuals there is often no clear-cut injury. These tears are likely largely degenerative and are often horizontal through the meniscus. There is localized pain along the line of the joint, perhaps a bit of swelling, and often waking at night because of knee pain. Plain X-rays often show coexisting changes of OSTEOARTHRITIS. MRI scanning confirms the diagnosis. Conservative treatment should be tried, but if not successful, a partial meniscectomy can be done. Total meniscectomies definitely predispose people to subsequent osteoarthritis. How great a risk factor partial meniscectomies will prove to be is not yet clear.

Milwaukee shoulder   This is a destructive arthritis affecting the shoulder and involving hydroxyapatite crystals. It affects mostly women over the age of 70 years, frequently has blood in the joint, and is sometimes known as *bloody old shoulders.*

Symptoms and Diagnostic Path

Pain, swelling, and loss of range of movement come on over weeks or months. The pain tends to be continuous, unlike OSTEOARTHRITIS where it is worse with movement. The swelling is cool, unlike GOUT or INFECTIVE ARTHRITIS. The joint rapidly becomes unstable, and X-rays show severe destruction of the joint with loss of bone on both sides of the joint. Ultrasound or MRI will usually show destruction of the rotator cuff, which is considered important in the development of this arthropathy.

Fluid taken from the joint is typically blood-stained and contains hydroxyapatite crystals. These are very small and can generally be seen only on electron microscopy. Because of this they were discovered in these severely damaged joints only in 1976 and are not routinely looked for. Their role in the joint destruction is still not clear. There is a tendency for the Milwaukee shoulder to settle down in time, although this may take one or two years. Because of this and the limited success of any treatment, it is often managed conservatively.

Treatment Options and Outlook

Injection of CORTICOSTEROIDS into the joint is best avoided since it has not been shown to be beneficial and may make the crystal deposition worse. Painkillers and NSAIDs are used where safe to do so but have only limited value. Using a long-acting local anesthetic to block the suprascapular nerve that runs over the top of the shoulder blade and supplies the shoulder joint may give good pain relief. Surgery is difficult because of the degree of damage to the tissues around the joint.

mixed connective tissue disease   The symptoms of rheumatic diseases often overlap, especially early in the course of the illness. When this happens and no specific diagnosis is obvious, the term OVERLAP SYNDROME, or undifferentiated connective tissue disease, is often used to describe the illness. In 1972, Dr. Sharp described a distinct subgroup of patients with overlapping symptoms of SYSTEMIC LUPUS ERYTHEMATOSUS (SLE), SCLERODERMA, and MYOSITIS who had an antibody to extractable nuclear antigen (ENA) and named the condition mixed connective tissue disease. The ENA antibody test has since been refined and is now named RNP (ribonuclear protein antibody). Mixed connective tissue disease was thought to represent a group of patients with a distinct illness and prognosis. However, it is not clear that this is the case. When patients with mixed connective tissue disease were followed for many years, their illness often evolved into classical SLE, scleroderma, or myositis. Furthermore, the RNP antibody test is not specific for mixed connective tissue disease and occurs in patients with SLE and other classical autoimmune diseases. Mixed connective tissue disease is probably best thought of as a subset of patients with overlap syndrome who have antibodies to RNP. It is not clear that there is any clinical usefulness in making this distinction.

As is the case for the autoimmune diseases that comprise mixed connective tissue disease, its cause is not known. The various theories proposed are described under systemic lupus erythematosus, scleroderma, and dermatomyositis.

Symptoms and Diagnostic Path

Patients have combinations of symptoms that overlap various autoimmune diseases. These symptoms include RAYNAUD'S PHENOMENON, trouble swallowing, and tightness of the skin that are typical of scleroderma; pleurisy, arthralgia, arthritis, mouth ulcers, rash, and pericarditis that are typical of SLE; and muscle weakness typical of myositis. The disease often starts slowly with non-diagnostic symptoms such as fatigue, aches and pains, and Raynaud's phenomenon. It may take several years before the characteristic manifestations evolve. The pattern of symptoms can change over time, and in many patients the illness evolves over time toward SLE, scleroderma, or myositis. Regardless of whether mixed connective tissue disease is regarded as a separate disease entity, there are still important associations with a strongly positive RNP antibody test. People with a strongly positive test are unlikely to develop the more severe kidney or brain problems that can occur in SLE. They are at high risk of developing pulmonary hypertension, and their arthritis is more likely to be erosive (cause bone damage around the joints) than other patients with connective tissue disease.

The diagnosis is clinical. All patients have a positive antinuclear antibody (ANA) test and by definition a positive test for RNP antibodies. The most suggestive clinical findings are swollen hands, inflammation of the joints, inflammation in muscles, Raynaud's phenomenon, and thickening of the skin in the peripheries.

Treatment Options and Outlook

The treatment of overlap syndrome involves aspects of the treatment of SLE, scleroderma, and myositis. The treatment for individual patients is selected according to the symptoms present. NSAIDs are often used to treat arthralgia and arthritis; corticosteroids to treat myositis, pleurisy, and pericarditis; immunosuppressive drugs to treat kidney disease; and antireflux drugs to treat difficulty swallowing. The treatment of PULMONARY HYPERTENSION is discussed elsewhere. Patients are monitored because their illness is likely to change over time and evolve toward one of the classical autoimmune diseases with a prognosis similar to that disease. Although mixed connective tissue disease was originally thought to have a good prognosis, it is clear that patients frequently suffer debilitating symptoms, especially quite severe aches and pains. They sometimes suffer poorly healing ulcers from severe Raynaud's phenomenon, swallowing difficulties, and arthritis that can be very difficult to treat. Studies are limited but probably about one in five patients has died from the disease within 10 years of diagnosis and about half die from pulmonary hypertension.

Risk Factors and Preventive Measures

There are no known risk factors or preventive measures for mixed connective tissue disease.

morphea   See SCLERODERMA.

MRI   See MAGNETIC RESONANCE IMAGING in Appendix II.

multicentric reticulohistiocytosis   A rare disorder in which cells called histiocytes and multinucleate giant cells are filled with fat and infiltrate into tissues, especially skin and joints. It is mostly a disease of middle age but can occur at any age. In 60 percent of patients the arthritis starts before the skin is involved and diagnosis is then very difficult.

Symptoms and Diagnostic Path

The typical appearance in the skin is of nodules up to 2 cm in diameter, reddish in color, and numbering from a few to several hundred. Hands, ears, face, chest, lips, and the inside of the mouth and throat can all be involved. The arthritis resembles that of RHEUMATOID ARTHRITIS, except that the joints at the ends of the fingers (distal interphalangeals) are often involved. It is often a highly destructive arthritis.

Other organs, including the lungs, heart, stomach, thyroid, and bone marrow may be affected. There may be a mild anemia, raised ESR, and moderately high cholesterol, but none of these help with the diagnosis. X-rays show destructive joint lesions that are difficult to differentiate from rheumatoid arthritis. Biopsy of the skin nodules or joint lining (synovium) shows the typical fat-filled cells. Many conditions are associated with multicentric reticulohistiocytosis. Nearly 50 percent of patients react positively to a skin test for tuberculosis (TB), and a few patients have had active TB. About a third have other skin lesions, suggesting raised cholesterol (xanthelasma), and a number have had autoimmune diseases. About a quarter have had cancers of various kinds. These have included cancer of the breast, stomach, lung, bowel, cervix, ovary, and blood and also melanoma.

Treatment Options and Outlook

Treatment is difficult. Successful treatment of a number of cancers and TB has improved the joint and skin disease in a few patients. However, lowering cholesterol levels, CORTICOSTEROIDS, and other medications used for rheumatoid arthritis as well as blind treatment for TB (i.e., without a definite diagnosis) have not been particularly useful. The powerful immunosuppressants CYCLOPHOSPHAMIDE and CHLORAMBUCIL were used with reasonable success until quite recently. Their significant side effect profile led to the trial of other agents, but because multicentric reticulohistiocytosis is rare it is not possible to set up adequate trials to compare treatments and come up with the best for different situations. Methotrexate is very effective in many patients and reasonably safe for longer term suppression. The TNF blockers, particularly INFLIX-IMAB, have recently been used in resistant cases with success. Recently, there are a few intriguing reports of the bisphosphonates, ALENDRONATE and PAMIDRONATE, being used with good results. CORTICOSTEROIDS, NSAIDs, and painkillers are also used.

myasthenia gravis An autoimmune disorder that results in muscle weakness and is caused by antibodies against receptors for a chemical messenger, acetylcholine, that transmits messages from nerves to muscles. Myasthenia affects about 10 people out of 100,000 and, although it can occur at any age, most often affects young or middle-aged adults and women more often than men.

Although about 80 percent of patients with myasthenia gravis have antibodies against acetylcholine receptors, the underlying cause of myasthenia is not known. Individual patients form antibodies against slightly different parts of the acetylcholine receptor, so it is not a case of a unique antibody causing the disease. The approximately 20 percent of patients who do not have antibodies against acetylcholine receptors by standard tests may have them if a more sensitive assay is used or may have antibodies against other muscle enzymes or receptors. There is an increased risk of myasthenia in patients with other autoimmune disorders such as thyroid disease, rheumatoid arthritis, and SLE. The reason for this is not known. One possibility is that T lymphocytes that have been activated by an underlying autoimmune disease stimulate B lymphocytes to produce antibodies against ace-

tylcholine receptors. The thymus gland, an organ that lies just underneath the sternum (breastbone), seems to play an important role in the cause of myasthenia. This observation was first made when physicians noticed that patients with a tumor of the thymus gland, called a thymoma, developed myasthenia much more often than other people did. The thymus plays an important role in programming lymphocytes to react, or not react, against various antigens. Another clue to the cause of myasthenia may be that PENICILLAMINE, a drug that was previously used to treat rheumatoid arthritis but has now been replaced by more modern drugs, can cause myasthenia as a side effect. The way in which penicillamine causes myasthenia is not clear, but it can also cause other autoimmune diseases such as glomerulonephritis, suggesting that it somehow activates autoimmune responses.

Symptoms and Diagnostic Path

The key symptom of myasthenia is weakness that comes on, or gets worse, when a muscle is used repetitively. Myasthenia often starts in a few muscles, a type of disease called localized myasthenia, and at this stage patients may not realize that symptoms are related to use. For example, myasthenia often starts in the muscles that move the eye or those that carry out the act of swallowing, and therefore a patient early in the illness may notice only occasional double vision, droopy eyelids, or difficulty swallowing. In about 80 percent of patients with myasthenia the first symptoms affect the eyes, but over time most develop generalized disease with symptoms in many muscles. In about 20 percent of patients the illness remains localized to a few muscle groups.

The clinical findings are helpful in diagnosing myasthenia and in distinguishing it from rheumatological causes of weakness. In myasthenia the eye muscles are often affected, causing droopy eyelids (ptosis) that fatigue easily. Ptosis can occur in other neurological diseases, but then it is almost always fixed and does not fluctuate. If a physician can make ptosis appear by keeping a patient looking up for a time to fatigue the muscles that keep the eyelids open, it is a valuable clue to the diagnosis of myasthenia. Other clues are double vision and difficulty swallowing that fluctuates in severity. DERMATOMYOSITIS AND POLYMYOSITIS are rheumatological conditions that cause muscle weakness and have to be distinguished from myasthenia. Although these conditions often affect swallowing, the proximal limb muscles (thigh and shoulder) are much more severely affected in dermatomyositis and polymyositis and the eye muscles are usually spared. In myasthenia, muscle strength typically fatigues rapidly, but later in the illness weakness may be present all the time, making it more difficult to distinguish from polymyositis.

Blood tests also help distinguish myasthenia from myositis. In myositis the levels of muscle enzymes (creatine phosphokinase) are often elevated, but in myasthenia they are usually normal. In myasthenia a blood test for acetylcholine receptor antibodies is positive in more than 70 percent of patients. The test is more likely to be positive in patients with severe generalized disease than those with localized myasthenia. False-positive tests are rare but can occur in other autoimmune diseases such as SLE.

The classical test for myasthenia is called the Tensilon test. Edrophonium (Tensilon) is a drug that increases the levels of the transmitter acetylcholine by inhibiting its breakdown. The increased concentrations of acetylcholine are able to overcome the blocking effects of the antibodies against the acetylcholine receptor, temporarily, and the symptoms of myasthenia improve dramatically. Edrophonium is injected intravenously and symptoms improve almost immediately, with the response lasting about 10 minutes. Mild side effects often occur, such as nausea, sweating, abdominal cramps, and lightheadedness from the test, but more serious problems such as low blood pressure, vomiting, asthma, slow heart rate, and worsening of weakness are unusual.

Electromyography (EMG) is a test in which thin needles are placed into muscles to measure their response to electrical stimulation. The height of the signal reflects the response and in myasthenia after repeated electrical stimulation the response decreases in amplitude.

A chest X-ray or CT scan is often performed to look for an enlarged thymus gland.

A combination of clinical findings, acetylcholine receptor antibodies, a Tensilon test, and an EMG is used to make the diagnosis.

Treatment Options and Outlook

There are several different treatments for myasthenia that can be divided into three groups: (1) drugs that increase the concentrations of the neurotransmitter acetylcholine; (2) drugs that modulate the immune response; and (3) surgical removal of the thymus gland. Several drugs such as aminoglycoside antibiotics, tricyclic antidepressants, and phenytoin can worsen the symptoms of myasthenia and should be avoided if possible.

Drugs that increase the concentrations of the neurotransmitter acetylcholine Acetylcholine is released by the nerve and acts on its receptor to stimulate muscle response. Several drugs, such as pyridostigmine and neostigmine, inhibit the enzyme acetylcholinesterase that breaks down acetylcholine. These drugs, also called anticholinesterases, therefore increase the concentrations of acetylcholine in the nerve terminal. Increased concentrations of acetylcholine can partially overcome the blocking effects of antibodies against acetylcholine receptors. Treatment with anticholinesterase drugs improves the symptoms of myasthenia, but it does not treat the underlying problem. If very high doses of anticholinesterases are prescribed, they can cause high levels of acetylcholine to accumulate in the nerve terminal and paradoxically cause weakness that is difficult to distinguish from myasthenia.

Modulation of the immune response Many drugs that alter the immune response have been used to treat myasthenia, but CORTICOSTEROIDS are the most widely used. Most patients treated with corticosteroids improve, usually within a few weeks, and about 30 percent go into remission. High doses of steroids can sometimes worsen myasthenia, so many physicians start with a medium or low dose and slowly increase it. If remission does not occur or if the disease relapses when the doses of cortico steroids are decreased, another immunomodulating drug such as AZATHIOPRINE is usually added. In some patients the combination of corticosteroids and azathioprine is not effective and alternative treatments such as CYCLOSPORINE, INTRAVENOUS IMMUNOGLOBULIN, or PLASMASPHERESIS are tried. The combination of corticosteroids and azathioprine or another immunomodulating drug controls myasthenia with lower doses of steroids than would otherwise be possible, thus avoiding the side effects that often accompany high-dose steroids.

Surgical removal of the thymus gland Thymectomy is usually performed to remove the tumor in patients who have a thymoma. If surgery is not possible for technical reasons or because the patient is in poor health, the tumor is treated with radiation therapy. Physicians noticed that the symptoms of myasthenia improved after thymectomy in patients who had a tumor, and this led to trials of thymectomy in patients with myasthenia that was not associated with a thymoma. There are no definitive trials, and experts differ in their assessment of the usefulness of thymectomy in myasthenia. Nevertheless, because the current consensus is that it is useful, thymectomy is frequently performed in younger patients with generalized myasthenia. Symptoms can worsen immediately after surgery, so it is important that the surgery be performed in a center with experience in the management of myasthenia.

Treatment of myasthenia can usually control symptoms or put patients into remission, but prolonged treatment is often needed. The symptoms of myasthenia can suddenly worsen, sometimes for no apparent reason and sometimes after an infection or some other illness, and cause severe weakness affecting the muscles needed for breathing. This is called a myasthenic crisis and needs urgent treatment. Sometimes this involves placing the patient on a respirator in an intensive care unit until the crisis has resolved.

Risk Factors and Preventive Measures

Apart from the use of penicillamine, there are no known risk factors or preventive measures for myasthenia gravis. Penicillamine is seldom used these days and the adverse effects will be well known to any doctors still prescribing it in special circumstances.

myocarditis Inflammation of the heart muscle (myocardium) that can occur as part of many infectious and autoimmune illnesses.

The most common cause of myocarditis is a viral infection. Why some viruses affect the heart,

and do so only in a few people, is not clear. Lyme disease is another infectious cause. Myocarditis is not common in autoimmune illness but can occur in patients with SYSTEMIC LUPUS ERYTHEMATOSUS, SCLERODERMA, DERMATOMYOSITIS AND POLYMYOSITIS, and VASCULITIS. Another cause of myocarditis, RHEUMATIC FEVER, falls somewhere between an infectious and an autoimmune disease. Rheumatic fever is an autoimmune reaction to a streptococcal infection, usually a strep throat, but by the time myocarditis occurs, the organism may already be gone.

Symptoms and Diagnostic Path

The symptoms of myocarditis vary and can include chest pain, tiredness, shortness of breath, rapid heart rate, low blood pressure, and symptoms of heart failure such as edema. Inflammation of the heart muscle can also be associated with inflammation of other parts of the heart such as the heart valves (endocarditis) and the outer lining of the heart (pericarditis).

The diagnosis is usually made clinically based on the symptoms, ECG, and ultrasound examination of the heart. Occasionally a biopsy of the heart is obtained by threading a catheter through one of the large veins in the groin or neck into the right side of the heart and using a tiny forceps to obtain a small amount of tissue. This technique, endomyocardial biopsy, is safe and is used to monitor patients who have had a heart transplant for signs of rejection but unfortunately provides only a minute sample of tissue that can be very difficult to interpret.

Treatment Options and Outlook

There is no generally accepted specific treatment for myocarditis. The symptoms of heart failure are treated with drugs to increase the elimination of fluid (diuretics) or increase the efficiency of heart muscle contraction (digoxin and angiotensin-converting enzyme inhibitors or vasodilators). In patients who have an autoimmune disease treatment with corticosteroids and other immunosuppressants is often tried. Some types of myocarditis last only a short time and resolve completely, but others can cause permanent heart muscle weakness and heart failure.

Risk Factors and Preventive Measures

Myocarditis is not a disease in itself but a possible manifestation of the illnesses discussed above. The risk factors are therefore having or developing one of these conditions, a systemic viral illness being the most common. There are no known preventive measures.

myopathy   The term myopathy indicates any disease of muscle that does not involve inflammation. Although not very common, there are many different causes of myopathy. Those involving a rheumatic disease or treatment are discussed elsewhere in this book. The more common causes are briefly discussed here. They all cause weakness as their main symptom. EMGs and muscle biopsies (see DERMATOMYOSITIS AND POLYMYOSITIS) are often essential in making the correct diagnosis. Muscle biopsies in particular can be difficult to interpret and should be examined by a pathologist with a special interest in muscle disease at a center that processes a large number of specimens.

Neuromuscular disorders   Normal nerve function is essential for healthy muscles, and anything affecting motor nerves will impact on muscle function. Many such disorders will present with obviously neurological symptoms.

• MYASTHENIA GRAVIS and Eaton-Lambert syndrome affect the junction between nerve and muscle.

• Diabetic amyotrophy, Guillain-Barré syndrome, and others affect proximal nerves as they leave the spine. Guillain-Barré syndrome is a fairly frequent cause of paralysis, affecting mostly young adults but also older individuals on occasion. Typically it starts with altered sensation in the feet and then progressive weakness that affects the legs first and steadily moves up the body. It can stop at any stage, but if it progresses to involve the chest, the patient may need ventilation to stay alive. Swallowing, bladder function, and nerves of the head and face may be affected. About 70 percent of patients have had an infectious illness just prior to onset of paralysis, and this is thought to trigger it. Diagnosis is made from the typical clinical picture, finding a high protein level but normal cell count in the cerebrospinal fluid (the fluid that surrounds the brain and spinal cord) and excluding other possible causes. Treatment involves care of a paralyzed patient, prevention of thrombosis, ventilation when necessary, and plasma exchange or intravenous immunoglobulin infusions in severe disease. Typically 80 percent of patients make a good recovery, 15 percent are left with some disability, and 5 percent die. A poorer outcome is suggested by older age of onset, preceding diarrheal illness, rapid onset of weakness, ventilation, and the presence of antiganglioside antibodies.

Muscular dystrophies   The muscular dystrophies are a group of inherited conditions that cause progressive muscle dysfunction. Each syndrome is unique in its genetic abnormality and presentation. Common muscular dystrophies include Duchenne's, Becker's, facioscapulohumeral, and limb girdle types. Many of these present in childhood or early adulthood, and there is frequently a family history to suggest the diagnosis. This group of diseases is not generally regarded as rheumatic and will not be dealt with in detail in this book.

Malignancy   Malignancy can cause muscle wasting and weakness because of poor nutrition, general debility, and the cytokines produced either by the tumor or against the tumor by the immune system. Certain tumors can also have specific effects on nerves and muscles, and the Eaton-Lambert syndrome mentioned above is one. Carcinoid tumors may cause weakness of proximal muscles (shoulders and hips). Malignancy is also sometimes associated with dermatomyositis and polymyositis.

Drugs   A long list of drugs can cause a myopathy, and only the more common or important ones will be listed here (see DRUG-INDUCED RHEUMATIC DISEASE). Drugs can cause a myopathy through different mechanisms. PENICILLAMINE, hydralazine, and procainamide can induce the immune system to attack muscle. Thiazide diuretics can lower potassium to the extent that it affects muscle function. Others like alcohol damage muscle directly. CHLOROQUINE, clofibrate, cimetidine, cocaine, COLCHICINE, gemfibrozil, CORTICOSTEROIDS, heroin, all the statins (cholesterol-lowering drugs), phenytoin, sulfonamides, valproic acid, vincristine, and zidovudine may all occasionally affect muscle function.

Metabolic

- Disorders of glycogen metabolism may be inherited and have their major effect on muscle. The best known of these is McArdle's disease, but there are many others.

- Disorders of fat metabolism are even less common but can cause similar problems.

- A number of inherited abnormalities of mitochondrial function may lead to myopathy (and other effects) occurring at different ages. Mitochondria are small organelles within cells that are crucial in energy processing.

- Myoadenylate deaminase deficiency causes problems in providing a source of energy (ATP) for the cell. It is the most common of the metabolic myopathies. It may occur as a primary deficiency but has also been described as occurring secondary to other muscle diseases.

- Many minerals capable of forming salts that are normally present in constant amounts in the body are essential for muscle function. High or low levels of these may lead to weakness or spasm and cramping of muscles. These include calcium, magnesium, phosphorus, potassium, and sodium.

- Kidney failure and liver failure may be associated with muscle weakness.

Endocrine   Although not common, muscle disease is well recognized in association with Cushing's disease, hyper- or hypothyroidism, hyperparathyroidism (a calcium disturbance resulting from an overactive parathyroid gland), Addison's disease (failure of the adrenal glands), and ACROMEGALY.

myositis   Inflammation of muscle has many causes. While the various causes may produce a range of symptoms, the effect on muscle is always weakness with or without pain and tenderness.

The enzymes contained in muscle cells are released into the blood in large amounts and can be measured to assist in the diagnosis and to evaluate the response to treatment. The most useful of these is CREATINE KINASE or CPK (see Appendix II). Muscle biopsy and sometimes EMG are important in making the diagnosis (see DERMATOMYOSITIS AND POLYMYOSITIS). The more important rheumatic diseases which present primarily as muscle disease that dermatomyositis, polymyositis, and INCLUSION BODY MYOSITIS, which are discussed under those headings. The connective tissue diseases, especially SYSTEMIC LUPUS ERYTHEMATOSUS, SCLERODERMA, and the OVERLAP SYNDROME may also be complicated by an inflammatory myositis, which is autoimmune in nature. Note that the differentiation between inflammatory and noninflammatory (see MYOPATHY) is to a degree artificial. Conditions associated with drug ingestion and malignancies listed above as causes of myopathy may also be inflammatory. There are several other causes of myositis; some are discussed below.

- Myositis ossificans results in sheets of calcium being laid down in or alongside muscle. This usually follows trauma or surgery. The affected muscle, often in the thigh, is painful and swollen with a woody feel. Treatment is difficult. BISPHOSPHONATES, diltiazem (a calcium channel blocker), and anticoagulants (blood-thinning medications) are often tried. Exercise and stretching should be avoided during the acute phase. Myositis ossificans sometimes resolves spontaneously.

- RHABDOMYOLYSIS.

- Viral infections are a common cause of muscle inflammation. This is usually mild and short-lived but can cause significant problems on occasion. The influenza viruses, infectious mononucleosis, coxsackie, and rubella viruses are all well-described causes of myositis. Bacterial infections, parasites such as trichinella, and toxoplasma can cause myositis. In addition, some bacteria such as staphylococcus and streptococcus may cause abscesses within muscle.

neonatal lupus   A rare condition in which some features of systemic lupus erythematosus develop in newborn babies.

It is thought that this autoimmune disease is transmitted from the mother to the child through autoantibodies that cross the placenta and affect the baby. This means that the disease lasts only as long as the mother's antibodies remain in the infant. Women with SLE have a greater chance of having a baby with neonatal lupus, particularly if the mother has a positive blood test for SSA or SSB antibodies (also called Ro and La antibodies). About half the affected pregnancies occur in women who have never had SLE or a similar illness, but many of the mothers of babies with neonatal lupus do have SSA and SSB antibodies. The risk of having a baby with neonatal lupus is about 2 percent in women with SLE who have SSA or SSB antibodies and may be higher, about 5 percent, in those who have both. If a woman has already had one affected child, then the chance that the next child will be affected is about 16 percent.

Symptoms and Diagnostic Path

Sometimes babies of women with SLE develop the typical skin rash of lupus. If this happens, it is usually not present at birth but develops a few weeks later. The rash is reddish, often affects the face and scalp, and is worse on parts of the body such as the face and scalp that are exposed to ultraviolet light. Neonatal lupus does not mean that the baby has chronic lupus, and symptoms resolve as the baby clears the maternal antibodies. In neonatal lupus other features of lupus are uncommon, but thrombocytopenia can occur because of autoantibodies to platelets.

A more serious and irreversible problem is heart block, a condition in which the electrical messages from the atria are not conducted to the ventricles.

The first indication of this problem is when a pregnant woman has routine checkup at about the 20th week of pregnancy and the baby's heart rate is found to be very slow. Heart block can lead to heart failure, and this can occur while the baby is still in the uterus or after birth.

All patients with lupus are usually closely monitored during pregnancy, but those who have SSA or SSB antibodies are monitored particularly carefully. This includes regular ultrasound examinations of the growing baby that provide measurements of how well the baby is growing and how the heart is functioning. The diagnosis of neonatal lupus affecting the heart is usually made by ultrasound. Neonatal lupus causing a rash is usually diagnosed when the rash appears a few weeks after the baby is born and has a typical appearance.

Treatment Options and Outlook

Antibodies that have crossed the placenta and affected the baby cause the symptoms of neonatal lupus. Symptoms such as skin rash resolve as the baby clears the antibodies and do not need any specific treatment. The developing heart of the baby can be seen on ultrasound. If inflammation of the heart (myocarditis) is suspected or if heart block is already present, treatment with dexamethasone, a corticosteroid that crosses the placenta, can be tried. If heart block develops, it is usually irreversible, and the infant will require a pacemaker soon after birth. Overall, approximately 20 percent of affected infants die, 5 percent before birth, 10 percent before three months of age, and 5 percent between three months and three years of age.

Risk Factors and Preventive Measures

Infants of mothers with SLE and anti-Ro antibodies have about a 2 percent risk of getting neonatal lupus, rising to 5 percent if their mother has both anti-Ro and anti-La antibodies. If the mothers have the antibodies but do not have SLE, there is still a risk of neonatal lupus but it is less. If a mother has already had a baby with neonatal lupus, the risk that her next baby will get it is 16 percent.

While neonatal lupus itself is not preventable, strategies have been tried to prevent heart block. As mentioned above, the powerful corticosteroid dexamethasone can be given to the mother as this crosses the placental barrier well. Studies so far are limited, but it appears this may be beneficial in less than half the cases. It had been hoped that frequent screening would pick up affected infants early before irreversible damage had been done, but often the heart block comes on suddenly and treatment at that stage is no longer effective. Careful monitoring and treatment is still warranted, however, as some infants will be able to be protected.

neuropathic arthritis (**Charcot's joint**)   A destructive type of arthritis that occurs in patients with neuropathy.

The health of a joint depends on the ability of the body to make small adjustments to absorb shock and prevent injury. Patients with nerve damage that affects their ability to feel pain or sense where in space the joint is can sustain damage to a joint during day-to-day activities. Repeated microtrauma is thought to be the most important cause of neuropathic arthritis, but the abnormal nerve function may also alter the blood supply to the joint and increase the risk of arthritis.

Chronic syphilis causing nerve damage was a common cause of neuropathic arthritis. Because there are effective antibiotics to treat syphilis, it is now seldom a cause of Charcot's joint. The most common disease causing neuropathic arthritis is diabetes. A rare condition called syringomyelia that affects the spinal cord and the nerves to the arms can cause neuropathic arthritis of the shoulder.

Symptoms and Diagnostic Path
The symptoms of neuropathy—numbness, tingling, decreased ability to feel pain and temperature, and poor position sense—precede neuropathic arthritis but may not have been noticed by the patient. The

arthritis typically occurs in a large weight-bearing joint such as the ankle or knee in the limbs affected by neuropathy. If the arms are affected by neuropathy, the shoulders can be damaged.

The symptoms are those of severe osteoarthritis with bony swelling, effusion, pain, instability, and loss of function. Because of nerve damage, pain may be less severe than would be expected from the severity of the arthritis.

The diagnosis is made from the symptoms and the X-ray. The X-ray shows destructive arthritis with bone debris. If the cause of neuropathy is not known, blood tests for syphilis and diabetes are performed.

Treatment Options and Outlook
No specific treatment is available for neuropathic arthritis. As far as possible the underlying neuropathy is treated, but nerve damage is often irreversible. The affected joint should be protected and weight bearing reduced. Symptoms are treated as for osteoarthritis, but intra-articular corticosteroid injections are avoided. Joint replacement surgery is avoided if possible because the prosthetic joint will also be damaged by microtrauma and there is a high failure rate.

Risk Factors and Preventive Measures
Any cause of impaired nerve supply to a joint or joints could lead to a Charcot joint, the common ones being discussed above. Prevention will vary depending on the cause of nerve damage. Excellent control of blood sugar in diabetes delays the onset of nerve damage.

nonsteroidal anti-inflammatory drugs (**NSAIDs**) A class of drugs that is anti-inflammatory and analgesic. Although NSAIDs effectively reduce pain and inflammation, they do not affect the overall outcome or progression of arthritis. Therefore, to treat rheumatoid arthritis, NSAIDs are often combined with disease-modifying drugs (DMARDs).

NSAIDs inhibit cyclooxygenase (COX) enzymes and thus decrease the production of prostaglandins. There are two COX enzymes, COX-1 and COX-2, that differ in their function. COX-1 is found in many tissues at a low level of activity and has important effects in promoting platelet aggregation and protecting against peptic ulcers. COX-2 is often present only in cells that have been stimulated, a process known as induction. COX-2 is induced in response to inflammation. Drugs that inhibit COX-2 decrease the formation of prostaglandins in cells where their production has been stimulated and are therefore anti-inflammatory. Drugs that inhibit COX-1 have two important effects. First, they decrease the production of thromboxane, a prostaglandin-like substance that makes platelets in the blood stickier. Thus aspirin, which inhibits COX-1, is used to prevent heart attacks. Second, because COX-1 helps maintain the health of the stomach lining and protect against ulcers, drugs that block COX-1 increase the risk of peptic ulcers and bleeding from the GI tract. NSAIDs are classified according to whether they nonselectively inhibit both COX enzymes (nonselective NSAIDs) or whether they are more selective for COX-2 and spare COX-1 (COX-2–selective NSAIDs).

Nonselective NSAIDs

Most of the older NSAIDs inhibit both COX-1 and COX-2 and thus have anti-inflammatory and antiplatelet effects and increase the risk of peptic ulcers. Some older drugs like meloxicam that were originally marketed as "safer" NSAIDs have subsequently been found to be largely COX-2 selective once testing for these differential actions became possible. Aspirin is a unique nonselective COX-inhibitor because in very low doses it binds to the COX-1 enzyme of platelets and irreversibly inactivates it, making those platelets less sticky for their life span, usually about a week. The antiplatelet effects of other nonselective COX inhibitors are much shorter because they only block the enzyme while the drug is present in the bloodstream. This is why aspirin is the drug used to prevent heart attacks and stroke and why physicians recommend that patients taking regular NSAIDs who need cardiovascular protection should still take low-dose aspirin. Recent studies have made this area even more complex. In those studies, researchers found that taking a regular NSAID, IBUPROFEN, before aspirin seemed to block the long-term effects of aspirin on platelets. This occurs because ibuprofen blocks the access site where aspirin binds to the COX enzyme. If patients took aspirin first and

then took ibuprofen, the long-term antiplatelet effects of aspirin were not altered. Interestingly, a COX-2-selective drug did not affect the antiplatelet effect of aspirin, whether it was taken before or after aspirin. There are many nonselective COX inhibitors such as ASPIRIN, ibuprofen, DICLOFENAC, PIROXICAM, NAPROXEN, and others.

COX-2 Selective NSAIDs

As gastrointestinal adverse effects such as heartburn, ulcers, and bleeding were the commonest adverse effects of the NSAIDs and were due to inhibition of COX-1, it was thought that drugs that only inhibited COX-2 (the inflammation-related enzyme) would be safer. CELECOXIB and rofecoxib were the first of these drugs to be brought to market and trial data certainly showed that they caused much less GI adverse effects. However data on rofecoxib soon emerged suggesting an increased risk of heart disease was associated with its use. As further evidence accumulated, first rofecoxib and then a newer drug, valdecoxib, were withdrawn by their manufacturers because of these concerns. Other COX-2 inhibitors etoricoxib and lumiracoxib are currently not approved by the FDA. In many countries, etoricoxib has been withdrawn from the market, owing to its association with liver problems.

Indications for NSAIDs

Almost any type of pain or inflammation has been treated with NSAIDs. Generally, pain caused by acute inflammation such as gout responds well, but that caused by nerve damage responds poorly. NSAIDs are used to treat pain and inflammation associated with many kinds of arthritis and soft tissue problems, including RHEUMATOID ARTHRITIS, OSTEOARTHRITIS, RHEUMATIC FEVER, Still's disease, JUVENILE IDIOPATHIC ARTHRITIS, GOUT, ANKYLOSING SPONDYLITIS, TENDINITIS, and BURSITIS.

There is no good evidence that one NSAID is more effective than another. A common misconception is that the newer COX-2-selective drugs are more effective than older, nonselective NSAIDs. On average this is not the case, but people do respond differently. Finding that different patients find particular NSAIDs more effective is not unusual. However, if a condition has not responded to treatment with two or three NSAIDs, it is unlikely to respond to others, and a different type of treatment may be more appropriate.

Side Effects of NSAIDs

Millions of people take NSAIDs and serious problems are relatively uncommon. Nevertheless, because NSAIDs are so widely prescribed, a significant number of people develop problems from taking them.

Allergy Some people are allergic to NSAIDs. This reaction can be serious, causing urticaria (a blotchy red raised rash), swelling of the face and tongue (angioedema), and wheezing. This type of allergy occurs more often in people who have asthma or nasal polyps. If someone has had a severe allergic reaction to one NSAID, he or she is likely to have a similar reaction to other NSAIDs.

GI Indigestion and heartburn are common and are often the reason people stop taking NSAIDs. Less common, but more serious, are peptic ulcers. These can be silent and occur without the usual warning symptoms of indigestion or abdominal pain. NSAIDs should be taken with food, but doing so does not necessarily prevent peptic ulcers. In many research studies endoscopy has been performed on patients treated with NSAIDs, and small superficial ulcers are often visible. These superficial ulcers do not usually cause problems and frequently heal on their own. However, some of them become deeper and can lead to complications such as bleeding or perforation of the stomach.

Bleeding from the GI tract can be slow or rapid. Slow loss of blood may cause no symptoms other than anemia occurring over several months. A large GI bleed will often cause vomiting of blood or passing altered blood in the stool. One of the signs of bleeding from the stomach is pitch-black bowel motions. Iron tablets that are used to treat anemia caused by iron deficiency often color the stool greenish black, and this can cause confusion. Bowel motions with altered blood, in addition to being black, are also often runny and very smelly. Patients who pass altered blood should seek medical attention immediately since significant blood loss can be serious and should be investigated and treated.

- A complicated ulcer can occur in anyone taking NSAIDs but there are several factors that increase the risk of GI complications. These include being older than 65 years, taking an anticoagulant, having had a previous peptic ulcer or bleeding from it, and taking an NSAID combined with a corticosteroid. The risk of a complicated ulcer with nonselective NSAIDs can be as high as three per 100 people per year.

- There are several ways to decrease the risk of GI side effects caused by NSAIDs. The most effective is to avoid NSAIDs entirely, but this is not often an option because limited alternative treatments are available to treat musculoskeletal pain. If avoiding NSAIDs is not possible, there are two choices. If the patient has a low risk of any cardiovascular event such as heart attack or stroke then a COX-2 selective drug like celecoxib can be used. In older patients or those with cardiovascular risk factors, then using a nonselective NSAID with minimal or no cardiovascular risk such as naproxen together with a gastroprotective agent would be safer. Gastroprotective agents are medications that at least partially prevent erosions and ulcers forming in patients taking NSAIDs and include proton pump inhibitors such as OMEPRAZOLE and the prostaglandin analogue MISOPROSTOL.

One controversy regarding the COX-2-selective drugs is an observation made in a subgroup of patients from the CLASS study, a clinical trial that examined the GI safety of celecoxib. Investigators found that patients taking celecoxib who continued to take low-dose aspirin for cardiovascular protection seemed to lose some of the GI benefits of taking a COX-2-selective NSAID. In other words, the risk of peptic ulcer in patients taking celecoxib and low-dose aspirin and those taking nonselective NSAIDs was similar. This information was obtained by breaking the original study group into subgroups, a statistical technique that is frowned upon because it has in the past led to conclusions that were not substantiated when larger studies specifically designed to focus on that particular subgroup of patients were performed. Therefore, until further information becomes available, the potential negative effects of low-dose aspirin on the GI risk reduction of COX-2-selective NSAIDs will be debated. The use of low-dose aspirin along with nonselective NSAIDs also increases the risk of ulcers and bleeding. Ibuprofen interferes with the action of aspirin and should be taken at least one hour after daily low-dose aspirin.

Several drugs appear to decrease the risk of GI complications associated with NSAIDs. MISOPROSTOL, a drug that is similar to a prostaglandin, protects the stomach against peptic ulcers. Its most common side effect, diarrhea, and the fact that it can cause abortion make it unpopular. Proton pump inhibitors such as omeprazole, lansoprazole, and rabeprazole that effectively decrease the production of acid in the stomach protect against ulcers caused by NSAIDs. Both ulceration and bleeding have been shown to be reduced in high-risk patients. Together with misoprostol they are therefore recommended in patients at significant risk of GI complications who need to take NSAIDs. Eradicating *Helicobacter pylori,* a bacteria that causes a very low-grade infection in the lining of the upper GI tract and predisposes to ulceration, with a course of antibiotics also reduces the risk of NSAID-induced bleeding. In general, patients who have had GI bleeding because of taking an NSAID should never take one again. However, a recent study showed that using a COX-2 inhibitor, celecoxib, with high-dose proton pump inhibitors safe. Further studies are required.

Cardiovascular All NSAIDs can cause some fluid retention. Usually this is mild and causes only a little ankle puffiness, but it can be severe and worsen symptoms such as shortness of breath in patients with heart failure. Blood pressure can also increase, usually by only a small amount, but in a few people by a lot. The VIGOR trial showed that the COX-2 inhibitor, Vioxx, caused less GI damage than the comparison nonselective NSAID, Naproxen. However slightly more patients in the Vioxx group had myocardial infarctions (heart attacks) than in the control group. This could have been because low-dose aspirin (protective against heart attacks) was not allowed in this trial or because naproxen protected against heart attacks or because Vioxx predisposed people to heart attacks. Gradually, more evidence accumulated that it was the Vioxx and in September 2004 it was withdrawn from the market. This obviously

focused attention on other COX-2 inhibitors and the nonselective NSAIDs. Another COX-2 selective drug, valdecoxib, was withdrawn in 2005 and apart from celecoxib no other COX-2 drugs are approved by the FDA. Celecoxib has been fairly extensively studied and appears reasonably safe at the doses usually prescribed for arthritis (100 to 200 mgs per day). It was used in very high dose (400 mg twice a day) to try to prevent adenomas from forming in the bowel of at-risk patients and at this dose was associated with an increase in cardiac events. Since 2004, large-scale population studies have suggested that the nonselective NSAIDs also increase the risk of heart attacks. This effect is relatively small and varies among the different drugs. A metaanalysis of these studies showed that of the most widely used NSAIDs diclofenac and then ibuprofen had the highest risk and naproxen did not convey any increased risk.

Patients with a cardiac history or over the age of 65 years should only take NSAID therapy, if there is no safer alternative. If going on NSAID therapy, careful attention should be paid to kidney function and blood pressure control. All these patients and any others in whom low-dose aspirin is indicated should continue their aspirin, recognizing that this increases their risk of GI adverse effects and thereby probably requiring a gastroprotective agent. Naproxen seems the safest NSAID from the cardiac point of view. If ibuprofen is used it should be taken at least one hour after low-dose aspirin as it physically interferes with the action of aspirin.

Renal NSAIDs decrease the blood flow through the kidney and can decrease function, sometimes severely. Both selective and nonselective NSAIDs can affect kidney function. NSAIDs do not cause significant renal effects in most patients. However, patients with diabetes, heart failure, kidney disease, and those taking diuretics or ACE inhibitors (angiotensin-converting enzyme inhibitors—a group of drugs that lowers blood pressure) have a higher risk. In these people serum creatinine levels are usually monitored to check kidney function.

Other Abnormal liver function tests, usually mild, occur in 1–15 percent of people. Rashes, ringing in the ears, and a feeling of lightheadedness can occur. Serious blood problems such as neutropenia are rare. NSAIDs are avoided in the late stages of pregnancy because they can cause premature closing of the ductus arteriosus, a blood vessel that is important for maintaining the fetal circulation. Experimentally in the laboratory, NSAIDs, especially COX-2 selective drugs, slow down bone healing, and it is prudent to avoid these drugs in people with healing fractures or after surgery to bones. About 10 to 20 percent of patients with asthma, especially atopic individuals (those with hayfever and nasal polyps as well), get worsening of their asthma when taking aspirin and very occasionally NSAIDs as well.

Drug Interactions

Nonselective NSAIDs, because they decrease platelet stickiness, can increase the risk of bleeding in patients taking warfarin and other anticoagulants. Taking two different NSAIDs together (other than low-dose aspirin for cardiovascular protection) is not recommended, because combining NSAIDs is not more effective and increases the risk of side effects.

Methotrexate often appears as an interacting drug on pharmacy computers when patients fill a prescription for an NSAID. This is because many NSAIDs can increase the concentrations of methotrexate but usually by only a small amount. In rheumatology practice, with the low doses of methotrexate used, this interaction is seldom clinically important and methotrexate is often prescribed together with an NSAID for RA.

NSAIDs can blunt the ability of drugs, particularly diuretics (water pills) and ACE inhibitors, to lower blood pressure.

Clinical Use

A simple analgesic such as acetaminophen is likely to have fewer side effects than an NSAID and is therefore usually the drug of choice for patients with pain that is mild and not associated with much inflammation, for example osteoarthritis. If there is significant inflammation, for example as in rheumatoid arthritis, an NSAID relieves pain and stiffness more effectively than acetaminophen.

In young healthy individuals with a transient painful musculoskeletal condition such as a tennis player with tendinitis, NSAIDs are effective and reasonably safe. In those over 65 years of age, at risk of GI hemorrhage or cardiac events, with high blood pressure or kidney dysfunction, a careful analysis has to be made of the risks of NSAID treatment versus the likely benefits and a decision made with the patient as fully informed as possible. The choice of NSAID is frequently made on which adverse effect to avoid rather than because of any difference in effectiveness and coprescribing to minimize adverse effects has become very common. For most of the adverse effects discussed above the lower the dose the safer the drug is.

Whichever NSAID is chosen, it is important to remember that NSAIDs treat symptoms and not the underlying disease. If the problem is a self-limited one that will heal over time, for example tendinitis, this may be all that is required. For an illness such as rheumatoid arthritis, though, treatment with an NSAID alone will allow joint damage to progress.

A number of observational studies have suggested that long-term NSAID therapy may protect against Alzheimer's disease and certain tumors, especially bowel cancers. The recent concerns about cardiovascular safety discussed above have largely put an end to long-term studies of currently available drugs as preventive agents, but research will no doubt proceed to find safer compounds that can be studied as preventive agents.

occupational therapy Occupational and physical therapists work with patients to maintain and restore function, reduce pain and deformity, and prevent deterioration and injury. There is a lot of overlap between occupational and physical therapy. However, physical therapy tends to focus on problems related to moving, walking, exercise, and muscle-strengthening. Occupational therapy places more emphasis on modifying the home or workplace to suit the patient or teaching the patient skills that will be useful in the dealing with day-to-day activities. Occupational therapists also provide advice about the many splints, orthoses, and aids that can significantly improve a patient's quality of life. Physical and occupational therapists both play important roles in the care of patients with rheumatic diseases.

olecranon bursitis The olecranon bursas are between the skin and the olecranon, which is the bony prominence at the back of the elbow. The bursa is a sac lined with synovial tissue and contains a small amount of synovial fluid that allows the bony part of the elbow to move with minimal friction against the many surfaces it comes up against. Perhaps because it is so exposed to trauma it is one of the most common of the body's many bursas to cause problems. This often occurs in young men in occupations such as carpet laying or car mechanics or at any age because of recreational activities ranging from skateboarding and wrestling to gardening. It may also occur as a result of an inflammatory arthritis.

A significant blow to the olecranon bursa can cause traumatic bursitis. If fluid is removed, it is usually bloodstained. Lesser, repeated trauma can also cause bursitis, but the fluid is less likely to be bloodstained. If symptoms are minor, treatment is with rest and elbow protection with or without NSAIDs. If more severe, the fluid can be aspirated and a compressive bandage applied. If the patient is going to return to a work or recreational setting where similar trauma is likely to happen again, a protective elbow guard should be recommended.

Because of the thin skin over the elbow and frequent trauma, it is relatively easy for infecting organisms to reach the bursa through breaks in the skin. Infection should always be excluded by aspirating fluid from the bursa if there is doubt. With established infection the skin is red and warm and very tender. The blood count may show a raised white cell count. Fluid from the bursa is thick and murky because of all the cells in it, and growing the organism from this fluid should be possible. These are commonly staphylococcal or streptococcal species from the patient's own skin, but many of other organisms may be introduced. Antibiotics and painkillers are used, but the fluid must be removed for successful treatment. This can be done as an outpatient as a simple daily aspiration in uncomplicated infections. If the patient has diabetes, HIV infection, or is otherwise immunosuppressed, then inpatient treatment is preferred. In resistant cases surgical drainage or even removal of the bursa may be necessary. Antibiotics are continued for two weeks.

Olecranon bursitis also occurs quite commonly in RHEUMATOID ARTHRITIS, psoriatic arthritis (see PSORIASIS AND PSORIATIC ARTHRITIS), and GOUT. These are usually sterile inflammatory lesions, but the patients are not immune to infection and this should be considered. Aspiration and injection of a small dose of CORTICOSTEROID can speed resolution.

opportunistic infection An infection that occurs with immunosuppression and is caused by an organism that would not normally infect healthy people. Immunosuppressed patients have a higher risk of becoming infected, both with the usual organisms that affect healthy people and with opportunistic organisms. The term nosocomial infection means an infection acquired in the hospital. Patients who are immunosuppressed have a high risk of nosocomial infection, and some of these are caused by opportunistic infections. The consequences of an infection are also often more serious. For example, chicken pox is seldom a serious condition in healthy people but can be fatal in immunosuppressed patients.

The underlying cause of opportunistic infection is suppression of the immune system. The normal immune response is a protective mechanism that prevents infection. Patients with immunosuppression, whether it be from AIDS, diabetes, cancer, or drugs used to suppress the immune system, have a greater risk of unusual infections. These include aspergillosis, tuberculosis, nocardiosis, and fungal and pneumocystis infections. Because their immune systems are suppressed, however, these individuals are also more likely to be infected with organisms such as streptococci and staphylococci that often infect healthy people.

Symptoms and Diagnostic Path
The symptoms of infection can be changed by immunosuppression. For example, corticosteroids will often suppress much of the acute inflammatory response to an infection. Fever, swelling, and pain may be less severe in immunosuppressed patients and may lead to the diagnosis of infection being overlooked.

The gold standard for the diagnosis of infection in immunosuppressed patients, as it is in healthy patients, is culture of the infecting organism. In spite of having a suppressed immune system, most patients can still mount enough of a response to an infection to cause symptoms such as fever and malaise. Physicians are particularly conscious of the risk of infection in immunosuppressed patients and often draw blood for culture in patients with symptoms such as fever that would otherwise be thought to be minor.

In patients with rheumatic diseases who are taking immunosuppressive drugs, the diagnosis of infection is often complicated by the possibility that the rheumatic disease, and not infection, could be causing the symptoms. For example, if a patient with vasculitis treated with the immunosuppressive drug cyclophosphamide develops a fever, the question arises whether this is due to an opportunistic infection or active vasculitis. If the cultures of blood and other body fluids are negative, the decision whether to treat someone for infection with antibiotics or for autoimmune disease with more powerful immunosuppression is often based on clinical judgment.

Treatment Options and Outlook
Distinguishing between infection and active autoimmune disease, although sometimes difficult, is important, because the treatment can have negative effects if the wrong diagnosis is made. Immunosuppressive drugs such as corticosteroids and cyclophosphamide could worsen an infection because they suppress the ability of the body to fight infection. To make matters more complicated, immunosuppressive drugs will often cause symptoms such as fever to improve, leading to the erroneous impression that the correct diagnosis has been made. On the other hand, antibiotics will not effectively treat a flare of an autoimmune disease, and they can sometimes cause fever.

If the specific cause of an opportunistic infection is identified, usually through culture of an organism, appropriate antibiotic or antifungal treatment can be started. Usually the infection responds to treatment and can be cured. However, if the patient has an irreversible cause of immunosuppression (such as HIV infection), opportunistic infections can recur.

Risk Factors and Preventive Measures
The common causes of immunosuppression such as AIDS, cancer, immunosuppressive drugs, and diabetes are discussed above and all increase the risk of opportunistic infections. There are relatively few preventive measures possible. Avoiding high-risk situations is important. As well as avoiding direct contact with people who have a current infection, immunosuppressed individuals should avoid hos-

pital admission if possible. If they have to be admitted, they should be nursed with special precautions in isolation, sometimes called reverse barrier nursing. It can be useful to vaccinate younger relatives for chicken pox if they are going to be around the immunosuppressed individual to prevent them from getting an active infection that they can pass on. The immunosuppressed person can receive killed vaccines and should get a flu jab every year. Their immune response to the vaccination may however be weak. Herpes zoster or shingles is a significant problem and can be mitigated by booster vaccination. It is common practice to treat patients receiving high-dose or prolonged cyclophosphamide therapy with an antibiotic, cotrimoxazole, to prevent pneumocystis pneumonia. For people taking immunosuppressive drugs, regular monitoring of the blood count will detect when the white cell count falls too low and allow appropriate adjustment of doses.

osteoarthritis (OA) This is the most common form of arthritis and is very ancient, being present in Neolithic skeletons. It is a major health problem for dogs, horses, and other animals as well as humans. The number of people suffering from OA increases with age and at 65 years of age 80 percent of people will have X-ray evidence of OA. However, X-ray changes do not necessarily mean that person will have problems from the OA, and only 10 percent of 65 year-olds will have symptoms. It is a major cause of pain and disability in the elderly and has significant socioeconomic importance. OA is the most common reason for JOINT REPLACEMENT surgery. People under the age of 65 years with OA will have double the medical costs as those not having OA. As the population ages, it is estimated that 18 percent of the U.S. population (59 million people) will have OA in 2020.

While the precise cause is not known, a lot is known about the processes and risk factors. Risk factors are any factor that is conclusively shown to be associated with an increased risk of getting the particular disease. It does not mean that the factor causes the disease. There are many ways of classifying (or subdividing) OA. This section will take the simple approach of dividing it into primary and secondary. In secondary OA, there is a clear-cut cause. In primary OA, no such cause is apparent, although there are well-known risk factors.

Whatever the cause, the processes are fairly similar in established disease. Indeed, OA has been described as the common final pathway of joint failure, resulting from various insults to the joint. The bones forming the vast majority of joints in the body are covered by a lining of cartilage where they come into contact with each other. The cartilage has no blood vessels, lymph ducts, or nerves and only very few cells, called chondrocytes. People therefore do not feel their cartilage, and it gets its nutrients from the fluid secreted by the joint lining cells (synovium). To the naked eye cartilage looks like hard, glistening whitish plastic.

The cartilage is made up of arcing strands of type II collagen that hold long, complex sugar and protein molecules tightly in place. These molecules attract water molecules very powerfully. When weight is applied to the cartilage some of the water is squeezed out, and then as the weight eases off, the water is sucked back into the cartilage. This gives joints their sponginess and protects the bones from the constant jarring to which they would otherwise be subjected. Normal joints contain a small amount of fluid, which provides nutrients to the cartilage and reduces friction between the cartilage on each side of the joint. This fluid contains hyaluronan, which has viscoelastic properties. This means that it is viscous at relatively low speeds, allowing smooth sliding while walking and running. At rapid speeds, however, it becomes elastic, providing give and bounce as, for example, when landing from a jump.

In early OA, the character of the synovial fluid changes so that there is more friction and less sponginess. The surface of the cartilage becomes worn and ragged, and strands of collagen are broken, allowing the water-attracting sugar and protein molecules to escape. As the disease progresses, cracks develop in the cartilage and it becomes thinner. Although traditionally regarded as a noninflammatory disease (see ARTHRITIS for classification), there is often low-grade inflammation, which contributes to the changes in cartilage and bone. The loss of shock absorption by cartilage puts increased stress on the underlying bone. This responds by developing a thickened surface, growing bony protrusions around the edges of the joint (called osteophytes), and later forming cysts in the bone.

Risk factors for primary OA   Obesity is an important risk factor for OA. Studies have shown that obesity contributes 21 percent of the risk for OA of the knee, compared with 9 percent for a family history, 8 percent for a previous knee injury, and 1 percent for a previous meniscectomy. The risk goes up with increasing weight. Over half the U.S. population is overweight. If the heaviest third reduced their weight to that of the middle third, there would be 20 percent fewer people with OA. Not only does weight loss reduce the risk of getting OA, but it also reduces the speed of progression once the disease is established. The strongest association with being overweight is with knee OA, but there is also an association with not only other weight-bearing joints but also with hand OA. This indicates that the effect of obesity is not purely through excessive loading of joints.

There are rare families who develop early OA with great frequency. A number of mutations have been identified in the genes for type II collagen and other cartilage constituents. Although there is clearly a hereditary influence on other more common forms of OA, especially hand and knee OA in women, the genetic basis for this has not been discovered and may be quite complex.

Certain occupations are associated with OA developing in particular joints. Examples include hip OA in farmers, finger OA in rock climbers, knee OA in builders, and midfoot joint OA in ballet dancers. Recreational exercise in people with normal joints is not a risk factor for OA, but joint injuries or biomechanical abnormalities do predispose athletes to OA, especially elite athletes.

It has been observed that women with OSTEO-POROSIS have a lower risk of developing OA and vice versa. While this is interesting in looking at mechanisms, it is not useful in treatment and prevention.

Despite interest in the impact of hormonal factors on OA, especially that of estrogen, there is no clear association.

Causes of secondary OA   Metabolic causes include ACROMEGALY, HEMOCHROMATOSIS, CPPD, and ALKAPTONURIA.

Skeletal abnormalities leading to OA include congenital dislocation of the hip, slipped femoral epiphysis, Perthes disease (all affecting the hip), developmental bony abnormalities, leg length abnormalities, and HYPERMOBILITY SYNDROME.

Trauma is a frequent cause of secondary OA. This may be from an acute injury such as a fracture through the joint or dislocation, following joint surgery, especially meniscectomy, at the knee (see KNEE PAIN) or from repeated minor trauma.

Any inflammatory arthritis can lead to secondary OA, the most common being RHEUMATOID ARTHRITIS. INFECTIVE ARTHRITIS very rapidly damages cartilage and leads to OA.

Symptoms and Diagnostic Path

Pain, crepitus (a grating in the joint), stiffness, instability, and loss of function are the symptoms of OA. The pain usually starts gradually and is described as a mild-to-moderate ache. It gets worse with exercise and feels better with rest. Pain at rest or at night can occur with advanced disease. Since people cannot feel their cartilage, the pain obviously comes from other structures. These include the synovium or joint lining, the joint capsule, tendons and ligaments around the joint, muscles that stabilize the joint, as well as bone and periosteum (the lining layer around bone). Because of all these different sources of pain, it is not surprising that the level of pain does not often agree with the severity of the changes seen on X-ray. It also explains why the pain can change in character and intensity from day to day.

The stiffness is mainly first thing in the morning and after resting for short periods during the day. It seldom lasts more than 20 to 30 minutes, unlike inflammatory arthritis. Loss of range of movement in a joint can cause many problems such as a poor grip (fingers), difficulty combing hair and dressing (shoulders), inability to reverse in a car (neck), difficulty getting in and out of a car (hips), difficulty descending stairs (knee), and limited ability to stride (ankle).

Hand OA often gives rise to bony swellings at the distal interphalangeal joints, called Heberden's nodes, and at the proximal called Bouchard's nodes. These may be intermittently painful, but the main problem is a slow loss of range of movement.

People with this nodal OA are at increased risk of getting knee OA. The base of the thumb joint is also often involved and leads to a weak grip. The wrist is involved in some forms of secondary OA and occupational OA. The spine, hips, and knees are frequently involved, but apart from MILWAUKEE SHOULDER syndrome, the elbows and shoulders are not. Hip OA can sometimes be deceptive because it can give rise to pain in the front of the knee.

Although OA is usually a slowly progressive disease, certain factors can make it progress more rapidly. In nodal OA of the hands, there is sometimes quite severe pain and swelling in one or two joints that subsides over a month or two but is associated with more rapid cartilage damage. This occurs in a form of OA called erosive OA because bone is slowly eaten away at the joints, leading to more deformity than usual. This needs to be differentiated from the crystal arthropathies, GOUT and CPPD. Gout in particular is much more likely to develop in joints that are already damaged, especially if they become cold. Gout is usually recognized when it occurs in the feet, ankles, or knees; it may not be suspected in the fingers. In addition if it occurs in the hips, diagnosis may be very difficult. CPPD frequently occurs in association with long-standing OA.

A typical history and examination is usually enough to make the diagnosis in established disease. This is then confirmed with the appropriate X-rays. The physical examination and sometimes the X-rays may show minimal abnormalities in early disease. In this situation it is important to exclude other causes of the symptoms. Blood tests are normal in primary OA. The physical examination may prompt investigation for one of the metabolic or inflammatory causes listed above. All patients under the age of 55 years should have screening tests to look for the excessive iron load found in hemochromatosis. The presence of chondrocalcinosis (calcium lining the joint cartilage) on X-ray suggests CPPD, and testing for causes of this is appropriate. Most patients with CPPD, however, do not have an underlying metabolic abnormality.

While the X-ray changes of OA are easily recognized, there are two confounding issues. First, pain does not correlate well with the degree of X-ray change, especially in the hand. Second, because OA on X-ray is so common, many people present-

ing with another form of arthritis will have OA changes that they may have had for years and that are not necessarily causing their problems. MRI scans can show the joint in great detail, including depth of the cartilage, inflammation in ligaments and other soft tissues, and so-called bone bruising in areas of bone under particular stress. They are not often indicated but are very good at sorting out exactly what is going on in difficult circumstances.

Treatment Options and Outlook

The aims of treating OA are to relieve pain, improve function, and slow down progression. Actual improvement of joint structure (for example, regrowing damaged cartilage) is an area of considerable interest and research but to date has not been achieved with any certainty.

Osteoarthritis is very common. It is painful and can have a major impact on an individual's quality of life but is not life threatening. It usually starts toward the end of a person's working life when he or she has some discretionary spending money. All these factors make it the ideal condition for swindlers to make a lot of money from selling "wonder cures." Needless to say, the authors are not the first people to come to this realization and there are many dubious treatments promoted for use in OA. The treatments listed below all have good evidence supporting their use in OA (see CLINICAL TRIAL for discussion of evidence). The text discusses their place in treatment as well as other alternative treatments that show promise.

Proven nonpharmacologic treatments:

- Education
- Aerobic and joint-specific exercise
- Joint protection and unloading
- Weight loss
- Footwear, orthotics, and appliances
- Heat and cold
- Self-help group telephone support

Proven pharmacologic treatments:

- Acetaminophen
- Topical counterirritants and capsaicin

- Nonselective nonsteroidal anti-inflammatory drugs
- COX-2 nonsteroidal anti-inflammatory drugs
- Weak narcotic drugs
- Intra-articular corticosteroid
- Intra-articular hyaluronan

Surgery:

- Osteotomy
- Joint replacement

Proven nonpharmacologic treatments Understanding a chronic disease helps someone gain control over it. Information and advice can be obtained from the patient's doctor, specialist nurses, the Arthritis Foundation, or relevant Internet sites (see Appendix III). Written material, self-help groups, and exercise classes are all helpful in this regard.

Exercise has been shown to be beneficial. This has been best studied in knee OA, where specific exercises to strengthen the quadriceps muscles improve function and reduce pain. Other stretches and exercises can be used to improve function when other joints are involved. They are best undertaken under the guidance of a physician or physical therapist specializing in this area. Aerobic exercise to improve fitness has a nonspecific effect on reducing pain levels. This also makes weight loss easier. Resistive exercise can also improve function and decrease pain (see EXERCISE).

A range of devices available make everyday activities easier (see ASSISTIVE DEVICES). These can improve function without actually altering the arthritis. The use of a walking stick reduces the load put through a weight-bearing joint and can improve mobility considerably if one knee or hip is the most limiting factor. Occupational therapists can help assess the likely utility of such a device before the patient buys it, can also provide training in joint protection, and can advise concerning safety issues around the house.

Weight loss improves pain and mobility by unloading weight-bearing joints. It has also been shown to slow progression of OA, and this may be through effects other than mechanical unloading. While weight loss may on the surface seem to be the most easily modifiable factor for the patient with OA, everyone who has tried to lose weight knows it is easier said than done. Those who join a program, whether that be a hospital-based multidisciplinary program or a community-based program such as is run by Weight Watchers, are far more successful than those who go it alone.

Cushioned insoles or specially constructed shock-absorbing shoes can reduce the impact of walking. Orthoses can be used to correct malalignment and to shift the line of weight bearing away from the more severely affected side in knee OA. Knee braces can occasionally relieve pain in severe disease. Taping the kneecap may relieve pain while appropriate exercises are being done.

The appropriate use of heat or cold packs can help relieve pain. Cold packs are generally most effective when there is a flare of pain in a joint (see ICE). Broken-up ice cubes in a cloth, a bag of frozen peas, or a proprietary ice pack may be used. The cold pack is applied for 20 minutes at a time, and the skin should be protected from direct contact to prevent frostbite. HEAT, traditionally a hot-water bottle but more commonly a wheat bag or gel that can be heated in a microwave, is more helpful in relieving the pain associated with stiff, immobile joints.

Acupuncture may give pain relief in OA. It re quires a course of treatments, and its effect lasts only for up to four weeks after the course is finished.

Some experimental evidence suggests that electromagnetism promotes cartilage growth, but there is no evidence in humans. Several small studies have suggested a weak benefit from pulsed electromagnetic fields in OA patients, but larger studies are needed. There is no evidence that the stationary magnets that are widely marketed are effective (see MAGNETS).

Proven pharmacologic treatments ACETAMINO-PHEN is the first line of treatment. It is an effective painkiller and very safe at usual doses. The most common side effect is nausea. It can be taken occasionally as required but is more effective when taken regularly. It can also be used just before undertaking activities that the patient knows will cause pain. Which method is used will depend on the severity of the pain. Patients need to be aware that some other drugs contain acetaminophen in combinations, and this needs to be taken into consideration in order not to exceed the maximum daily dose.

Many patients not responding adequately to acetaminophen will find improved relief from NSAIDs. There are short-acting and long-acting forms of these, and they may also be used as required, although regular use is more effective. The most common side effect is irritation or bleeding from the upper gastrointestinal tract. This can be partially prevented by the use of either MISOPROSTOL or a proton pump inhibitor such as OMEPRAZOLE, RABEPRAZOLE, PANTOPRAZOLE, or LAN-SOPRAZOLE. Unfortunately, one of the main risk factors for GI bleeding is increasing age (over 65 years particularly). Therefore, taking NSAIDs can be risky for older people with OA. The COX-2 inhibitor CELECOXIB minimizes this adverse effect, but in older patients at risk of heart disease should be taken with low-dose aspirin and a gastroprotective agent (see NONSTEROIDAL ANTI-INFLAMMATORY DRUGS for full discussion).

Weak narcotic analgesics such as TRAMADOL or acetaminophen combined with CODEINE, HYDRO-CODONE, or dextropropoxyphene are also a useful step up from acetaminophen for more severe pain. They can all cause drowsiness in some people and constipation if taken regularly. They are often taken at night with plain acetaminophen during the day for these reasons.

Injection of small amounts of CORTICOSTEROIDS into the joints can relieve pain effectively. This is most often used in the knees and at the base of the thumb. Injections are generally limited to two or three per year in any one joint. There is slight leakage out of the joint, and a number of patients (especially women) experience flushing after the injection. This may last from six to 48 hours. There is a very slight risk of introducing infection with any injection, and they should not be done if the patient has an active infection elsewhere.

Injections of hyaluronan substitutes were first developed to replace that substance in the altered synovial fluid in OA (see under Cause above). Two such substitutes, HYALGAN and SYNVISC, have been approved by the U.S. Food and Drug Administration for use in knee OA. Both are given as a course of injections, have a small risk of local reactions, and a very small risk of introducing infection. They provide some pain relief in roughly 70 percent of patients but in a smaller percentage as the OA becomes increasingly severe. The relief lasts for between six weeks and 12 months. Since they can be demonstrated to be in the joint for only a few days (Synvisc longer than Hyalgan), this effect must be for reasons other than the replacement of hyaluronan. These reasons are not clear. There is no evidence that they slow down progression of the disease, although research is in progress looking at this.

GLUCOSAMINE AND CHONDROITIN SULFATE are both constituents of normal cartilage. They have become very popular among arthritis sufferers over the past few years and are often marketed in combination. Some studies show pain relief that is moderate but better than placebo (see CLINICAL TRIAL for explanation of placebo) when using them. Other studies indicate no effect.

Investigational treatment Glucosamine and chondroitin are both constituents of normal cartilage. They have become very popular among arthritis sufferers over the past few years and are often marketed in combination. A number of trials of varying quality have shown that glucosamine reduces pain in OA. However when an analysis of the eight double-blind randomized trials was done there was no greater benefit than with placebo. A well-designed trial of glucosamine and chondroitin alone or in combination, celecoxib, and placebo showed no benefit of glucosamine or chondroitin or the combination of these above placebo in reducing pain, improving function, or slowing cartilage loss. Celecoxib was significantly more effective than placebo in reducing pain. A two-year follow-up study has failed to show any reduction in joint space loss in any group compared to placebo. It has been argued by proponents of glucosamine that the glucosamine hydrochloride used in this U.S. study is different and inferior to glucosamine sulphate. Currently, there is no good evidence that these agents are useful in OA, and accumulating evidence that they are not.

Tetracyclines are antibiotics that have also been shown to inhibit some of the breakdown enzymes found in cartilage called metalloproteinases. The activity of these enzymes is increased in the cartilage of people with OA. One 30-month trial of the tetracycline, doxycycline, has shown a significant slowing in the rate of cartilage loss but no difference in pain. The expected side effects of this antibiotic were moderately frequent. Systematic review of the trials of diacerein has shown pain-relieving effects similar to NSAIDs and one study suggested it may slow cartilage loss. Diarrhea is a frequent adverse effect, and more longer term study is required to know whether this will be useful. Topical NSAID gel that can be rubbed onto troublesome joints could prevent the side effects of the larger doses that have to be taken by mouth. There is some short-term effect in relieving pain, but it is not great and these are unlikely to be helpful to most people with significant OA. CAPSAICIN is derived from chili peppers and depletes pain fibers of substance P thereby interfering with their ability to transmit pain signals to the brain. It is effective in reducing pain in OA when rubbed onto affected joints regularly but remains expensive.

Surgery Lavage (washing the joint out with salty water) is not infrequently performed for patients with severe OA. This can be done in the office using a needle or in theater using an arthroscope. In the latter case, the surgeon may trim a meniscus or protruding bits of synovium as well. Two controlled studies have failed to show any worthwhile benefit from these procedures. There does not appear to be any advantage in combining lavage and steroid injection. Debridement, or removing the abnormal cartilage during arthroscopy, is controversial. Two well-controlled studies have produced opposite results, one positive and one negative. Drilling into the bone where the cartilage is very worn so that bleeding and healing with cartilage (but not proper articular cartilage) occurs does not seem beneficial.

Osteotomy involves taking a wedge of bone out to alter the lie of the joint surfaces so that more weight is taken through the least damaged areas. This is done most often at the knee in young patients who want to delay a total joint replacement.

JOINT REPLACEMENT is an excellent treatment for advanced OA of the hip or knee. The vast majority of OA patients express great satisfaction with this form of surgery. Other joints can also be replaced, but the results do not match those of hip and knee replacements.

ARTHRODESIS still has a place in the management of severe OA associated with incapacitating pain. It gives excellent pain relief but with loss of all movement at that joint. It is most often used at the ankle and the base of the thumb in OA.

Risk Factors and Preventive Measures

The risk factors for OA are discussed in some detail in the preceding sections. For primary OA, these are chiefly genetic and increased weight. Losing weight is the single most effective preventive measure for primary OA. It reduces the risk of getting OA, and for those people who already have OA it slows progression of the disease. As mentioned above, if the heaviest third of the U.S. population reduced their weight to be the same as the middle third, there would be 20 percent less people (about 10 million) with OA.

In secondary OA, trauma is seldom avoidable but surgical trauma can be mitigated. Meniscectomy (cartilage operation) is a major risk factor for later OA of the knee. If this is necessary, it makes sense to remove the least tissue possible. Early diagnosis and effective treatment of the metabolic causes of secondary OA may delay the development of OA. There has for some years been debate about whether to screen the general population for hereditary hemochromatosis and the official consensus is that this would not be cost effective. It is absolutely necessary, however, to screen relatives of someone known to have hemochromatosis and anyone presenting with suggestive signs or symptoms at an early age for the common hemochromatosis genes. People with hypermobility syndromes should be counseled about appropriate activities, exercise, and stretching program. Good control of the inflammation in the inflammatory arthritides will delay the development of secondary OA.

osteochondritis dissecans When a fragment of joint cartilage with its underlying bone becomes detached and sometimes breaks off into the joint, it is known as osteochondritis dissecans. This affects mainly children and adolescents and is more common in boys. The child complains of an aching pain, especially during or after vigorous exercise. The joint may click or even lock if a loose body jams between the two bones. The joint is usually slightly swollen and may be tender. Although any joint may be affected, the knee is by far the most common joint involved. The inner surface of the medial (inner) condyle of the femur (thighbone) is the usual site.

The exact cause is not known, but trauma seems to be involved with nearly half the patients reporting an injury before the symptoms start. There is often a family history and these individuals are often short. X-rays may provide the diagnosis, but if not, CT or MRI scans will with great accuracy. They will also show if the fragment is still in its correct place if this is not clear on X-ray.

If the fragment is in place, it may heal with rest and avoiding vigorous activity, especially in younger children. Maintaining good muscle tone in the quadriceps (muscles in front of thigh) is very important if this course is taken. If the pain continues or the fragment seems to be coming off, it can be wired or screwed into place. This is usually done by arthroscopic surgery (see ARTHROSCOPY AND ARTHROSCOPIC SURGERY). Small loose fragments are removed from the joint. If this leaves a bare patch on the joint surface, it can be cleaned and drilled. It will then heal over with hyaline cartilage. Although this is not as resilient as normal articular (joint) cartilage, symptoms will resolve. Younger children in whom the osteochondritis heals without intervention have the best outcome.

In the institutionalized elderly, the combination of proximal muscle weakness and weak bones leads to an increased tendency to fall and high fracture rate. Hip fracture in this group of patients is not uncommonly a terminal or preterminal event, and some have argued for routine vitamin D supplementation in this situation. Recent studies in the UK showed that patients with low vitamin D levels were more likely to have had a fracture than those with normal levels. Patients with chronic pain not only limit their activities (and therefore their sun exposure) compared to pain-free peers, but some may actually have pain and weakness because of vitamin D deficiency. A study of people attending a multidisciplinary pain clinic showed that 18 percent had vitamin D levels consistent with OSTEOMALACIA (that is, observable bone abnormalities) and 32 percent had vitamin D deficiency. Whether patients like this respond to vitamin D supplementation is not yet known. Another group at particular risk of vitamin D deficiency are dark-skinned immigrants to temperate countries because of the reduced penetration of sun rays through dark skin. Among these, women who cover themselves almost completely in public for cultural reasons are at particular risk.

osteomalacia (rickets) A disorder in which bone does not calcify normally, is weak, and deforms. It is known as rickets in children.

Normal bone is formed when cells called osteoblasts lay down a matrix called osteoid that then calcifies when calcium and phosphate are laid down to form hydroxyapatite. This process requires good-quality osteoid and normal concentrations of calcium and phosphate in the body. One of the most important regulators of calcium and phosphate levels is vitamin D. Any condition that leads to decreased calcium, phosphate, or vitamin D levels, or affects the mineralization of bone can cause osteomalacia.

Vitamin D deficiency Vitamin D deficiency is the most common cause of osteomalacia and can occur in several ways. In many developing countries dietary intake of vitamin D may be inadequate, but in developed countries this rarely happens, except in the elderly. More common is poor absorption of vitamin D. This can happen in people who have had part of their stomach and duodenum removed to treat peptic ulcer and people with CELIAC DISEASE or any other disorder that affects the ability of the bowel to absorb food and nutrients. Patients with liver disease can get osteomalacia because they are less able to transform vitamin D to 25-hydroxy vitamin D, the precursor of the active form 1,25-dihydroxy vitamin D. Similarly, patients with kidney disease can get osteomalacia because the kidney is an important site where 25-hydroxy vitamin D is converted to 1,25-dihydroxy vitamin D. Sunlight aids the formation of active vitamin D. People who have borderline vitamin D levels can develop osteomalacia if they spend a lot of time indoors and are not exposed to sunlight.

Rare inherited types of osteomalacia are caused by lack of the enzymes needed to make the active form of vitamin D or by tissues not being able to respond to it. These usually cause osteomalacia in childhood.

Phosphate deficiency This is not a common cause of osteomalacia because phosphate is conserved efficiently by the kidneys, but there are rare inherited disorders in which the kidneys leak phosphate into the urine. Osteomalacia caused by phosphate loss is usually diagnosed in childhood. Rarely soft tissue tumors, most often in the abdomen, can cause phosphate loss in the urine and osteomalacia in adults.

Poor mineralization Occasionally even if supplies of calcium, phosphate, and vitamin D are adequate, osteomalacia can be caused by rare conditions that decrease the ability of bone to mineralize (lay down the calcium and phosphate normally). Hypophosphatasia is a rare inherited condition associated with low or absent levels of alkaline phosphatase, an enzyme that plays an important part in mineralization of bone. This type of osteomalacia usually presents in early childhood. Another cause of poor bone mineralization was treatment with older bisphosphonates such as ETIDRONATE. Bisphosphonates, a group of drugs that inhibit bone resorption and formation, are used to treat osteoporosis and Paget's disease. The newer preparations do not cause osteomalacia.

Symptoms and Diagnostic Path

Mild osteomalacia may not cause any symptoms, but more severe disease can cause dull aching bone pain, particularly at the ends of long bones, that can be mistaken for arthritis. Osteomalacia in children can result in soft bone that deforms as the child grows and leads to deformities such as bow legs. In adults and children, affected bone is weak and fractures more easily. Weakness and pain of the muscles of the thighs and shoulders, a condition called proximal myopathy, is often associated with osteomalacia. In children, inability to walk caused by a combination of bone pain and muscle weakness may be the presenting symptom of osteomalacia. The diagnosis of osteomalacia or vitamin D deficiency is unfortunately too often not made until some complication such as a fracture occurs and even then may be missed. The increased ease of measuring vitamin D levels in recent years should improve this situation. The diagnosis may be made incidentally or after a fracture. It is hoped that increased awareness of the importance of vitamin D and at-risk groups will lead doctors to increased screening for low vitamin D levels. Sometimes an X-ray performed for another reason shows poorly mineralized bone or findings such as pseudofractures that are typical of osteomalacia. Pseudofractures are narrow cracks in the bone. If a bone scan is performed, they light up on the scan much as a fracture would. No one is certain what causes pseudofractures, but they may be may be stress fractures that heal more slowly than usual. Routine blood tests may also give a clue to the diagnosis of osteomalacia. In contrast to osteoporosis in which all blood tests are normal, moderate or severe osteomalacia is almost always associated with abnormal blood tests. The alkaline phosphatase level is usually elevated in most types of osteomalacia except the rare hereditary disease hypophosphatasia. In patients with poor intake or absorption of vitamin D the blood levels of the vitamin, as well as calcium levels, are low. Osteomalacia caused by phosphate loss is associated with low levels of phosphate in the blood and an abnormally high amount in the urine. Rarely a bone biopsy is performed to diagnose osteomalacia. Once a diagnosis of osteomalacia has been made, further tests will be required to find out what the underlying cause is.

Treatment Options and Outlook

The treatment of osteomalacia depends on the underlying cause but usually includes vitamin D and calcium. Patients who are unable to make the active form of vitamin D are treated with calcitriol, an active form of vitamin D. Patients who are losing phosphate may also need phosphate supplements. Osteomalacia responds rapidly to treatment. However, patients need to have their blood levels of calcium monitored because treatment with too much vitamin D can cause a high blood calcium concentration.

Risk Factors and Preventive Measures

Vitamin D deficiency should be suspected in at-risk groups and be tested for. These groups include dark-skinned people living in temperate countries, the elderly, especially those living in institutions, people with chronic pain, and those with a variety of GI disorders that can lead to vitamin D malabsorption including gastrectomy, biliary cirrhosis, intestinal resection, pancreatic insufficiency, and nephrotic syndrome (protein leakage through the kidneys), as well as people taking certain antiepileptic drugs. Once a low vitamin D level is identified and the cause ascertained, supplementation will prevent osteomalacia from developing. This can be done as a low-dose daily combination tablet of calcium and vitamin D in mild cases. Monthly vitamin D tablets are recommended in moderate or severe cases and there is a long-acting injectable form for those with severe malabsorption. Routine supplementation in the institutionalized elderly without investigation is quite reasonable as so many of this group will be deficient.

osteomyelitis Infection of bone, most often affecting the long bones. Chronic or partially treated osteomyelitis can persist for months or years and cause destruction of normal bone architecture.

The most common cause of osteomyelitis is bacterial infection with organisms such as staphylococci and streptococci. Other bacteria seldom cause osteomyelitis, but gram-negative bacteria such as salmonella can do so, particularly in patients with SLE, HIV, or another cause of immunosuppression. In some countries tuberculosis is a common cause of osteomyelitis.

Bone is usually sterile. Therefore to cause osteomyelitis, infecting organisms have to gain access. Usually bacteria spread to bone through the bloodstream from an infection at some other site. This is called hematogenous spread. Another way bacteria gain access to bone is by spreading from an infection in nearby tissues such as skin or a joint. This is called contiguous spread. The third way bacteria can get to bone is directly if there is penetrating trauma or a fracture that exposes bone.

Anyone can get osteomyelitis, but patients with DIABETES MELLITUS, SICKLE-CELL DISEASE, and immunosuppression have a higher risk. Foot ulcers are common in patients with diabetes because they can affect both the blood supply to tissues and the nerves that provide sensation to the foot. The combination of poor blood supply and decreased feeling in the foot often leads to ulcers caused by injuries or pressure. These ulcers can become infected, and this can spread to bone.

Patients with RHEUMATOID ARTHRITIS are also at high risk, partly because the higher than normal blood through the joints predisposes them to hematogenous spread of infection. Repeated surgical procedures to joints and immunosuppressive treatment will also increase risk.

Symptoms and Diagnostic Path

The first symptom is severe pain, usually in a leg. Osteomyelitis often affects the ends of bones close to joints, and distinguishing osteomyelitis from INFECTIVE ARTHRITIS can sometimes be difficult. In both conditions the patient will not want to move the affected limb because of pain. The limb is often swollen, warm, and excruciatingly tender. In young children and infants who cannot complain of pain, the only symptoms may be crying and refusing to move a limb. Other symptoms of acute infection such as fever and malaise are common.

Apart from long bones, osteomyelitis most often affects the vertebrae. If this occurs the main symptom is severe localized back pain. Clues that osteomyelitis rather than the more common slipped disk is the cause of back pain are fever, continuous pain, localized pain, pain at rest, and pain at night.

The diagnosis of osteomyelitis is usually suspected clinically. Deciding if a superficial skin infection such as cellulitis has penetrated bone and caused osteomyelitis is sometimes difficult. X-rays are not helpful early in the illness because they are normal. After the infection has been present for a week or two, the X-ray may show elevation and thickening of the outer lining of the bone—called a periosteal reaction. Later in the illness X-rays may show areas of bony destruction and areas of increased density. Radionuclide bone scans are often performed to try and differentiate soft-tissue and bone infection but tend to light up with both. Magnetic resonance imaging (see Appendix II) is more helpful.

Blood cultures are performed routinely and may be positive. Laboratory tests such as the white blood cell count and ESR are often elevated, but this is not specific and occurs with any cause of infection or inflammation.

Treatment Options and Outlook

Antibiotics and surgery are important. The choice of antibiotics is based on the organism isolated, and combinations are often used. Before the results of cultures are available and if no organism is isolated, the antibiotic selection usually covers staphylococcal infection and, if clinically suspected, gram-negative infection. Antibiotics are usually administered intravenously for several weeks to ensure high concentrations of drug in the bloodstream. Once the infection is controlled, patients often complete a four to six week course of antibiotics at home. They receive either intravenous drugs, given by a home health service, or oral antibiotics. Surgery is usually performed early in the course of osteomyelitis, particularly in adults. Surgery involves draining any collections of pus in the soft tissues, removing dead tissue, clearing the bone of infection, and obtaining a bone biopsy for culture.

If the general health of the patient is good and the infected bone was previously healthy, osteomyelitis usually responds to antibiotics and surgery, particularly if these are provided early in the course of the illness. If osteomyelitis is partially treated or if dead bone remains and acts as a reservoir for bacteria, infection can recur. If osteomyelitis is severe or not treated early, it can cause death of part of the bone, leading to weakness and instability. Chronic osteomyelitis can be very difficult to treat because eradicating the bacteria from areas of dead bone where antibiotics do not penetrate well is difficult. Some patients require antibiotic treatment for many months and repeated surgery before the infection is cured.

Risk Factors and Preventive Measures

The risk factor for osteomyelitis is any situation that facilitates the entry of bacteria into the bone, be that via the bloodstream, from neighboring tissues, or through trauma. These events are seldom preventable. However needle exchange programs are likely to reduce the frequency of osteomyeli-

tis and septic arthritis in intravenous drug users although this has not been studied. Diabetics with any loss of sensation in their feet should visually inspect their feet, especially the soles, regularly, for example when drying their feet after showering. Intermittent inspection of diabetics' feet by their health-care provider should also be part of their management.

osteopath Dr. Andrew Taylor Still established the first school of osteopathy in Kirksville, Missouri, in 1892. He emphasized the importance of treating the whole person as opposed to concentrating on the disease. This was at a time when the scientific basis of modern medicine was making huge advances, especially in the discovery of bacteria as a cause of distinct illnesses and in the classification of disease. Still reacted against this disease-oriented approach. Although mainstream medicine has since swung back to taking a holistic approach, Dr. Still was ostracized at the time. Some of his beliefs, for example that spinal dysfunction caused infections, were certainly difficult to accept and contributed to the reaction against him.

There are now a number of schools of osteopathy in the United States and graduates (DOs) practice medicine with the same rights and privileges as graduates from traditional schools of medicine. DOs are all trained in osteopathic manipulative treatment and will use it if considered appropriate but will also prescribe antibiotics or other pharmaceuticals if these are considered appropriate. The use of mainstream therapies by DOs does not pertain outside the United States.

The osteopath examines the patient for evidence of somatic dysfunction. This is revealed by changes in tissue texture, asymmetry of bony landmarks, restriction of motion, or tenderness. Manipulative therapy is aimed at restoring normal body mechanics, lymphatic drainage, and autonomic nervous system activity.

Some evidence supports the use of manipulation by an osteopath or other practitioner for acute low BACK PAIN, neck pain, CARPAL TUNNEL SYNDROME, FIBROMYALGIA, and possibly OSTEOARTHRITIS. However, there are relatively few well-controlled studies (see CLINICAL TRIAL) of osteopathy.

osteoporosis A condition in which bone mass and strength is decreased, resulting in fragility and increasing the chance of a fracture. Many patients mistakenly use the terms osteoarthritis and osteoporosis interchangeably. These are two unrelated medical problems. Although someone could have both osteoarthritis, a degenerative arthritis, and osteoporosis, it is important to recognize that these are different problems.

Bone is a rigid, calcified connective tissue that protects and supports people's bodies. There are two types of bone. Cortical bone is hard and dense, and it forms the outer layer. Trabecular or cancellous bone forms a scaffoldlike structure within the outer cortical layer. Bone, in contrast to what one would think, is not inert but is constantly being resorbed and replaced. Bone also acts as a reservoir for calcium stores. If the supply of calcium in the body decreases, bone can be resorbed to supply the mineral. The cells that are important regulators of bone turnover are osteoblasts, which lay down new bone, and osteoclasts, which resorb bone. The remodeling of bone can be affected by hormones, drugs, and physical activity. Hormones such as cortisol and the closely related group of drugs CORTICOSTEROIDS increase bone resorption. On the other hand, estrogens and weight-bearing exercise decrease bone resorption. Women are more likely to develop osteoporosis and fractures than men because they have a lower peak bone mass, lose bone more rapidly after menopause, and live longer.

Osteoporosis affects millions of people in the United States and is a major public health concern, causing 1.5 million fractures and 250,000 hip fractures annually. The chance of a 50-year-old woman having a hip fracture during her lifetime is 14 percent for Caucasians and 6 percent for African Americans. It is estimated that it costs $10–15 billion annually to treat these fractures. Osteoporosis can be divided into two types, primary and secondary. Primary, unlike secondary osteoporosis, is not associated with any underlying illness and is not caused by a drug.

Primary osteoporosis There does not seem to be a single cause of primary osteoporosis, but several factors contribute. Bone mass differs even in healthy people. Age has a major effect. Bone mass increases until people are in their 30s. The peak bone mass an individual reaches is an important determinant of bone mass in later life. Good nutrition, calcium intake, and physical activity in childhood will increase peak bone mass. Smoking in adolescence and early adult life will decrease it. After people achieve peak bone mass in their 30s, it slowly decreases as they age. In women there is a period of rapid bone loss around menopause when the effects of estrogen on bone are lost.

Apart from age, several other factors are associated with low bone mass and osteoporosis. Smoking, low body weight, inactivity, inadequate calcium intake, heavy alcohol use, early menopause, and a family history of osteoporosis all increase the risk.

Secondary osteoporosis The most common cause of secondary osteoporosis is treatment with corticosteroids. The risk is related to the dose and duration of steroid treatment. High doses of corticosteroids, say 30 mg or more of prednisone a day, will cause osteoporosis in most people, but even low doses such as 7.5 mg a day or less increase the risk. Patients taking long-term corticosteroids should be monitored for osteoporosis. Often corticosteroids are prescribed for a chronic illness such as rheumatoid arthritis or SLE, illnesses that can themselves predispose to osteoporosis.

Another common cause of osteoporosis is failure of the ovaries or testes to produce the sex hormones estrogen and testosterone. Menopause usually occurs naturally, often around the age of 50, but a young woman whose ovaries are removed surgically will go through menopause prematurely and start to lose bone. In some young women the ovaries stop functioning. For example, the ovaries can shut down in elite athletes and ballet dancers who follow a rigorous exercise program. These people can develop osteoporosis even though they are young and extremely physically active. Menstrual irregularity or complete disappearance of cycles (amenorrhea) can be warning signs that a young female athlete is at risk for accelerated bone loss and osteoporosis. In athletes osteoporosis increases the risk of stress fractures. Most of the bone loss is reversible if ovarian function returns to normal, but this often does not happen until the athlete decreases or stops competitive training. In men sex hormones are also important for maintaining bone health. Men whose testes are removed or stop producing the male hormone testosterone have a much higher risk of developing osteoporosis.

An overactive thyroid (hyperthyroidism or thyrotoxicosis) can cause osteoporosis. Replacement doses of thyroid hormone prescribed for patients with an underactive thyroid (hypothyroidism) can also cause osteoporosis, particularly if the dose is too high.

Other illnesses, for example hyperparathyroidism (overactive parathyroid glands), can cause secondary osteoporosis, but these are unusual causes. Any severe illness that decreases mobility increases the risk of osteoporosis. Patients at highest risk are those who are confined to bed and receiving high doses of corticosteroids.

Fractures   The reason osteoporosis is an important health problem is that it increases the risk of fractures. Some of these fractures, for example vertebral fractures, can occur with normal everyday activities, but hip, arm, and leg fractures are caused by falls. Therefore, for an individual the risk of fracture is affected not only by bone mass but also by the chance of falling. Anyone can fall and fracture a bone. In fact, children often sustain fractures. However, as people age, the risk of fracture increases because physical capacity declines and bone becomes osteoporotic and fragile. Balance, strength, vision, and coordination all decrease with aging and increase the risk of falling and therefore fracture.

Symptoms and Diagnostic Path

Osteoporosis is usually silent, and most people have no acute symptoms until they have fracture. The first noticeable sign of osteoporosis is loss of height. This shrinking is often ascribed to aging but is often a marker of significant osteoporosis. Patients with severe osteoporosis may lose some of the height of their vertebrae so that the spine becomes curved forward, a posture that was sometimes called a *dowager's hump* because of the propensity for osteoporosis to occur in elderly women. Apart from loss of height and curving of the spine, osteoporosis does not cause symptoms unless a fracture occurs. Because the bone is thin and weak, it is more likely to fracture after minor stress or trauma. A com-

pression fracture in a vertebra, sometimes called a crush fracture or wedge fracture, often occurs with coughing or ordinary day-to-day activities such as lifting a heavy object. The first symptom of a compression fracture is often acute back pain. The pain is felt in the back over the vertebra affected and can be severe, limiting regular activities and even making sleeping or changes in posture difficult. In contrast to chronic back pain that often affects the lower back for years, an osteoporotic fracture causes sudden severe pain, often affecting the upper back. The pain from an osteoporotic fracture can last for weeks and usually improves slowly. After someone has had several compression fractures of the spine, though, there is often residual dull aching pain. More serious fractures involving the hip or radius usually occur only after a fall, and the symptoms—pain, swelling, and inability to use the limb—are usually obvious. Typically women with moderate-to-severe osteoporosis have Colles' fractures (just above the wrist) in their 50s, vertebral fractures in their 60s, and hip fractures in their 70s. Colles' fractures should therefore be taken as a warning of potentially severe osteoporosis.

Because osteoporosis causes so few symptoms, it is difficult to diagnose unless people who are at risk are screened routinely and the diagnosis made before a fracture has occurred. No blood or urine tests are helpful for diagnosing osteoporosis, although a lot of research is directed at developing such tests. In fact, all the standard tests of bone health such as calcium, phosphate, and alkaline phosphatase are usually normal in patients with osteoporosis. Increased levels of biochemical markers of bone resorption can be detected in the urine of patients with osteoporosis. These tests do not tell enough about an individual's actual bone density or risk of fracture to use them for diagnosis but can be helpful to monitor response to treatment.

Osteoporosis is often not diagnosed until an X-ray, often performed for an unrelated reason, shows thin bones and perhaps partial collapse of a vertebra. Regular X-rays are not a very good way to diagnose osteoporosis because approximately 40 percent of the bone mass has to be lost before bones appear thin on X-ray. A diagnosis of osteoporosis can be made much earlier by obtaining a measurement of bone mass. There are several techniques for measuring bone density, the best estimate of bone mass (see DEXA in Appendix II).

The diagnosis of osteoporosis is made by comparing an individual's bone density with that of the average healthy young adult, and this is expressed as a T score. The lower the T score, the thinner the bone and the greater the risk of a fracture. A T score of -2.5 is regarded as the point at which the risk of fracture rises steeply and has been determined by the World Health Organization as indicating a diagnosis of osteoporosis. It is important to remember that fractures can occur in anyone if bone is sufficiently stressed by a fall. Therefore the concept of a threshold is a little artificial because the risk of breaking a bone is affected not only by how thin the bone is but also by the chance of falling. The T score was developed to provide a standardized measure of bone density because many different techniques are used to measure bone density. It represents the relationship between a person's bone density and that of the average young adult. A T score of -2 means that a person's bone density is two standard deviations below average. People are not all exactly the same, and a standard deviation is a statistical measurement of the normal spread for any measurement, be it weight, height, or bone density. For any measurement, for example height, weight, or bone density, only 2.5 percent of people will fall below two standard deviations from the average.

The risk of fracture almost doubles for a decrease in bone density of one standard deviation (i.e., a T score of -1). A T score of -2.5 was selected, somewhat arbitrarily, as the bone density score at which the risk of fracture was increased enough for all patients to be treated for osteoporosis. Most techniques for measuring bone density report the result as both a T score and a Z score. The Z score represents how far a person's score is from the average of other people of the same age and sex. The Z score is not as useful as the T score for deciding when a person needs treatment but may indicate that a search for a cause of secondary osteoporosis is required.

Once osteoporosis has been diagnosed, a careful history and physical examination should be performed to make sure that there is no underlying cause, in other words, to exclude causes of secondary osteoporosis.

Treatment Options and Outlook

The most effective way to treat osteoporosis is to prevent it. Lifestyle changes that prevent osteoporosis are also helpful for treating it.

- *Avoiding Causes of Osteoporosis* People who have osteoporosis or want to prevent it should alter their lifestyle to avoid smoking and drinking a lot of alcohol since these decrease bone density. Avoiding drugs that cause osteoporosis is not always possible. For example, if someone needs high doses of corticosteroids to control an illness, then avoiding these drugs may not be possible. Most physicians agree that the lowest dose of corticosteroid that controls a condition should be used, and in this way the negative effects of this class of drugs on bone is kept to a minimum.

- *Increasing Peak Bone Mass* If peak bone mass is high, then even if it decreases as the person ages, it will remain higher than in a person who started with less bone and lost the same amount. Young adults can improve their peak bone mass by ensuring an adequate intake of calcium and by exercising regularly.

- *Exercise* Marked inactivity such as bed rest decreases bone density. This is because the stresses placed on bone by exercise help remodel and strengthen it. Weight-bearing exercise such as jogging, tennis, and weight lifting increases bone density. Exercise such as swimming that does not place much load on bones does not improve bone mass. The importance of weight bearing on bone health is illustrated by the fact that astronauts lose a lot of their bone mass while they are weightless in space even though they perform exercises. Regular strenuous exercise can increase bone density. However, when the person stops training hard, bone density quickly falls to its previous level. In other words, regular moderate exercise several times a week will maintain bone mass better than irregular bursts of intense exercise.

- *Calcium and Vitamin D* Two key requirements for healthy bones are calcium and vitamin D. Calcium is a major constituent of bone, and vitamin D regulates calcium absorption from the gut. The modern diet tends to be low in calcium, which is found in high concentration in milk and milk products such as yogurt and cheese. Because people worry that cholesterol in their diet may increase the risk of heart disease, they have cut down on milk products, and consequently their calcium intake has decreased. For most people a daily intake between 1,000 and 1,500 mg of calcium is recommended. A cup of milk, one of the richest sources of calcium, provides about 300 mg of calcium. For many people diet alone does not provide enough calcium and a supplement is needed. The amount of calcium in a person's diet, combined with the amount in their supplement, should add up to their recommended daily intake.

Many different calcium supplements are available. The amount of calcium they provide varies. So that everyone understands exactly how much calcium a particular tablet provides, the label provides information in milligrams (mg) of elemental calcium per tablet. Calcium carbonate is a cheap, effective, and widely available preparation. Some patients who do not have acid in their stomachs do not absorb calcium carbonate well and calcium citrate may be more effective for them. Calcium is absorbed better if it is taken at the same time as food.

Recent studies of calcium supplements have suggested that women taking the calcium as opposed to the placebo tablets had a slightly higher incidence of heart disease. It should be noted that these studies were not designed to test this relationship and therefore the finding should serve as a cautionary note rather than proof of the relationship. In these studies, women took two calcium tablets a day equal to or more than 1,200 mg of calcium. To complicate matters, there is some evidence that calcium supplements will improve cholesterol levels and thereby lessen the risk of heart disease. We also know that good levels of vitamin D (which promotes calcium absorption) are associated with a lower risk of heart disease. The current recommendation is therefore that calcium supplementation should be about 600 mg a day (equal to one standard tablet although contents do vary) to bring the total calcium intake into the 1,000 to 1,500 mg a day range.

A deficiency of vitamin D causes a bone disorder called OSTEOMALACIA. This is different from osteoporosis, which is not caused by vitamin D deficiency. However, an adequate intake of vitamin D is needed to ensure adequate calcium absorption and healthy bones. The recommended daily intake of vitamin D is 400–800 international units (IU) and most multivitamins designed for daily use contain this amount.

Medication   As an individual's risk of fracture increases or if they have already had a fracture, the benefit of using medication to strengthen their bones increases. Medication use should always go hand in hand with the lifestyle changes discussed above. The World Health Organization has recently developed a computerized tool for predicting someone's risk of major osteoporotic fracture and specifically hip fracture. This uses the DEXA score but can use height and weight instead and a number of well-recognized clinical risk factors such as age, family history of fracture, previous fracture, tobacco and alcohol use, rheumatoid arthritis, and corticosteroid use. The tool gives the risk of having a fracture in the next 10 years, and studies so far suggest that treatment is cost effective at any age if the risk is more than 7 percent. Most drugs currently used to treat osteoporosis slow the resorption of bone but usually do not increase bone formation. Treatment usually stabilizes bone density or increases it slightly. Three groups of drugs are commonly used to treat osteoporosis: estrogen and the closely related selective estrogen receptor modulators (SERMs), bisphosphonates, and calcitonin.

- *Estrogen and SERMs*   After menopause women have a high risk of developing osteoporosis because the beneficial effects of natural estrogen on bone metabolism are lost. This can be reversed by estrogen replacement therapy. The effects last only while the patient takes the treatment. Men cannot take estrogens to prevent or treat osteoporosis because the female hormone causes breast enlargement and other side effects. Supplementing the male hormone testosterone has been tried as a treatment for osteoporosis but has not been useful, except in men who have a low testosterone level.

Many women find that the other effects of estrogen, for example decreasing the number of hot flashes and improving mood, make it an attractive treatment for osteoporosis. On the other hand, others gain weight, feel bloated, and dislike the uterine bleeding that comes with estrogen treatment. Recent studies have shown that women taking some forms of estrogen replacement have a slightly increased risk of developing clots. This is similar to the risk of taking oral contraceptives. There is also an increased risk of breast cancer. For these reasons estrogen replacement is no longer considered a first-choice treatment for osteoporosis. Drug companies have now developed a class of drugs, SERMs, that stimulate some of the estrogen receptors in the body, particularly the receptors in bone, without stimulating estrogen receptors in other places, like the breasts or uterus. These drugs increase bone density without causing uterine bleeding and do not increase the risk of breast cancer. In fact, RALOXIFENE (trade name: Evista) has been shown to be equal to tamoxifen in preventing breast cancer in women. However, it does only appear to be effective in those women who have had estrogen receptor positive breast cancer. Tamoxifen, originally developed and used for many years to prevent recurrence of breast cancer, is also a SERM and has some bone protective effect. SERMs do not alleviate the other symptoms of estrogen deficiency such as hot flashes.

Observational studies performed in large groups of women seemed to show that estrogen replacement decreased the risk of myocardial infarction. If true, this would be a very important reason to prescribe estrogens, because ischemic heart disease is the most common cause of death in women, as it is in men. However, a large randomized, controlled trial called the HERS study did not find any benefit of estrogens on the risk of heart attack. In fact, in the early part of the study there were more cardiovascular events in the estrogen than in the placebo group. This was probably because estrogens (and SERMs) increase the risk of blood clotting. Some experts believe that the wrong type of estrogen was studied and that the study did not continue long enough to show the beneficial cardiovascular effects of estrogen. However, others believe that the original observational studies were wrong because they selectively studied women who took more care of their health and took more estrogens. These same people believe that the results of the HERS study, a double-blind, randomized controlled study that found no benefit, represent the true effect of estrogens. A recent meta-analysis combined all 31 randomized controlled trials addressing this issue in an attempt to resolve it. This found that the risk of stroke and deep-vein thrombosis was significantly increased in users of estrogen-containing hormone replacement therapy (as most people accept), but that the risk of heart disease was not. However there is equally no evidence that estrogen prevents heart disease. Because estrogens and SERMs increase the risk of clotting, they are usually avoided in women who have had a deep-vein thrombosis.

- *Bisphosphonates* This group of drugs binds strongly to bone and prevents it from being resorbed. There are now several bisphosphonates including ETIDRONATE, ALENDRONATE, RISEDRONATE, IBANDRONATE, and zoledronate. Many studies have shown that the newer bisphosphonates such as alendronate and risedronate increase bone density and reduce the risk of fractures by about 50 percent in people with low bone density.

Bisphosphonates are not absorbed from the stomach very efficiently. Therefore they should be taken on an empty stomach so that food and other drugs do not interfere with their absorption. They can also cause ulcers in the esophagus if they stick or reflux back up into the esophagus. To reduce the risk of this happening, the instructions for taking bisphosphonates usually advise patients not to lie down after taking them.

If patients cannot swallow or have an esophageal problem that makes it likely that tablets will stick, there are bisphosphonates that can be given intravenously. Generally these are used only in patients too sick to take tablets by mouth. The instructions for taking a bisphosphonate are usually as follows:

1. Take your tablet with a full glass of water first thing when you get up in the morning.

2. Do not eat or drink anything, other than water, for at least 30 minutes after you have taken the tablet. Even coffee or fruit juice stops the drug from getting into your body. Waiting an hour before eating or drinking anything else will enhance the absorption of the drug.

3. After you have taken the tablet stay upright and do not go back to bed. This is so that the tablet does not reflux back up your esophagus.

4. Take the tablet by itself, not with your other medicines. Delay taking your other medicines for at least an hour.

These instructions are difficult for many patients to follow regularly. Because these drugs bind so avidly to bone, most manufacturers have produced a tablet that can be taken once a week (alendronate or risedronate) or even monthly (risedronate or ibandronate). A rare adverse effect of the bisphosphonates is osteonecrosis of the jaw where a small part of the jaw bone dies. This is very painful and difficult to treat. Most cases have occurred in cancer patients receiving high doses of intravenous bisphosphonates rather than the doses used to treat osteoporosis. However, if significant dental work such as extraction or root canal work is not urgent it is prudent to withhold bisphosphonates for two to three months before having it done.

- *Calcitonin* This hormone produced by the body slows bone resorption. Drug companies have been able to manufacture calcitonin, and it is an effective treatment for osteoporosis. Unfortunately, as occurs with most hormones, calcitonin is destroyed by acid in the stomach. Therefore, to get it into the body, it has to be given by an injection under the skin or else as a nasal spray. The nasal spray is much more convenient to use than injections but is probably less effective than bisphosphonates in reducing the risk of osteoporotic fractures. One advantage of calcitonin is that if a patient has pain caused by an osteoporotic fracture, it may reduce pain.

- *Other Drugs* A number of other agents have been used either when there are contraindications to the above medications or experimentally. None of these are first-line therapy. Parathyroid hormone functions in the body to remove calcium from bone to maintain normal levels of calcium. Surprisingly then, intermittent use of recombinant parathyroid hormone has been shown to increase bone density and reduce fracture rate. Calcitriol, an activated form of vitamin D, has been effective in some but not all trials and may be more effective in preventing corticosteroid-related bone loss than in uncomplicated postmenopausal osteoporosis. Vitamin K is essential for normal clotting of the blood but also has effects on bone and several studies in Japanese women have shown that supplementation reduces the fracture rate. This has not been demonstrated in Caucasians, and there may be dietary or genetic factors that account for the effect in the Japanese women. DENOSUMAB is a monoclonal antibody (see BIOLOGICALS) that inhibits the action of bone-resorbing osteoclasts. It is given as an injection under the skin every six months and is at least as effective in increasing bone density as alendronate and probably slightly more effective. However, it has effects on the immune system, and there are more infections in people using it. This will require further study before it becomes an accepted treatment.

Strontium ranelate has been shown to increase bone density and reduce fractures but is not available in the United States currently. Tibolone is a synthetic steroid that has been shown to be effective in a few trials but there are concerns about its safety, in particular whether it causes strokes. Fluoride initially showed great promise as it increased bone density dramatically. However, traditional doses actually increased the fracture rate. The lower doses used in more recent studies suggest reduction in vertebral fracture in some but not all studies.

- *Preventing Fractures* Many people, including scientists, forget that the point of treating osteoporosis is not to increase bone density but to decrease the number of fractures. The two often go hand in hand, but not always. Early studies with fluoride showed that it was able to increase bone density substantially, even more than bisphosphonates, but unfortunately fracture risk was not decreased. There were two important lessons from these studies: First, not all drugs that increase bone density automatically reduce the risk of fractures. Second and perhaps more importantly, fractures are more important than bone density. So it is important not to forget that the aim of treating osteoporosis is to prevent fractures and that many fractures are caused by falls that could be prevented.

Simple things can reduce the risk of falling. Some of these are common sense: getting rid of loose throw rugs and other objects that can trip someone, having nonslip surfaces, using a cane for support, not hurrying (for example to answer the telephone), and keeping a night-light on to see the way to the bathroom. People with poor vision are more likely to fall, so it makes sense for everyone to have their vision checked from time to time. Alcohol and medicines that affect balance, such as sleeping pills, increase the risk of a fall. So if someone has osteoporosis and is at risk of falling, he or she should try to avoid these drugs. Studies performed in nursing homes have shown that the risk of serious fractures, particularly hip fractures, was reduced if patients at high risk wore hip protectors. These are appliances that provide padding around the hip to protect the fragile bones. Unfortunately, most people who have a high risk of falling do not want to wear bulky padding all the time to provide protection on the few occasions when they do fall. Therefore, these protective devices are not popular. It may be useful to remember that skateboarders, a group of people who often break bones, have recognized the value of protective padding and to explore the best way to use padding and shock-absorbing devices to protect the elderly against hip fractures.

osteosarcoma This is a highly malignant tumor that starts within bone and spreads outward to the periosteum (lining of the bone) and surrounding soft tissues. It affects mainly children and adolescents but may be increasing in frequency in adults. Most osteosarcomas developing in people over the age of 50 arise in bone affected by PAGET'S DISEASE. This is the most feared complication of Paget's disease.

Symptoms and Diagnostic Path

The first symptom is usually pain that is constant and may be worse at night. There is often tenderness over the area. Later on there may be a swelling, and occasionally a fracture may occur through the weakened bone. Blood tests often show a raised ESR and alkaline phosphatase (see Appendix II). The early X-ray changes may be difficult to interpret, with vague areas of bone destruction (dark on the X-ray) alternating with denser-than-usual bone. Lifting of the periosteum and radiating streaks of new bone are the most typical X-ray changes but may also be seen in other rapidly growing tumors. Both CT and MRI scans are very good at showing the extent of the tumor, and CT scans are usually done to look for spread into the lungs. A careful biopsy should be done to confirm the diagnosis.

Treatment Options and Outlook

Osteosarcoma had a bad outcome up till the 1970s, with only one in five patients surviving five years from the time of diagnosis. Recent reports show 70 percent of patients surviving five years. This dramatic improvement is due to the development of adjuvant chemotherapy to supplement surgical removal of the tumor and the aggressive removal of secondary tumors (usually from the lungs). Chemotherapy is usually begun before surgery. The ideal regimen is not yet clear, and several different ones are in use. If a limb is involved, it usually has to be amputated through or just above the joint above the tumor. Although this is less radical than some of the surgery done before chemotherapy, removing just the bone around the tumor in order to avoid amputation leads to a higher recurrence rate. Radiotherapy is used only in special circumstances. The removal of nodules of tumor that have spread to the lungs or bone definitely improves the outcome and may require repeated operations in the early years. There is no known strategy for prevention of osteosarcomas.

overlap syndrome The symptoms of rheumatic diseases commonly overlap, particularly early in the course of the illness. The term overlap syndrome or undifferentiated connective tissue disease is often used loosely to mean that a patient has a connective tissue disorder with clinical features of several different autoimmune diseases without being typical of one. Some patients with overlap syndrome may not fulfill the strict diagnostic criteria for any one connective tissue disorder, and others may fulfill the criteria for more than one diagnosis. Overlap syndrome is most often used to describe an illness with some features of lupus, scleroderma, and dermatomyositis. Mixed connective tissue disease (MCTD) is another condition with features that can overlap several autoimmune conditions. Patients with MCTD have a positive test for antibodies against ribonuclear protein (RNP), and patients with overlap syndrome do not.

It is not usually difficult to separate SLE and RA because their symptoms are usually different. However, there are a few patients who have features that are common to both diseases. This array of symptoms has sometimes been called *rupus*, a term derived from the amalgamation of the abbreviations RA and lupus. Some rheumatologists would call this illness an overlap syndrome or undifferentiated connective tissue disease.

As is the case for most autoimmune diseases, the cause of overlap syndrome is not known and is discussed under the individual conditions.

Symptoms and Diagnostic Path

In the early phases of many autoimmune diseases the clinical features can be similar. Rather than make a diagnosis that may later turn out to be incorrect, many rheumatologists make a diagnosis of undifferentiated connective tissue disease or overlap syndrome. As time passes the clinical fea-

tures of the illness may evolve so that a clear diagnosis of lupus, scleroderma, dermatomyositis, or another autoimmune disease can be made. Patients with overlap syndrome have combinations of symptoms that can occur in various autoimmune diseases. These include Raynaud's phenomenon, difficulty swallowing, and tightness of the skin that are typical of scleroderma; pleurisy, arthralgia, mouth ulcers, rash, and pericarditis that are typical of SLE; and muscle weakness, typical of myositis.

The diagnosis is clinical. Many patients have a positive antinuclear antibody (ANA) test. If patients with overlap symptoms have a positive test for RNP antibodies, the diagnosis is mixed connective tissue disease.

Treatment Options and Outlook

The treatment of overlap syndrome involves aspects of the treatment for SLE, scleroderma, and myositis, with individuals treated according to the symptoms they have. NSAIDs are often used to treat arthralgia and arthritis; CORTICOSTEROIDS to treat myositis, pleurisy, and pericarditis; immunosuppressive drugs to treat kidney disease (which is rare); and antireflux drugs to treat difficulty swallowing. Patients are monitored because their illness is likely to change over time and evolve toward one of the classical autoimmune diseases with a prognosis similar to that disease.

Risk Factors and Preventive Measures

Although there may be a genetic component to the overlap syndrome as with other connective tissue diseases, the mechanism is unknown, and most patients will not have a family history. There are no effective preventive measures.

Paget's disease Although Sir James Paget first described this bone disease with "chronic inflammation and deformity" in the 19th century, there is evidence that it has existed since prehistoric times. It is common in the United States, Britain, Australia, and New Zealand but rare in Asia. Not only does its occurrence vary in frequency between countries but also between areas within a country. Paget's disease becomes increasingly common with increasing age, being rare before the age of 40 years and then doubling in frequency every 10 years after the age of 50. It affects 2–3 percent of those aged over 50 years in the United States with men being affected more than women.

Paget's disease is characterized by areas of bone being resorbed by large cells called osteoclasts and then replaced with new bone by cells called osteoblasts. This process occurs in normal bone all the time in a highly controlled manner so that bones can adjust, for example to changes in weight, and repair. What distinguishes Paget's disease is that the osteoclasts are hyperactive, resorbing bone faster than normal and in a disorganized fashion. The result is that affected bone is enlarged, is weakened, and has an unusually large blood supply. This increased blood flow causes the warmth often felt over pagetic bones. The cause of this disordered bone behavior is not certain. However, small viral inclusion bodies have been found in the osteoclasts, suggesting a viral cause. Research has shown links with measles, respiratory syncytial, or canine distemper viruses. It is thought that viral infection of the osteoclasts early in life results in their abnormal behavior many years later. There is an aggregation in families, with 30 percent of patients having at least one affected relative, indicating a possible genetic component to the disease.

Symptoms and Diagnostic Path

Many patients have no symptoms when they are diagnosed. This usually occurs when routine blood tests show a raised ALKALINE PHOSPHATASE level (see Appendix II) without any obvious cause. X-rays are then taken and show the Paget's disease. Other patients may be diagnosed when the typical changes are seen on an X-ray taken for an unrelated reason. Paget's disease may present in a number of ways.

The skull, spine, sacrum, pelvis, and lower limbs are most frequently involved. Although seldom seen these days because of earlier treatment, the skull may become enlarged in a rather characteristic fashion with a large, bulging forehead. Deafness still commonly occurs and may be due to involvement of the skull with pressure on the auditory nerves or involvement of the small conducting bones (ossicles) in the middle ear. Rarely, the base of the skull may be softened by pagetic involvement and move upward under pressure. This can cause pressure on the upper spinal cord and cerebellum and block the flow of cerebrospinal fluid, causing increased pressure within the skull. Paget's disease affecting the spine may cause pain of its own accord or by compression of nerve roots as they leave the spine. Very rarely, there may be pressure on the spinal cord itself. Involvement of the pelvis often causes pain or discomfort, and some patients complain of a feeling of increased heat. In time this often affects the gait. If the bone around the hip joint is affected, the head of the femur (thighbone) may gradually push through into the pelvis (protrusio acetabuli). The long bones of the legs are often affected. They can frequently be felt to be warm and may bend because the bone is softer than usual. If bone close to a joint is affected, secondary OSTEOARTHRITIS often develops after a few years. The long bones are at increased risk of fracture. This may occur after a fall or motor vehicle accident with a complete break in the bone or as pseudofractures. Pseudofractures do not extend right across the bone and occur particularly on the outer surface of long bones that have bent. They are typically quite painful but do not otherwise prevent the patient from mobilizing.

The most feared complication of Paget's disease, OSTEOSARCOMA, is fortunately very rare. Less than 1 percent of people with Paget's disease develop this highly malignant tumor of the bone that is very difficult to treat. Patients may note an increase in pain in one particular area with swelling, and the alkaline phosphatase level usually rises dramatically. Occasionally less malignant tumors, giant cell tumors, may develop. If a patient with Paget's has an unrelated cancer that spreads, it not infrequently spreads to pagetic bone because of the increased blood flow there. Sometimes with widespread disease the blood flow can increase to such an extent that it causes heart failure or makes angina difficult to control.

The characteristic X-ray appearance of enlarged bones with alternating areas of increased resorption and formation of bone together with a raised alkaline phosphatase level is usually sufficient to make the diagnosis. Differentiating Paget's disease from secondary bone tumors, especially prostate cancer can be difficult. Several very characteristic X-ray findings support a diagnosis of Paget's disease. However, if there is no history to help, it can sometimes be impossible to differentiate on X-ray. In these situations a biopsy is usually required. Radionuclide bone scans are useful in showing the extent of bone involvement but do not differentiate Paget's from other bone diseases. CT and MRI scans are often used to show nerve or brain abnormalities. Audiological testing can differentiate between nerve deafness and involvement of the conducting ossicles. Blood and urine tests can give more information about the rate of bone turnover but are seldom required. Alkaline phosphatase, type I procollagen carboxyterminal peptide, and osteocalcin all reflect bone formation. Urine hydroxyproline or pyridinium cross-linked peptides reflect resorption of bone. In general, the level of alkaline phosphatase reflects both the extent of bony involvement

(the more bones involved, the higher the level) and the activity of disease. It is useful for monitoring treatment in most patients, but is less helpful in those with skull involvement.

Treatment Options and Outlook

Treating asymptomatic Paget's disease is not always necessary. However, the available treatments have improved so much over the past 15 years that many patients are now treated at an earlier stage. Indications for treatment include:

- Pain from the Paget's disease itself
- Preventing increasing deformity around a joint and therefore delaying the development of osteoarthritis
- Nerve entrapment, either present or impending; this should include any involvement of the base of the skull or temporal bone (the auditory nerve passes through this)
- If surgery to an affected area is planned, the patient should receive medical therapy first to limit intra- and postoperative bleeding
- Heart failure or difficult-to-control angina; treatment reduces blood flow and thereby reduces the workload of the heart
- Fractures that have either occurred or are likely to occur given the extent of involvement of the bone
- High calcium levels, although this is rare unless patients are immobilized, as might occur for example when they are hospitalized for an unrelated illness

Painkillers and NSAIDs should be used appropriately for pain, but they do nothing to alter the disease process itself. This is achieved with either CALCITONIN or one of the BISPHOSPHONATES. Calcitonin has been used for many years and is reputed to have pain-relieving effects as well as shutting down the activity of the osteoclasts. Both human and salmon calcitonins are available. Salmon calcitonin is more effective and is more commonly used. Calcitonin is administered by injections under the skin either daily or every other day. Its use is limited by side effects, principally flushing and diarrhea. A nasal calcitonin spray has recently become available but is not approved for use in Paget's disease.

The first bisphosphonate to be used was ETIDRONATE (trade name: Didronel). At the doses required to treat Paget's disease this interfered with normal bone growth and was of limited use. The newer generation bisphosphonates have, however, revolutionized the treatment of Paget's disease. These include PAMIDRONATE (trade name: Aredia) which has to be given as an intravenous infusion, ALENDRONATE (trade name: Fosamax), and RISEDRONATE (trade name: Actonel). These are all highly effective in normalizing markers of bone turnover and reducing pain. Pamidronate may cause short-lived flulike symptoms but is well tolerated. There are a number of different regimens for giving these drugs. Giving a course and then following a marker of Paget's disease such as the alkaline phosphatase is usual to see when retreatment is required.

Risk Factors and Preventive Measures

Although a slow virus infection in early life is strongly suspected as a cause of Paget's disease, no such virus has been isolated and grown and its origin therefore remains unknown. Therefore, no preventive measure is possible at this time.

palindromic rheumatism   A rare type of inflammatory arthritis that causes symptoms in one or a few joints for a few hours or days and then resolves completely, only to recur days, weeks, or months later.

The cause is unknown. In less than 50 percent of patients with palindromic rheumatism the illness evolves into classical rheumatoid arthritis (RA) and a few patients develop SLE. In many patients though, the illness does not evolve into another rheumatic disease.

Symptoms and Diagnostic Path

Acute attacks of severe arthritis causing pain, swelling, and redness in one or a few joints are usual. Knees, wrists, shoulders, and small joints of the hands are often affected. The symptoms can be severe initially, stopping patients from working or performing day-to-day activities, and then often settle over a few days, even without any treatment.

The attacks recur without warning and can be separated by days, weeks, or months. The patient usually has no symptoms between attacks. If the illness evolves into RA, the attacks become more frequent and never resolve completely.

The diagnosis is usually made from the history. By the time the patient sees the physician, the joint symptoms have usually resolved completely. Gout is another cause of acute attacks of arthritis that should be considered. The acute attacks of gout classically start in the big toe and take longer to settle, usually a week or two. Blood tests do not provide conclusive information but may be helpful in two regards. First, persistently normal uric acid levels even when the patient is well make GOUT less likely. Second, it has been known for many years that those patients who will go on to develop RA often have a positive test for RHEUMATOID FACTOR (see Appendix II). More recently, a more specific test for RA, ANTI-CYCLIC CITRULLINATED PROTEIN (anti-CCP) antibodies (see Appendix II) have been shown to be positive in 83 percent of people who went on to develop RA. The ESR may be raised during an acute attack.

Treatment Options and Outlook

Palindromic rheumatism does not cause joint destruction or deformity, but the symptoms can be incapacitating while they are present. Treatment with an NSAID, particularly if started when the patient notices the first symptoms of an attack, can be effective. If NSAIDs alone do not control the attacks, CORTICOSTEROIDS such as prednisone for a few days will help. If the attacks are frequent, regular treatment with an NSAID or a low dose of prednisone may decrease their frequency. If not, HYDROXYCHLOROQUINE, a DMARD used to treat RA, is often effective. If palindromic rheumatism evolves into RA, it is treated as RA. The figures vary somewhat in different studies, but one long-term follow-up study showed that 29 percent of patients with palindromic rheumatism went on to develop RA and 6 percent developed a connective tissue disease. In this study, the authors showed that those treated with antimalarials such as hydroxychloroquine were slightly but significantly less likely to go on to develop a chronic rheumatic disease. Although this is an interesting result, it is a nonrandomized retrospective study and therefore subject to numerous possible sources of error. However, palindromic rheumatism is not common and randomized controlled studies are therefore difficult to perform, leaving doctors and patients to make decisions based on incomplete evidence.

Risk Factors and Preventive Measures

Palindromic rheumatism is a poorly understood syndrome (i.e., collection of symptoms and signs), and there are no known risk factors or preventive measures. The ability of hydroxychloroquine therapy to prevent progression to a well-defined chronic inflammatory arthritis as discussed above is interesting but remains unproven. Nevertheless, hydroxychloroquine is a reasonably safe medication and may well be worth a trial for the individual patient.

panniculitis A rare condition that causes inflammation of fat just under the skin and causes painful red lumps. Most panniculitis is caused by one of four conditions.

1. ERYTHEMA NODOSUM
2. SYSTEMIC LUPUS ERYTHEMATOSUS (SLE) or VASCULITIS. The panniculitis in SLE is sometimes called lupus profundus and causes painful nodules that can ulcerate.
3. Weber-Christian disease. This is a rare illness that causes recurrent attacks of panniculitis with arthralgia, abdominal pain, and fever, mostly in young women.
4. Pancreatic disease. Serious conditions such as pancreatitis or cancer of the pancreas can cause panniculitis. One of the functions of the pancreas is to secrete enzymes that digest dietary fat. Panniculitis may be caused by high levels of pancreatic enzymes in the bloodstream that damage fatty tissue.

parvovirus Parvoviruses are small DNA viruses with only limited genetic capabilities. They therefore rely on host cells for certain functions. For this reason, the only parvovirus that infects humans, the human parvovirus B19 (HPV-B19), has a pre-

dilection for rapidly dividing cells such as activated lymphocytes. HPV-B19 is the cause of the illness, erythema infectiosum, also known as *fifth disease* or *slapped cheek syndrome*. This is a common infectious disease causing fever and rash mainly in children and often spreading rapidly throughout small communities. Outbreaks often start in elementary schools where up to 60 percent of susceptible children may be infected.

Symptoms and Diagnostic Path

The acute illness starts as a flulike illness with fever, muscle aches, and headaches. The bone marrow virtually stops producing red cells, and white cell and platelet production is also affected. In most healthy people this is not serious since it lasts only about two weeks. However, HPV-B19 can cause life-threatening aplastic crises in patients with hemolytic anemias such as the thallassemias. These patients have red cells that break up after a shorter time than normal, and to maintain a reasonable level, they have to manufacture new red cells much faster than usual. When red cell production stops because of HPV-B19 infection (an aplastic crisis), these patients can become profoundly anemic.

Antibodies to HPV-B19 appear after about 10 days, and these will clear the virus from the blood. They also allow diagnosis of the infection. IgM antibodies are detectable for up to five months after infection and need to be present to identify a particular illness as being due to HPV-B19. The IgG antibodies are detectable for the rest of that individual's life and indicate only exposure to the virus some time in the past. In different populations, between 40 and 80 percent of people have evidence of being exposed at some time. As the level of IgM antibody rises, the rash, joint pain, and arthritis may appear. The patient is no longer infectious at this stage. Children often get an irregular red rash on the cheeks leading to the name, slapped-cheek syndrome. Joint pain is common in the acute infection, occurring in 8 percent of children and 80 percent of adults. There are four areas in which HPV-B19 is important in rheumatic diseases:

1. Acute B19-associated arthritis
2. As a trigger of JUVENILE IDIOPATHIC ARTHRITIS

3. As a possible trigger of RHEUMATOID ARTHRITIS
4. As a possible trigger of connective tissue diseases

Acute B19-associated arthritis The acute illness is typically short-lived in children. Up to 80 percent of adults get joint pain or arthritis. Arthritis is more common in women and on average lasts six to nine months. About two-thirds of those with joint pain describe joint swelling, most often affecting the hands, feet, and knees.

B19 and juvenile arthritis Although usually short-lived, acute arthritis has been reported as persisting for over a year in a few children. The pattern of joint involvement has been variable, resembling rheumatoid arthritis in some and pauciarticular juvenile arthritis in others. There is in addition some evidence that HPV-B19 may trigger juvenile arthritis. A report from India showed that many more patients with juvenile arthritis had evidence of previous B19 infection than controls (see CLINICAL TRIAL for explanation of controls). A Scandinavian study found that more than a third of juvenile arthritis patients undergoing joint replacement had B19 DNA in the joint lining of the affected joints. These and other similar studies are interesting but do not show proof of causation.

B19 and rheumatoid arthritis There are many difficulties proving that an infection triggers rheumatoid arthritis or other chronic arthritis. Researchers have tackled the problem in different ways and, although there are interesting findings, they are far from conclusive and not all the studies are consistent. One approach is to follow up a group of patients who develop B19-related arthritis and see if any of them develop typical rheumatoid arthritis (i.e., a chronic, rheumatoid factor-positive arthritis that erodes joints). There are several such studies, but none of them have shown progression to rheumatoid arthritis. Isolated reports discuss patients developing typical rheumatoid arthritis after HPV-B19 infection, but these do not exclude a chance occurrence. Another approach is to examine groups of rheumatoid arthritis patients for evidence of B19 infection. A number of studies using sophisticated techniques have shown that the virus persists, particularly in the bone marrow and joint lining of some patients with rheumatoid arthritis,

despite blood tests being negative. The numbers of patients so affected are not great, however. A very detailed study found B19 DNA in nearly 80 percent of joint lining specimens from rheumatoid arthritis patients. This was far more than in controls. The study went on to show that the virus was alive and infectious, and it could stimulate the type of immune response likely to cause rheumatoid arthritis. If these findings could be repeated, it would provide strong evidence for HPV-B19 involvement in triggering rheumatoid arthritis. It is thought from historical evidence that HPV-B19 is a New World virus, reaching Europe only in the 16th century. This would fit with the emergence of rheumatoid arthritis.

B19 and connective tissue diseases There are a number of reports of patients with HPV-B19 infection that is very difficult to differentiate from SYSTEMIC LUPUS ERYTHEMATOSUS (SLE). These patients have had facial rashes, fever, joint pain and arthritis, muscle pain, low white blood cell and platelet counts, and reduced COMPLEMENT levels, features all typical of SLE. They also developed a number of autoantibodies. Most of these patients had positive ANA tests, some were positive for anti-DNA, Ro, and La antibodies (also found in SLE) and others for rheumatoid factor or Scl-70 (found in SCLERODERMA). Many of these patients have had short-lived illnesses lasting weeks to months and settling with only symptomatic treatment, but a few have lasted for one to two years. This, however, indicates that HPV-B19 can cause an illness very like SLE or other connective tissue diseases, not that it can cause these diseases. In a study of 99 SLE patients who had just been diagnosed, there was no evidence of recent HPV-B19 infection.

To summarize these findings, HPV-B19 infection can mimic both early rheumatoid arthritis and connective tissue diseases and has provided some interesting insights for researchers. However, research has not yet shown that B19 can trigger these diseases.

Risk Factors and Preventive Measures

The human parvovirus is common and so easily transmitted that 70 percent of the population have been exposed to it by the third decade of life. Most people are infected as children and either have a short-lived feverish illness with a rash or no symptoms at all. There is therefore no great drive for mass vaccination. A vaccine has been developed, but no population studies have been done and it is not in common clinical use. A safe effective vaccine would be of most use to patients with hemolytic anemias who can develop life-threatening illnesses upon infection. Early in an infant's life, the antibodies to parvovirus obtained from its mother would make a vaccine less effective. As infections start in relatively young children, such a vaccine would have to be given at around one year of age.

patellofemoral disorders The powerful muscles in front of the thigh (the quadriceps muscles) join to form a strong tendon (patellar tendon) that passes over the front of the knee joint to attach a few inches down the front of the tibia (the larger of the two lower leg bones). Within the tendon is a small, roughly heart-shaped bone, the patella, that forms a joint with the femur (thighbone), running in a groove between the two curved condyles at its lower end. This bone provides a mechanical advantage to the quadriceps muscles in straightening the knee. This patellofemoral joint lies within the same joint cavity as the main knee joint (tibiofemoral) and is not uncommonly a source of pain (see KNEE PAIN).

Infants can occasionally be born with a dislocated patella. The patella is usually small and the knee is in valgus (knock-kneed). The tissues attaching to the outside of the patella are very tight, and the patella slips over the outer or lateral condyle of the femur while the baby is still in the uterus. Surgery is required to release these tight tissues and realign the patella. Older children can get habitual dislocation of the patella. The muscle and tendon attaching to the outside of the patella are again too tight, and in order to bend the knee, the patella has to slip over the lateral condyle. Unless very mild, this also has to be treated surgically with release of the tight tissues.

Recurrent dislocation or subluxation usually occurs in adolescents, girls more frequently than boys. This is different than habitual dislocation in cause and is generally less severe. Typically, these individuals have a larger-than-usual angle between the thigh and the patella tendon (called the Q angle) and will thus appear knock-kneed. This may be because of true genu valgum (knock-knee), the femur may be twisted inward slightly (persistent femoral anteversion), or the tibia may be turned slightly out. Some patients also have a small high patella (patella alta) or a small, lateral femoral condyle, making it easier for the patella to slip over the condyle. Some patients have a degree of HYPERMOBILITY. Complete dislocation is easily diagnosed even if the patella has slipped back into place, but subluxation can be more difficult. Here the patella does not actually leave the groove between the two condyles but hits up against the inside of the lateral condyle, causing pain. A careful examination and X-rays usually lead to the correct diagnosis. Initial treatment is by strengthening the quadriceps muscle, particularly the one on the inner lower aspect of the thigh that controls the patella movement and prevents it from moving outward. If this muscle is strengthened and the problem persists, surgery may be necessary. The lateral tissues may be released as in habitual dislocation, or more radical procedures can be done to correct the alignment of the patella.

Another cause of knee pain in adolescent girls is usually known simply as anterior knee pain. The pain is often felt during or after sports and may wake the child at night. These girls tend to be more knock-kneed than average, but no dislocation or subluxation can be demonstrated. They generally have weak quadriceps. Some patients have tight hamstrings (the back of the thigh muscles) that may be brought on by wearing high-heeled shoes. Both of these latter conditions increase the pressure between the kneecap and the thighbone in the patellofemoral joint. The treatment is a combination of stretching the hamstring and strengthening the quadriceps muscles. Surgery should be avoided.

The nail-patella syndrome is a rare, inherited disorder in which there is abnormal development of the nails, abnormal bony development around the elbows, and very small or sometimes absent patellae. The autosomal dominant gene responsible for this syndrome has been identified. Although there is no treatment, it is important to recognize the syndrome in order to start screening for the glaucoma and kidney disease that frequently occur as part of the condition. Bipartite patella refers to a condition where the two bone centers in the patella do not grow together as normal and leave a thin layer of cartilage between them. Because cartilage is weaker than bone, this can fracture following repetitive stress. It heals well with splinting. Chondromalacia patellae describes softening of the cartilage at the back of the patella. This gives rise to an aching pain in the front of the knee, especially when it is kept bent for long periods (e.g., in the cinema) or climbing stairs or cycling. It may result from poor alignment of the patella with the femur so that there is increased shear force on the cartilage during movement or from tight hamstrings. Treatment is primarily with strengthening the quadriceps and stretching the hamstrings.

pericarditis The heart is enveloped in two membranes. The inner one, lying right against the heart, secretes a small amount of fluid so that the two layers move easily against one another, thereby reducing any friction to the constantly moving heart. The outer layer is relatively tough and prevents excessive expansion of the heart, for example during exercise. It also creates negative pressure that does not allow the heart to empty completely when it pumps out blood. These two layers of membrane are together called the pericardium. Inflammation of the pericardium is called pericarditis.

Although pericarditis is not very common, there are many conditions that can cause it. Only some of these are rheumatic diseases, but a brief list is as follows:

Infections Viruses, bacteria, TUBERCULOSIS, fungi, and very rarely other infections such as syphilis can all cause pericarditis.

Ischemic heart disease A few patients develop an autoimmune pericarditis after a heart attack or cardiac surgery (Dressler's syndrome), while others may have pericarditis as part of the damage of a heart attack.

Uremia Patients with severe kidney failure often develop pericarditis.

Tumors Many tumors will occasionally spread to the pericardium. Most commonly a lung cancer spreads directly to involve the pericardium.

Conversely, radiotherapy of the chest for cancer is another cause of pericarditis.

Trauma This may be either an injury that penetrates the chest and directly damages the pericardium or a blunt blow to the chest wall as in a motor vehicle accident.

Drug-induced lupus Procainamide and hydralazine were well-known causes but are seldom used now. Isoniazid used to treat tuberculosis and minoxidil used to treat hypertension are still used and may cause pericarditis.

Miscellaneous Other diseases such as hypothyroidism, SARCOIDOSIS, FAMILIAL MEDITERRANEAN FEVER, and severe anemia are occasional causes.

Rheumatic diseases The best-known rheumatic causes are SYSTEMIC LUPUS ERYTHEMATOSUS (SLE), SCLERODERMA, and RHEUMATOID ARTHRITIS. Pericarditis may also occur in Still's disease or systemic-onset JUVENILE IDIOPATHIC ARTHRITIS, MIXED CONNECTIVE TISSUE DISEASE, and the OVERLAP SYNDROME.

Symptoms and Diagnostic Path

Chest pain is the most common symptom and is usually present when a rheumatic disease is the cause. The pain may be severe and is maximal behind the breastbone but may also be felt in the left chest and through to the back. Sometimes it can radiate into the arms as in a heart attack. Typically sitting up or leaning forward relieves the pain somewhat. Pain is not always present. Mild painless pericarditis likely occurs more commonly than diagnosed. Pericarditis is diagnosed in 20–30 percent of SLE patients at some time, although it is not a major problem in all of these patients. If the space between the two membranes fills with a lot of fluid (termed a pericardial effusion), the heart will be unable to fill normally (tamponade) and the patient may be breathless and weak. When severe, this is a life-threatening disorder. Tamponade is not common in the rheumatic disorders, occurring in less than 4 percent of SLE patients with proven pericarditis. With long-standing inflammation the pericardium may tighten around the heart again, restricting its ability to fill and pump blood (constrictive pericarditis). Occasionally in the CREST syndrome, this may occur as a result of calcification of the pericardium.

There is often a crunching sound as the two membranes rub against each other in pericarditis. This *pericardial friction rub* is the most important sign of the disease. If tamponade is present, there will be signs of increased pressure of blood in the veins of the neck. The ECG will often show characteristic changes of widespread raised *ST segments.* A chest X-ray may show an enlarged heart shadow. An echocardiogram (ultrasound scan of the heart) is very good at demonstrating fluid in the pericardial sac. It should be remembered that patients with rheumatic diseases may also get pericarditis due to infections, drugs, or trauma. When the cause is in doubt, and especially if infection is likely, fluid may be removed from the pericardial sac. This is an invasive procedure and should be done under controlled conditions.

Treatment Options and Outlook

Pericarditis of rheumatic origin usually responds to anti-inflammatory treatment with CORTICOSTE-ROIDS. This may be given in large intravenous pulses for a rapid effect. All patients with recent onset of pericarditis should be carefully observed for the development of tamponade. If this develops, removal of pericardial fluid may be lifesaving. This is done by inserting a needle into the pericardium (usually from under the left-sided ribs close to the lower end of the breastbone). Either an ECG lead is attached to the needle so that a signal can be seen when it touches the heart or an ultrasound technician can assist in placing and monitoring the position of the needle. When effusions keep recurring it may be necessary to cut windows in the pericardium to allow free drainage. If long-standing inflammation has led to significant tightening or constriction of the heart, the only treatment is to peel the pericardium off surgically. In rheumatic diseases if the pericarditis is diagnosed and treated promptly, the outcome is usually very good.

pharmacogenetics The terms *pharmacogenetics* and *pharmacogenomics* are often used interchangeably and describe an area of intense medical research that seeks to predict how an individual will respond to a drug based on his or her genetic makeup. This contrasts with most other medical uses of genetics that seek to find the genes that predispose people to develop a particular illness or to intervene in a disease by inserting modified genes (gene therapy).

There is a lot of variability between people in their response to the same dose of a drug. A few are allergic, some have little or no response, some have a good response, and some have such a strong response that they develop side effects. This means that when a new drug is marketed, the standard dose chosen is the one that suits most people. This standard dose will, however, be too low for some people and too high for others. Many factors affect response to a drug, some of these such as diet, smoking, alcohol intake, body weight, and kidney and liver function are environmental, but genetic variations also alter responses. The ultimate aim of pharmacogenetics is to identify the genes that affect responses to drugs and use this information to select the best drug, and the correct dose, for each individual. Pharmacogenetics can be divided into two big areas: genes that affect the concentration of drugs and genes that affect the response to drugs.

Genes that affect the concentration of drugs Most drugs, after they are absorbed, are metabolized in the body. Usually this is a way of breaking down the active drug and excreting it. Sometimes, though, an inactive drug, called pro-drug, is metabolized to an active drug. Drugs are metabolized by enzymes. Genetic variation in these enzymes can result in increased or decreased activity compared with the usual enzyme activity found in most people. A group of enzymes called cytochrome P450 (CYP), found in the liver and intestinal wall, metabolize more than half of all drugs. The CYP enzymes are broken down into families labeled 1, 2, 3, and so on. These are further subdivided into subfamilies labeled A, B, C, and so on and then into genes labeled 1, 2, and 3.

There are several genetic variants of CYP drug-metabolizing enzymes that affect how active they are. For example, approximately 5–10 percent of most Caucasian populations have a variant of CYP2D6 that is either inactive or poorly functional. This means that these people poorly metabolize drugs that are substrates for this enzyme. Sometimes this means that they will not respond to a drug. For example, codeine is activated to morphine by CYP2D6. Therefore, people with an enzyme that functions poorly do not activate codeine well and do not receive the analgesic benefits of codeine when they take it. More often, having a defective enzyme means that people accumulate high levels of a drug. For example, the older antidepressants such as amitriptyline and nortriptyline are also metabolized by CYP2D6, but in this case they are inactivated by it. Therefore, people with the inactive enzyme have higher blood levels of these antidepressants and are more likely to have side effects if they are given standard doses of the drugs.

Important genetic variations have been discovered in CYP3A, CYP1A2, CYP2C9, and CYP2C19. The clinical importance of a variation depends on the drug affected. If the drug is effective and safe over a wide range of concentrations, genetic variation is unlikely to be clinically important. On the other hand, if the concentrations of a drug that are effective and those that cause side effects are close, a small increase or decrease in concentration can result in side effects or lack of effect. For example, CYP2C9 is the enzyme responsible for metabolizing most of the active component of warfarin, a drug used to prevent blood clotting. The concentration of warfarin is critically important. If it is slightly too low a blood clot can result, and if it is too high the patient may bleed. Genetic variants of CYP2C9 called *2 (star 2) and *3 are less effective and result in a greater concentration and therefore greater effect of warfarin in people who have these variants. At this stage it is not clear if genotyping people before they start warfarin will provide information that improves outcomes compared will the usual way warfarin is dosed and monitored.

Not all drugs are metabolized by CYP enzymes. A genetic variation in an enzyme called thiopurine methyltransferase (TPMT) slows the metabolism of azathioprine and causes a substantial increase in sensitivity to it. The homozygous form (both strands of DNA are affected) of the gene associated with impaired TPMT activity occurs in approximately one in 300 people. Although this is a relatively rare variant, its consequences can be devastating. If someone with a defective TPMT enzyme takes standard doses of AZATHIOPRINE (trade name: Imuran), bone marrow failure is likely to result because very high levels of the drug accumulate. Genetic testing for TPMT variants is now available.

The concentration of a drug in the body is affected by many factors. Obvious ones are the dose of drug taken and the rate at which enzymes eliminate it, but less obvious are transport systems that move a drug across different barriers. Some cells have transporters that move drugs and other substances across their membranes. One of the best known is the multidrug resistance (MDR), also called P-glycoprotein (PgP), transporter. The MDR transport system was discovered when scientists noticed that some cancer cells became resistant to anticancer drugs because they had a protein, PgP, which enabled them to pump the drugs out of the cells. The MDR system is present not only in cancer cells but also in healthy cells in the gut, kidney, and brain. In the gut MDR pumps drug out of cells back into the lumen and thus decreases absorption of some drugs such as CYCLOSPORINE that use this transporter. In the brain MDR helps form what is called the blood-brain barrier, a barrier that prevents drugs from entering the brain. There are many variations in the MDR gene that can alter the activity of the transporter and thus affect concentrations of drugs in different parts of the body.

New genetic variations in enzymes and transporters are still being discovered. To make matters more complex, there can also be variations in the promoter area of genes. This area drives the activity of the gene. Therefore, promoter variants can result in the transporter or enzyme being more or less active even though the gene coding for it is normal.

Genes that affect response to drugs Drugs act in different ways, but many bind to receptors that then activate a cascade of messengers. This means that two people who have the same concentration of a drug can have different responses if they have different receptors. Genetic variants in receptors that mediate the effects of drugs used to treat asthma appear to have clinical effects, but there is much less evidence that receptor variants alter responses to antirheumatic drugs. For example, there is speculation that genetic variability in the TNF receptor may explain why some patients respond well to TNF-blocking drugs and others do not but the evidence is preliminary.

Summary Pharmacogenetics has had a limited effect on the way antirheumatic drugs are used. To decrease the risk of side effects, some clinicians test for TPMT enzyme deficiency before prescribing azathioprine. There is limited data that genetic variation is helpful in predicting responses to antirheumatic drugs such as TNF-antagonists and methotrexate, and genetic tests to predict the effects of these drugs remain research tools.

photopheresis (extracorporeal phototherapy) A patient's blood is removed, the white blood cells are separated by centrifugation and exposed to ultraviolet light, and then they are infused back into the patient. To enhance the response to light, either the patient takes a photosensitizing drug such as methoxypsoralen before the white cells are separated or the photosensitizing drug is added directly to the white blood cells before they are exposed to light. Photopheresis has been used to treat several autoimmune diseases including SYSTEMIC LUPUS ERYTHEMATOSUS, RHEUMATOID ARTHRITIS, and SCLERODERMA and some types of skin lymphoma.

Photopheresis modulates the immune system, but how it does so is not clear. Lymphocytes affected by phototherapy are rapidly removed from the circulation. Because only about 10 percent of lymphocytes are affected, depletion of lymphocytes is not the main mechanism of action. More likely the altered lymphocytes induce an immune response when they are reinfused.

Photopheresis is usually performed on two days every four weeks for six to 12 months. There are few side effects. However, drawing blood and reinfusing it can sometimes be difficult if a patient has fragile veins.

Anecdotal responses to photopheresis have been reported in autoimmune disease, but there is not much scientific information to support the use of this treatment outside of clinical trials. One study reported modest benefits on skin-thickening in patients with scleroderma, but the design of the trial was criticized and more studies are needed.

physical therapy Modern physical therapy has become quite diverse and specialized. Giving a concise definition that will usefully inform the reader is difficult. In addition, many schools of thought have pursued particular philosophies and become identifiable as separate from mainstream physical therapy. The American Physical Therapy Association includes four general activities in their 1995 definition of care and services provided by or under the supervision of a physical therapist:

1. Examining patients with impairments, functional limitations, or disability in order to determine a diagnosis, prognosis, or outcome and therapeutic intervention
2. Alleviating these impairments or functional limitations by designing, implementing, and modifying therapeutic interventions, which might include the following:
   (a) Therapeutic exercise
   (b) Manual therapy or manipulation
   (c) Prescribing or making ASSISTIVE DEVICES, protective devices, and other equipment
   (d) Using airway clearance techniques
   (e) The use of physical, mechanical, or electrotherapeutic modalities
   (f) Patient education
3. Prevention of injury, impairment, or functional limitation including the promotion of fitness and health
4. Engaging in consultation, education, and research

For patients with rheumatic disorders, therapeutic exercise is perhaps the most important physical therapy intervention. The underlying philosophy here is to identify the patient's functional limitation. In other words, what in his or her daily life is difficult or impossible to do? The reason for this inability (the impairment) can then be determined from a careful examination. With this knowledge the best way of alleviating the impairment (and thereby improving function of daily activities) through appropriate exercise can be determined and implemented. EXERCISE in this sense might include activities and techniques to improve mobility, muscle strength and force, neuromuscular control, cardiovascular fitness, muscle endurance, balance, coordination, breathing patterns, posture awareness, and/or movement patterns. Hydrotherapy or exercise in water has particular advantages for people with severe arthritis. Water provides buoyancy, unloading painful joints, and at the same time provides all-around resistance. This allows a range of strengthening exercises to be done with very little stress to the weight-bearing joints. In addition, many people find warm water soothing.

Manual therapy (manipulation) can be used to improve the range of movement at joints or relieve pain in dysfunctional joints but should be used with care in the inflammatory forms of arthritis because the connective tissues are often in poor condition. Physical therapists frequently use heat and cold, massage, ultrasound, or electrotherapeutic modalities such as faradic stimulation or transcutaneous electrical nerve stimulation (TENS) to relieve pain or promote healing.

pigmented villonodular synovitis (PVS) A rare disease that causes the synovium to proliferate and invade bone.

The cause of PVS is not known. It behaves like a benign tumor and causes the synovium to proliferate in frondlike strands (villi) or form nodules that can invade and destroy adjacent bone. The proliferating synovium is rich in blood vessels, and small amounts of bleeding cause hemosiderin, a type of pigment, to accumulate.

Symptoms and Diagnostic Path

PVS almost always affects one joint, most often the knee or hip. The affected joint gradually becomes painful, stiff, and swells from time to time. If synovial fluid is present it may be heavily bloodstained. This is a clue to the diagnosis because only a few conditions cause bloodstained synovial fluid.

There are no specific clues to the diagnosis on physical examination. The most important clue is the presence of bloodstained synovial fluid in a patient with arthritis affecting one joint. An X-ray may show early changes such as thinning of the cartilage or late changes such as bony erosions. MRI can show characteristically decreased signal intensity on both T1 and T2 images, a finding thought to be caused by the accumulation of hemosiderin in the synovium. The definitive diagnosis is made by ARTHROSCOPY with biopsy of the synovium.

Treatment Options and Outlook

Treatment is surgical resection. Arthroscopic or open synovectomy is often successful, but the disease can recur and require repeated surgery or radiation therapy. INFLIXIMAB has been used in resistant disease to control but not eradicate the disease. This raises the possibility of PVS being an inflammatory process, which is considered to be the case by some health workers.

Risk Factors and Preventive Measures

There are no known risk factors or preventive measures for PVS.

plantar fasciitis This is a very common cause of pain in the heel or foot, especially in middle-aged or elderly individuals. It is more common in the overweight and in those with flat feet.

Shortly after the heel strikes the ground in normal walking, the foot goes into pronation to absorb the force of impact. Pronation involves a loosening of the joints of the midfoot so there is more give and a slight turning out of the forefoot while the calcaneus or heel bone itself tilts over to the inside and dips its nose down. This results in the force of landing and weight bearing being spread through a number of bones, joints, ligaments, and muscles rather than just in a direct line through the heel to the ground. One of the important structures in this mechanism is the plantar fascia. This is a tough, flat fibrous tissue that spans the sole of the foot from the front lower edge of the calcaneus to the base of the toes supporting the long arch of the foot like an unusually wide bowstring. It also sends further slips along the toes that serve to tighten the plantar fascia when the toes are curled up (as when taking off from that foot). As the foot goes into pronation the long arch tends to collapse slightly, and the plantar fascia is stretched and stressed. This is a normal event. However, if the stresses are suddenly increased by, for example, rapid weight gain or large increase in distance walked, then microtears can develop in the plantar fascia. This results in small areas of inflammation that can accumulate and cause pain. This commonly affects the middle section of the plantar fascia or its attachment to the calcaneus.

A similar process can occur with normal or minimal stresses if the structures themselves are abnormal. This can occur in patients with inflammatory arthritis such as RHEUMATOID ARTHRITIS who are prone to develop *overpronation* or in people who are naturally flat-footed. Patients with SPONDYLO-ARTHROPATHIES are also prone to develop inflammation at the attachment of the plantar fascia to the calcaneus with relatively little stress.

Symptoms and Diagnostic Path

People usually complain of pain underneath the foot just in front of the calcaneus. The pain often comes on after unaccustomed standing, walking, or athletic activity. The pain is often worst in the morning or after a rest and eases a bit with walking.

The typical pain should suggest the diagnosis that is confirmed on physical examination. Tenderness can be produced by pressing on the front end of the calcaneus toward the inner border of the sole or toward the middle of the long arch of the foot. Pain will also be felt when the toes are pulled upward since this tightens the plantar fascia. X-ray may show a heel spur, but this seldom affects treatment.

Treatment Options and Outlook

Relieving the pressure over the attachment of the plantar fascia may improve pain on walking, especially if there is a spur. This is achieved by using a heel pad either with a cutout below the tender area or a softer gel material in this area. However, this does not address the cause. Since pronation is an important factor in most cases, an insole that supports the long arch along the inner border of the foot and acts to limit pronation is often used. This can be combined with a pressure-relieving cutout. Weight loss and appropriate footwear are important for some people. Injection of a local anesthetic and CORTICOSTEROID around the attachment of the plantar fascia is helpful in settling the inflammation down quickly. Occasionally surgical release of the fascia is necessary, and sometimes removing a troublesome spur is helpful.

Risk Factors and Preventive Measures

Risk factors for plantar fasciitis are discussed above. A number of preventive strategies are tried, although few have been studied in a controlled manner. Semi-rigid orthoses supporting the long arch of the foot have been shown to significantly prevent symptoms in at-risk people. They can however be quite uncomfortable to wear, especially for athletic activities. Stretching is widely and appropriately practiced. The muscles at the back of the calf lack both strength and flexibility in athletes with plantar fasciitis. During the rehabilitation phase, a common stretch is to hook a towel around the toes and forefoot and pull back on this, thus stretching both the plantar fascia itself and the muscles at the back of the calf. For prevention, however, a better stretch is to stand on a step on the ball of the foot, rise up on the toes and slowly lower the heel until it is below the level of the rest of the foot and the calf muscles feel tight. This is also an excellent strengthening exercise for the calf muscle. Good footwear is important for those people at the ends of the normal spectrum who either overpronate or have a high-arched, stiff midfoot. A common mistake is for overpronators to get athletic shoes with a lateral (outside of the heel) flare around the heel. Normal heelstrike is just lateral to the midline, and if there is a flare here exaggerating the normal shape of the heel it will tend to throw the foot into overpronation with increased force and make things worse. These individuals should look for a shoe with a cutaway on the lateral half of the back of the heel.

plasmapheresis (therapeutic plasma exchange) Removal and replacement of a patient's plasma in order to remove large molecules such as antibodies and other proteins. The rationale for plasmapheresis is simple—if a disease is caused by antibodies, removing them should improve the disease.

Plasmapheresis is performed by drawing blood out of a vein and passing it into a centrifuge that separates cells from plasma. The patient's plasma is removed and replaced with saline and albumin or plasma from the blood bank. The reconstituted blood is infused back into the patient through another vein. Removing the entire plasma volume takes about two hours, and doing this reduces the concentration of large proteins in the circulation by about 60 percent. Usually three to five exchanges are performed over seven to 10 days, removing 90 percent of the patient's own antibodies.

Side effects of plasmapheresis The side effects of plasmapheresis are usually temporary and minor. Obtaining venous access in patients with small veins can sometimes be difficult. Unsuccessful attempts to place a needle in a vein can cause local bruising. Removing blood during plasmapheresis can lower the blood pressure to the extent that the person becomes dizzy or faints. This can be treated by infusing more fluid to replace the volume that has been removed from the circulation. If too much fluid is replaced, it can cause shortness of breath due to heart failure. This is treated by slowing down the rate of fluid replacement or treating with a diuretic that increases urine production.

Blood will clot in the plastic tubes used to remove it unless it is mixed with an anticoagulant. The anticoagulant used, citrate, can bind calcium in the patient's blood and cause muscle cramps and numbness or tingling around the mouth and in the hands and feet. Calcium supplements will improve these symptoms but are seldom needed.

Allergy to the replacement plasma is rare but can cause a rash or a more severe allergic reaction. Patients taking ACE inhibitors (angiotensin-converting enzyme inhibitors), a class of drug used to treat high blood pressure or heart failure, may flush and have low blood pressure during the procedure. The reason is that ACE inhibitors slow the breakdown of a bradykinin, a chemical produced when the blood is processed during plasmapheresis. Patients are asked to discontinue ACE inhibitors for at least 24 hours before plasmapheresis.

Viral infections such as hepatitis C can be transmitted in the replacement plasma, but this is rare because donors are screened. Plasmapheresis is expensive.

Indications for plasmapheresis Plasmapheresis is used as an emergency treatment for patients who have a serious illness caused by a circulating antibody or protein. The procedure reduces the amount of antibodies, but only temporarily. Therefore treatment with immunosuppressive drugs to decrease production of new antibodies is often started at the same time.

The indications for plasmapheresis are controversial. Generally GOODPASTURE'S SYNDROME, MYASTHENIA GRAVIS, Guillain-Barré syndrome, and a closely related disease, chronic inflammatory demyelinating polyneuropathy, as well as thrombotic thrombocytopenic purpura (see THROMBOCYTOPENIA), CRYOGLOBULINEMIA, and hyperviscosity syndrome are accepted indications.

Controlled trials show that plasmapheresis had no benefit in rheumatoid arthritis, kidney disease due to SYSTEMIC LUPUS ERYTHEMATOSUS (SLE) and polymyositis. The SLE trial was criticized be cause plasmapheresis alone was compared with standard immunosuppressive drugs. Plasmapheresis, although it temporarily decreases proteins, can cause a rebound increase in antibody production if it is used without immunosuppressive drugs. Plasmapheresis is used empirically in critically ill patients with SLE or VASCULITIS.

podiatrist A doctor of podiatric medicine (D.P.M. degree), specializing in the treatment of foot and ankle disorders. Podiatrists train for four years at a podiatric school and then spend several years in a residency program.

Podiatrists deal with problems such as bunions, corns, calluses, ingrown toenails, hammertoes, claw toes, foot pain, flat feet, diabetic foot problems, and foot and ankle injuries. Treatment usually involves orthotics, devices designed to correct or improve foot and ankle biomechanics. Examples of orthotics are wedges to correct uneven leg length or adjust the angle of the ankle or forefoot, shoe inserts to provide greater shock absorption and decrease pressure on painful areas, arch supports, braces, and fitted shoes. Podiatrists also perform foot and ankle surgery.

polyarteritis nodosa This was the first form of VASCULITIS described, in 1866, in Germany. It is uncommon, affecting about five per million persons per year in England, nine per million in Minnesota, but up to 77 per million in Alaskan Eskimos. All ages and races are affected, but it is more common in men than women and usually affects those in middle age.

In most patients with polyarteritis nodosa defining the precise cause is difficult. Circulating immune complexes are often found in the blood system. These are complexes of antibodies or immunoglobulins together with sometimes identifiable antigens that can become large enough to lodge in vessel walls. Here they may initiate an immune attack on the vessel wall that is the primary manifestation of the disease. Small- and medium-sized arteries are affected in polyarteritis nodosa. Biopsy specimens show localized destruction of the vessel walls, particularly by neutrophils. These areas are weakened and may bulge as they heal, giving rise to small nodules that could be felt along the course of arteries and the origin of the earlier name, periarteritis nodosa. Feeling these today is unusual because the disease is diagnosed and treated much earlier.

There is a strong association with chronic HEPATITIS B infection in some parts of the world. Evidence of hepatitis B infection is found in 10–50 percent of polyarteritis patients and probably accounts for the higher incidence in Alaskan Eskimos in whom this infection is very common. Hepatitis B may be the antigen that drives the development of immune complexes. Antibodies directed against the vessel wall have also been found. It is possible that antigens on an infectious agent are similar to those on the endothelium of the vessel wall. The antibodies against the one may therefore crossreact against the other and direct the immune attack against the endothelium. Other infections that have been linked to the development of polyarteritis include hepatitis A, cytomegalovirus, PARVOVIRUS, and HTLV1. In developed countries, polyarteritis nodosa is more frequently associated with malignancy. The tumors involved are usually those affecting the blood-forming cells, including myelodysplastic syndrome and lymphomas, but many other tumors have been reported. In these cases, the activity of the vasculitis usually mirrors the state of the tumor.

At the site of damage in the vessel wall, is often overgrowth of endothelial cells and fibrous tissue, presumably in an attempt to repair the damage. This sometimes leads to blocking off of the artery. In addition, many factors promote coagulation (clotting) during a vasculitic illness. Clots may occur not only in damaged arteries but also in veins, whose slower blood flow makes them susceptible to this.

Symptoms and Diagnostic Path

As with many forms of vasculitis, polyarteritis nodosa can start and progress in many different ways. The most frequently involved organ is in fact the kidney (70 percent), although this is seldom what leads to the diagnosis. More commonly the joint, skin, or nerve manifestations lead to investigation and diagnosis. Most patients will experience a degree of fever, weight loss, loss of energy, and generalized aches. More specific symptoms include the following:

Skin Half of all patients develop skin lesions. The earliest lesions are often small purplish black spots on the feet and legs that can easily be felt to be lumpy (palpable purpura). This may progress to ulceration or even gangrene, usually affecting one or several toes. LIVEDO RETICULARIS is common.

Joints More than 50 percent of patients have joint symptoms. This may be widespread joint pain or arthritis of the lower-limb joints. Occasionally polyarteritis presents with a POLYMYALGIA RHEUMATICA-like syndrome. There is seldom damage to the joints.

Kidney There is commonly a protein leak into the urine, indicating damage to the filtering part of the kidneys (glomeruli). Occasionally this can be severe and cause nephrotic syndrome. Red blood cells in the urine also signal glomerular damage. High blood pressure may be due to glomerular damage or narrowing of the artery taking blood to the kidney and affects 25 percent of patients.

Nerves Most patients, 50–70 percent, develop nerve damage. Classically, this involves one or several peripheral nerves in the arms or legs. It starts with pain and altered sensation in the distribution of the nerve followed by weakness, developing hours or days later. Less commonly there is loss of sensation in both legs in the area short socks would cover. Very occasionally blood vessels in the brain may be affected, leading to seizures or a stroke.

Gut The gallbladder and appendix are most likely to be affected, but blood vessels supplying the intestines (mesenteric arteries) may also become narrowed or clot. If severe these are surgical emergencies. The liver is seldom affected except where there is chronic hepatitis B infection.

Other Virtually any organ may be affected, but apart from the above, this is rare. Myocardial infarction and heart failure have been reported. Lung lesions presumably due to vasculitis may be found. Testicular and eye involvement are also well recognized but uncommon.

Associated diseases A variant of polyarteritis nodosa called microscopic polyarteritis or microscopic polyangiitis affects the kidneys in almost all patients and the lungs in many. Unlike classical polyarteritis nodosa, it does not usually affect medium-sized blood vessels in the gut or other parts of the body. Microscopic polyangiitis can also cause eye and ear symptoms and can sometimes be mistaken for WEGENER'S GRANULOMATOSIS.

A polyarteritis nodosa-like syndrome can occur in patients with other rheumatic diseases such as RHEUMATOID ARTHRITIS, SJÖGREN'S SYNDROME, CRYO-GLOBULINEMIA, hairy cell leukemia, and other blood disorders. Metastatic cancer that is usually highly malignant and septicemia (infection in the bloodstream) can mimic polyarteritis nodosa, although the mechanisms of disease are different.

When a patient presents with weight loss, malaise, joint pain, and several nerve lesions, the diagnosis is usually suspected immediately and soon confirmed. However, polyarteritis can present in so many diverse ways that the diagnosis is not uncommonly delayed. Blood tests will show a marked inflammatory response with raised ESR and C-reactive protein. There is mild anemia, sometimes a raised white cell count, and low albumin, but none of these findings are specific to polyarteritis nodosa. Rheumatoid factor may be positive, complement levels reduced, and hepatitis B markers positive.

A biopsy of involved tissue showing the typical pattern of destruction of the vessel wall of a small artery is the usual confirmatory test. Skin, muscle, testes (if involved), or a sensory nerve, the sural nerve, may be biopsied. If none of the involved tissue is accessible, an angiogram is performed. This involves the injection of dye into the arteries supplying the gut, liver, and kidneys and taking X-rays that show the arterial system very clearly. In polyarteritis nodosa affected arteries have an irregular diameter and typically appear beaded. The classical small aneurysms (localized dilatations along the arteries) are seen less often these days because of earlier diagnosis and treatment. It is important to rule out the possibility of infection and consider the presence of an underlying malignancy in all patients.

Treatment Options and Outlook

The initial treatment should be vigorous to try to prevent irreversible organ damage from this potentially devastating disease. Over 85 percent of patients will die within five years without treatment. Initial treatment is with high doses of CORTICOSTEROIDS. This may be given as intravenous pulses of methylprednisolone every day or every other day for three doses initially and changed to daily PREDNISONE thereafter. Although they are effective in controlling the inflammation, corticosteroids may increase the tendency for arteries to thrombose. For this reason many rheumatologists also use an antiplatelet agent at the same time. Low-dose ASPIRIN is usually used, although other agents are becoming available.

When the disease is severe or does not respond rapidly to corticosteroids, cytotoxic drugs such as CYCLOPHOSPHAMIDE or CHLORAMBUCIL are usually used. These drugs may have some additional benefit in preventing the overgrowth of endothelium and fibrous tissue that frequently leads to arteries being persistently narrow once the acute disease is settled. They are also highly effective in settling the inflammatory response. If these are not effective or contraindicated, INTRAVENOUS IMMUNOGLOBULIN (IVIG) is a further option in the initial phase of the illness. The mechanism of its action remains unclear, but it has been shown to be effective in a number of forms of vasculitis.

Once the acute inflammatory phase is controlled, ongoing treatment is required, first to prevent relapse and second to manage longer-term consequences of the disease and treatment. Because the side effects of corticosteroids and the alkylating agents cyclophosphamide and chlorambucil are mostly related to long-term use, it is common to try switching to another agent for longer-term control. This is either METHOTREXATE or AZATHIOPRINE, which are often combined with a small dose of prednisone.

Hypertension and other factors that might promote atherosclerosis (the common age-related arterial narrowing) must be extremely well controlled in these patients who have suffered widespread damage to their arteries. Antiplatelet therapy should probably be continued for life. Anti-OSTEO-POROSIS treatment may be used to protect against the effects of the corticosteroids, especially in postmenopausal women. Infection is a concern in patients receiving powerful immunosuppression drugs as described above and should be promptly treated. With modern treatment approximately 70–80 percent of patients can be expected to be alive five years after diagnosis.

Risk Factors and Preventive Measures

In developing countries where chronic hepatitis B infection is a major risk factor it would be possible to reduce the incidence of both hepatitis B and polyarteritis nodosa with universal vaccination against hepatitis B. A safe reliable vaccine is available and is usually given in childhood or at any later age in at-risk groups.

polymyalgia rheumatica (PMR) This syndrome affects middle-aged and elderly people. It is characterized by pain and stiffness in the shoulders and hips. There are European paintings depicting the associated condition, TEMPORAL ARTERITIS, together with good written descriptions of polymyalgia rheumatica going back 600 years. However, it was only in the 1950s that the name polymyalgia rheumatica came into being. It is common in people of northern European origin, although it has been described in many parts of the world. In northern Europe and the northern states of the United States, approximately 18 in 100,000 people over the age of 50 years develop the disease, making it a fairly common rheumatic disorder. Between 10 and 15 percent of patients with PMR develop a distinctive form of VASCULITIS, temporal arteritis.

Despite considerable research, the cause of PMR remains obscure. Since nearly all patients are aged over 50 years, there is clearly some relationship to age. However, the relevance of this is unclear. There is an increased frequency of the genetic allele HLA-DR4 in patients when compared with controls (see HLA). This may indicate that patients have a genetically determined way of responding to antigens that predisposes them to getting the disease.

There are certainly a number of families where two or more members have developed PMR. However, there are also reports of husbands and wives developing PMR that would support exposure to the same antigen rather than hereditary factors as a cause.

The walls of affected arteries in temporal arteritis (and sometimes in uncomplicated PMR) are affected in patches. A chronic immune attack which classically leads to organized clumps of immune cells arranged in what is termed a granuloma. Only arteries with elastic layers in their walls are attacked, and the attack seems to be centered on or close to this elastic layer. The smaller arteries lose the elastic layer, so mostly large or medium-sized arteries are affected. There have been a number of postulated antigens that might initiate the immune response, but none have stood up to further investigation.

Symptoms and Diagnostic Path

Typically an older individual in good health develops a low-grade fever and loses some weight. Transient aches and pains may be present for weeks or months. The pain and stiffness settles in a shoulder and then moves to both the hip and the shoulder region within a few weeks. Less commonly a patient wakes up one morning unable to get out of bed because of the pain and stiffness. Lethargy and depression are common. Severe stiffness on rising in the morning is characteristic, and several hours may pass before the patient is able to move about reasonably normally. This characteristic stiffness often returns when the individual sits down to rest during the day. Pain and waking at night are common. Although movement makes the pain worse, the pain usually described as being in the muscles rather than the joints. Muscle strength is normal, although pain may make it difficult for the patient to be sure of this.

Some patients do have an associated arthritis, usually affecting the knees, wrists, or sternoclavicular (between the collarbone and breastbone) joints. Between 10 and 20 percent of patients with PMR develop temporal arteritis. On the other hand, between 20 and 40 percent of patients with temporal arteritis have symptoms of PMR. Temporal arteritis is discussed separately.

No diagnostic test is available for PMR. Biopsy of a temporal artery can confirm temporal arteritis if this is present and may occasionally be positive in uncomplicated PMR. However, in the absence of a diagnostic test it is important to exclude other conditions that can present in a similar way. This is particularly important when the onset is atypical in some way. The ESR is almost always raised. Although polymyalgia with a normal ESR is frequently discussed, this is very rare. Typically the ESR will be raised to between 50 and 100 mm per hour. Other markers of inflammation such as C-reactive protein will also be raised, and a rise in alpha globulins is common but nonspecific. Many studies have shown a selective reduction in CD8+ T cells in patients with PMR that returns to normal after about one year of treatment. Researchers have hoped that this might provide a more specific test for PMR, but confirmation is awaited. The enzymes released by an inflamed or damaged liver (especially alkaline phosphatase) are frequently mildly raised, and liver biopsies have shown mild inflammatory changes in PMR (see Appendix II for description of tests). The important characteristics in making the diagnosis are some combination of the following: a Caucasian patient aged over 50 years with persistent (more than a month) pain in the shoulders and pelvic girdle, marked morning stiffness, no true muscle weakness, an ESR over 40 mm per hour, and excellent relief with a small dose of PREDNISONE.

The fewer of these characteristics that are present, the less typical the illness is and the more likely it is to be another illness presenting like PMR. RHEUMATOID ARTHRITIS starting for the first time in an older individual is well known to mimic PMR. Multiple myeloma and lung cancer are the two malignancies most likely to produce this type of syndrome, but a number of other malignancies that have spread to bone can also do this. Osteoarthritis (OA) of the neck is very common. When combined with the lethargy, loss of appetite, and raised ESR caused by an unrecognized low-grade infection, OA may lead to an erroneous diagnosis of PMR. Leukemias and lymphomas may occasionally cause confusion as can MYOPATHIES, MYOSITIS, hypothyroidism, infective endocarditis, and the rare ATRIAL MYXOMA.

Treatment Options and Outlook

CORTICOSTEROIDS are almost always required. With mild disease it is possible to try NSAIDs first. However, these drugs have greatly increased toxicity in the elderly. It is therefore often safer and more effective to use corticosteroids, usually prednisone. The majority of patients will experience marked-to-miraculous relief with 15 mg of prednisone daily. Occasionally patients will need higher doses, but this should prompt a careful consideration of whether the diagnosis is correct. The dose may be reduced to 10 mg per day over two months and then very gradually reduced as symptoms and the ESR allow. Too rapid a reduction results in more relapses, and these patients end up taking more prednisone than they would have with a more gradual reduction. Treatment is usually required for between two and five years, when it may be stopped without any recurrence of the PMR. A very small number of patients continue to take a small dose of prednisone for many years. If it is not possible to reduce the prednisone without a recurrence of symptoms or the corticosteroid side effects are too great, another medication is usually added. This is usually AZATHIOPRINE or METHOTREXATE.

Once the initial inflammation is controlled, the patient usually feels very much better. The most difficult aspect of treatment is in limiting the corticosteroid side effects. The risk of OSTEOPOROSIS should be evaluated. Most patients will benefit from preventive treatment, at least for the duration of the prednisone therapy. Corticosteroids and inflammation may promote atherosclerosis. Since many PMR patients are at an age where they are at risk of cardiovascular events, they should take an antiplatelet agent such as low-dose ASPIRIN. This has not been submitted to controlled trial and is unlikely to be because of the cost of such a trial. Protection from bruising and limiting weight gain are also important in long-term corticosteroid therapy.

Although there is some variation between different studies, at least 50 percent of patients should be able to stop treatment within two years and the vast majority by four to five years. Between 20 and 50 percent of patients will suffer significant adverse effects from the long-term prednisone therapy. The risk of adverse effects is related to higher initial doses, total dose taken, and longer duration of treatment.

Risk Factors and Preventive Measures

There are no proven risk factors or preventive measures.

polymyositis See DERMATOMYOSITIS AND POLYMYOSITIS.

pregnancy Patients with rheumatic diseases face four major questions during pregnancy.

1. What is the effect of drugs used to treat rheumatic disease on pregnancy?
2. How can pregnancy affect rheumatic illness?
3. How can rheumatic illness affect the pregnancy?
4. Pregnancy-related rheumatic condition.

These questions are difficult to answer because each individual's situation is different and there is not much information available from clinical trials. The treatment of rheumatic disease in pregnancy is complicated and best performed by a team of physicians bringing together obstetric and rheumatology expertise.

What Is the Effect of Drugs Used to Treat Rheumatic Disease on Pregnancy?

A few drugs are generally considered safe when taken in pregnancy because many women have taken them and the rate of congenital abnormalities has not been increased. A few drugs are also known to be unsafe in pregnancy because they are teratogenic—often causing abnormalities in the unborn baby. For most drugs, though, very little is known about risks in pregnancy because, as a general principle, drug exposure is avoided in pregnant women. Therefore limited information accumulates. The information provided by manufacturers is often not very helpful, and the package insert for most drugs contains the phrase "this drug is not recommended for use in pregnancy and should not be used unless the benefits are

thought to outweigh the risk." Because the risks and benefits differ in every patient, there are few rigid guidelines. For example, anticancer drugs are almost always avoided in pregnancy because they are teratogenic. However, if a pregnant woman has cancer that needs to be treated immediately to protect her life, physicians will usually recommend treatment, even though this might require termination of the pregnancy.

Known teratogenic drugs include METHOTREXATE, CYCLOPHOSPHAMIDE, all the anticancer drugs, warfarin, and THALIDOMIDE. LEFLUNOMIDE is teratogenic in animals and has the disadvantage that it stays in the body for many months after a person stops taking it. There is very little information about the effects of leflunomide on human pregnancy, but it is avoided. In fact, many rheumatologists try not to use it in women of childbearing age. If a woman who is able to bear children is treated with leflunomide and stops it for any reason, many rheumatologists will prescribe a course of cholestyramine to speed up the elimination of leflunomide. If a woman taking leflunomide wants to become pregnant, the drug is stopped, cholestyramine is prescribed, and blood levels of leflunomide are measured to make sure they are almost undetectable before the woman tries to become pregnant.

MISOPROSTOL is teratogenic and also stimulates prostaglandin receptors on the uterus, causing it to contract. Misoprostol is used in some countries to induce abortion.

NSAIDs are not teratogenic in the classical sense. However, if they are used in the last trimester of pregnancy, they can cause premature closure of the patent ductus arteriosus, a small blood vessel that joins the circulatory systems of the lung and the body in the fetus and normally closes only after birth. Premature closure of the patent ductus arteriosus can cause PULMONARY HYPERTENSION in the fetus. NSAIDs can also have other harmful effects at the end of pregnancy and may prolong labor and increase the risk of bleeding in the fetus. There is some recent evidence that NSAIDs increase the rate of miscarriage if they are taken at the time of conception. Women planning to become pregnant should not therefore take them, but they may be taken in the second trimester once the pregnancy is well established. Low-dose aspirin on the other hand appears safe throughout pregnancy.

CORTICOSTEROIDS are probably not teratogenic but can cross the placenta and suppress the adrenal glands of the unborn baby so that after birth it cannot make enough cortisol. This is easily treated by prescribing corticosteroids for the newborn baby. Corticosteroids can also affect the growth of the unborn baby. Prednisone does not cross the placenta very well and is the preferred drug for treating the mother. Dexamethasone, on the other hand, crosses the placenta very well and is the preferred drug in the rare situations where the corticosteroid is prescribed for the fetus. Corticosteroids are often used to control SLE and other inflammatory rheumatic diseases in pregnancy. It has been known for some time that corticosteroids during pregnancy increase the incidence of cleft palate in animals. Neither this nor other malformations have been shown to occur in humans with increased frequency. Corticosteroid use during pregnancy does on the other hand increase the incidence of diabetes of pregnancy, hypertension, and premature labor.

For some drugs such as HYDROXYCHLOROQUINE and SULFASALAZINE, there are case reports of fetal abnormalities. However, none of the studies of groups of women taking these drugs during pregnancy demonstrates an increased risk of birth defects, and the drugs appear reasonably safe, although it would take impossibly large studies to say they are completely safe. As the inflammation of RHEUMATOID ARTHRITIS often improves during pregnancy, it is reasonable to stop these drugs during pregnancy if the arthritis is well controlled. However, SLE flares in pregnancy can be very dangerous to mother and infant and hydroxychloroquine is usually continued through pregnancy to prevent this. AZATHIOPRINE is another drug that has been used extensively during pregnancy in women with SLE. It crosses the placenta and is an antimetabolite suggesting it may be harmful to the fetus. However it is a prodrug and needs to be activated by human enzymes before it has its antimetabolic effect. The fetal liver lacks the enzyme to do this, and this may explain its relative safety during pregnancy. There probably is a slight increase in the incidence of fetal abnormalities with its use, and

the risks of the disease flaring need to be weighed against this.

METHOTREXATE certainly causes fetal abnormalities when used at the high doses used to treat malignancies. Whether this is the case with the much lower doses used for arthritis is unclear. Because methotrexate is used so commonly, there have been a number of accidental pregnancies in women taking low doses, and there does not appear to be any increase in fetal abnormalities in their children. While this does not mean that methotrexate should ever knowingly be taken by a pregnant woman, it does mean that accidental ingestion while pregnant does not inevitably mean the pregnancy should be aborted. There are small numbers of women with Crohn's disease and rheumatoid arthritis who have been treated with anti-TNF agents (see BIOLOGICALS) without an obvious increase in fetal abnormalities. However, the potential effects remain unknown, and all biologicals should be avoided during pregnancy.

There are several important principles regarding medicines in pregnancy:

- The time when most medicines are most likely to harm the unborn baby is in the first weeks or months of pregnancy, often before most women know they are pregnant. This means that if a patient is taking medicines regularly and wants to become pregnant, she should discuss this with her physician and plan the pregnancy.

- If a woman is taking a teratogenic drug, she and her partner should use reliable contraception to ensure that she does not become pregnant.

- If a woman taking medicines becomes pregnant unexpectedly, she should notify both her rheumatologist and obstetrician immediately.

- Some of the drugs used to treat rheumatic diseases can have effects for weeks or months after a woman stops taking them. They may need to be stopped several months before trying to become pregnant.

- Generally to protect the baby, as few medicines as possible are used in pregnancy. However, they are often needed to control serious rheumatic diseases. For example, uncontrolled SLE can be more dangerous to the unborn baby than some of the medicines used to control it. Many women with different types of arthritis who have needed treatment in pregnancy have had healthy babies.

- Smoking and drinking alcohol, sometimes not considered drugs, can have harmful effects on the baby. Pregnant women should avoid them.

How Can Pregnancy Affect Rheumatic Illness?

Rheumatoid arthritis improves in about 75 percent of pregnant women and sometimes goes into temporary remission. This does not last, and the arthritis often flares after pregnancy. There are a few women whose disease remains unchanged or even worsens during pregnancy. Physicians do not understand why rheumatoid arthritis (RA) may improve in pregnancy. One theory is that the increase in levels of hormones such as progesterone is responsible. Another is that pregnancy induces a state of immunological tolerance. In other words pregnancy suppresses the mother's immune system so that it does not reject the unborn baby. As a result of the altered immune response, the arthritis improves.

The choice of drugs to control RA is affected by pregnancy. Luckily, because RA usually improves during pregnancy, many women are able to stop DMARD therapy during pregnancy and manage on just a low dose of prednisone.

Women with SLE were traditionally advised not to become pregnant because the risks to the mother and the baby were considered to be too high. This advice has changed, and many patients with SLE have had healthy babies. Pregnancy was thought to worsen SLE. Several recent studies have shown, though, that there is no increased frequency of lupus flares in pregnancy. Others have reported that a third of patients get worse, a third stay the same, and a third improve. Pregnancy affects the choice of treatment for SLE, and teratogenic drugs such as cyclophosphamide are avoided. This means that ideally SLE should be under good control before pregnancy. A common complication of pregnancy is preeclampsia, a condition characterized by edema, high blood pressure, and proteinuria. Untreated preeclampsia can progress to seizures. Preeclampsia is more common in women with SLE. When it occurs it can be confused with a flare of lupus nephritis that causes identical symptoms. Eclamptic seizures can be confused with CNS lupus-causing seizures.

How Can Rheumatic Illness Affect the Pregnancy?

RA does not usually have any direct effects on pregnancy. However it, and any chronic arthritis that affects the hips and pelvis, can make it more difficult for a woman to deliver vaginally. SLE can have direct effects on pregnancy. Women with SLE have more difficulty conceiving, more frequent abortions and stillbirths, and a greater risk of premature delivery and babies with a low birth weight. Difficulties with conception may be caused by the effects of SLE on ovulation. Women who have been treated with cyclophosphamide have a risk of ovarian failure, causing premature menopause. Spontaneous abortions (miscarriages) are more frequent, particularly in women with the ANTIPHOSPHOLIPID ANTIBODY SYNDROME. If SLE decreases blood flow to the placenta, it affects the growth and development of the baby. This is monitored closely using ultrasound to measure the blood flow across the placenta and to monitor growth. About 80 percent of pregnancies in patients with well-controlled SLE are successful, resulting in the delivery of a live baby. The biggest risk factor for a poor outcome is active lupus before pregnancy. Other factors associated with fetal loss, are renal disease, previous fetal loss, and antiphospholipid antibody syndrome.

Women with lupus have a greater chance of having a baby with NEONATAL LUPUS, particularly if the mother has a positive blood test for SSA or SSB antibodies (also called Ro and La antibodies). The risk of having a baby with neonatal lupus is about 2 percent in women with SLE who have SSA or SSB antibodies and may be higher, about 5 percent, in those who have both. Neonatal lupus can cause a serious and irreversible problem called heart block, a condition in which the electrical messages from the atria are not conducted to the ventricles. The first indication of this problem is when a pregnant woman has routine checkup at about the 20th week of her pregnancy and the baby's heart rate is found to be very slow.

Pregnancy-Related Rheumatic Conditions

A few rheumatic conditions are more common or particular to pregnancy. CARPAL TUNNEL SYNDROME commonly occurs in late pregnancy and resolves with or without treatment within a few months of delivery. DE QUERVAIN'S TENOSYNOVITIS usually occurs after delivery and requires treatment to resolve it. Low back pain and pelvic pain are common in pregnancy due to the natural softening of ligaments and altered posture due to the shift in the center of gravity. To a certain extent, this can be minimized by maintaining physical fitness prior to and during pregnancy. One condition that is particular to pregnancy is transient osteoporosis. This is a rare but important condition where there is localized loss of calcium and phosphate from bone associated with severe pain. The two most common sites are the hip and spine, but many other areas have been reported. Affected bone is fragile, and many women have fractured their hips spontaneously. Although X-rays can confirm the diagnosis, they are avoided in pregnancy. MRI scanning shows characteristic changes that cannot however be distinguished from infection, and the diagnosis therefore remains a clinical one. Avoiding stress to the affected area is the only treatment during pregnancy, although sometimes a metal rod is inserted into the femur to prevent hip fracture, particularly if the other hip has already fractured. The cause is unknown.

prepatellar bursitis Bursas are small, flat sacs that develop where friction is likely to occur. They are lined by synovial cells that secrete a small amount of fluid into the sac that then allows free movement between the body parts on either side of it. Bursas just beneath the skin such as the prepatellar bursa actually develop after birth. This bursa lies between the skin and the lower half of the patella or kneecap, an area where there would be considerable friction during crawling or kneeling.

Symptoms and Diagnostic Path
When the prepatellar bursa becomes inflamed, it fills with fluid and can be seen to bulge in front of the knee. There may be warmth and redness and kneeling becomes very painful.

Trauma either in the form of a significant blow as in falling onto concrete or recurrent trauma from an occupation requiring considerable kneel-

ing is the most common cause. Previously known as housemaid's knee it is now usually seen in carpet layers and builders. Because it is so close to the skin surface, there is a risk of penetrating injury introducing infection. GOUT, CALCIUM PYROPHOSPHATE DIHYDRATE DEPOSITION DISEASE, and RHEUMATOID ARTHRITIS can also cause prepatellar bursitis.

Treatment Options and Outlook
Treatment with NSAIDs may relieve pain. While the bursitis settles protective devices should be worn by those with occupational exposure. Aspiration of the fluid may speed resolution and culturing the fluid may ensure that there is no infection. If it is persistent, a small amount of CORTICOSTEROID may be injected, especially if it is associated with an inflammatory arthritis. Occasionally recurrent or resistant bursitis may require surgical removal of the bursa.

psoriasis and psoriatic arthritis Psoriasis is a common scaly rash affecting about 2 percent of the population in developed countries. There are areas of high incidence such as northern Russia and Norway (5–10 percent of the population) and low incidence such as Latin America (less than 0.5 percent). The connection between psoriasis and arthritis was recognized as long ago as the 1850s. For many years, however, this was thought to be RHEUMATOID ARTHRITIS occurring in patients with psoriasis. Research in the 1950s clarified the distinction between rheumatoid arthritis and psoriatic arthropathy, which is now classified as one of the spondyloarthropathies. Estimates vary, but around 10 percent of patients with psoriasis will develop an associated arthritis. Men and women are equally affected, although men predominate in the spinal arthritis type and women in the rheumatoid type (see Symptoms for discussion of different types). Onset is most commonly between the ages of 20 and 40 years. The HUMAN IMMUNODEFICIENCY VIRUS (HIV) is changing the rates of occurrence of both psoriasis and associated arthritis, especially in sub-Saharan Africa.

Most research has looked at the cause of the skin disease psoriasis rather than the occurrence (usually later) of the arthritis. Unless arthritis is specifically mentioned, this discussion refers to psoriasis. There is a strong genetic component in its causation, and there are also a number of well-known factors that initiate the rash or make it worse.

Roughly 30 percent of patients have a first-degree relative with psoriasis. In one large study a child's risk of developing psoriasis was 4 percent if neither parent had the disease. This increased to 28 percent if one parent had psoriasis and to 65 percent if both parents were affected. If one identical twin develops psoriasis, then the other has a 70 percent chance of doing so as well. This risk drops to 20 percent if the twins are not identical. There is therefore a very strong hereditary component to psoriasis. The nature of this, however, remains unknown.

Genetic studies have shown that in patients who develop psoriasis before the age of 20 years, the psoriasis susceptibility gene is close to the Cw6 allele on chromosome 6 (see GENETIC FACTORS for an explanation of terms). Ongoing studies are trying to unravel this area and find the precise gene involved. This area, however, is unlikely to be important in all patients. For example, West Africans have a high rate of Cw6 but very low incidence of psoriasis. There are numerous weak associations between psoriasis and other alleles, but much work is required before the associations will be clear.

A genetic association with psoriatic arthritis as distinct from psoriasis has been looked for without any clear results. There is a strong association between HLA-B27 and the spondylitic form of psoriatic arthropathy, as there is in ANKYLOSING SPONDYLITIS and SPONDYLOARTHROPATHY.

Psoriasis is largely a cell-mediated disease (see IMMUNE RESPONSE for an explanation). This means that a population of lymphocytes called T cells is driving the immune attack directed at the skin, joints, and entheses (where tendons, ligaments, or joint capsules attach to bone). The CD8 T cells are much more prominent in this than in other forms of arthritis like rheumatoid arthritis. Careful examination of these CD8 T cells suggests that they are responding to a small number of antigens. These antigens (thought to come from infectious agents) are similar in the skin and joints but frequently differ in different patients.

Infection with bacteria called streptococci (a common cause of a sore throat and fever) is well known to initiate psoriasis or make it worsen. Evidence indicates that other infections may also do this.

Trauma to the skin may result in psoriasis appearing in the injured area in 25 percent of patients. This is known as the Koebner phenomenon. Interestingly, other patients sometimes have a *reverse Koebner phenomenon*. Here trauma to a psoriatic plaque may lead to the skin clearing in the injured area. The mechanisms underlying the Koebner phenomenon are unknown.

Drugs such as beta-blockers, HYDROXYCHLORO-QUINE, and lithium may cause flares of the disease. Stopping CORTICOSTEROIDS is also well known to do this. Psychological stress has been reported to worsen psoriasis or be associated with its onset. Sunlight usually makes psoriasis better but in about 10 percent of patients may make it worse.

HIV infection is associated with severe psoriasis and psoriatic arthritis. The HIV epidemic in sub-Saharan Africa has lead to a dramatic increase in both psoriasis and psoriatic arthropathies. Previously both diseases had been rare. There are two main theories why this has occurred. The first relates to the increased susceptibility to infection that HIV-positive people have. This leads to a much greater load of organisms in people living in Third World conditions. The second theory revolves around an immunological mechanism whereby dendritic cells (professional antigen-presenting cells) can bypass CD4+ T cells and stimulate CD8+ cells.

Symptoms and Diagnostic Path

Psoriasis Typical skin plaques are reddish raised areas covered with thick silvery scales. Both sides of the body are usually affected. Frequently affected areas include elbows, knees, scalp, and buttocks. Similar plaques may occur at sites of trauma or surgical scars (Koebner phenomenon). The nails may be affected with small pits on their surface or heaping up of layers of skin underneath the nail (subungual hyperkeratosis) and lifting of the nail off its bed (onycholysis). This can look very like a chronic fungal infection.

Apart from the typical appearance described above, there are several well-known variations.

Guttate psoriasis is a form that usually comes on suddenly in teenagers, often after an infection. There are many small plaques of 1–2 cm diameter scattered all over the body. Flexural psoriasis affects the back of the knees and front of the elbows (opposite to the usual form) and is particularly likely to develop into generalized pustular psoriasis. In palmoplantar psoriasis, the soles of the feet and palms of the hand are studded with small non-infective pustules.

There are three main complications of psoriasis. Generalized pustular psoriasis is characterized by sheets of small pustules that are not infective. This is often associated with a fever and generalized illness and can be a life-threatening condition. Generalized exfoliative dermatitis with erythroderma is another life-threatening complication. More than 80 percent of the skin becomes inflamed, the skin peels off, and there may be widespread weeping of serous fluid. The third complication is psoriatic arthritis.

Psoriatic arthritis   In 75 percent of people with psoriatic arthritis, the arthritis follows the rash by a variable period. In 15 percent they start at the same time, and in the remaining 10 percent the arthritis precedes the rash. In this last case the diagnosis may be more difficult. Five different forms of arthritis associated with psoriasis are distinguishable.

1. *Oligoarthritis*   This is the most common form. A common pattern of involvement might be one knee and several proximal interphalangeals (PIPs). The metacarpophalangeals, PIPs, and metatarsophalangeals as well as any of the lower-limb joints may be involved, although typically only two to four joints are affected at any one time. Trauma to a joint can result in it becoming inflamed. Dactylitis is often associated with this form. This is due to inflammation of the joints of a toe or finger as well as the tendon sheaths, giving rise to a diffusely swollen digit, the so-called sausage digit.
2. *Rheumatoid Pattern*   Almost as common is symmetrical arthritis affecting the small joints of the hands, wrists, elbows, knees, ankles, and feet. This is indistinguishable clinically from rheumatoid arthritis. However, the rheumatoid factor is

negative and the patient has psoriasis. Research has shown subtle differences between the two diseases in the inflammatory joint lesions when carefully examined, but this is not usually of practical use in diagnosis and treatment. MRI scanning shows that the inflammation is localized around the attachment of tendons and ligaments with edema of the underlying bone. This is different from rheumatoid arthritis but is not yet in clinical use to differentiate the two.

3. *DIP Arthritis*   A very characteristic appearance is the swollen inflamed distal interphalangeal joint (DIP), the last joint in the fingers. MRI scanning shows that the inflammation extends from the DIP joint into the nail bed although it is not yet known which starts first. This is often associated with psoriatic nail lesions in the nail of the same finger. MRI scanning shows that the inflammation extends from the DIP joint into the nail bed although it is not yet known which starts first. Sausage digits may occur. This form of psoriatic arthritis may occur alone or be associated with one of the other forms.
4. *Spondylitis*   This form is very similar to ankylosing spondylitis (AS). However, peripheral arthritis, especially of the knees, ankles, and hands, is more common than in AS. Involvement of the sacroiliac joints (where the spine joins the pelvis) is more likely to be one-sided or predominantly one-sided than in AS. The neck is often severely affected in psoriatic spondylitis and may become quite rigid, causing difficulty with driving, among other activities. Arthritis in the neck is commonly associated with scalp psoriasis.
5. *Arthritis Mutilans*   Although rare, this is a very typical manifestation of psoriatic arthritis. The small joints of the hand become severely eroded. In one or more fingers destruction of the joints becomes so advanced that the finger shortens and there are redundant folds of skin. In the absence of a joint the finger is floppy and almost useless.

A characteristic of all forms of psoriatic arthritis is the inflammation at entheses. It is also seen in AS. Inflammation of tendons is also very common. About a third of patients with psoriatic arthritis develop EYE PROBLEMS. Two-thirds of these develop conjunctivitis (inflammation of the most superficial covering layer of the front of the eye), and nearly one-third develop iritis. Iritis is inflammation of a deeper layer, also in the front of the eye, that can lead to significant problems if not treated promptly.

As mentioned above, people with DIP arthritis almost always have nail involvement on the same finger, and those with severe neck involvement often have scalp psoriasis. Apart from these, there is no particular association between the type of psoriasis and the type of arthritis. There is, however, one further association that should be mentioned. Pustular psoriasis of the palms and soles appears distinct from the more typical forms of psoriasis and is not associated with the above forms of arthritis. It is, however, associated with a hyperostosis affecting the chest wall and a noninfective form of osteomyelitis. This is described under the heading SAPHO SYNDROME.

Although the most common age of onset of psoriasis is between five and 15 years, psoriatic arthritis usually starts much later. However, children may get psoriatic arthritis. Unlike the figures given above for adults, in children 50 percent get the arthritis first, 40 percent get the rash first, and 10 percent get both at the same time. The oligoarthritis and spondylitis forms are the main ones to affect children.

The diagnosis is made on the clinical grounds described. Most patients will have the rash of psoriasis as an obvious clue. The rash, however, may be very subtle. Minor scaling around the scalp may have been thought by the patient to be dandruff for many years. The rash of psoriasis is not always irritating, and patients can be relatively unaware of small patches around the buttocks or belly button or, not seeing their relevance, not tell their physician about these patches. Sometimes the arthritis is characteristic enough to be diagnosed as psoriatic even in the absence of a rash, but this is not always possible. Sausage digits, enthesitis, and marked tendon involvement are all in favor of psoriatic arthritis. Skin psoriasis is usually distinctive enough to be diagnosed clinically. When there is doubt a biopsy will confirm the diagnosis.

X-rays may give valuable information in differentiating the arthritis from clinically similar but distinct forms of arthritis. Characteristics when x-raying peripheral joints include the asymmetry and involvement of the DIPs (unlike rheumatoid arthritis), a characteristic appearance of erosive disease aptly termed *pencil in cup* appearance, the development of new bone along the outer margins of bones (periostitis) and at entheses, and a tendency for joints to fuse. In the spine features that differentiate psoriatic from ankylosing spondylitis include asymmetrical sacroiliac involvement, fewer syndesmophytes, less disease of the small facet joints at the back of the spine, severe neck involvement with relative sparing of the lower spine, and fluffy new bone formation along the front of the vertebrae. MRI changes showing the focus of inflammation at the enthesis (tendon or ligament attachment) or the extensive bony edema seen in a sausage finger can be highly suggestive of psoriatic arthritis.

Treatment Options and Outlook

The treatment aims in psoriatic arthritis may include the following:

1. Controlling the rash
2. Suppressing joint and tendon inflammation
3. Maintaining and improving musculoskeletal function
4. Preventing and minimizing disability
5. Providing psychosocial support in living with a chronic rash and arthritis

Patients with milder disease may obtain most of their care from their primary health care provider. Those with severe disease, though, will need input from a number of specialist providers at different times. These may include rheumatologists, dermatologists, orthopedic surgeons, physiotherapists, rehabilitation specialists, and counselors. Treatment in many areas needs to be highly individualized and is difficult to generalize. This particularly includes rehabilitation and counseling. Note that a number of studies have shown that more patients with psoriasis use alcohol excessively than the general population. The reason for this is unknown, but support in this area may be required. Another difficulty in generalizing about treatment is that psoriatic arthritis is very variable. Some people have intermittent, troublesome problems and others have unremitting, highly destructive disease. Of all forms of chronic arthritis, psoriatic arthritis is most likely to go into remission, often for periods of two to four years at a time. It is often possible to come off all medication during these periods, although a later relapse is not uncommon. With these provisos, a brief, general discussion of the treatment of rash and musculoskeletal problems follows.

Skin psoriasis   Topical treatments are tried first because of their greater safety. They may include the following.

- Various preparations of coal tar. This is safe and effective for the common plaque psoriasis. It is used less often these days because it is messy when applied to the skin, although some newer preparations are easier to use. It can also stain skin or cause irritation. Coal tar shampoos and preparations used in the bath are effective and commonly used.
- Dithranol, often combined with salicylic acid, is another older medication that still has a useful role in treatment. It is started at a low dose and gradually built up to avoid skin irritation.
- Salicylic acid preparations are useful in getting rid of excessive scale.
- Corticosteroid creams and ointments are very effective and easy to use. There are many preparations that are generally classed as mild, moderate, potent, or very potent. Once the psoriasis is controlled, it is important to step down the potency and then reduce the frequency of use to prevent the rebound flare that occurs when these preparations are suddenly stopped. They may cause marked thinning of normal skin, and if applied to large areas, systemic corticosteroid side effects can develop due to absorption. For these reasons potent and very potent preparations are best avoided in psoriasis.
- Calcipotriol (calcipotriene) is used as a cream or ointment to the skin or as a lotion to the scalp. It is effective in mild-to-moderate psoriasis. It is important to limit the amount used since it is a

vitamin D derivative and large doses may cause raised blood calcium levels. It is odorless and does not stain but may cause some irritation to the skin.

- Phototherapy is used in two forms: UVB light by itself is effective in mild-to-moderate psoriasis; UVA light can be used with a psoralen to potentiate it. A psoralen, usually methoxsalen, may be given two hours before exposure to UVA light or the patient can bathe in psoralens before exposure. This form of treatment is given twice a week for four to six weeks only. It is delivered by specialist centers and is closely controlled because of the increased risk of squamous cell skin cancers.

Systemic therapy is used for widespread or very troublesome psoriasis. Because of the increased risk of adverse effects, some monitoring and specialist supervision is required for these therapies. For these reasons as well as the fact that psoriasis is often not very irritating, many patients, usually after a number of years of trying various treatments, choose to live with their psoriasis, using treatment only when there is a flare. Systemic therapies include the following.

1. METHOTREXATE is very effective in all forms of psoriasis. It may be taken by mouth or as intramuscular injections and is usually built up gradually from a low dose.
2. Acitretin (trade name: Soriatane) is a retinoid used in severe or extensive psoriasis. It is a metabolite of the older etretinate, which is a derivative of vitamin A. Acitretin is a teratogen (may induce abnormalities in the unborn fetus). Reliable methods to prevent pregnancy must be in place for at least one month before and for three years after treatment with acitretin. Tetracyclines and vitamin A should be avoided, and liver function and lipid (cholesterol) levels need to be monitored. Dryness of mucous membranes and poor tolerance of contact lenses are quite common, and aches and pains may occur. Abnormal calcification of soft tissues may complicate treatment, and X-rays should be taken to look for this if the patient suffers unusual musculoskeletal symptoms.

3. CYCLOSPORINE is effective for severe and otherwise difficult-to-control psoriasis. It is a powerful immunosuppressant, and adverse effects are not uncommon with long-term use. These include tremors, increased hair growth especially on the face, high blood pressure, and less commonly, kidney damage and infections. Intermittent cyclosporine therapy has been tried to limit the occurrence of side effects. While studies so far have shown it to be reasonably effective in controlling the psoriasis, it is not clearly safer.

4. Anti-TNF agents are effective in skin psoriasis.

Psoriatic arthritis First-line therapy comprises NSAID therapy and local corticosteroid injection. NSAIDs are effective in many patients with spondylitis and/or mild peripheral arthritis. Early reports suggested that some NSAIDs might be better than others, but current evidence suggests that they are all potentially helpful. The individual agent should therefore be chosen more on the likelihood of adverse effects in the individual patient than on efficacy. While there is a theoretical concern that NSAIDs might lead to worsening of the rash, this has not been borne out in practice. When one or two joints are resistant to treatment with NSAIDs or the patient has experienced adverse effects, then injection of local corticosteroids into the joint is highly effective. Depending on the activity of the disease, this may give very long-lasting relief. It also does not seem to produce any rebound flare, perhaps because of the small dose used and the fact that there is a gradual washout of effect as the body metabolizes the drug. Injections should not be given through psoriatic plaques as getting good antisepsis on a plaque is not possible.

Second-line therapy or DISEASE-MODIFYING ANTIRHEUMATIC DRUGS are indicated when the arthritis is severe and unresponsive to the measures above or deformity is developing as a result of the arthritis. Many drugs have been used to treat psoriatic arthritis. Evidence of varying strength shows that SULFASALAZINE, AZATHIOPRINE, cyclosporine, methotrexate, LEFLUNOMIDE, and TUMOR NECROSIS FACTOR (TNF) ANTAGONISTS are effective. Other DMARDs are used because of evidence for their use in treating other forms of inflammatory arthritis. Note that the lack of scientific evidence does not necessarily

mean a drug does not work. It may just be that the appropriate study has not been done. The more commonly used medications and some newer medications are listed below.

- Sulfasalazine is a relatively safe, well-tolerated medication effective in some patients with psoriatic arthritis. It is, however, less often effective than when used to treat rheumatoid arthritis. In moderate disease it is often tried first because of its good safety profile. Rashes, headaches, nausea, and occasional liver toxicity are the main adverse effects. Starting at a low dose and gradually increasing to 2–3 g per day in divided doses and taking the tablets with food lessens the nausea and headaches. Sulfasalazine may be used in HIV-associated disease since it does not suppress the immune system.

- Methotrexate given in doses ranging from 7.5–30 mg once a week is the drug used most frequently in moderate-to-severe psoriatic arthritis. It is effective for both skin and joint problems. The main concern is the liver cirrhosis that may occur with long-term usage. This was a significant problem when methotrexate was given in three divided doses over 24 hours for skin psoriasis but was less frequent when used in rheumatoid arthritis as a single dose. It remains to be seen whether using it as a single dose in psoriatic arthritis has a similar low rate of cirrhosis. That is, the difference could be due to the different dosage or the different diseases. Other problems include lung inflammation, acute liver inflammation, sun sensitivity, and subtle mental disturbances such as impaired memory. Taking a small supplement of folic acid slightly reduces the number of adverse effects. Although the nature of psoriatic arthritis lends itself to the intermittent use of DMARDs (as opposed to rheumatoid arthritis), methotrexate in particular is likely to be followed by a flare if stopped.

- Azathioprine has been used for many years and is effective for both skin and joints. It is relatively well tolerated, although a few people lack the enzyme to metabolize it and cannot tolerate it at all. Liver toxicity, allergy, and a dose-related reduction in bone marrow activity are seen. The main limiting factor in its use, however, is a slight increase in malignancy with long-term use. This is mainly skin cancers and lymphomas.

- Cyclosporine is very effective in both skin and joint disease. It works rapidly and would be used more but for the relatively frequent occurrence of adverse effects (see above under Treatment). For this reason it has been used in combination with other drugs (usually methotrexate) to try to get by with a lower dose. While this is certainly effective, it is not clear that combination treatment will provide a safer form of long-term treatment. Stopping cyclosporine also has the tendency to be followed by a flare.

- Leflunomide has been shown to be effective in a randomized study but is not as frequently successful in psoriatic arthritis as it is in rheumatoid disease. Diarrhea, skin rashes, and liver abnormalities are the most frequent adverse events.

- Etretinate is effective for the arthritis as it was for the rash until largely superseded by its metabolite acitretin (see above). Relatively frequent adverse effects limited the use of etretinate.

- PUVA therapy, when used for skin psoriasis, has been found to improve arthritis in some patients, especially those with spondylitis.

- Hydroxychloroquine and PENICILLAMINE have been used but are not generally recommended. Hydroxychloroquine has made psoriasis worse in some patients, and penicillamine causes frequent side effects. Somatostatin, zinc, vitamin D derivatives, colchicine, and many other treatments have been tried with either little success or limiting adverse effects.

- Recently TNF antagonists have shown remarkable efficacy in psoriasis and associated arthritis. ETANERCEPT, INFLIXIMAB, and ADALIMUMAB have all been studied in randomized placebo-controlled trials (see CLINICAL TRIAL) and shown to be highly effective in reducing joint inflammation, improving skin psoriasis, slowing X-ray changes due to the arthritis, and improving patients' quality of life. Although there have been some significant side effects, in a follow-up of the etanercept trial, 80 percent of patients continued on etanercept after three years, and nearly half were in remis-

sion. These TNF antagonists seem to be effective in all subtypes of psoriatic arthritis, and their use is limited largely by cost and the potential for significant side effects. A number of other BIOLOGICALS are under investigation in psoriatic arthritis. Alefacept has been approved by the FDA for the treatment of psoriasis.

Psoriasis is a chronic skin condition that remits and relapses over many years. Cure is not possible. Psoriasis can vary from a tiny patch that the patient forgets about to an itchy, profusely scaling rash covering most of the patient's body. Treatment is aimed at achieving a level of control that the individual finds acceptable. Many people benefit from belonging to the Psoriasis Association or similar support group.

Psoriatic arthritis too is very variable in its severity. Apart from the fortunately rare arthritis mutilans form, joint destruction tends to be less severe than with, for example, rheumatoid arthritis. There is a marked tendency for inflamed joints to fuse, especially when spondylitis involves the neck. Remission for years at a time is not uncommon. HIV-associated disease is more rapidly progressive, although some lessening of the inflammation has been noted with the onset of AIDS. Patients who are older at the time of onset (over 60 years of age) appear to have a more severe and destructive arthritis than younger patients. The oligoarthritis form of arthritis may progress over years to a more rheumatoid pattern with many joints involved, but the frequency of this varies considerably among different studies.

Risk Factors and Preventive Measures

The risk factors for developing psoriatic arthritis are not only having psoriasis but also having someone in the family with psoriasis. There are no known preventive measures and, in particular, aggressive treatment of skin psoriasis does not seem to reduce the frequency or severity of the arthritis.

pulmonary hypertension (PH) A pressure in the pulmonary arteries of 25 mmHg or higher. The pressure in the pulmonary arteries that carry blood from the right ventricle to the lungs is much lower than the pressure on the left side of the heart that supplies blood to the rest of the body. When abnormally high pressures are in the blood vessels on the right side of the heart, this is called pulmonary hypertension, a rare condition. When the pressure is elevated in the blood vessels in the rest of the body (the left side of the heart), this is called systemic hypertension or more often just hypertension or high blood pressure, a common clinical condition familiar to most people.

Pulmonary hypertension can be classified into one of two types, primary or secondary. Primary pulmonary hypertension or PPH is when the main abnormality is in the medium-sized arteries in the lungs themselves. Secondary pulmonary hypertension is when other conditions such as severe heart or lung disease cause a secondary increase in the pulmonary artery pressure. Several connective tissue diseases, most often SCLERODERMA and SYSTEMIC LUPUS ERYTHEMATOSUS (SLE), are associated with a type of pulmonary hypertension very similar to PPH.

Dr. D. T. Dresdale first coined the term primary pulmonary hypertension and described the clinical entity, an almost uniformly fatal illness more common in young women, in 1951. Since then there have been major advances. PPH is rare in the population, affecting about one to two people per million. There are now more effective treatments available that have improved the prognosis.

The medium-sized arteries in the lungs of patients with PPH have very thick walls and a narrow lumen, often with a small amount of clot in them. The basic cause of PPH is obstruction of the medium-sized arteries, but the underlying mechanism of this is not known. Researchers noticed that about 6 percent of cases of PPH tracked in families, suggesting that in some patients there was a familial or genetic cause. In others, though, the disease was sporadic. Dr. John Newman and his colleagues have identified a gene that predisposes certain families to developing PPH. By studying families affected by PPH, these and other scientists linked the disease with mutations in a gene that codes for bone morphogenic receptor II (BMP II), a receptor activated by a growth factor. Most patients with PPH do not have the familial type of disease. However, the discovery

of the genetic cause of the familial type may help scientists identify the other causes of PPH. Since the discovery that there are abnormalities in the BMP II gene in 50 percent of patients with familial PPH, new data show that 25 percent of patients with what was thought to be sporadic PPH also have abnormalities. This suggests either that they developed a new mutation of the gene or that the familial PPH is often incorrectly diagnosed as sporadic PPH. Recent work also shows that only about 20 percent of people in an affected family who have the abnormal BMP II gene go on to develop PPH. In other words, one abnormal gene alone is not enough to cause the disease. There are likely to be other genes or environmental triggers that determine who gets PPH.

A PPH-like illness can occur in patients with scleroderma, SLE, and HIV and after treatment with dexfenfluramine and fenfluramine, drugs used to suppress appetite and treat obesity. Some experts classify these types of pulmonary hypertension as variants of PPH, although there is an underlying predisposing illness. Others, though, classify them as causes of secondary pulmonary hypertension. Secondary pulmonary hypertension can occur as a result of any chronic lung or heart disease. These are summarized in the following table. Scleroderma can cause pulmonary hypertension of both types. The PPH type of disease occurs more often with the CREST type of scleroderma and may affect up to 10 percent of patients. Secondary pulmonary hypertension with systemic sclerosis occurs in patients with severe lung scarring.

Symptoms and Diagnostic Path

The first symptom is unusual shortness of breath when exercising. This tends to come on gradually over a few years. When the illness is more severe chest pain, fainting, heart failure, and rhythm abnormalities occur.

Patients with limited scleroderma or CREST are much more likely to develop PPH-like pulmonary hypertension than patients with what is usually considered the more severe type of scleroderma—generalized disease or systemic sclerosis. Pulmonary hypertension develops only in some patients with CREST and usually does so after many years. The severity of CREST symptoms is not related to the

CAUSES OF PULMONARY HYPERTENSION

Primary Pulmonary Secondary Pulmonary Hypertension	Primary Pulmonary Hypertension-like Disease	Hypertension
Familial PPH	CREST/scleroderma	Heart valve abnormalities
Sporadic PPH	SLE	Heart failure
	HIV	Any chronic lung disease
	Appetite suppressants	Sleep apnea
	Chronic liver disease	Repeated pulmonary emboli

risk of developing pulmonary hypertension. Some patients with CREST and pulmonary hypertension have such minor scleroderma symptoms, only a few telangiectasia, some skin tightening across the fingers, and occasional Raynaud's phenomenon, that these symptoms are overlooked and an incorrect diagnosis of sporadic PPH is made. In patients with CREST, a decrease in exercise tolerance can be the first clue that pulmonary hypertension has developed.

In the CREST syndrome, systemic sclerosis, SLE, or undiagnosed PPH, the diagnosis is suspected when the patient complains of shortness of breath on exertion and is found to have a loud second heart sound when listening to the heart. Initial investigations may show a right shift in the electrical axis of the heart on electrocardiogram and a fairly normal-looking chest X-ray and CT scan of the chest (except when secondary to lung disease). However, the most useful test is a full lung function test that shows marked reduction in the ability of gases to cross from the air to the blood in the lung (DLCO) relative to the ability to move air in and out of the lung. Once the diagnosis is suspected, pressure in the pulmonary artery can measured by ultrasound. In some patients the pressure is measured more accurately by placing a catheter in the right side of the heart by threading it up through a large vein in the leg. A chest X-ray can show an enlarged heart, but in PPH and PPH-like conditions, the lung tissue is normal. In patients with secondary pulmonary hypertension caused by lung disease, the lungs are abnormal on chest X-ray. A lung biopsy is usually avoided because there is a risk of bleeding. No blood tests are helpful.

The DLCO provides prognostic information in that those patients with a DLCO result of less than 50 percent do less well than those with higher readings. It is also useful in following the progress of patients. When large groups of patients with systemic sclerosis not thought to have pulmonary hypertension have been screened for it using ultrasound examinations of the heart (echocardiogram), between 10 and 15 percent have been found to have raised pulmonary pressure. Most rheumatologists will therefore screen high-risk patients, although the ideal time to do this is not clear yet.

Treatment Options and Outlook

Pulmonary hypertension has no cure, and the treatment options are limited. Because more research information is available about treating PPH than PPH-like pulmonary hypertension, physicians often use information about PPH to decide how to treat pulmonary hypertension associated with SLE or scleroderma.

Anticoagulation Although most types of pulmonary hypertension are not caused by blood clots, most experts believe that damage to the lining of blood vessels makes it more likely that small clots will form in the blood vessels in the lungs and aggravate the obstruction. Therefore, most patients with PPH receive warfarin, a drug that decreases the ability of blood to clot.

Vasodilators The blood vessels in PPH are very thick with narrow channels. At some stages of the disease these blood vessels can still respond to drugs that dilate them. Calcium channel blockers such as nifedipine and diltiazem are drugs developed to treat systemic hypertension. By dilating arteries in the lungs, they can also decrease the pulmonary artery pressure in some patients with PPH.

Prostanoids have very powerful effects on blood flow and in dilating arteries. The naturally occurring prostaglandin prostacyclin and a number of analogues have been used to treat PH. EPOPROS-TENOL is a stable form of prostacyclin but is still very short-lived and is given by continuous intravenous infusion. Prolonged therapy requires a special long-term catheter with its attendant complications. Functional ability is significantly improved on treatment, but there are fairly frequent side effects including nausea, diarrhea, and jaw pain. TREPRO-STINIL can be infused under the skin by a very small pump and is therefore more convenient than epo-prostenol, although most patients get pain at the infusion site. Walking ability and breathlessness are improved. Iloprost is a stable analogue of prostacy-clin which been used to treat severely impaired circulation in the hands or feet of systemic sclerosis patients for many years but is not FDA-approved for use in the United States yet. Many other drugs intended to work primarily on the lungs have been developed into aerosols that can be inhaled directly into the lungs and thereby use smaller doses and get less side effects. An inhaled form of iloprost has been developed and shows reasonable short-term responses. It does need to be used six to 10 times a day and causes fairly frequent headache, cough, and faintness. In a two-year study, most patients stopped its use for a variety of reasons before the end of follow-up.

The FDA approved bosentan (trade name: Tra-cleer) for the treatment of PPH. Bosentan is taken as a tablet and blocks receptors for endothelin, a very potent vasoconstrictor produced by the body. The most common side effect is abnormal liver function tests. Bosentan improves walking ability in patients with PPH but not much in those with secondary PH. It may also prolong survival, but this needs further study. Bosentan blocks both endo-thelin type A and B receptors. There are also now two type A receptor blockers, of which ambrisen-tan is approved for use in the United States.

Nitric oxide, a gas produced in small amounts in the body, is one of the strongest vasodilators discovered. Several research groups are using nitric oxide gas inhaled for several hours a day as an experimental treatment for PPH. Nitric oxide works through a messenger, cyclic GMP. A drug, sildena-fil (trade name: Viagra), slows the breakdown of cyclic GMP in the blood vessels of the penis and is a useful treatment for impotence in men. It also does so in the lungs and has produced some prom-ising early results in treating PH. Small studies have shown that it improves blood vessel function about as much as bosentan and epoprostenol, and a larger study showed that it increased walking time but had little effect on breathlessness. Side effects include flushing, heartburn, and diarrhea but are not very troublesome.

It is not clear if drugs such as epoprostenol, nitric oxide, and bosentan work entirely through their vasodilating effects. Patients who do not vasodilate when they receive the drugs acutely still seem to respond after a few months of treatment, sug-gesting that the drugs may have long-term effects helping the thickened arteries to remodel. Because of the difficulty in treating PH and the modest responses obtained even with these new medica-tions discussed above, it is becoming increasingly common to combine medications. There is some evidence that adding sildenafil to bosentan or either to a prostanoid may improve the response. Patients with PH will usually also be treated with oxygen, usually via a concentrator that looks like a small fridge and from which concentrated oxygen can be piped around the patient's house. This not only relieves breathlessness on exertion, but oxy-gen itself can dilate the blood vessels in the lungs.

Surgery   A heart and lung transplant, or more often a single lung transplant, is used to treat PPH that is not responding to medical treatment. A lim-ited number of organs are available. Many patients with PPH associated with connective tissue diseases are not placed onto the transplant list because of their associated illness. Transplantation usually cures PPH but requires long-term immunosuppres-sion to prevent rejection.

Outcome

The prognosis of PPH is poor. Most studies show that only about half of affected patients survive three years. The new treatments improve symp-toms, but they have not been available for long enough to know how much they improve the overall outcome.

In a study comparing patients treated with bosentan as well as the older treatments to those treated prior to the availability of bosentan, 70 per-cent of the bosentan-treated patients survived two years as compared to only 47 percent of the earlier patients. Although this is promising, it is not conclusive evidence. In clinical trials the effects of the drugs have, on average, been small, for example a 15 percent increase in the distance that patients could walk in six minutes. Many experts believe that the main role of the new treatments will be to act as a bridge to lung transplant surgery rather than to provide an effective medical alternative to surgery.

Risk Factors and Preventive Measures

Excellent treatment of heart failure, chronic lung disease, and sleep apnea will mitigate against but often not completely prevent the development of PH in these disorders. Anticlotting treatment should theoretically prevent PH developing due to recurrent pulmonary emboli. However, the problem here is recognizing this often difficult-to-diagnose condition. The appetite suppressants that caused a primary PH-like disease are no longer available. There are no preventive measures for PPH or PH associated with connective tissue diseases, but the hope is that with earlier recognition and more effective treatment the outcome for these patients will improve.

pyoderma gangrenosum A rare skin rash that causes deep punched-out ulcers and can be associated with rheumatic diseases.

The cause of pyoderma gangrenosum is not known. In about half of affected people it occurs alone. In the other half it is associated with a chronic inflammatory illness such as INFLAMMATORY BOWEL DISEASE, RHEUMATOID ARTHRITIS, SYSTEMIC LUPUS ERYTHEMATOSUS, or less often, hepatitis C, HIV, sarcoidosis, and leukemia.

Symptoms and Diagnostic Path

The first symptom is a skin ulcer. This can start as a small nodule or blister that ulcerates and increases in size rapidly. The lesions can occur anywhere but are more common on the lower legs, often at a site of minor trauma. Characteristically, the ulcers have a purple- or violet-colored border and have a punched-out appearance with the edge of the ulcerated skin overhanging the base of the ulcer. The ulcers of pyoderma gangrenosum can be extremely painful. Nonspecific systemic symptoms such as fever, arthralgia, and myalgia are common.

The appearance of the ulcer is often classical, but a skin biopsy is usually performed to exclude other causes of ulcers such as malignancy or infection. The biopsy appearance of pyoderma gangrenosum, although not specific, is helpful because it shows a large number of neutrophils infiltrating the tissue. No laboratory tests are helpful for making the diagnosis.

Treatment Options and Outlook

Pyoderma gangrenosum can be very difficult to treat. No specific treatment is always successful. Local wound dressing, elevating the leg, rest, and topical antiseptics are usually tried, but most patients also require systemic therapy. Many drugs that modulate the immune system have been tried. CORTICOSTEROIDS are the primary drug treatment, but many patients are treated with additional immunomodulators such as METHOTREXATE, AZATHIOPRINE, DAPSONE, COLCHICINE, CYCLOSPORINE, and INTRAVENOUS IMMUNOGLOBULIN. The ulcers respond slowly and often take a year or more to heal. Most dermatologists try to avoid surgery if possible because trauma appears to spread the lesions.

Risk Factors and Preventive Measures

The associated diseases discussed above are risk factors for developing pyoderma gangrenosum, although very few people with these conditions will. No risk factors are known for isolated pyoderma gangrenosum, and there are no preventive measures. If someone has pyoderma gangrenosum or has had it in the past, it is well described to occur in the wound after surgery. This appears less likely if the stitches are subcuticular (that is, they do not pierce the skin).

RA See RHEUMATOID ARTHRITIS.

radiculopathy See BACK PAIN.

Raynaud's phenomenon A progressive color change of an extremity (usually a hand or fingers) from white to blue to red in response to cold or emotion. Exactly how many people suffer from Raynaud's phenomenon is unknown, but it is probably about 5 percent of the population.

Blood flow to the skin is vitally important for conserving or losing body heat. The greater the blood flow through skin, the more heat is lost and vice versa. For this reason, blood flow through skin at normal room temperature is 10 to 20 times greater than required to keep the skin healthy, and the blood vessels have the ability to alter blood flow enormously. Closing down the small arteries taking blood to the fingers, for example, is a normal response on walking out into the cold so that the individual does not lose too much heat. If the cold is severe or prolonged enough, anybody's hand can go white due to the marked reduction in blood flowing just below the surface of the skin. The change to blue occurs when there is some blood flow but not quite enough. Because the tissues are starved of oxygen and the blood is moving slowly, more than usual oxygen is extracted from the blood, turning it blue. When the spasm of the arterial walls relaxes there are compensatory mechanisms that result in excessive blood flow through the area, giving a dusky red appearance. People with primary Raynaud's phenomenon have the same physiological response, but it is exaggerated and occurs with much less cold provocation than normal and also occurs with emotion. Those

with secondary Raynaud's phenomenon also have this exaggerated response but occurring on a background of disease processes present in the blood vessels that make the Raynaud's more likely to occur and more severe.

In diseases such as SCLERODERMA in which Raynaud's phenomenon is a hallmark, permanent changes occur in the blood vessels. In particular, there is a buildup of collagen and fibrous tissue in the walls of small arteries leading to permanent narrowing that can be severe. When the smooth muscle in the vessel wall contracts, such a narrowed artery can block off altogether. The small blood cells called platelets are activated and release large amounts of substances such as thromboxane A2 and serotonin that can overwhelm the protective mechanisms (such as prostacyclin secretion) of the endothelium (inner lining of blood vessel) and lead to contraction following little or no stimulus.

Many conditions can cause Raynaud's phenomenon or similar constriction of peripheral blood vessels:

Primary Raynaud's phenomenon This term is used when there is no recognized cause and no associated disease. It is customary to wait two years before calling it primary because Raynaud's may be the first manifestation of a disease. Typically people with primary Raynaud's phenomenon have intermittent attacks affecting both hands and/or feet but do not develop any scarring on the fingertips, have normal nail fold blood vessels, and have a normal ESR and, often, a negative ANA test. They are often young and the Raynaud's disappears after five to 10 years in about half of them.

Secondary Raynaud's This can be associated with several conditions.

Connective tissue disease Systemic sclerosis, DERMATOMYOSITIS AND POLYMYOSITIS, SYSTEMIC LUPUS

ERYTHEMATOSUS (SLE), RHEUMATOID ARTHRITIS, and OVERLAP SYNDROME are all associated with Raynaud's phenomenon. About 95 percent of patients with systemic sclerosis have Raynaud's, as do up to 80 percent of overlap syndrome patients, 60 percent of SLE patients, and smaller percentages of patients with polymyositis and rheumatoid arthritis.

Occupational People who operate vibrating machinery sometimes develop Raynaud's phenomenon. This can also be produced by inappropriate use of a crutch, causing pressure on the blood vessels in the armpit. There is no proven tendency for this condition to develop into a connective tissue disease. A few patients have developed connective tissue diseases after use of vibrating machinery, but because they are so few this could be by chance.

Thoracic outlet An extra rib at the lower end of the neck or its fibrous remnant can cause the hand and arm to turn cold and white during certain positions due to pressure on the large blood vessels traveling toward the arm.

Drugs or toxins A number of medications cause constriction of peripheral blood vessels as part of their normal action, including most beta-blockers (used for high blood pressure and angina) and ergot preparations (used for migraine). Some patients will be very sensitive to these effects, and others may already have poor circulation to the feet and hands. These patients will probably not tolerate these drugs. Some drugs can cause Raynaud's phenomenon as a toxic effect (e.g., bleomycin, an anticancer drug) as may other toxic substances, particularly polyvinyl chloride. Amphetamines, cocaine, and even nicotine can cause Raynaud's phenomenon in susceptible people.

Hyperviscosity Conditions such as CRYOGLOBU-LINEMIA, polycythemia, and paraproteinemia can cause sludging of the blood in smaller arteries and precipitate constriction of the arteries.

Symptoms and Diagnostic Path

Raynaud's phenomenon is usually seen in the fingers but can also occur in the toes, ears, nose, and tongue. There is often pain and numbness with the white and blue color change and a sensation of burning warmth with the redness. Only part of a finger may be affected, or several fingers, or it may be more widespread. The whiteness may come on very suddenly. Primary Raynaud's may be precipitated by emotion as well as cold, but the other secondary forms do not usually occur with emotion. Critical loss of blood supply such that tissues actually die or are severely damaged does not occur in primary Raynaud's under normal conditions.

Small areas of tissue death at the tips of the fingers that form small scarred pits are, however, very typical of systemic sclerosis. Gangrene can also occur with complete absence of blood flow. This is usually associated with severe permanent narrowing of the blood vessels that do not then respond to treatment. Sometimes the tip of a toe or finger develops dry gangrene, shrivels, and drops off. This is, fortunately, rare. In systemic sclerosis there is strong evidence that a very similar process of intermittent severe narrowing of arteries taking blood to internal organs such as the heart and kidneys occurs. Certainly, the severe crises of high blood pressure and kidney failure that used to cause the death of many systemic sclerosis patients before effective treatments were discovered occurred more frequently in winter.

The diagnosis is made on the typical three-color change in response to cold or emotion. The patient's description is usually enough, although provocation tests can be done. The simplest is just to soak an affected hand in cold water and allow it to dry in the air. A careful history should be taken to exclude the other causes listed above. An examination will be directed at finding signs of connective tissue diseases and assessing the state of peripheral arteries. Smoking dramatically worsens the arterial damage. This should be asked for in the history and measures taken to encourage the patient to quit.

Treatment Options and Outlook

The treatment of Raynaud's phenomenon depends on the severity. Many patients with primary Raynaud's will manage very well with simple measures and not require any regular medication. Others with severe secondary Raynaud's may need hospitalization for intravenous therapy or surgery. Prolonged ischemia (lack of blood supply) can be extremely painful, and appropriate pain relief may be required.

Mild Giving up smoking and avoiding cold exposure are the keystones to self-management. It is vital that the person's whole body be warm and not just the hands. Avoidance of cold may involve giving up outdoor winter sports, having a range of gloves for different situations, using the various proprietary pocket hand warmers, and not getting wet when it is cool or windy.

Moderate Almost patients with secondary Raynaud's phenomenon should take low-dose ASPIRIN as an antiplatelet agent. One group of the family of calcium channel blocking drugs (the dihydropyridines) is particularly effective in dilating peripheral arteries. These include nifedipine, amlodipine, felodipine, and isradipine. They are usually used to lower blood pressure. In that situation the warmth in the hands and feet that they produce is sometimes regarded as an adverse effect. Headache, flushing, and dizziness are possible adverse effects. The drugs may be used continuously or just during the colder months. About two-thirds of patients will experience a decrease in frequency and severity of attacks with one of these medications. The long-acting preparations should be used to avoid rebound constriction of blood vessels.

Nitroglycerin is traditionally used as a tablet or spray under the tongue for angina. It is very effective at dilating both arteries and veins. A gel form can be applied to fingers or toes affected by severe Raynaud's that does not ease with warming. Since it has a short action it is practical to use only to resolve an attack rather than regularly to prevent attacks. The treatment involves rubbing 1–2 cm of the gel into the affected skin. A headache is the only common adverse effect and occurs if too much is used.

Severe This includes ulcers, critical reduction in blood flow with intractable pain or threatened gangrene, or gangrene itself. Ulcers should be kept clean, and antibiotics do have some effect if there is infection, although their penetration into the ischemic area is poor. Some people apply topical antibiotics directly onto the infected area in this situation. Surgical removal of infected tissue may be necessary. The above treatments are used with full doses of the calcium channel blockers.

Prostacyclin is a substance that endothelial cells produce to counteract the effect of activated platelets. It is a very potent dilator of blood vessels and an antiplatelet agent. Several forms can be administered as a drug. Intravenous prostacyclin and a more stable analog, iloprost, have been shown to heal ulcers and relieve symptoms. The period of symptom relief after stopping the infusion varies from a couple of weeks to three months. A number of oral forms have been trialed, currently with only modest or no effect. See the treatment section of PULMONARY HYPERTENSION for further discussion of these drugs. The intravenous forms unfortunately also cause headaches, vomiting, and diarrhea when used in pharmacological doses. These adverse effects limit how much can be given. The dose is gradually increased over three days to see what level the patient can tolerate, and then this maximum tolerated dose is continued for a variable course.

Studies with angiotensin-converting enzyme inhibitors (usually used to control high blood pressure) have shown variable results. Fluoxetine (trade name: Prozac), usually used to treat depression, has shown some promise in two small trials but needs further study. Sildenafil (trade name: Viagra) has also shown some promise but larger well-controlled studies are needed. BOSENTAN (see treatment section of pulmonary hypertension) reduces ulceration in patients with systemic sclerosis but did not reduce the frequency of Raynaud's attacks. The antiplatelet drug, dipyridamole, has some theoretical advantages to aspirin but in practice does not seem effective.

The nerve messages to arteries to constrict come along sympathetic nerves that form a fine network along the outer wall of the artery. Removing this sympathetic nerve supply often results in good dilatation of the artery. The sympathetic nerves can be divided at the level of the neck, or the fine network can be stripped off each individual artery at the level of the hand. Some surgeons feel that this is more effective because some of the constricting tissues around the artery are stripped off as well. Results are better if at least 2 cm of artery are stripped. These small sympathetic nerves can also be temporarily blocked by injection of a long-acting anaesthetic agent, bupivacaine, at the wrist or base of the finger to assist with healing of a resistant ulcer as well as relieving the pain. Occasionally, surgical amputation is required.

Primary Raynaud's phenomenon is a common troublesome condition that can usually be managed with sensible lifestyle changes and intermittent medication. Although studies vary, about 10 to 20 percent of people thought initially to have primary Raynaud's phenomenon go on to develop a connective tissue disease. Having abnormal nail fold blood vessels or abnormal blood tests at the outset are the best predictors of a later connective tissue disease, although they are still not very accurate in this regard. Fewer patients who are less than 20 years of age when they develop Raynaud's will have an underlying disease than those who develop it later. In its severest form, usually when part of systemic sclerosis, Raynaud's phenomenon can cause intractable pain, cause loss of fingers and toes, and possibly contribute to heart and kidney failure.

Risk Factors and Preventive Measures

The risk factors for secondary Raynaud's are discussed above. Bleomycin is hardly used anymore because of its adverse effects and occupational polyvinyl chloride exposure has been much reduced since the 1970s and 1980s when it was a significant cause of Raynaud's phenomenon. The use of nicotine, amphetamines, and cocaine are voluntary. Both vibrating machinery and protective clothing have improved, but this is still an occasional cause. Workers who develop this should be moved to another job not involving vibrating machinery. There is no preventive measure for primary Raynaud's phenomenon.

reactive arthritis Joint inflammation develops as a result of an infection in some other part of the body, usually the throat, gut, or urinary and genital organs. The arthritis is not infectious and gets its name from the assumption that the immune system is reacting to an infection and, in doing so, causes the arthritis. An initiating infection cannot always be found. The term reactive arthritis only came into being in the 1970s but is now widely used and incorporates those patients with Reiter's syndrome (see Symptoms below). Hans Reiter described the syndrome in an army officer in 1916, although reactive arthritis had probably been rec-

ognized 200 years previously. The clear link to diarrhea was established by Paronen after an outbreak of shigella infections in Finland toward the end of the Second World War. Together with other SPONDYLOARTHROPATHIES, reactive arthritis is frequently misdiagnosed if patients are not seen by rheumatologists. A recent study showed that 36 percent of reactive arthritis patients diagnosed at a specialist center had not had the correct diagnosis made before being seen there. Also many patients have mild and transient disease. For these reasons it is difficult to know how common reactive arthritis is. An estimate is that 10 in every 100,000 people will develop the disease each year. Outbreaks of particular infections can dramatically alter this.

There is no doubt that infections cause reactive arthritis. However, reactive arthritis is not infectious. While there remains much to be learned about how reactive arthritis develops, there is a generally accepted broad outline of events. First an infection develops. Particular organisms are involved (although the list is steadily increasing), and the infection usually involves a mucosal surface. Mucosal surfaces include the mouth, nasal passages, throat, gut, and genital and urinary tracts. As a result of this infection the immune system becomes sensitized (or immunized) to parts of the organism. This enables the immune system (both cells and antibodies) to attack and destroy the infecting organism (see IMMUNE RESPONSE). During the infection either live organisms or fragments of organisms are seeded into joints. In many cases it seems likely that cells of the immune system actually carry fragments or bacterial products into the joints. Some time later, after the infection has resolved, sensitized immune cells (lymphocytes) recognize the presence of these bacterial products in the joints and instigate an inflammatory response in an attempt to destroy them. This is reactive arthritis.

Although a number of different organisms may cause reactive arthritis, many of them have similarities. They are gram-negative (a staining property that has been used to identify organisms for many years), their cell membranes are rich in molecules called lipopolysaccharides and peptidoglycans and they can enter the human host's cells and survive there. The most frequently implicated organisms are *Chlamydia trachomatis, Clostridium difficile, Campylobacter, Salmonella, Shigella,* and *Yersinia.* These organisms typically cause HLA-B27-associated arthritis (see below). Other less frequently described organisms include *Streptococci, Escherichia coli,* and treatment with bacillus Calmette-Guérin (BCG) (see DRUG-INDUCED RHEUMATIC DISEASE). This latter organism is instilled into the bladder of patients with bladder cancer to stimulate the patient's immune response to the cancer. A benign organism that does not cause serious disease, it was originally used to protect against tuberculosis. It has been shown to improve the outcome of bladder cancer, but a few patients do develop a reactive arthritis as a result. LYME DISEASE may be considered a reactive arthritis but is discussed separately. Viruses, including those causing HEPATITIS, PARVOVIRUS, and RUBELLA, cause a reactive arthritis but are discussed separately since they are fairly distinct from this group of diseases.

Patients with reactive arthritis are much more likely to be HLA-B27 positive than the general population (see ANKYLOSING SPONDYLITIS for a discussion of HLA-B27). This is, however, not as common as in ankylosing spondylitis. Clearly many people without this gene develop reactive arthritis that is indistinguishable from those with HLA-B27. There may be some broad differences in the type of arthritis people develop, but this is not due to HLA-B27 alone (see Symptoms below).

Chlamydia trachomatis DNA and RNA have consistently been found in the joint fluid or lining in a significant proportion (up to 30 percent in some studies) of reactive arthritis patients. This indicates that the organism is alive in the joint. Finding other organisms implicated in causing reactive arthritis in the joint, has been very difficult. There may be some differences between chlamydia and the other organisms.

Of the five classes of immunoglobulin or antibodies, IgA antibodies are most involved in fighting infection at mucosal surfaces and are, in fact, secreted out onto these surfaces. A characteristic finding in reactive arthritis patients is persistent IgA antibody formation. These antibodies are directed against many antigens on the causative organisms. Their persistence suggests that the organism or at least large parts of it remain within the body, stimulating further antibody production.

During outbreaks of infections with a relevant organism, not everyone develops a reactive arthritis. HLA-B27-positive people are at increased risk, but this accounts for only part of the risk. For example, in a recent outbreak of salmonella diarrhea, 12 percent of affected people developed reactive arthritis. Just less than half of these were HLA-B27 positive. Ongoing research is looking at whether some people's immune systems may be more likely to allow these organisms to persist in the body and therefore result in reactive arthritis.

Symptoms and Diagnostic Path
Within the broad grouping of the term reactive arthritis, three fairly distinct clinical presentations can be observed.

Oligoarticular reactive arthritis This causes pain and swelling in a few joints, sometimes only one. The knee is the joint most frequently affected. If more than one joint is involved, it is usually asymmetrical, e.g., the ankle of one leg and knee of the other. Over 60 percent of this group is positive for HLA-B27 and they may develop spondylitis. This form of arthritis typically follows infection with *Campylobacter, Chlamydia, Clostridium difficile, Salmonella, Shigella,* and *Yersinia* organisms. If looked for (it is a research procedure only), bacterial products are often detectable in the joints.

Typically there has been some sort of illness days or weeks before the arthritis, sometimes affecting several people in the family. This presumed infection may be quite mild. Abdominal pain in the days before the arthritis starts is common. Many patients feel generally unwell with fatigue and mild fever. Knees, ankles, and hips are most commonly affected, then shoulders, elbows, or wrists. Fingers are only occasionally affected, although the presence of dactylitis is typical. Dactylitis describes inflammation of the small joints of a finger as well as the tendons running along it. This results in a generally swollen finger with limited movement, sometimes described as a *sausage finger.* Affected joints are swollen and warm but often with much less pain and tenderness than their appearance suggests. The arthritis can move from one joint to another over several days. Inflammation of the sacroiliac joints where the spine meets the pelvis can lead to low-back pain and stiffness. Occasionally the spine may also be affected, but severe spinal disease is very unusual. Inflammation of tendons (tendinitis) and their attachments to bone (enthesitis) are very common and may cause marked disability.

Several skin conditions may occur with reactive arthritis. Keratoderma blenorrhagicum is a scaly thickening of the skin on the soles of the feet or palms of the hand similar to palmo-plantar PSORIASIS. Indeed, this form of the disease is very similar to the oligoarticular form of psoriatic arthritis. Circinate balanitis (a rash on the penis) as well as inflammation of the mucous membranes of the mouth, throat, and urinary tract may occur. When present this does not imply that the cause was a sexually transmitted disease. Similarly, although gut infections commonly set off the arthritis, noninfectious inflammation of the gut can clearly occur long after the infection has resolved.

Inflammation in the eye is a part of reactive arthritis, although not everyone gets it. Conjunctivitis is the most common manifestation, followed by uveitis (see EYE PROBLEMS). These quite commonly recur. The heart is only occasionally affected, with breakdown of the electrical conduction system being the most common occurrence. The kidneys may be affected very occasionally, usually in the presence of high IgA levels.

Reiter's syndrome This is often described as a separate entity. It is in fact a form of reactive arthritis just as described above. By convention, however, the term Reiter's syndrome is used when there is arthritis, conjunctivitis, and urethritis occurring altogether. Urethritis is inflammation of the tube carrying urine out of the bladder. Skin manifestations are more common with Reiter's than without, but otherwise there are no major differences.

Reactive arthritis This may present as a polyarthritis resembling RHEUMATOID ARTHRITIS. This form is not associated with HLA-B27, the patients do not develop spondylitis, and finding bacterial remnants in their joints has been difficult. Many organisms seem to able to induce this form of arthritis, with streptococci being typical. Interestingly, BCG has been reported to cause both this form and the oligoarticular form of arthritis.

The symptoms suggestive of a preceding infection or treatment for bladder cancer are important in leading to a search for the causative organism. However, especially when only one joint is involved, ruling out INFECTIVE ARTHRITIS or GOUT by aspirating joint fluid for laboratory examination is important. Frequently nothing in the physical examination alone can differentiate these. When several joints are involved in the oligoarthritic form, it needs to be differentiated from the other spondyloarthropathies. This may be very difficult, especially if back pain is present. Sometimes a period of follow-up is necessary to differentiate reactive arthritis from ankylosing spondylitis or even psoriatic arthritis if the latter rash is not obvious. In the polyarthritis form it is likely that many patients are in fact diagnosed with rheumatoid arthritis if the initiating infection is mild. The rheumatoid factor, however, is negative.

Nonspecific tests reflecting inflammation such as the ESR, C-reactive protein, and white cell count may be raised early on. The HLA-B27 test may be positive but does not assist in the diagnosis. Early on in the disease X-rays are unlikely to show any abnormalities. Later on small bony outgrowths at the previously inflamed attachments of ligaments and tendons (entheses) are common. The use of MRI has increasingly shown the importance of inflammation at these entheses in reactive arthritis. Where there is doubt, such a finding on MRI may support the diagnosis of reactive arthritis. However, MRI scanning should not be necessary in most patients. Urine examination may show the presence of white cells but no organisms. This indicates a noninfective inflammation of the urinary tract. An attempt should be made to grow the organism presumed to have initiated the arthritis, recognizing that the infection may be over and that this may no longer be possible. Cultures may be taken of stool, urine, and throat swabs. Because it is often too late to grow the organism by the time the arthritis is present, the more useful tests are often those that look at the body's response to infections. By measuring the patient's own antibodies, it is sometimes possible to tell that there has recently been an infection with a certain organism. Such serological tests are available for *Salmonella, Yersinia, Neisseria gonorrhoeae, Campylobacter, Chlamydia,* and beta-hemolytic streptococci. A positive test for one of these in a patient with reactive arthritis strongly suggests but does not prove that the organism initiated the arthritis.

Treatment Options and Outlook

The treatment of reactive arthritis will vary considerably, depending on the stage and severity of the disease. At different stages the goal of treatment may be to prevent arthritis from occurring, to abort the arthritis by treating the cause, or to control inflammation in established disease.

When there is a reasonably high risk of arthritis occurring after particular infections, it seems logical to hope that early treatment may prevent arthritis from occurring. For example, scientists know that about 12 percent of northern European populations will develop reactive arthritis if infected during an outbreak of salmonella diarrhea. Normally only seriously ill patients would be treated with antibiotics for this infection since it is a self-limiting disease and antibiotics may cause more harm than good. Could physicians, however, prevent most cases of reactive arthritis by very early antibiotic treatment? Two good studies in this situation involving salmonella outbreaks have shown no benefit from early antibiotic treatment. Against this there is some evidence that treating urinary and genital infections caused by *Chlamydia trachomatis* reduces the likelihood of reactive arthritis developing.

If the arthritis is caused by the immune system reacting against the presence of an organism, treating that organism with antibiotics might be expected to improve the arthritis or settle it altogether. Many studies have now been done using appropriate antibiotics for six to 12 months. Studies on patients with reactive arthritis due to gut infections have shown no positive result. As mentioned above, *Chlamydia trachomatis* may be slightly different in that evidence of living organisms in the joint can frequently be found. Two studies suggest that there may be some benefit of antibiotic treatment in chlamydia-induced arthritis. However, not enough patients had a good response to be sure, and a further study showed no benefit. Therefore, the answer at this stage is still unknown.

Treatment for established arthritis varies according to severity. One or two swollen joints will often respond well to injections of CORTICOSTEROIDS into the affected joints. As long as infection has been ruled out, this is a very safe procedure. Corticosteroid injections are also very useful in managing enthesitis and sometimes tendinitis. For more widespread joint pain and arthritis, NSAIDs are effective. Since many patients are relatively young, NSAIDs are fairly safe. For many patients this is all that is required.

For more severe or sustained arthritis, DMARDs are used, most commonly SULFASALAZINE. This drug was in fact designed over 60 years ago by a doctor who believed that most arthritis was due to infections. She therefore thought that a combination of the newly discovered sulfa antibiotics and a form of aspirin (the *sala-* in sulfasalazine) would be an effective treatment. An early trial was negative. It was hardly used for treating arthritis until the late 1970s, although it was found to be very successful in treating inflammatory bowel disease. However, it is now a well-established DMARD in many forms of arthritis and in controlled trials has been shown to be effective and safe in treating reactive arthritis. Sulfasalazine is usually used first, but if not successful METHOTREXATE or AZATHIOPRINE may be used.

Ice can give good relief to inflamed joints and tendons, and flexible splints can provide support, but the joints should not be immobilized. Conjunctivitis is treated with corticosteroid drops. Deeper inflammation in the eye (uveitis) is usually treated with corticosteroid drops and drops to dilate the pupils. However, uveitis can have serious consequences and patients may need specialized attention from an ophthalmologist. The urinary tract disease is usually mild and seldom requires specific treatment. The skin conditions are treated in a similar way to psoriasis.

Most patients with reactive arthritis can expect a good outcome. The arthritis will often settle relatively soon, sometimes within a few weeks. There may, however, be recurrences that can be set off by infections or other stresses. Studies of outcome vary considerably, but probably 70 percent of patients can expect to be free of arthritis five years after diagnosis.

Risk Factors and Preventive Measures

The main risk factor for developing reactive arthritis is getting one of the infections discussed above.

However, it is likely that the minority who develop the arthritis are genetically primed to do so. The organisms are widespread, and it may not be possible to avoid infection. However, *Salmonella* and *Campylobacter* infections are often from eating chicken, and careful food hygiene would prevent a number of these infections. In particular, uncooked chicken should not be allowed to sit in the fridge too long, and frozen chicken should be thawed before cooking to ensure that the center is thoroughly cooked. *Chlamydia* infections are sexually acquired and can be prevented by condom use. Once the infection is acquired, there is some evidence that treating *Chlamydia* but not the other infections will reduce the frequency of arthritis.

reflex sympathetic dystrophy (RSD, shoulder-hand syndrome, Sudeck's atrophy, posttraumatic sympathetic dystrophy, algodystrophy, causalgia, complex regional pain syndrome) A rare condition that causes continuous, severe, unremitting pain, usually in one limb. It affects women more often than men and can occur at any age, including childhood. Complex regional pain syndrome is now the official term, but the authors have used RSD since it is the most widely used term. Complex regional pain syndrome or CRPS is divided into type I and type II on the basis of type II having definite nerve damage as part of the cause.

The cause of RSD is not known. It often occurs after an injury, for example after a fracture or gunshot wound. After an injury there is a natural tendency to protect the injured limb, or it may have been immobilized in a cast, causing the hand or foot to swell, turn blue and blotchy, and feel abnormal. These responses to immobilization can be precursors of RSD. For example, frozen shoulder or stroke, which cause someone to keep his of her arm still, is often associated with swelling of the hand on the affected side. This occasionally progresses to RSD. The severity of the injury does not seem to affect the chance of developing RSD, and sometimes RSD can follow a minor injury. RSD usually affects only one limb but can be bilateral.

Some experts have argued that RSD is a poor name for this condition because it is not a reflex and the sympathetic nervous system may not play an important part. The proposed alternative name, complex regional pain syndrome, describes the condition without inferring its cause but is not yet widely used. RSD affects pain perception. Whether this is caused by abnormal nerve circuits in the brain or spinal cord or by abnormal regulation of sympathetic nerve fibers in the affected limb is not known.

Dogma suggests that abnormal sympathetic nerve activity plays an important part in the cause of RSD. The sympathetic nervous system is responsible for automatic biological functions such as sweating and temperature control. There is some evidence in support of this theory because many responses that are regulated by the sympathetic nervous system are abnormal in RSD. For example, the affected limb often has abnormal sweating and temperature regulation. In addition, blocking sympathetic nerves by injecting a drug can improve symptoms. On the other hand, studies of sympathetic nerve activity yielded conflicting results and abnormal conduction in nerves that carry pain sensations, which may also be important.

Symptoms and Diagnostic Path

There are three major groups of symptoms: pain, autonomic nerve dysfunction, and dystrophic changes. Steinbrocker suggested that there were three stages. Stage 1 is marked pain and swelling, stage 2 is dystrophic changes, and stage 3 is atrophy. Many patients do not pass through all three stages.

Pain This is the major symptom of RSD. If there was a preceding injury, the pain is out of proportion to the severity of the injury or the physical findings. Pain in RSD is often constant, burning, and difficult to localize, occurring both on the surface and in the deep tissues. The patient may feel pain in response to a stimulus such as light touch that would not normally be painful (allodynia) or may feel much more pain than would be expected after a slightly uncomfortable stimulus (hyperalgesia). There is often exquisite tenderness so that a patient cannot bear to have the affected limb touched.

Autonomic nerve dysfunction This leads to changes in blood flow, temperature, and sweating. Compared with the opposite limb the affected one can be pale, cold and clammy, or warm and dry. There is often swelling of the soft tissues with edema.

Dystrophic changes   Later in the illness are dystrophic changes so that the skin becomes thin and shiny, the nails thick and brittle, and the muscles smaller and weaker. Involuntary muscle spasms, muscle contractures, and atrophy can occur late in the illness.

Diagnosis   The diagnosis is clinical, and there is no specific diagnostic test for RSD. Blood tests are normal. Early in the illness a radionuclide bone scan of the affected limb shows increased blood flow, and late in the illness, decreased flow. Late in the illness an X-ray often shows osteoporosis in the bones of the affected limb.

Treatment Options and Outlook

Patients with a fracture affecting the movement of a limb, for example a wrist fracture, have a high risk of developing RSD. Exercises to keep the fingers moving and prevent swelling in the hand may prevent RSD. Two randomized, controlled studies have now found that vitamin C supplementation for 50 days after a wrist fracture significantly reduces the occurrence of RSD. How this works and what the best dose is remains unknown, but 500 mg a day is generally recommended. Once RSD has occurred, the sooner treatment is started the better. The mainstay of early therapy is aggressive physical therapy to restore movement and pain control. Early in the development of RSD a course of CORTICOSTEROIDS can help to decrease pain and swelling. NSAIDs are seldom very effective. A sympathectomy, removing the sympathetic nerve supply to a limb, is often tried. This can be achieved surgically by cutting the nerve or chemically by injecting a drug around the nerve. The results of a sympathectomy are variable. Many other drugs are used to treat RSD, including drugs that block the adrenergic receptors that mediate sympathetic nerve responses, and calcitonin, administered either as an injection or as a nasal spray. Several small studies have shown BISPHOS-PHONATES to significantly reduce pain. Treatment of RSD is difficult, and there have been few good clinical trials to evaluate how effective different treatments are. Many patients with established RSD have persistent symptoms. Low doses of tricyclic antidepressants such as AMITRYPTILINE can be helpful for the pain, and psychological counseling may improve the outcome.

Invasive treatments are reserved for patients with resistant symptoms. These include ablating the sympathetic nerves either surgically or chemically as mentioned above, injecting clonidine (an antihypertensive drug) around the spinal cord in the epidural space, injecting baclofen (a muscle relaxant) around the cord, or stimulating the spinal cord electrically. While there is some evidence for using these techniques, the numbers of patients having these forms of treatment are small and it is difficult to draw firm conclusions. Spinal cord stimulation seems to improve pain but not functional ability.

In one study 36 patients with RSD for at least six months received spinal cord stimulation and physical therapy and 18 received physical therapy alone. To stimulate the spinal cord, surgery is performed to insert an electrode close to the nerves as they exit the spine. A pulse generator provides a current that the patient can regulate. The current produces a feeling of pins and needles that overrides the pain. The investigators found that stimulation decreased pain by about 25 percent, but function did not improve. The study was criticized because patients were selected to receive spinal cord stimulation only if they responded to it, and the placebo effects of surgery and using high-tech hardware was not controlled (see CLINICAL TRIAL).

In the baclofen study only six women with RSD and troublesome muscle spasms were studied. The baclofen was injected into the epidural space around the spinal cord on abnormal muscle spasms. Baclofen was administered continuously by a small pump for up to three years, and most of the women improved with reduced spasms and pain. Injection of baclofen into the epidural space and spinal stimulation are expensive and invasive treatments but may be options for selected patients.

Risk Factors and Preventive Measures

Prolonged immobility and smoking are risk factors for the development of RSD. Early and active mobilization should be practiced in all at-risk settings including after fractures, surgery, heart attacks, and strokes. Stopping smoking may help. Although it is a risk factor, studies to see whether stopping at the time of the incident reduces RSD development have not been done. Prescribing 500 mgs of vitamin C after at-risk fractures (especially wrist and lower leg) will prevent a significant number of RSD cases.

Reiter's syndrome   See REACTIVE ARTHRITIS.

relapsing polychondritis   This is a rare disease in which there are intermittent bouts of inflammation affecting cartilage. The first patient was reported in 1923, but even by 1960 there were only 10 patients reported. It can start at any age but usually does so between 40 and 50 years. Relapsing polychondritis occurs in all races and affects men and women equally. It is estimated that about three people in every million develop the disease every year in the United States.

The cause is unknown. There is good evidence for an immune attack directed against type II collagen, the main constituent of cartilage in a number of areas in the body. Immune cells are found at the sites of cartilage damage as are antibodies and COMPLEMENT components. Further, antibodies directed against type II collagen are found in many, although not all, patients. Levels of these antibodies parallel activity of the disease in some patients. Approximately a third of patients have another autoimmune condition that usually starts before the polychondritis. All the connective tissue diseases, many other inflammatory arthritides (see ARTHRITIS), inflammatory bowel disease, diseases of blood cells and the immune system, as well as PSORIASIS and DIABETES have been associated with relapsing polychondritis.

Symptoms and Diagnostic Path

Cartilage containing type II collagen provides structural strength to a number of widely separated organs. The distribution of these structures indicates the main areas of damage in polychondritis. About 10 percent of patients also get a VASCULITIS. The following describes roughly in order of frequency the typical manifestations of relapsing polychondritis.

Ear   The outer ear, or pinna, becomes intermittently inflamed in over 80 percent of patients. Because there is no cartilage in the lower flap of ear (where earrings are normally worn), this gives a very characteristic appearance. The rest of the ear becomes red and swollen, with the lower flap appearing normal. After repeated attacks the ear softens and looks smaller and floppy. The canal leading to the eardrum can also be affected, closing off and causing hearing loss. However, deafness more commonly follows small-vessel vasculitis affecting the inner ear. This can cause dizziness, severe nausea that does not respond well to medication, and eventually profound deafness. This affects about 30 percent of patients.

Nose   The cartilage of the bridge of the nose is involved in 30 percent of patients at some stage of the disease. It becomes mildly swollen, red, and warm, and this lasts from days to weeks. After repeated attacks the cartilage collapses, causing a depression in the midpart of the bridge of the nose. This is known as a saddle nose deformity.

Respiratory tract   The main windpipe or trachea that can be felt in the front of the neck takes air into the lungs, where it is distributed by smaller airways. Because of the pressure differences inside and outside of the chest wall, it is necessary to have something keeping the trachea open or it would collapse. This is achieved by having C-shaped rings of cartilage that can easily be felt regularly spaced all the way down the trachea. If these are affected by the chondritis they may soften and start to collapse, leading to wheezing, coughing, choking, and shortness of breath on exertion. These patients are at increased risk of chest infections. Collapse of the trachea can lead to death.

Joints   Ankles, wrists, and elbows are most frequently involved, and over 70 percent of patients will get arthritis during the course of the disease. Other joints may be affected. Attacks may last weeks to months and do not parallel inflammation elsewhere in the body. Despite the severe pain, joint swelling is slight and there is relatively little damage to the joints.

Heart and arteries   Abnormalities of electrical conduction in the heart may occur. Inflammation of the attachment of the heart valves leads to their becoming leaky. When this affects the aortic valve (through which blood is pumped around the body), it can cause heart failure. Surgical replacement of the valve is often required and the surgery can be difficult. The walls of the large arteries, especially the aorta, can become weakened and enlarge.

Eyes Many eye problems can occur, with 50 percent of people having some problem. These can include swelling behind (causing a bulging eye) or around the eye. Inflammation of the white coating layer in front of the eye can occur, and occasionally this is severe enough to cause destruction and bulging of the eye contents. Inflammation of other parts of the eye (iridocyclitis, chorioretinitis, and keratitis) may occur but are not common (see EYE PROBLEMS). Vasculitis may affect the vessels at the back of the eye.

Kidneys A few patients develop inflammation of the filtering part of the kidneys (glomerulonephritis).

Skin A range of rashes have been described, but none are specific for relapsing polychondritis. Palpable purpura (purple-black spots that can be felt) and urticaria (hives) may be signs of vasculitis. ERYTHEMA NODOSUM, LIVEDO RETICULARIS, and thrombophlebitis (inflammation of veins just under the skin) are all described.

Nervous system This is usually a result of vasculitis causing loss of blood supply to an area of brain or nerves. Strokes, peripheral nerve lesions, or spinal cord lesions may occur.

Fever Nearly 50 percent of patients will have a fever at some time. This frequently causes diagnostic confusion, with a variety of infections being suspected.

Other Relapsing polychondritis is associated with an unusually high incidence of malignancy. This can occur before, at the same time, or after the relapsing polychondritis and has been reported in up to 10 percent of patients. Myelodysplastic syndrome is the commonest, but lymphomas and other cancers also occur.

Diagnosis In its full-blown state relapsing polychondritis is not difficult to diagnose. It is a rare disease, however, and many doctors will not have previously encountered it. This may lead to the diagnosis not being considered. The various manifestations of the disease may also not occur together. Many other conditions can mimic isolated effects of polychondritis that may therefore not be diagnosed until a pattern of disease becomes apparent. Commonly used criteria for diagnosis require three of the following seven features: (1) typical inflammation of both ears; (2) an arthritis as described above; (3) inflammation of the cartilage of the nose; (4) eye inflammation; (5) inflammation of the cartilage of the trachea or voice box; (6) disturbance of inner ear function, e.g., dizziness, nausea, and hearing loss; and (7) biopsy of cartilage showing typical mild inflammation.

It is very important to evaluate the upper airways by breathing tests (spirometry) and usually CT scanning since disease here can be rapidly fatal. Spiral CT scans are particularly useful in giving a three-dimensional picture of the inside of the trachea and main airways without the need for invasive procedures. Echocardiography (an ultrasound examination) is used to examine the heart, the valves, and the first part of the aorta. CT or MRI scanning can accurately image the rest of the aorta and other large vessels. Usually the ESR, C-reactive protein, and white cell count will be raised, reflecting the inflammation. These are not, however, specific for relapsing polychondritis. Anticollagen type II antibodies cannot be measured in routine laboratories and are not always positive. Those patients with other coexisting diseases may have abnormal investigations because of those diseases.

Treatment Options and Outlook

The aims of treatment are to minimize the pain and disability caused by the less dangerous manifestations and to try and prevent damage to those organs that may result in death or severe disability. NSAIDs and low-dose CORTICOSTEROIDS are effective in treating the arthritis and mild inflammation of the ears and nose. If the attacks are very severe or when there is involvement of the heart, major blood vessels, kidneys, or there is a vasculitis, then high-dose corticosteroids are used. Ideally this can be tapered off after the attack settles and discontinued. Relapsing polychondritis does not always respond to corticosteroids, however, and does not always settle within a reasonable time period. In these situations immunosuppressive treatment is used. CYCLOPHOSPHAMIDE, AZATHIOPRINE, CYCLOSPORINE, methotrexate, and plasmapheresis have all been reported to be successful, and DAPSONE and COLCHICINE have been used in milder disease. In recent years the anti-TNF agents INFLIXIMAB and ETANERCEPT have been reported to be very effective in small numbers of patients whose disease has not responded to these medications. It should be pointed out, however, that relapsing polychondritis is such a rare disease that controlled trials of treatment will probably never be done. The rationale for treatment will be borrowed from diseases that are more frequent and have some similarities.

The trachea and major airways present special problems. If there is narrowing or collapse high up in the trachea, a tracheotomy tube can be inserted to prevent obstruction. For obstruction of airways lower down it is possible to put stents in that hold the airway open. However, there have been problems with these devices. People with mildly collapsible airways may benefit from using a pump that forces air into the lungs at night. This is known as continuous positive airways pressure or CPAP and is quite frequently used in patients with SLEEP APNEA. Leaking heart valves can be surgically replaced, but the tissues may be weak and repeat surgery may be required.

Profound deafness is not uncommon and is a major cause of disability. Respiratory and heart complications contribute to the reduced life expectancy of patients with relapsing polychondritis. About three-quarters of these relatively young patients will be alive five years after diagnosis. However, in those with vasculitis only 45 percent will be alive at five years.

rhabdomyolysis Severe muscle damage causing tissue necrosis (death).

Rhabdomyolysis is not a specific disease, and it can be caused by any condition that results in severe muscle damage. Such damage can occur from direct injury, for example if a person is crushed in a motor vehicle accident; after unusually severe exertion, for example in new recruits starting military training; or after repeated seizures. Muscle damage and rhabdomyolysis can be associated with metabolic abnormalities such as a very low serum potassium level. Muscle inflammation associated with viral infections is usually mild, but occasionally severe muscle damage can occur. Other causes of muscle inflammation, and occasionally rhabdomyolysis, are alcohol, cocaine, heat stroke, statin cholesterol-lowering drugs, and polymyositis or dermatomyositis.

Symptoms and Diagnostic Path
Severe muscle pain and swelling are common. This contrasts with DERMATOMYOSITIS AND POLYMYOSITIS where pain and swelling are seldom prominent. The patient may notice dark urine. This is caused by myoglobin, a pigment produced by muscle breakdown. Affected muscles are weak and painful to move.

In addition to the symptoms, a clue to the correct diagnosis is a marked increase in the concentration of creatine phosphokinase (CK or CPK), an enzyme elevated when muscle is inflamed or damaged. Myoglobin can be detected in the plasma and in the urine.

Treatment Options and Outlook
There is no specific treatment for rhabdomyolysis. The most serious complication is kidney failure. This occurs because high concentrations of myoglobin are toxic to the kidney. Kidney function can be protected by ensuring that the patient has plenty of fluids and that the urine remains dilute. If renal function deteriorates, some patients need dialysis for a few weeks until the kidneys recover. Rhabdomyolysis usually settles spontaneously.

rheumatic fever An immunological reaction to a streptococcal infection that causes fever and arthritis acutely but leads to chronic damage of the heart valves. Rheumatic fever was common in the United States until the introduction of penicillin, when the incidence declined. However, it has not been eradicated, and episodic cases, or clusters of cases, still occur. Rheumatic fever is much more common in developing countries and seems to thrive under conditions of poverty and crowding. Children younger than 15 years of age are at greatest risk.

Rheumatic fever is caused by an immunological reaction to an infection with a group A beta-hemolytic streptococcus. In some people this organism is part of the bacterial population normally living in the nose and throat, but it can be invasive and is the cause of strep throat. Streptococcal throat infection itself is often self-limiting, even without treatment. However, one cannot predict which infections are likely to precipitate heart disease, and therefore all are treated with antibiotics.

Scientists do not know why the streptococcus sometimes lives happily as part of the usual bacterial population and at other times causes streptococcal throat infection that can lead to rheumatic fever. Only about 1 percent of streptococcal infections lead to rheumatic fever. The genetic makeup of both the patient and the streptococcus seem to be important determinants of the type of infection and who goes on to develop rheumatic fever. Rheumatic fever is caused by antibodies against the streptococcus reacting against the patient's own tissues.

Symptoms and Diagnostic Path

Rheumatic fever occurs two to five weeks after a streptococcal throat infection. The throat infection may have been minor and by the time rheumatic fever occurs has usually resolved. Fever and arthritis are common symptoms. The fever can be very high and responds to treatment with aspirin. Arthritis tends to affect large joints such as the knee, hip, ankle, wrist, and elbow. Arthritis tends to be flitting, moving from one joint to another, or additive, adding a new joint to the one that is already affected. Arthritis in rheumatic fever causes severe pain that is out of proportion to the amount of swelling or obvious inflammation. The pain can be so severe that the child is unable to walk.

Other less common findings are a rash called erythema marginatum, subcutaneous nodules, a movement disorder called Sydenham's chorea, and carditis. Erythema marginatum is usually a flat, pinkish rash with a clear margin, sometimes with clearing in the center. It can be very subtle and evanescent. Subcutaneous nodules are found in rheumatic fever but are rare. These nodules are usually smaller than a pea and are found over tendons. Sydenham's chorea is a movement disorder that causes abnormal movements of the hands and face. The patient often disguises these involuntary movements by turning the movement into a semi-purposeful action. The result is that sometimes children with chorea are thought to be very fidgety or unable to sit still. Sydenham's chorea can recur years later during pregnancy without any symptoms of another attack of rheumatic fever. Carditis is inflammation of the heart. During acute rheumatic fever myocarditis, pericarditis, and endocarditis can occur. Myocarditis, inflammation of the heart muscle, often causes an increased heart rate and can cause heart failure. Pericarditis, inflammation of the outside lining of the heart, can cause chest pain and a pericardial effusion (fluid around the heart). Endocarditis, inflammation of the heart valves, causes a murmur, a noise caused by blood flowing across an abnormal heart valve.

Repeated attacks of rheumatic fever can cause chronic, permanent damage to heart valves. This can cause heart rhythm problems, enlargement of the heart, and heart failure.

The diagnosis of acute rheumatic fever is clinical. The Jones criteria are used for classification, but some patients with rheumatic fever do not fulfill the criteria. The Jones criteria require laboratory evidence of a streptococcal infection and the presence of two major criteria or one minor and one major criterion. The major criteria are carditis (myocarditis, pericarditis, or endocarditis), erythema marginatum, subcutaneous nodules, chorea, and arthritis. The minor criteria include fever, an elevated erythrocyte sedimentation rate (ESR), arthralgia, and a history of a previous attack of rheumatic fever.

A throat swab may still be positive for streptococcus when rheumatic fever develops, or if it is negative, an elevated antistreptolysin antibody level will suggest a recent streptococcal infection. The ESR is usually elevated, but other blood tests are not helpful. An electrocardiogram can show an increased PR interval, a widening of the distance between the P and R waves. An echocardiogram may show pericarditis or abnormalities of the heart valves.

Treatment Options and Outlook

Preventing rheumatic fever is possible by treating streptococcal throat infections, particularly in children. If rheumatic fever develops, an NSAID, most often high doses of aspirin, relieves fever and arthritis. Penicillin is used to eliminate any remaining streptococci, and occasionally if there is carditis, a course of corticosteroids is prescribed. The acute attack subsides within a few months, However, if a patient has had one attack of rheumatic fever preventing further attacks is important. The risk of permanent damage to the heart valves is much higher after repeated attacks of rheumatic fever. A long-term antibiotic, most often a monthly injection of long-acting penicillin, is prescribed to prevent this. If there is permanent damage to heart valves, surgery to repair or replace these may be required. Heart valves that have been damaged by rheumatic fever have a greater risk of becoming infected (INFECTIVE ENDOCARDITIS).

Risk Factors and Prevention

Crowding and poor hygiene are the major risk factors for acute rheumatic fever. Community or societal moves to reduce these will reduce the incidence as well as bring other advantages. In developed countries, the increased use of antibiotics to treat infective sore throats has played some part in the lower incidence of rheumatic fever. There is some controversy over whether the streptococcal strains prevalent now are less able to induce rheumatic fever than those 40 or more years ago.

Secondary prevention refers to the prevention of repeated attacks in children who have already had an attack of rheumatic fever. This is very important in order to prevent further heart damage. Either daily low-dose antibiotics or three or four weekly injections of long-acting penicillin can be used and are proven to be effective although not completely so. Generally, patients without heart involvement will have this antibiotic prophylaxis until they are 18 to 20 years of age as long as they have not had an attack for at least five years. Those with heart involvement will take prophylaxis until they are 25 years old as long as they have not had an attack for at least 10 years. These guidelines are not universally accepted because people can get repeat attacks when they are much older, although this becomes increasingly rare.

rheumatoid arthritis (RA) A chronic inflammatory autoimmune disease that fluctuates in sever-

ity and affects the joints, causing swelling, pain, loss of function, and eventually deformity. It can also affect other organs. Purists maintain it should therefore be called rheumatoid disease rather then rheumatoid arthritis. RA has a major socioeconomic impact, not only by causing disability and decreasing the earning capacity of affected people but also by increasing use of medical resources such as doctor visits, hospital admissions, and surgery. In the last 20 years improvements in the drugs available to treat RA and recognition that early control of the disease is important have improved outcomes.

RA affects about 1 percent of the population in most countries. It is rare in some populations such as rural West Africans and more frequent in some, such as Pima Indians. The cause of RA is not known. Several ideas have been proposed—most often that it is either an infectious or genetic disease.

Infection An infectious cause has been suspected and hunted for decades but has never been convincingly or reproducibly proven. Patients with RA make antibodies to a wide range of antigens which has sometimes led researchers down misleading trails.

One of the first organisms suggested as a cause of RA was the Epstein-Barr virus (EBV), the organism that causes infectious mononucleosis (mono). In the 1970s, it was found that many patients with RA had antibodies against the virus, and speculation mounted that the virus played a role in the cause of RA. This was an attractive theory because it was known that EBV activated B lymphocytes and was associated with rare types of cancer, suggesting it could interact with the immune system. Most adults have been infected with EBV at some time. Many experts think RA stimulates the B lymphocytes to produce many antibodies, one of which is the antibody against EBV, and that the virus does not cause RA.

Several viral illnesses such as RUBELLA, PARVOVIRUS, HEPATITIS, and HUMAN IMMUNODEFICIENCY VIRUS (HIV) (see VIRAL ARTHRITIS) can cause arthritis, but efforts to isolate a specific virus from patients with RA have not been successful. Similarly, infection with Mycoplasma, Chlamydia, and Proteus have been considered as causes of RA, but the evidence is not convincing.

Genetic causes Undoubtedly genetic factors play a part in determining who gets RA, because it tends to run in families. If someone has a parent or sibling with RA, that person's risk of getting the disease is doubled. However, genetic factors are not the whole answer. If RA were entirely genetic, one would expect that identical twins would have 100 percent concordance. If one identical twin gets RA, though, there is about a 20 percent chance that the other twin, who has exactly the same DNA, will develop RA.

The genetic factors that increase the risk of RA are not clear (see HLA and GENETIC FACTORS). Rheumatoid arthritis has been known to be associated with HLA tissue types since the 1970s, with the risk of RA increased fourfold in individuals with the HLA-DR4 tissue type (new nomenclature HLA-DRB1 0401, 0402, and so on, for the different variants of the 04 tissue type). The strength of the association varies in different populations and is weaker in African-American than in Caucasian populations. Several research groups are performing genome-wide scans where the whole DNA sequence is examined in families with RA for markers that track with RA to try to localize the search to smaller areas of the genome. So far, other than confirming the association with the HLA region, the results have not been reproducible.

Other possible risk factors Women develop RA three times as often as men and RA often seems to improve in pregnancy, suggesting that hormones may influence the immune system in ways that alter the risk of developing RA.

Cigarette smoking is associated with about a 50 percent higher risk of developing RA, and RA is more severe in smokers. The mechanism is not clear, but smoking stimulates many liver enzymes that metabolize drugs and chemicals. These enzymes possibly convert an unidentified chemical into a by-product that affects the risk of RA.

RA is much less common in West Africa than it is in the United States, although critics argue that scientists are not certain about this because so few studies have been done in Africa. Observational studies from Africa also suggest that as people move into urban areas, where the risk of infections such as malaria is decreased, the risk of RA increases.

It has been proposed that chronic infection with an organism such as malaria may stimulate the immune system and protect against RA and that the Western-type lifestyle with excellent hygiene may increase risk. An argument against this is that recent evidence suggests that the incidence of RA is decreasing in developed countries such as the United States.

How RA Causes Disease

Although scientists do not know what causes RA, they do have an excellent understanding of how RA causes disease. Inflammation of the synovium is central to the pathogenesis of RA. The synovium that is normally thin becomes thickened, hypertrophied, and filled with fibroblasts and inflammatory cells such as lymphocytes and macrophages. Small new blood vessels form (angiogenesis). The proliferating synovium, called a pannus, replaces normal synovium and is locally invasive, damaging the underlying bone and cartilage.

Several cell types play an important role. T lymphocytes were thought to be the key cell driving RA, and drug companies produced antibodies that effectively depleted T cells in patients with RA. Surprisingly, this had little effect on disease activity, suggesting that perhaps T cells were not critical to the development of RA. Current opinion is that T cells do play a role in the pathogenesis of RA, but other cells such as macrophages, which produce cytokines, are also important. B lymphocytes produce antibodies, including rheumatoid factor, which is discussed later. Many mediators such as the cytokines tumor necrosis factor (TNF) and interleukin-1 and the chemokines amplify and sustain the inflammatory process. The strategy of developing drugs to block cytokines has led to effective new drugs for RA.

Symptoms and Diagnostic Path

The key symptoms and laboratory findings in RA are shown in the Table.

General symptoms RA is an illness that affects much more than just the joints, and systemic symptoms are common. Symptoms often start gradually, over months. Patients often experience difficulty pinning down exactly when their illness

COMMON SYMPTOMS AND LABORATORY FINDINGS IN RHEUMATOID ARTHRITIS

General	Joint	Extra-articular	Laboratory
Morning stiffness	Pain	Rheumatoid nodules	Anemia
Fatigue	Symmetrical swelling	Pleurisy	High platelet count
Low-grade fever	Stiffness	Lung disease	High ESR
Lack of energy	Warmth	Pericarditis	Rheumatoid factor
Depression	Loss of function	Eye inflammation	Normal white cell court
Loss of weight	Deformity	Felty's syndrome	Erosions on X-ray
Lymph nodes	Fusion	Sjögren's syndrome	Inflammation on imaging

started. The first symptoms are often vague and include fatigue, lack of energy, feeling depressed or washed out, and stiffness in the morning that lasts longer than 30 minutes. The stiffness in most noninflammatory causes of arthritis such as osteoarthritis lasts only a short time and improves once the patient is moving, whereas the stiffness in inflammatory diseases is much more severe and long lasting. It is not unusual for patients to say that their morning stiffness lasts until they take a hot bath or place their hands under running hot water. Loss of weight can occur with more severe RA and is part of the systemic illness. Lymph nodes can increase in size. This does not usually cause symptoms. However, if a physician notices the enlarged nodes, it may trigger a series of tests to make sure the patients does not have cancer, infection, or lymphoma.

Joint (articular) symptoms Typically RA affects many small joints in a symmetrical distribution at the same time. The metacarpophalangeal and proximal interphalangeal joints (knuckles) of both hands and wrists are most often affected. In some patients, though, the illness first causes symptoms in the small joints of the feet. Affected joints show signs of inflammation such as warmth, swelling, pain, and reduced movement. In a few patients joint swelling and other symptoms can occur in short, sharp attacks that resolve completely until they recur. This is called PALINDROMIC RHEUMATISM. More frequently, however, RA causes persistent symptoms in joints that may fluctuate in severity.

RA has a predilection for the small joints of the hands and feet, but most joints can be affected.

Listing those that are seldom or never affected is easier. RA seldom affects the distal interphalangeal joints (the last joint of the fingers) and does not affect the lower back. It can affect hips, knees, shoulders, wrists, ankles, cervical spine (neck), and temporomandibular joint (jaw). The joints of the small bones in the larynx (voice box) can become inflamed, causing hoarseness or narrowing of the airway. Symptoms vary in severity. Some patients are so severely affected that they are unable to function, and others are able to continue their day-to-day activities with some limitations.

Early in the illness swelling predominates, and this may lead to restricted movement of a joint and affect the patient's ability to make a fist or grip objects. Later in the illness permanent deformities can occur. One of the most common is called ulnar deviation. If a patient stretches out his or her fingers with the palms facing the ground, the fingers angle away to the side rather than pointing straight forward. Early in the disease the patient can correct the deformity by using other muscles to pull the fingers straight, but later the deformity becomes fixed and permanent. Other common deformities affect the fingers and wrist. A *boutonniere* (buttonhole) deformity affects the middle knuckle of the finger so that the joint is permanently flexed. It is called a boutonniere deformity because the joint sticks out between two slips of a tendon so that the anatomy looks like a button popping out of a buttonhole. A *swan neck* deformity is when the end joint of the finger is flexed and the middle joint is hyperextended, so the finger ends up resembling a swan's neck. If the wrist is chronically inflamed the whole hand can migrate downward off the wrist, resulting in a step-down or dinner fork deformity. These deformities can be corrected surgically, but such procedures do not necessarily improve function.

Late in the disease affected joints permanently lose their ability to move through a normal range of motion or even fuse and lose their ability to move at all. Fusion is a mixed blessing because while joints that cannot move do not fulfill their normal function, they are also frequently less painful. In fact, a common surgical treatment for chronic pain in a joint that does not respond to medical treatment and where movement is not vital is surgical fusion (ARTHRODESIS).

Joints move, stabilize, absorb shock, and help with balance. The major symptom of arthritis, apart from pain, is loss of function. This may affect daily activities such as walking, eating, dressing, and bathing but can also affect a person's ability to hold a particular job. A concert pianist and a bricklayer may seem to require very different tasks from their joints, but both jobs demand hands that can function effortlessly. Frequently patients with RA have to modify their lifestyle, hobbies, and employment because of limitations imposed by their arthritis.

Extra-articular symptoms   RA affects not only the joints but can also affect almost any organ. For this reason many experts prefer to call it rheumatoid disease rather than rheumatoid arthritis.

Rheumatoid nodules   Nodules ranging in size from smaller than a quarter-inch to larger than an inch (RHEUMATOID NODULES) are a frequent manifestation of extra-articular disease and are a marker of more severe and aggressive RA.

Pleurisy   The main symptom of pleurisy is chest pain that gets worse on taking a deep breath or coughing. These symptoms can also occur in patients who have a broken rib or inflammation or infection of the lung. Many patients with RA have mild pleurisy without knowing about it. More severe disease causes symptoms of pleurisy and sometimes a collection of fluid in the space between the lung and its lining (pleura). This is called a pleural effusion, and because it can be caused by cancer, pneumonia, infection, and many other diseases, it often starts a train of tests to try and find the cause. Unfortunately, there is no specific test that differentiates between a pleural effusion caused by RA and other diseases. The pleural fluid in RA often has a very low glucose concentration, but this finding is not specific.

Lung disease   In addition to causing pleurisy, RA can affect the lungs in several other ways. The most common is called interstitial fibrosis, which causes streaks of scarring throughout the lung tissue. Many patients with interstitial fibrosis do not have any symptoms early on. However, if a chest X-ray is taken, it can show scarring even at this stage. Why RA causes interstitial fibrosis is not clear, but male sex, severity of RA, and smoking increase the risk. Severe interstitial fibrosis causes shortness of breath and cough, and it decreases exercise capacity. Tests of lung function usually show what is called a restrictive defect, in other words, the volume of the lungs is decreased. Very occasionally lung disease can occur before arthritis symptoms occur, resulting in confusion about the diagnosis.

RA can cause rounded nodules within the lung. This used to occur more commonly in people with pneumoconiosis, an occupational lung disease usually acquired from working in coal mines, but nodules can occur in any patient. When only one or a few nodules are seen it can be very difficult to differentiate this from cancer, and a biopsy is often required.

Pericarditis   Just as fluid can accumulate between the lung and its lining layer, it can also accumulate between the heart and its lining layer, the pericardium. Again, many patients with RA have mild pericarditis that does not cause major symptoms or problems, and they are not aware of it. Mild asymptomatic pericarditis does not need any specific treatment. More severe disease that causes chest pain and a large pericardial effusion should be treated. The symptoms of a pericardial effusion are variable but can include chest pain or tightness, edema, and shortness of breath. Typically the chest pain from pericarditis is felt in the middle of the chest, varies with position, and can get worse with breathing. Other heart problems are rare, but rheumatoid nodules have been found in the heart, where they may cause rhythm problems.

Eye inflammation   Dry eyes, as a component of Sjögren's syndrome accompanying RA, are common but serious inflammation of the eye that threatens vision is uncommon. Scleritis, or inflammation of the fibrous layer of the eye, can cause pain, redness, and more seriously, thinning and weakness of the eyeball. If this happens, the white part of the eye looks blue or black because thinning of the lining allows the darker interior to show. Inflammation of the sclera usually causes a red, painful eye. The pain is deeper, more severe, and more aching in character than the superficial scratchiness caused by conjunctivitis or episcleritis. Vision can be affected, and scleritis should be treated by an ophthalmologist. Treatment involves management of the underlying RA and may require CORTICOSTEROIDS and immunosuppressive drugs. In patients with severe RA, rheumatoid nodules can occur in the eye and cause the sclera to become thin, and if inflammation is not controlled, to weaken so that the inside of the eye ruptures through the wall and blindness results. (See also EYE PROBLEMS.)

Felty's syndrome   This rare complication of RA is discussed separately (see FELTY'S SYNDROME).

Sjögren's syndrome   See SJÖGREN'S SYNDROME.

Other symptoms   RA rarely affects other organs such as the liver, kidneys, or peripheral nerves, but RHEUMATOID VASCULITIS can occur and affect these organs. If symptoms of kidney disease such as proteinuria develop, they are more likely to have been caused by drugs used to treat RA than the disease.

Diagnosis   The formal diagnostic criteria for RA were revised by the American Rheumatism Association (now the American College of Rheumatology) in 1987 and are shown in the table. These criteria were developed mainly for research purposes to make sure that researchers in different countries were studying the same disease and are not always helpful clinically. Since there is now more emphasis on diagnosing and treating RA as early as possible, before nodules and erosions are present, some patients treated for RA may not fulfill the diagnostic criteria.

AMERICAN RHEUMATISM ASSOCIATION 1987 REVISED CRITERIA FOR THE CLASSIFICATION OF RHEUMATOID ARTHRITIS

- Morning stiffness. This must affect the joints and last at least an hour. Many patients with noninflammatory rheumatic diseases such as osteoarthritis have morning stiffness, but this lasts for only a short time. Many patients with uncontrolled RA say that they are stiff all day, but generally stiffness improves after a few hours.
- Arthritis affecting three or more areas at the same time.
- Arthritis affecting the wrists, metacarpophalangeal (MCP), or proximal interphalangeal (PIP) joints.
- Symmetrical arthritis.
- Rheumatoid nodules.
- A positive blood test for rheumatoid factor.
- X-ray changes such as erosions that are typical of RA.

According to these criteria, a patient who fulfills four criteria has RA. The first four criteria must have been present for at least six weeks, and a person who has any four criteria at the same time can be classified as having RA.

Laboratory findings in RA   Laboratory tests can be helpful, but there is no specific diagnostic test for RA.

- A blood test called a rheumatoid factor (see Appendix II) is often, but not always, positive. Patients, and some physicians, often make the error of thinking that the test can definitively make or exclude the diagnosis of RA. About 80 percent of patients with RA do have a positive rheumatoid factor at some time in their illness. This means that at least 20 percent of patients with RA would be given the wrong diagnosis if physicians relied exclusively on the test. For most laboratory tests, the upper limit of normal is set so that between 2.5 and 5 percent of normal people fall outside of the normal range. This means that about 5 percent of healthy people have a positive RA factor, a number much higher than the approximate number of people with RA, which is about 1 percent of the population. To complicate matters, a positive rheumatoid factor occurs more frequently in the elderly, in patients with other autoimmune diseases such as SYSTEMIC LUPUS ERYTHEMATOSUS (SLE), and in those with chronic infections such as HEPATITIS C, TUBERCULOSIS, or INFECTIVE ENDOCARDITIS. In other words, the test for rheumatoid factor is useful but must be interpreted with the other clinical findings. Antibodies to cyclic citrullinated peptides (anti-CCP antibodies) are as effective as RA factor in diagnosing RA and have fewer false positive results.

- Many blood tests become abnormal in RA because of inflammation. These tests are not helpful in making the diagnosis of RA because they are not specific and can be abnormal with virtually any infection or illness that causes inflammation. An elevated erythrocyte sedimentation rate (ESR) or C-reactive protein (CRP) are such tests. However, they can be useful in differentiating an inflammatory illness such as RA from noninflammatory ones such as osteoarthritis or fibromyalgia.

Anemia is common in RA, and it is usually a type of anemia called anemia of chronic disease. The white blood cell count is usually normal, sometimes useful in differentiating RA from SLE, where the white cell count is often low. The platelet count is often elevated (thrombocytosis) when RA is active.

Imaging findings   An X-ray of the hands or feet is often ordered. If RA is severe, this may show the typical changes of narrowing of the joint space and erosions of bone around the joints. These X-ray changes are usually irreversible, so it does not make sense to wait for them to occur before making the diagnosis of RA. Later in the illness the X-rays may show deformity and destruction of joints. Regular X-rays are not very sensitive for detecting joint damage, and many researchers have studied imaging techniques designed to detect joint inflammation and damage early. Radionuclide bone scans are very sensitive, and any joint or bone that has infection, damage, or inflammation lights up. Unfortunately, the test does not separate noninflammatory causes of arthritis such as osteo-

arthritis from RA. This means that a bone scan in any person with arthritis usually lights up in the joints that are hurting—something that could largely have been determined by simply asking the patient. More recently ultrasound and magnetic resonance imaging (MRI) have been studied. Ultrasound has the advantages that it does not expose patients to radiation and is easy to perform. The disadvantages are that the quality of the images depends on the person doing the test and can be difficult to interpret. Ultrasound can also be used to measure the blood flow to a joint. If a joint is inflamed the blood flow increases, and therefore, this technique has been explored as a way of determining which drugs are effective for treating RA. Ultrasound is still mostly an experimental way of studying how a drug is affecting a joint. MRI is much more expensive but gives very clear images of joint inflammation and erosions. Other than in research studies, it is not used in clinical practice to diagnose or monitor RA. MRI shows erosions before they become apparent on plain X-rays, perhaps indicating the need for more aggressive treatment to slow the disease process down.

Making the diagnosis   The diagnosis of RA is usually made from the clinical findings. High-tech tests such as MRI and ultrasound are not part of the diagnostic workup. Blood tests can be helpful, but most rheumatologists will diagnose RA based on the clinical findings, irrespective of the results. X-rays are usually performed when a patients is first seen but are often not helpful for making a diagnosis because they can be normal in patients with early disease. They are helpful because they provide baseline information so that the presence of new erosions or joint deformities and response to treatment can be tracked. The appearance of erosions early in the disease signals aggressive destructive RA and may influence the patient's and physician's approach to treatment.

RA can be confused with most other illnesses that cause arthralgia or arthritis. However, SLE, OSTEOARTHRITIS, REACTIVE ARTHRITIS, VIRAL ARTHRITIS, FIBROMYALGIA, VASCULITIS, and polyarticular GOUT are most often mistaken for RA.

Treatment Options and Outlook
The goals of treating RA include the following:

- To relieve pain
- To maintain and restore function
- To preserve muscle strength
- To prevent progression of disease

The treatment of an individual patient depends on the severity of disease, the patient's response to treatment, and the presence or absence of other conditions that may limit the drugs a patient can take. To achieve the goals of treatment, a multidisciplinary approach is needed. This involves several approaches:

- Rehabilitation (see EXERCISE, OCCUPATIONAL THERAPY, PHYSICAL THERAPY).
- Surgery (see JOINT REPLACEMENT).
- Drug therapy. Examples of the different analgesics, nonsteroidal anti-inflammatory drugs (NSAIDs), disease-modifying drugs (DMARDs), and corticosteroids used to treat RA are shown in the following table.

Analgesics ACETAMINOPHEN, because it appears to be less likely to cause GI ulcers than NSAIDs, is often the drug chosen first for many patients to control pain. However, it does not have any anti-inflammatory effects and therefore is not helpful for controlling joint swelling or the pain that results from it in RA. In most patients with RA, NSAIDs are more effective than acetaminophen for relieving symptoms caused by inflammation. However, late in the course of RA, damaged joints can cause pain, even though there is little or no inflammation. In this situation drugs to relieve pain can help someone perform day-to-day activities, sleep comfortably, and have a reasonable quality of life. The first priority is to control inflammation, and usually if this is controlled, pain decreases.

If acetaminophen or an NSAID and adequate control of RA with a DMARD do not control pain, the next step is to use a narcotic analgesic. Usually physicians start with a weak narcotic such as TRAMADOL or CODEINE, often combined with acetaminophen or aspirin. If this does not work, the patient and physician need to consider the risks and benefits of stronger analgesics such as morphine and meperidine. These analgesics are more addictive than weaker narcotics, but they can enable patients with severe end-stage disease that

EXAMPLES OF DRUG CLASSES USED TO TREAT RA (TRADE NAMES IN PARENTHESES)			
Analgesics	**NSAIDs**	**DMARDs**	**Corticosteroids**
Acetaminophen (Tylenol)	Aspirin (Anacin and many others)	Methotrexate (Rheumatrex)	Prednisone (Deltasone, Orasone)
• with Codeine (Tylenol #3)	Indomethacin (Indocin)	Hydroxychloroquine (Plaquenil)	Methylprednisolone (Medrol)
• with hydrocodone (Lortab, Lorcet, Vicodin)	Ibuprofen (Motrin, Advil)	IM gold (Solganal)	
• with oxycodone (Percocet, Roxicet, Tylox)	Naproxen (Naprosyn, Aleve)	Oral gold (Auranofin)	
• with propoxyphene (Darvocet N50, Darvocet N100)	Diclofenac (Voltaren)	Penicillamine (Cuprimine)	
	Etodolac (Lodine)	Sulfasalazine (Azulfidine)	
Tramadol (Ultram)	Flurbiprofen (Ansaid)	Minocycline (Minocin)	
	Ketoprofen (Orudis)	Azathioprine (Imuran)	
	Nabumetone (Relafen)	Cycloporine (Neoral)	
	Meloxican (Mobic)	Leflunomide (Arava)	
	Celecoxib (Celebrex)	Etanercept (Enbrel)	
		Infliximab (Remicade)	
		Anakinra (Kineret)	
		Adalimumab (Humira)	
		Rituximab (MabThera, Rituxan)	
		Certolizumab (Cimzia)	
		Golimumab (Simponi)	

has not responded to other treatment to function. If a patient has severe pain from arthritis, surgery to replace or fuse a joint is often more helpful than drugs.

Nonsteroidal anti-inflammatory drugs   NSAIDs are part of the symptomatic treatment of most types of arthritis because they have analgesic and anti-inflammatory effects and are more effective than pure analgesics such as acetaminophen in relieving the symptoms of RA. In most patients with RA, NSAIDs alone are not sufficient. Although they improve pain, stiffness and swelling, and enhance quality of life, they do not treat the underlying autoimmune problem nor do they alter the course of RA. NSAIDs therefore are almost always used in combination with a DMARD. There is no good evidence that one NSAID is more effective than another, but individual patients often find one drug more helpful than another. The newer COX-2-selective NSAIDs cause fewer peptic ulcers and other serious GI side effects but are no more effective in relieving the symptoms of arthritis than the older drugs. They also have potentially more cardiovascular adverse effects (see NONSTEROIDAL ANTI-INFLAMMATORY DRUGS for discussion of these and other adverse effects). The response to NSAIDs varies among patients. Although pain and swelling improve by approximately 30 percent on average, some patients have a better response and some no response at all. Many patients with RA cannot take an NSAID, either because of allergy or other side effects such as decreased renal function. Their illness can be treated effectively using DMARDs, corticosteroids, and analgesics.

Disease-modifying antirheumatic drugs   DMARDs are used specifically to modify the long-term course of RA by decreasing inflammation. There is no standard treatment for RA. Most but not all patients take DMARDs, and many patients with similar disease receive different drugs.

• *Which Patients with RA Should Take a DMARD?* The approach to DMARD therapy has changed completely over the last 20 years. Originally the approach was to treat RA with NSAIDs alone for as long as possible and to reserve DMARDs for patients with more severe disease. This was understandable, because the DMARDs available at that time, GOLD and PENICILLAMINE, often caused serious side effects, and there was little evidence to show that DMARDs changed the outcome of RA. The modern approach to treating RA is to use one or more DMARDs early in the course of the illness and to try to control the inflammation. There are at least three compelling reasons for this change in approach.

1. There is good evidence showing that the earlier RA is treated the easier it is to control.
2. DMARDs, if started early in the illness, improve long-term outcomes in RA.
3. The side effects of DMARDs no longer outweigh the problems caused by poorly controlled RA. Also, there are now many more DMARDs available so that most patients can find an effective drug that does not cause side effects.

The presence of rheumatoid nodules, a positive rheumatoid factor, many swollen joints and X-ray changes are markers for severe disease with an aggressive course and are indications that a DMARD should be used early in the illness. These days, most rheumatologists, once they have made a firm diagnosis of active RA, will recommend treatment with a DMARD. RA is said to be active when joints are warm, swollen, and tender. In other words, most patients with RA take DMARDs. There are a few exceptions. Rarely patients with RA go into remission on an NSAID alone and there is little benefit to be gained from adding a DMARD. However, over time most of these patients will flare and need a DMARD. Some patients who have had RA for 20 years or more have severely deformed joints but little active inflammation. This is sometimes called burned-out RA. In these patients the risks of DMARDs may outweigh the benefits.

• *Which DMARD Should Be Used?* The choice of DMARD is based on several factors. The most important are the characteristics of the individual DMARDs, the patient, and the severity of the RA.

DMARDs have different characteristics that affect choice. Some are more effective than others, some cost more, and their side effects (discussed in Appendix II) differ. The antitumor necrosis factor (anti-TNF) drugs such as ETANERCEPT, adalimumab, and INFLIXIMAB are at least as effective as METHO-TREXATE, the standard to which other DMARDs are compared. Also anti-TNF drugs act rapidly, within weeks, whereas most other DMARDs act more slowly. However anti-TNF drugs are expensive, costing about $12,000 a year, and increase the risk of infections. Anti-TNF drugs have also been on the market for a shorter time so their long-term side effects are not fully known.

The three anti-TNF agents, infliximab, etanercept, and adalimumab, have now been in use in RA for some years and have shown good efficacy in controlled trials. When added to methotrexate, they are effective at reducing inflammation, slowing joint damage, and improving physical functioning, and many patients report an improvement in their sense of well-being. Although combination with methotrexate is recommended, they have also been used successfully in combination with other DMARDs when methotrexate is contraindicated. Interestingly, although they all target the same molecule, patients who do not respond to one agent frequently respond to one of the others. ANAKINRA is also a biological agent, but one that interferes with the action of IL-1 rather than TNF (see CYTOKINES). Although it produces an improvement when added to methotrexate, it is less effective than the anti-TNF agents.

In clinical trials, SULFASALAZINE, LEFLUNOMIDE, and methotrexate are all about equally effective. Sulfasalazine is widely used in Europe but not in the United States. No one is sure why this difference in practice occurred. In Europe, the feeling is that although sulfasalazine causes more minor side effects than methotrexate, it is not an immunosuppressant, it does not cause liver scarring or methotrexate lung, and alcohol is not prohibited. On the other hand, U.S. physicians feel that methotrexate is better tolerated and more effective than sulfasalazine, and avoiding alcohol is not a great hardship. Leflunomide, as is the case with methotrexate, can also cause liver disease, but it has the disadvantage that it stays in the body for weeks or months after a patient stops taking it. This is particularly important for young women planning to have a family, because leflunomide is harmful to the unborn baby. Leflunomide often causes loose stools, so if a patient already has diarrhea, it is not a good choice.

MINOCYCLINE, AURANOFIN, and HYDROXYCHLO-ROQUINE are not as effective as methotrexate but seldom cause serious side effects. They are usually used to treat milder, early disease. Auranofin often causes diarrhea, and many patients cannot take it.

CYCLOSPORINE is expensive and the patient's kidney function must be monitored closely. It is no more effective than other DMARDs and is usually reserved for patients who cannot take other DMARDs.

RITUXIMAB is a newer biological that depletes B-cells (see IMMUNE RESPONSE). Early studies suggest it is very effective in patients whose RA has been resistant to other medications. Some patients respond to one course of treatment for periods of more than 12 months. It has also been used in combination with methotrexate. More long-term studies are required to fully evaluate its safety and place in the treatment of RA. ABATACEPT is a biological agent that interferes with the full activation of lymphocytes (see immune response and BIOLOGICALS). In a large well-designed trial of patients with resistant RA, it has been shown to be very effective in achieving ACR 50 and 70 responses. However, further experience is required to know where it will fit into the treatment armamentarium.

Gold injections and d-penicillamine are seldom used because they often cause side effects and have been replaced by more effective drugs. A few patients respond very well to gold injections, but most develop side effects.

Rheumatologists vary in their approach to DMARD treatment. Some would use a cheap, relatively nontoxic drug such as hydroxychloroquine first; others would choose methotrexate or sulfasalazine as their first-line agent. Except for anti-TNF drugs, it takes at least eight weeks to determine if a patient is responding to a DMARD. If there is a poor or partial response, the options are to increase the dose of the first DMARD, to switch to another DMARD, or to use a combination of DMARDs.

- *Which DMARD Combinations Are Used?* Most patients with RA receive combination therapy with an NSAID, a DMARD, and sometimes low-dose prednisone, but many also receive more than one DMARD. Aggressive combinations of DMARDs are used to improve control of RA. Many combinations used in clinical practice have not been fully evaluated in clinical trials. The risk of increased side effects has to be weighed against the benefit of improved disease control.

Hydroxychloroquine is used in combination with most other DMARDs. Other combinations include the following:

Methotrexate + cyclosporine
Methotrexate + sulfasalazine + hydroxychloroquine
Methotrexate + TNF antagonists
Methotrexate + leflunomide
Methotrexate + anakinra

The combination of methotrexate and leflunomide has been associated with severe liver disease in a few patients, and experts are debating the future of this combination. Combinations of biological (anti-TNF agents, anakinra, and rituximab) should not be used because of the markedly increased risk of serious infections.

Corticosteroids   Corticosteroids are used in three ways to treat RA.

1. *High Doses for Flares*   Some rheumatologists believe that a single high-dose pulse of an IV corticosteroid such as methylprednisolone is useful to control a disease flare. More often rapidly tapering oral dose packs or a long-acting intramuscular depot corticosteroid are used to control flares. A typical steroid dose pack starts with 40–60 mg of prednisone a day and then steps down to 0 mg over a week or two. People who take a steroid dose pack usually feel much better, and this happens very quickly. Often unless something else is done, this is a temporary solution and the symptoms come back at the end of the steroid treatment. Depot intramuscular corticosteroid injections have an effect that lasts about three to four weeks.
2. *Local Corticosteroid Injection*   A corticosteroid injection into an inflamed joint will often improve symptoms, sometimes for weeks or months (see JOINT INJECTION).

3. *Low Dose Oral Corticosteroids*   The place of steroids in the treatment of RA has changed. Initially when corticosteroids were first discovered, physicians thought that they were the cure for RA. However, the long-term side effects of steroids soon became obvious and there was a swing away from their use. In Europe, most patients with RA do not receive steroids, but in the United States approximately 50 percent of patients with RA take low doses of steroids. The reason for this difference in practice is not clear. In the United States, a low dose of a steroid such as prednisone 2–10 mg is often started early in the illness to try to control the disease rapidly. Steroids have the advantage that they work almost immediately. The plan is usually to taper the steroids slowly once a DMARD has started to work, but many patients remain on prednisone 2–5 mg a day in addition to a DMARD and an NSAID.

Several studies have shown that there are benefits and risks from low-dose steroids. The benefits are a rapid improvement in symptoms and perhaps a slowing in the rate of joint damage. The major risks are an increased rate of osteoporosis and cataracts. Some studies have found an increased risk of infection and even increased mortality associated with corticosteroid treatment in RA. These studies are controversial because patients were not randomly allocated to treatment with or without steroids. In clinical practice patients with more severe RA are treated with steroids, and some physicians believe that some of the apparent risks of low-dose steroids are in fact just markers of more severe RA. In spite of the controversy, rheumatologists agree that if steroids are needed, the lowest effective dose should be prescribed, and the patient must be monitored for side effects such as osteoporosis.

Outcome   Patients with RA frequently suffer silently, and the long-term effects of the disease were not fully understood for many years. The pioneering research of rheumatologists such as Drs. Fred Wolfe and Theodore Pincus who followed cohorts of patients over a long time and carefully measured what happened to them has changed this. Physicians now know that severe RA is associated with functional disability and increased mortality. More than half of the patients with RA who are working when the diagnosis is made will no longer be doing so in 20 years time, and approximately 25 percent will need joint replacement surgery. Physicians now also know that RA is a chronic disease that rarely goes into spontaneous remission, and there is no drug that provides a permanent cure. This means that most patients need lifelong treatment. Recent evidence showing that good control of RA improves long-term outcomes and improves survival.

Historically, the treatments for RA have not been very effective. In clinical trials a measurement called the American College of Rheumatology criteria for 20 percent improvement, or ACR20, is used to determine if a new drug is effective. The ACR20 requires a 20 percent improvement in the number of tender and swollen joints and a 20 percent improvement in three of five measurements (the patient's global assessment of disease activity, the physician's global assessment of disease activity, the patient's assessment of pain, the degree of disability, and the ESR or CRP). Most DMARDs achieve an ACR20 response in about 50 percent of patients, and these patients are considered to have responded to treatment. Thus, RA is often not well controlled in patients who are classified as responding to a DMARD in clinical trials. In clinical practice the results of treatment are often better than in research trials. This is because patients with severe, long-standing disease are more likely to be enrolled in research studies. In clinical practice, though, patients with early disease that responds well to treatment for RA are more frequent. Also in clinical practice combinations of DMARDs are used, whereas in clinical trials that seldom happens.

Many experts believe that the modest goal for RA therapies in clinical trials, a 20 percent improvement, is inappropriate and that research should focus on findings treatments that frequently result in a 50 or 70 percent (ACR 50 and ACR 70) response.

Risk Factors and Preventive Measures

Women and particularly women who do not become pregnant are at increased risk of getting RA as compared to the rest of the population. There are genetic risk factors as discussed above, both as far as possessing the so-called shared epitope on DR4, DR14, and some DR1 beta chains and other less well-defined genes. An example of this is that identical twins will both have RA 15 percent of the time and nonidentical twins only 3.5 percent of the time. These risk factors, however, are not generally subject to modification. Despite the general feeling that infections are implicated in triggering RA, there is insufficient evidence to make any recommendations.

Moderately heavy smokers for more than 20 years have a 1.4 times greater risk of getting RA. Smoking is also associated with more severe RA. The risk of smoking has been shown in many different types of study. One small but interesting study was of 13 twin pairs in whom only one of the pair had RA and only one of the pair smoked. In 12 out of 13, it was the smoking twin who had the RA. This is currently the only obvious modifiable risk factor for RA. Women who breast-feed for more than one year appear to have a slightly lower risk of getting RA.

rheumatoid nodule   Between 25 and 40 percent of patients with RA develop rheumatoid nodules at some time in the course of the disease. These nodules can occur anywhere. However, they are often found just under the skin in areas of the body where there is pressure or friction such as the elbows, hands, and feet. Rarely a patient can have rheumatoid nodules without any arthritis.

The nodules seem to be caused by a combination of RA and some local factor such as friction, pressure, or injury that acts as a trigger.

Symptoms and Diagnostic Path

RA nodules can be seen and felt, but they do not usually cause any symptoms. The nodules are usually firm and movable but can be very hard and fixed to the underlying bone. They are not usually tender. Because they get in the way, they sometimes become painful if they are bumped or irritated by repeated friction. Most patients have between one and four nodules varying in size between that of a dime and a quarter. Some patients, though, particularly those taking METHO-TREXATE, develop many small nodules about the size of a pea on their fingers.

RA nodules can rarely occur in other sites such as the lung or heart. They do not usually cause symptoms in the lungs but in the heart can cause rhythm abnormalities.

The appearance and distribution of the nodules and the fact that the person has RA make the diagnosis easy and a biopsy is seldom needed. A rheumatoid nodule in the lung shows as a spot on a chest X-ray and is difficult to distinguish from cancer or infection without a biopsy. Virtually all patients with rheumatoid nodules have a positive blood test for rheumatoid factor. If this test is negative, the diagnosis of rheumatoid nodule should be reconsidered.

Several other causes of skin nodules can be mistaken for a rheumatoid nodule. GOUT, another illness that causes arthritis and subcutaneous nodules, can be misdiagnosed as RA. The nodules in gout are called tophi and can be mistaken for RA nodules. If a tophus and a rheumatoid nodule cannot be distinguished clinically, a rheumatologist may insert a needle into the nodule and try to aspirate. An RA nodule is fibrous and there is no fluid or tissue in the needle. However, a tophus is made of uric acid crystals and there may be a white, toothpaste-like substance in the needle. Under a microscope this white substance is seen to consist of tightly packed uric acid crystals.

Treatment Options and Outlook

RA nodules are associated with more severe RA. As the disease responds to treatment the nodules, can become smaller or disappear. The response to methotrexate is a little unusual because, although it is an effective drug for controlling RA, patients can develop new nodules while taking it. Nodules do not need any specific treatment. If they ulcerate or become too much of a nuisance, a surgeon can remove them. Unfortunately, they sometimes come back in the same spot. Occasionally rheumatologists try to inject nodules with corticosteroids to make them shrink, and this can be helpful.

rheumatoid vasculitis   Rheumatoid arthritis (RA) can cause inflammation of blood vessels (VASCULITIS). This is rare and affects about 1 percent of patients. Rheumatoid vasculitis appears to have

become less common over the past 30 years in some developed countries, but not the United States.

Virtually all patients with RA and vasculitis have a positive rheumatoid factor. Vasculitis occurs in patients who have had severe disease for a long time, but why some patients get vasculitis and others do not is unclear.

Symptoms and Diagnostic Path

There is a limited form of rheumatoid vasculitis that just causes damage to small blood vessels under the nails, so-called nail-fold vasculitis, which does not cause significant problems and seldom progresses to involve other areas. This does not need any specific treatment. The more severe systemic form of rheumatoid vasculitis particularly affects blood vessels to the skin, nerves, white of the eyes (sclera), heart, and gut.

The first symptoms of systemic vasculitis are usually a rash or skin ulcers. The rash, caused by vasculitis of small blood vessels, is typical of LEUKOCYTOCLASTIC VASCULITIS, with raised purplish spots, usually on the legs, and small hemorrhages around the base of the nails. If larger blood vessels are affected, this causes leg ulcers. Vasculitis can affect the blood vessels that supply the peripheral nerves. If this occurs, it can cause mononeuritis multiplex, a syndrome that causes symptoms in isolated nerves in different parts of the body. The nerves that extend (bend back) the wrist and ankle are often affected and cause symptoms known as foot drop and wrist drop.

The diagnosis is often clinical. However, if there is a rash a biopsy is usually performed because it is an easy and noninvasive way of confirming the diagnosis.

Treatment Options and Outlook

The treatment for rheumatoid vasculitis is as for RA, but if vasculitis is progressing in spite of aggressive treatment, then high doses of CORTICOSTEROIDS, sometimes with CYCLOPHOSPHAMIDE are used. Of the newer agents, RITUXIMAB appears the most effective in patients who have not responded to traditional treatment, but no proper trials have been done due to the small number of patients with this condition. Rheumatoid vasculitis can usually be controlled with treatment, but damaged nerves may not recover.

rheumatologist   A physician specializing in the diagnosis and treatment of rheumatic illness. Rheumatologists first train in internal medicine and then subspecialize in rheumatology. Pediatric rheumatologists are trained in pediatrics and rheumatology. Some rheumatologists also act as internists for their patients and take care of all their other medical problems, but many treat only rheumatic illness. Rheumatologists not only diagnose and treat all types of arthritis but also conditions such as VASCULITIS, where arthritis is not the main problem. Several studies have shown that patients with RA treated by a rheumatologist receive better care and have better outcomes than those who are not. Rheumatologists aspirate and inject joints but do not perform surgery. This is done by orthopedic surgeons who often specialize in one area such as hand surgery or hip and knee replacement.

rotator cuff syndrome   See also SHOULDER PAIN for a description of shoulder function and associated conditions. The rotator cuff consists of a group of four muscles and their tendons that pass outward from the scapula (shoulder blade) to attach to the head of the humerus (upper arm bone). Their attachments start from in front of the humeral head and then pass over the top to just behind so that they grip the head rather like four fingers reaching out to hold it in place. The central muscle, supraspinatus, helps raise the arm to the side and the others help rotate the humerus. However, their most important physiological role is to control the movement of the ball-like humeral head as it rolls and slides on the shallow saucer-shaped glenoid (part of the shoulder blade) as the arm is moved by the more powerful outer muscles. The supraspinatus has to pass beneath the bony tip of the shoulder (the acromion) and its fibrous extension to attach to the top of the humeral head. The supraspinatus is particularly prone to getting squeezed or trapped there. Rotator cuff problems are reasonably common at all ages, but the cause differs at different ages. The term rotator cuff syndrome includes tendinitis and tears that may be partial or full thickness.

In younger patients the rotator cuff may be torn during overhead sports such as swimming, tennis, volleyball, or throwing. Patients under the age of 40 years usually have a partial tear. People taking part in throwing sports who have even minor instability are at high risk of getting rotator cuff tears. Tendinitis or inflammation of the tendon occurs in a similar manner, and in many instances both are present. Complete tears are usually the result of a violent fall with the arm stretched out.

Tendinitis comes on more slowly in the middle-aged patient and is associated with early degenerative or wear and tear changes in the tendon. In addition, loss of scapulohumeral rhythm becomes more common and frequently causes impingement on the rotator cuff tendons. Dislocation of the shoulder in a middle-aged patient is usually associated with a complete tendon rupture. In the older patient the pain tends to be less severe and of a more gradual onset. Many older patients first complain of the loss of range of movement rather than the pain. They are very frequently found to have tears without a specific history of injury.

Symptoms and Diagnostic Path

Younger patients have a rapid onset of pain and can usually relate it to a specific event or activity. There is aching in the shoulder and a sharp pain with lifting activities. The shoulder can usually be moved through a full range despite the pain with tendinitis or partial tears. With a complete supraspinatus tear the arm cannot be lifted away from the side.

Middle-aged patients have a more gradual onset of pain and have some limitation of movement, especially reaching behind their backs. They are often aware of the activities that make it worse. Working above shoulder height is painful and may become impossible. Night pain is common when rolling onto the affected shoulder. As time goes on there is often some associated weakness and loss of scapulohumeral rhythm. Elderly patients present with similar symptoms but often without any obvious injury or repetitive activity that might have caused it.

Rotator cuff tendinitis is suspected from the history and confirmed by showing that the pain occurs as the affected tendon is moved under the bony tip of the shoulder (acromion). The arm is raised above the head and then brought down slowly to the side. There is an arc of movement during which there is pain, and then the pain is relieved as the arm gets close to the body again and the swollen inflamed part of the tendon passes beyond the acromion. With a complete tendon tear the arm cannot be lifted away from the side by the patient. However if the examiner starts to lift the arm, the patient can then continue to raise it using the deltoid muscle. Degenerative changes in the cuff may be suspected when the head of the humerus is seen to ride up underneath the acromion. This suggests that the rotator cuff is no longer competent to hold it down in place. The biceps tendon is injured in many rotator cuff problems and may be tender to touch as it crosses the front of the shoulder.

Ultrasound examination is the best way to confirm the diagnosis. It can show the swelling of the tendon that occurs in tendinitis as well as the tendon crumpling up as it sticks when moved under the acromion. It will also demonstrate tears accurately. X-rays may show bony spurs below the acromioclavicular joint that can impinge on the supraspinatus tendon, glenohumeral joint damage, or other bony changes. An MRI scan will show the changes in the tendon just as well as ultrasound, but the arm cannot be moved during this to show that the tendon is catching.

Treatment Options and Outlook

A certain amount of rest and alteration of activities is necessary to allow healing of tendinitis to take place. With mild tendinitis NSAIDs may improve the pain and settle the inflammation. In more severe tendinitis a CORTICOSTEROID injection into the subacromial bursa is very effective in settling the inflammation. If there is an ongoing cause this must be addressed or the condition will simply recur. This may be faulty swimming technique in the young athlete or loss of normal scapular movement due to a functional scoliosis (curvature in the spine) in the older patient. Even when the initiating event was traumatic, rehabilitation is often required to restore normal movement of the shoulder complex as a whole. Younger patients with instability need an intensive stabilization program. Sometimes severe instability will require surgical intervention. Occasionally patients do not respond to these measures, particularly if they are unable to participate fully in a rehabilitation program. In this situation the tip of the acromion can be surgically removed and any inflammatory tissue cleaned away from the tendon. Bony spurs can also be removed from the underside of the acromioclavicular joint. This surgery is usually done by ARTHROSCOPY these days.

Partial tears of the rotator cuff tendons are initially managed as for tendinitis, except that corticosteroid injections are best avoided for the first four to six weeks to allow healing to take place. Complete tears in active young patients are usually repaired surgically. In older patients rehabilitation is often tried first and surgery used only if the outcome is not good. If the biceps tendon and the supraspinatus tendon are ruptured, then surgical repair should be undertaken since these patients often develop a severe destructive form of arthritis at the shoulder if repair is not undertaken.

Risk Factors and Preventive Measures

Work and sports involving overhead actions are the major risk factors in young and middle-aged people. Training to maintain good core stability and therefore the ability to stabilize the body and shoulder in the optimum position for movement is of prime importance in preventing injury. Balanced strength and flexibility at the shoulder are important, especially in athletes undertaking weight training to boost their performance. Those with instability of the gleno-humeral joint or generalized hypermobility may need specialized training or activity modification to prevent injury. In older people, maintenance of general fitness, ideal body weight, and avoidance of falls will reduce the risk of rotator cuff problems.

rubella (German measles) A viral illness common in childhood. In developed countries such as the United States rubella is now rare. Routine vaccination of children against rubella has decreased the incidence of disease. Rubella, and the vaccine used to prevent it, can cause arthritis and arthralgia.

The illness is caused by the rubella virus that is transmitted from person to person by contact or by droplets when an infected person coughs, sneezes, or talks.

Symptoms and Diagnostic Path

After someone has come into contact with an infected person and becomes infected, the virus incubates for two to three weeks. The first symptom is usually a red, blotchy rash on the face, trunk, and arms. The lymph nodes behind the ear and at the back of the head are often enlarged, and many patients have headache and a runny nose. The symptoms of rubella may be so mild that many patients do not notice them. Some patients, particularly adults, develop arthritis. The rash and arthritis often occur together at the time the patient is making antibodies against the virus, suggesting that the arthritis is due to antigen-antibody complexes. Rubella arthritis can affect large or small joints, and because it is often symmetric it can be mistaken for RA. However, rubella arthritis settles within a few weeks without any specific treatment. There are a few reports of more persistent arthritis after rubella infection. Arthralgia and myalgia are common after rubella vaccination, but arthritis is not. If it does occur, the pattern of arthritis is the same as that occurring after natural rubella infection.

Blood tests for antibodies against rubella are elevated in infected patients. If someone has recently been infected the IgM antibody is elevated, but if only the IgG antibody is elevated it means that the person was immunized against rubella or was infected in the past. The rubella virus has been isolated from inflamed joints in patients with arthritis, but this test is seldom performed.

Treatment Options and Outlook

There is no specific treatment for rubella or rubella arthritis. NSAIDs will relieve arthritis symptoms, which usually last only a few weeks and resolve spontaneously. The most serious complications of rubella are birth abnormalities in unborn babies. If a pregnant woman who is not immune to the disease becomes infected with rubella, the chance that she will have a baby with abnormalities of the heart, brain, or other organs is high. This was the impetus for recommending routine vaccination for all children. As a result of widespread vaccination, rubella is now very uncommon in the United States.

S

SAPHO syndrome (sternoclavicular hyperostosis, acne arthritis) Synovitis, acne, pustules, hyperostosis, and osteitis comprise the SAPHO syndrome. This is a rare illness that affects young adults who have arthritis or osteitis associated with acne or skin conditions that cause pustules.

The cause of SAPHO syndrome is not known. Some rheumatologists believe that it is a type of REACTIVE ARTHRITIS triggered by acne or acnelike skin problems; others believe that it is an infective arthritis caused by an unidentified organism. Most attempts to culture an organism have failed. In a few cases, though, *Propionibacterium acnes,* the organism that causes acne, has been isolated. In some studies there was a small increase in the frequency of the HLA-B27 tissue type, suggesting a genetic component. SAPHO syndrome can occur in association with pustular PSORIASIS and INFLAMMATORY BOWEL DISEASE.

Symptoms and Diagnostic Path

Arthritis is usually asymmetrical and affects large joints, a pattern characteristic of a reactive arthritis. Acne or some other skin condition that forms pustules is usually present, but the bone lesions can antedate the skin problems. If acne is the underlying skin condition, there are many large and deep pustules that cause painful lumps. Hyperostosis, thickening of a bone, often affects the collarbone (clavicle) and can resemble an infection (osteitis). Patients often develop pustules on their palms and soles.

The diagnosis is clinical. X-rays may show hyperostosis or osteitis of the clavicle or another affected bone. The X-ray appearance of the bones often suggests the diagnosis of OSTEOMYELITIS, and biopsies may have to be done to exclude this. Osteitis can affect the clavicle, pelvis, ribs, jaw, and other bones. The ESR is usually high, and patients may become anemic. Immunoglobulins (see IMMUNE RESPONSE) are usually raised, especially IgA. This is in keeping with an ongoing immune response at a mucosal border or skin surface.

Treatment Options and Outlook

Part of the treatment is to control the pustular skin condition, often with antibiotic ointments or tablets, but this seldom controls musculoskeletal symptoms. NONSTEROIDAL ANTI-INFLAMMATORY DRUGS (NSAIDs) often work remarkably well, reducing pain, increasing energy, and improving abnormal blood tests. However, in severe disease, this improvement is only for as long as the NSAID is taken regularly at good doses, and long-term NSAID use poses its own problems. SULFASALAZINE, COLCHICINE, METHOTREXATE, and, more recently, INFLIXIMAB have been used with at least some success. However, the most successful treatment seems to be with BISPHOSPHONATES. The bisphosphonate most frequently used has been intravenous PAMIDRONATE. Because SAPHO syndrome is rare, there are no randomized trials of treatment, but from the reports available pamidronate appears to be successful in virtually all patients. It resolves bony pain, corrects blood abnormalities, improves patient well-being, improves the appearance of the bone on X-ray, and even temporarily resolves palmar-plantar pustulosis, one of the associated skin conditions. Other bisphosphonates have also been reported to work. As most of these patients are young, it is best to limit the dose of bisphosphonate to the minimum required to control symptoms so as not to interfere with normal bone growth.

sarcoidosis   An illness that causes inflammation in many organ systems, primarily the lungs. Arthralgia or arthritis occurs in approximately 25 percent of patients. Sarcoidosis is more common in African Americans than in Caucasians and usually affects young adults, most often women.

The cause of sarcoidosis is not known. The similarity of the illness to tuberculosis and the observation that sarcoidosis has been transmitted by organ transplantation suggest an infection, but many researchers have tried unsuccessfully to identify an infectious cause. Characteristically sarcoidosis causes granulomas in tissue. Granulomas, visible under a microscope, are clusters of inflammatory cells arranged in a pattern. Tuberculosis also causes granulomas, but these have areas of dead tissue (caseation), whereas those in sarcoidosis are do not caseate.

Symptoms and Diagnostic Path

The symptoms of sarcoidosis depend on the organs involved. The lungs are affected in 90 percent of patients. The first symptom is often ERYTHEMA NODOSUM and enlargement of lymph nodes at the root of both lungs (bilateral hilar lymphadenopathy). The enlarged lymph nodes do not cause symptoms and may be discovered only incidentally if a chest X-ray is performed for some other reason. In most patients with enlarged lymph nodes the illness resolves. Some do progress and develop inflammation and scarring of the lung tissue that causes coughing and shortness of breath. Later in the disease the lymph nodes in the lung are no longer enlarged, but the scarring persists.

Sarcoidosis can involve almost any other organ. Rash; eye inflammation (see EYE PROBLEMS); enlarged parotid glands (the salivary glands in the cheeks); and heart, liver, nerve, and brain involvement can occur. Arthritis in early sarcoidosis occurs at the same time as erythema nodosum. This usually affects ankles, knees, or hands. There may be dactylitis, causing sausage digits as in REACTIVE ARTHRITIS. If a joint is biopsied, granuloma may be seen. The constellation of erythema nodosum, bilateral hilar lymphadenopathy, and ankle arthritis is called Lofgren's syndrome. There is often swelling, warmth, and tenderness around the joint (periarthritis) as well as directly over it. The arthritis associated with early sarcoidosis usually resolves over several months. A few patients develop chronic arthritis, which usually does not damage joints or cartilage.

Sarcoidosis can cause bone cysts, most often in the small bones of the fingers in an area affected by skin rash. Muscle involvement is common, but most patients do not have symptoms. A few can develop painful nodular swellings in muscle or weakness with elevated levels of muscle enzymes, resembling polymyositis (see DERMATOMYOSITIS AND POLYMYOSITIS).

The diagnosis of sarcoidosis is usually suspected clinically and confirmed by biopsy of affected tissue that shows granulomas without caseation. A biopsy is performed not only to confirm the diagnosis of sarcoidosis but also to exclude infection and malignancy. Some physicians will accept a clinical diagnosis in patients with bilateral hilar lymphadenopathy and erythema nodosum without a biopsy because the pattern is so classical. A blood test that measures levels of angiotensin-converting enzyme (ACE) is often elevated in patients with active sarcoidosis, but it is not sensitive or specific enough to make or exclude the diagnosis.

Treatment Options and Outlook

Many patients with sarcoidosis do not need any specific treatment because the disease remits. In patients with eye, lung, joint, or other organ involvement, CORTICOSTEROIDS are the first line of treatment. Many other drugs are used to treat patients who do not respond or who need high doses of corticosteroids to control their disease. METHOTREXATE is one such drug, but patients with sarcoidosis may be more sensitive to side effects and be more likely to develop hepatitis. Other drugs used to treat sarcoidosis are AZATHIOPRINE, HYDROXYCHLOROQUINE, and CYCLOSPORINE. NSAIDs are prescribed to control pain, but there is no specific treatment for arthritis associated with sarcoidosis. The treatment is usually determined by the effects of the disease on other organs.

scleroderma (systemic sclerosis, progressive systemic sclerosis)   A chronic illness characterized by increased fibrous tissue in the skin and internal organs, damage to small blood vessels, and the presence of autoantibodies. Scleroderma is rare. There are approximately 10 new cases per million people per year. Women get it three times more often than men, and people aged 30–50 years are most often affected. Scleroderma is divided into two major subgroups, diffuse and limited scleroderma, depending on how much skin is involved. The two groups have different clinical symptoms and treatment.

Diffuse scleroderma (diffuse systemic sclerosis) This involves rapid onset of skin changes that affect the hands, face, and central parts of the body such as the trunk, back, and abdomen within a year of developing RAYNAUD'S PHENOMENON. Organs such as the lungs, GI tract, and kidneys are often affected. Very rarely scleroderma can affect the internal organs and not the skin. This is called *scleroderma sine scleroderma.*

Limited scleroderma (limited cutaneous systemic sclerosis, CREST syndrome) This involves gradual skin tightening limited to the hands, forearms, face, and feet that develops after a patient has had Raynaud's phenomenon for many years. Apart from PULMONARY HYPERTENSION internal organ involvement is much less common than in diffuse scleroderma.

In addition, there are rare variants of scleroderma such as morphea or linear scleroderma that affect only the skin and underlying tissue. Morphea consists of reddish patches of scleroderma-like skin scattered over the body. If it affects the whole body it is called generalized morphea. Linear scleroderma is usually limited to one area and looks like a scar or tight band of skin. It was called coup de sabre when it affected the face because it looked as if the face had been scarred by a blow from a sword.

The cause of scleroderma is not known. Different mechanisms such as increased production of fibrous tissue, activation of the immune system, and damage to small blood vessels play a role. Why they become activated, though, is not known.

There is some evidence suggesting an autoimmune cause. Most patients with scleroderma have a positive blood test for autoantibodies such as antinuclear antibodies (ANA) (see Appendix II). Early in the disease there is some infiltration of lympho-

cytes in affected organs. Considering the amount of tissue damage, the amount of immunological activation is unimpressive. Many trials attempting to treat scleroderma with immunosuppressive drugs have failed. This suggests that although an early immunological trigger may be important, once the disease is established, other factors take over. The usual response to an injury is a rapid movement of inflammatory cells to the injured site, resulting in the release of cytokines and growth factors that activate fibroblasts that form scar tissue and then become inactive. This is probably the same process that is active in scleroderma, but for reasons that are not understood, the fibroblasts remain active and continue to produce fibrous tissue.

The key abnormality in scleroderma is that fibroblasts, cells that produce fibrous tissue, are activated so that normal tissue is replaced by fibrous tissue. Fibroblasts are part of normal connective tissue. They are usually inactive but can produce exuberant amounts of fibrous tissue when stimulated. Cytokines such as interleukin-1 and growth factors such as transforming growth factor-β (TGF-β) and platelet-derived growth factor (PDGF) can activate fibroblasts. Why this occurs much more exuberantly in scleroderma than in other inflammatory diseases is not clear. Interestingly, fibroblasts obtained from skin biopsies of patients with scleroderma maintain their ability to produce excessive amounts of fibrous tissue when cultured in the laboratory. These fibroblasts have no contact with the patient's immune system and therefore must somehow have been reprogrammed to produce excessive amounts of fibrous tissue independent of immune regulation. This observation suggests that in scleroderma perhaps the immune system has long-lasting effects on fibroblasts. The implication is that in established scleroderma drugs that decrease fibrosis may be more likely to help than drugs aimed at the immune system.

Symptoms and Diagnostic Path
Diffuse Scleroderma

Skin Virtually all patients with scleroderma have Raynaud's phenomenon. It is important to remember that this symptom is common, even in healthy people, and does not imply a diagnosis of scleroderma. In diffuse scleroderma skin changes usually follow soon after the onset of Raynaud's. In early disease the skin may be more puffy and edematous than fibrotic, but it soon progresses to become thick and inelastic. As people age the skin loses tone and becomes baggier so that lifting a pinch of skin from virtually anywhere on the body is easy. In patients with scleroderma the skin becomes tight and is difficult to lift by pinching gently. In patients with severe disease the skin is totally immobile and is called *hidebound*. In clinical trials the severity of skin involvement in patients with diffuse scleroderma is scored by grading how difficult it is to pinch the skin at several defined sites. This is called the Rodnan score, after Dr. G. P. Rodnan.

Scleroderma can affect skin in virtually any part of the body but most often the hands, arms, face, and trunk. The skin and soft tissues of the hands can become so tight that the fingers can hardly move. Small ulcers can develop at the tips of the fingers. Tight skin on the face can make someone look younger because his or her wrinkles disappear. If the skin around the mouth is tight, it can be difficult to open widely. Over several years the skin may improve a little, but most of the changes are permanent. This spontaneous improvement in skin tightness is a feature of scleroderma that has made it difficult for researchers to assess the true effect of drugs.

Joints, tendons, and muscles Arthralgia is common but arthritis is rare. Fibrosis can affect tendons and cause a symptom called a friction rub. This is a squeaky, rasping, scratchy noise that occurs when the tendon moves. Sometimes it is audible without a stethoscope. The patient can often feel the friction rub by placing a hand over the tendon when it is moving. Fibrosis of tendons, skin, and the soft tissue underneath the skin can limit or sometimes prevent movement at a joint (contractures). Patients often lose muscle bulk and become weak because of poor mobility and deconditioning rather than the disease itself. However, inflammation of muscle causing weakness of the thighs and shoulders can also occur. This proximal myositis can be difficult to diagnose unless muscle enzymes are checked.

Gastrointestinal system Scleroderma can occur in any part of the gastrointestinal tract but most often affects the esophagus. Fibrous tissue in the esophagus impairs its ability to coordinate the muscle contraction and relaxation that is needed to swallow efficiently. Difficulty swallowing, reflux of acid and food from the stomach into the mouth, and heartburn are common symptoms of gastro esophageal reflux disease (GERD). This affects more than 80 percent of patients. Poor motility can cause reflux esophagitis (inflammation of the lower part of the esophagus), and this can lead to narrowing (stricture) that further impairs swallowing.

Scleroderma can affect the stomach and small intestine, causing decreased motility that results in delayed emptying. This causes symptoms such as bloating, nausea, vomiting, loss of weight, abdominal pain, and constipation. The motility of the bowel can be slowed so much that it leads to symptoms such as severe pain, abdominal swelling, and vomiting, a clinical situation that resembles obstruction of the bowel and is called *pseudoobstruction*. Paradoxically, partial obstruction of the bowel can cause diarrhea. The decreased emptying of loops of bowel allows bacteria to flourish, and this results in diarrhea. This is called the *blind loop syndrome* and can lead to malabsorption of essential nutrients, particularly fat and the fat-soluble vitamins A, D, E, and K. Severe constipation can also occur and sometimes paradoxically cause diarrhea. The bowel becomes semiobstructed with hard stool, and the only stool that can squeeze past is liquid. This is called *overflow diarrhea*.

Scleroderma can sometime cause areas of weakness in the wall of the bowel, and small pockets form. These fill with air and gas produced by bacteria which show as many small air pockets on an X-ray. This is called *pneumatosis intestinalis*.

Respiratory system The lungs are often involved in systemic scleroderma. Inflammation in the lungs leads to formation of scar tissue, called interstitial lung disease. This can be mild and cause no symptoms or more severe, causing shortness of breath and cough. Shortness of breath, particularly when the person performs moderately strenuous activities, is usually much more of a problem than coughing. If a lot of fibrosis is in the lungs it may lead to infections that worsen the scarring. Severe lung disease can lead to failure of the right side of the heart, which pumps blood to the lungs. It does so by elevating the pressure in the pulmonary arteries, a condition called secondary PULMONARY HYPERTENSION.

Renal disease One of the most serious complications is scleroderma renal crisis. This usually occurs early in the illness in patients with severe diffuse scleroderma and consists of sudden onset of high blood pressure and renal failure. The cause is not known, and if a biopsy is performed, the kidney tissue itself is relatively normal. In contrast with SLE, there is little inflammation and no deposits of immunoglobulins clogging up the filtration mechanism. In scleroderma renal crisis the small arteries of the kidneys are narrowed and do not carry enough blood through the kidneys. Patients with scleroderma renal crisis may not have symptoms until kidney function is severely affected and causes symptoms such as nausea, vomiting, fatigue, and anemia.

Heart Scleroderma often affects the heart, but this seldom causes symptoms. Occasionally fibrosis of the heart can cause heart failure or an abnormal rhythm. Inflammation of heart muscle (myocarditis) and pericarditis can occur and seem to be more common in patients who also have myositis.

Limited Scleroderma Many patients with limited scleroderma have the five classical symptoms that comprise the CREST syndrome: calcinosis, Raynaud's phenomenon, esophageal dysmotility, sclerodactyly, and telangiectasia. The term CREST syndrome is derived from the first letter of each of these symptoms, but it is also often used to describe patients with limited scleroderma who have only three or four of the symptoms of CREST. Some physicians use the terms CREST syndrome and limited scleroderma interchangeably.

Skin Virtually all patients with limited scleroderma have Raynaud's phenomenon, and this is often present for many years before skin changes develop. Severe Raynaud's leading to painful, poorly healing ulcers on the tips of the fingers, called digital ulcers, is more common in patients with limited scleroderma than in those with diffuse scleroderma. Digital ulcers are very painful and heal over several months. The skin changes of limited scleroderma often affect only the hands and face but can be severe, leading to tight, shiny, poorly mobile fingers, or very subtle with just a little skin thickening. Tightness of the skin on the fingers is called sclerodactyly. Many patients also have telangiectasia. These are small red spots, about the size of a freckle, that consist of a network of blood vessels. Calcinosis (deposits of calcium in the skin and soft tissues) is less common.

Respiratory system In addition to the mildness of the skin and internal organ involvement, a major feature that characterizes limited scleroderma and differentiates it from diffuse disease is pulmonary hypertension. Patients with limited scleroderma have a predisposition to develop pulmonary hypertension that is virtually identical to primary pulmonary hypertension. Patients with diffuse scleroderma can also develop pulmonary hypertension, but this is usually milder and due to fibrosis of the lungs. In patients with limited scleroderma and pulmonary hypertension, the lungs themselves are fairly normal and the problem is in the small blood vessels of the lungs. The walls of these small blood vessels become thick and fibrotic, and the channel through which blood can flow is narrowed. Pulmonary hypertension develops in about 5 percent of patients and causes symptoms of fatigue, shortness of breath, fainting, and heart failure.

Gastrointestinal system Limited scleroderma usually affects only the esophagus and causes the same symptoms as diffuse scleroderma.

Diagnosis

The diagnosis of diffuse and limited scleroderma is clinical and depends on an astute clinician noticing the typical skin changes. These can be very subtle, particularly in patients with limited disease. On the other hand, diffuse scleroderma is usually easy to diagnose because the skin changes are severe and often progress rapidly. A skin biopsy is sometimes performed but is seldom needed to diagnose scleroderma. Other symptoms can be helpful in making the diagnosis. For example, virtually all patients with scleroderma also have Raynaud's phenomenon, and many have symptoms of GERD.

Blood tests are not particularly helpful; there is no specific blood test to diagnose scleroderma. Almost all patients with scleroderma have a positive ANA test, a test usually thought of for SLE. The pattern of the ANA test can give a clue to the diagnosis. A nucleolar pattern is more common in diffuse scleroderma and a centromere pattern in limited scleroderma. These patterns, however, are not diagnostic for scleroderma. Blood tests can be helpful in following a patient with Raynaud's phenomenon and no other features of autoimmune disease. Someone who has a positive ANA test and Raynaud's phenomenon would be followed more closely than someone with a negative ANA.

Tests for other autoantibodies are not specific or sensitive enough to make them helpful for most patients in clinical practice but are sometimes performed. An autoantibody, Scl-70, is found in about 50 percent of patients with diffuse scleroderma, and another, anticentromere antibody, in about 70 percent of patients with limited scleroderma. Another autoantibody, Jo-1, is found in approximately 20 percent of patients and is associated with a higher risk of developing lung disease.

Blood tests are helpful in diagnosing complications of scleroderma. Anemia and a rise in the serum creatinine concentration are typical of scleroderma renal crisis, and elevated creatine kinase levels are typical of myositis.

Other tests are often performed to diagnose complications of scleroderma. For example, if a patient has trouble swallowing, a barium swallow or an upper GI endoscopy will provide information about the function of the esophagus. X-rays can help diagnose lung disease in patients with diffuse scleroderma, but telling from X-rays if the lung disease is currently active or not is difficult. A high-resolution CT of the chest can be helpful in this situation. Active inflammation shows up as a uniform, smooth opaque area on the scan, called a *ground glass appearance*. Old scarred areas show up as streaky dense opacities. The CT scan can be very important in helping physicians decide how to treat scleroderma lung disease. If there is active inflammation, cyclophosphamide is the recommended treatment. If there is irreversible old scarring, the drug may cause more harm than good. Many physicians are uncomfortable relying entirely on the results of the CT scan to make this decision and order a bronchoscopy. This involves passing a thin fiberoptic instrument through the mouth or nose, between the vocal cords and down into the lungs and using it to flush sterile saline into a segment of lung and aspirate the fluid. This process is called bronchoalveolar lavage or BAL. If the BAL fluid contains many inflammatory cells such as neutrophils, it is a good indicator that there is active inflammation in the lung.

If pulmonary hypertension is suspected, the diagnosis can be made and the pressure in the pulmonary artery estimated by ultrasound. In some patients the pressure is measured more accurately by placing a catheter in the right side of the heart by threading it up through a large vein in the leg. The chest X-ray may show an enlarged heart, and in patients with CREST and pulmonary hypertension the lungs are normal. In patients with diffuse scleroderma and secondary pulmonary hypertension the lungs are abnormal and the chest X-ray shows a lot of scarring. A lung biopsy is usually avoided because there is a risk of bleeding.

Treatment Options and Outlook

There is no specific treatment for scleroderma. This is not because of lack of research effort. Virtually every drug used to treat other rheumatological conditions has been tried. Clinical trials are difficult to perform and interpret because scleroderma is rare, varies in severity and outcome, and few patients are willing to take a placebo (see CLINICAL TRIAL). Before researchers realized that the skin changes of scleroderma often improved spontaneously over time, many drugs tested in open-label studies acquired an undeserved reputation for being effective. Another important consideration is that most clinical trials have focused on measuring skin changes. The effects of scleroderma on the skin are cosmetically important and, if severe, can affect function, particularly of the hands, but do not shorten life. Thus many trials measured an outcome that was mainly of cosmetic significance. In short, many of the early studies on scleroderma were not helpful.

Skin symptoms The treatment of Raynaud's phenomenon is discussed under that heading. D-PENICILLAMINE is a drug that was regarded, on the basis of open-label studies, as an effective treatment for the skin changes of scleroderma. A placebo-controlled study compared two doses, 1,000 mg a day (an average therapeutic dose) and 125 mg every other day (a dose much lower than the one usually prescribed). The reason for comparing a therapeutic dose with one that was thought to be ineffective was that it avoided randomizing some patients to placebo. Therefore all patients received penicillamine, but some received a dose that was so small it was virtually a placebo. The study found little difference between the two doses. Many rheumatologists interpret these results as showing that penicillamine is not effective, but others interpret them as supporting low-dose penicillamine as a treatment for scleroderma. The use of penicillamine decreased after this study was published.

METHOTREXATE was effective in two uncontrolled studies. However, a double-blind, placebo-controlled study of 71 patients with diffuse scleroderma published by Dr. J. E. Pope and her colleagues in 2001 reported no statistically significant effect. There was a trend favoring methotrexate above placebo, but the benefits of methotrexate, if any, appear to be small.

Relaxin is a chemical produced in pregnancy that decreases the production of collagen, allowing skin and soft tissues to stretch and accommodate the growth and delivery of a baby. Preliminary studies with relaxin in scleroderma were promising, but this was not borne out in later studies.

CORTICOSTEROIDS can improve the swelling and edema that are part of early scleroderma. Because scleroderma renal crisis occurs more often in patients taking corticosteroids, though they are usually avoided if possible.

Several other treatments have been tried with mixed results. These include PHOTOPHERESIS, COLCHICINE, gamma interferon, and CYCLOSPORINE. No treatment has been convincingly effective. Cyclosporine often causes renal side effects such as decreased renal function and high blood pressure, problems that are already common in patients with scleroderma, and is seldom used outside of clinical trials. A small preliminary study found that patients responded to MINOCYCLINE, but larger studies were negative. Studies with TNF antagonists and BONE MARROW TRANSPLANTATION are under way.

Respiratory symptoms Both major causes of lung disease in scleroderma, interstitial fibrosis and pulmonary hypertension, can be treated. If interstitial lung disease causes lung fibrosis, this is irreversible. If there is inflammation, aggressive immunosuppression can stabilize lung function and improve the prognosis. CYCLOPHOSPHAMIDE has stabilized lung function in several small studies. Two recent randomized, placebo-controlled trials did show some benefit of treatment with cyclophosphamide, but not a great deal. Because prolonged treatment with cyclophosphamide is dangerous, treatment was stopped after one year, and a two-year follow-up was done in one of these studies. Apart from the patients feeling less breathless, all the other lung-function tests had relapsed to be similar to the placebo-treated patients by the end of the second year. In another study, treating the 60 percent of patients who either improved or stabilized on cyclophosphamide with ongoing AZATHIOPRINE did maintain the improvement. These studies have shown that the CT findings predict response to treatment reasonably, but bronchiolar lavage hardly at all. Research continues on developing strategies with drugs such as MYCOPHENOLATE MOFETIL, pirfenidone, gamma interferon, and ETANERCEPT, but without any clear breakthroughs as yet. Treatment of pulmonary hypertension, both secondary as usually seen in diffuse scleroderma and of the primary vascular type seen in the CREST syndrome, has made some progress and is discussed under pulmonary hypertension.

Gastrointestinal symptoms GERD is managed with general measures such as elevating the head of the bed, not eating or drinking for several hours before bedtime, and eating small meals, but most patients also require medications. Proton pump inhibitors such as OMEPRAZOLE, LANSOPRAZOLE, and RABEPRAZOLE decrease acid production in the stomach and improve reflux symptoms. Metoclopramide (trade name: Reglan) can improve symptoms by decreasing spasm in the lower esophagus. CISAPRIDE (trade name: Propulsid) stimulates esophageal motility, but a serious, sometimes fatal heart rhythm problem called torsade de pointes has severely restricted its use. If there is a stricture in the esophagus, the patients may require esophageal dilation.

Agents that increase the motility of the bowel such as cisapride, erythromycin and ocreotide improve symptoms of pseudoobstruction. The combination of erythromycin and cisapride must be avoided because the risk of torsade de pointes is increased. If there is a blind-loop syndrome, rotating courses of different antibiotics such as amoxi-cillin, tetracycline, and ciprofloxacin decrease bacterial overgrowth and improve symptoms. In some patients with severe malabsorption, nutrition is provided intravenously. This is called total parenteral nutrition or TPN.

Constipation can be very difficult to treat. It usually requires a special diet, drugs to increase the motility of the bowel, and laxatives.

Renal symptoms Scleroderma renal crisis is a serious complication and can lead to permanent renal failure requiring dialysis or lead to death. Blood pressure should be monitored carefully in all patients with diffuse scleroderma, and hypertension should be treated with an angiotensin-converting enzyme (ACE) inhibitor, a class of drug that has improved the outcome substantially. Blood pressure should be controlled with some urgency, and if there is any deterioration in kidney function the patient should be admitted to the hospital for intensive treatment and monitoring. Other drugs may be required in addition to the ACE inhibitor and, where available, continuous infusion of prostacyclin is sometimes effective. Accelerated hypertension that is not controlled can lead to renal failure. If this happens, dialysis is often needed, but sometimes if blood pressure is controlled, renal function recovers slowly over several months and some patients can come off dialysis.

The overall prognosis of scleroderma depends on the severity of organ involvement and tracks with the severity of skin involvement. Severe vascular pulmonary hypertension has a worse outlook when associated with scleroderma than when it is an isolated disease entity. Even with the newer therapies, there is probably only a 50 percent two-year survival currently. Patients going into a renal crisis now have a greater than 80 percent survival at one year compared to the 15 percent they would have had 25 years ago. Fibrotic lung disease and heart involvement also indicate a worse prognosis.

Risk Factors and Preventive Measures

Although there is an increased risk of getting scleroderma in the relatives of a patient, this is much less than most other connective tissue diseases, and the overall risk is still small. Infection with human cytomegalovirus (CMV) and other viruses has been linked to the onset of disease, but there is no definite proof as yet. A number of scleroderma-like diseases have resulted from drug or toxin ingestion. The anticancer drug, bleomycin, and cocaine can cause scleroderma-like disease, as can radiation therapy given to treat cancers. In Spain, ingestion of contaminated rapeseed oil led to an outbreak of a scleroderma-like disease called toxic oil syndrome. Despite these occurrences, careful study of true scleroderma patients has failed to find any common environmental link.

septic arthritis See INFECTIVE ARTHRITIS.

septic bursitis Bursas, or small sacs lined with synovial cells close to joints and tendons, can become inflamed as part of most types of inflammatory arthritis but can also become infected with bacteria. Usually bacteria gain access to the bursa through superficial skin abrasions that can occur as part of usual day-to-day activities. The olecranon (over the elbow) and the prepatellar (in front of the kneecap) bursas become infected most frequently.

Symptoms and Diagnostic Path
The symptoms of warmth, redness, exquisite tenderness, and decreased range of motion of the joint are similar to those that occur with other inflammatory causes of olecranon bursitis such as gout or repetitive trauma. Usually septic bursitis causes more severe symptoms, but infective and inflammatory bursitis can be difficult to distinguish.

Any activity that causes friction or repeated minor trauma to a bursa can cause bursitis and increases the chance of inflammation and infection. For example, patients in nursing homes who cannot walk often develop olecranon bursitis because they rest their weight on their elbows. Occupations such as carpet laying or roofing can also cause prepatellar bursitis. If bacteria gain access to the inflamed bursa, this can turn into a septic bursitis.

Because of the difficulty in knowing whether the bursa is infected, a needle is often inserted into the bursa, fluid is aspirated and then sent to the laboratory for culture. Infective bursitis is most often caused by *Staphylococcus aureus* infection.

Treatment Options and Outlook

The infection often responds to a course of oral antibiotics that cover this organism. If the clinical response is delayed, intravenous antibiotics, repeated aspiration of the bursa, or surgical drainage of the pus may be needed. (See also BURSITIS.)

shingles   See HERPES ZOSTER.

shoulder pain   The shoulder joint is a very complex joint with numerous potential causes of pain. The design of the joint is such as to allow the greatest possible range of movement of the arm. There is a trade-off between stability and range of movement, and the shoulder joint is therefore inherently one of the least stable joints in the body.

The shoulder joints   Strictly speaking, the shoulder joint should be referred to as complex since there are in fact four joints that all move together to allow normal shoulder movement.

The glenohumeral joint   This joint exists between the upper arm bone, the humerus, and a shallow saucer-shaped flattening of the shoulder blade or scapula. This is what is commonly called the shoulder joint. The different joints will be referred to by their correct anatomical names to avoid confusion. Although sometimes called a ball-and-socket joint, the scapular saucer (glenoid) is far too flat to be a socket and allows the head of the humerus to slide across the surface to a certain extent during normal movement. The joint has a circular cartilage called the labrum that increases the saucer shape of the rather flat glenoid. The joint capsule that attaches to both bones, surrounding the joint and helping hold it together, has to be quite loose to allow the huge range of movement possible at the shoulder. Without muscles to hold them together the humerus would therefore simply fall away from the scapula.

The scapula   To enable a greater range of movement than would exist at the glenohumeral joint itself, the scapula also moves. It does this by sliding and rotating against the back of the chest wall under the guidance of muscles that attach either to the spine or, on the other side, the humerus or upper arm bone. This is not a true joint but functions as one.

The acromioclavicular joint   The scapula is joined to the main skeleton by the clavicle. The powerful upper trapezius muscle (felt as a curve when running your hand down from neck to shoulder) comes from the spine in the neck and attaches along the upper surface of the clavicle and the spine of the clavicle. The upper trapezius holds them up in the manner of one-half of a suspension bridge. The joint between the scapula and clavicle is called the acromioclavicular joint and can be felt as a hard lump and groove on top of the shoulder. The acromioclavicular joint does not move very much and has short, powerful ligaments crossing it to give good stability.

The sternoclavicular joint   The clavicle (often called the collarbone) attaches to the skeleton of the chest at the sternoclavicular joint that lies just underneath the chin if this is pushed down against the chest wall. The sternoclavicular joint has to rotate quite a bit to allow normal shoulder movements to take place. It too has powerful ligaments holding it in place.

While the shape of the bony glenohumeral joint, the ring of cartilage (labrum) in it, and the surrounding joint capsule and ligaments do provide support and limit the range of movement of the humerus, muscular support is more important at this joint than at any other in the body. The muscles acting on the glenohumeral joint can be seen as being in two layers.

1. An inner ring made up of relatively small muscles holds the head of the humerus in place, rotates it, and initiates or counterbalances movements produced primarily by larger muscles. These are known collectively as the rotator cuff muscles.
2. The outer ring comprises a number of larger and longer muscles known as prime movers. Contraction of these muscles produces powerful movement of the arm. They often work in combination to produce the full range of movement and rely on the rotator cuff muscles to control movement of the head of the humerus.

Causes

Clearly there are many potential causes of shoulder pain. Many of these can be diagnosed by a skilled physician on examination alone. However, shoulder pain can sometimes be very difficult to diagnose. MRI scans, ultrasound examinations, X-rays, and ARTHROSCOPY may all be helpful. The main causes of pain are discussed below.

Rotator cuff syndrome   ROTATOR CUFF SYNDROME is the most common disorder seen, especially in those of middle age or the elderly. While most commonly seen as an isolated condition, it not infrequently complicates other forms of arthritis, especially RHEUMATOID ARTHRITIS. It is discussed elsewhere.

Calcific tendinitis   Calcific tendinitis causes quite different symptoms than rotator cuff syndrome. Although some patients may have had intermittent catching at the shoulder for some time, calcific tendinitis typically presents with sudden severe shoulder pain restricting all movement at the shoulder. This condition usually affects people aged 40 to 60 years, and the supraspinatus tendon is most frequently involved. An X-ray will show calcified tissue in the area of the rotator cuff tendons. Note that people may have calcification here without any symptoms, in which case it is best left alone. Ultrasound or MRI scans may show degeneration in the affected tendons. Blood tests are typically normal. Painkillers, NSAIDs, ice, and resting the arm in a sling may all help relieve pain in the early stages. Corticosteroid injections may help if there is an associated rotator cuff syndrome. Exercises to improve the rotator cuff function should be started once the pain has settled. Surgical removal of the calcium and repair of the rotator cuff tendons is occasionally required.

Biceps tendinitis   The biceps muscle has two tendons at the shoulder level. One of these (the long head of the biceps) passes through the glenohumeral joint over the head of the humerus. This, along with the rotator cuff muscles, is very important in controlling the movement of the head of the humerus. For this reason bicipital tendinitis usually occurs when there is an injury to other parts of the shoulder complex or instability of the glenohumeral joint. There are therefore usually other abnormalities as well. Most commonly this is rotator cuff impingement. Athletes performing overhead activities are particularly likely to develop this combination of injuries. Tendinitis of the long head of the biceps can occur by itself, for example as an overuse injury in weight lifters. Pain is felt in front of the shoulder, and the tender, swollen tendon can often be felt as it crosses the front of the head of the humerus in its groove. X-rays may show abnormalities of the groove but are seldom done these days. Ultrasound is excellent for showing the swelling around the tendon as well as the small tears in it that often set off the inflammation. MRI or ARTHROSCOPY are used to examine that part of the tendon lying inside the joint. Rest, NSAIDs, ice, and physical modalities such as ultrasound may help settle tendinitis early on. A CORTICOSTEROID injection alongside but not into the tendon is very helpful in resistant or chronic cases. Occasionally surgery is required, usually combined with other procedures such as repair of the rotator cuff. A gradual return to activities with appropriate exercises will prevent recurrence. The most important aspect of treating bicipital tendinitis is to diagnose any other disorders that may have lead to it and address them. The most common are rotator cuff problems and instability.

Biceps tendon rupture   Complete rupture of the long head of the biceps occurs occasionally. In this case the muscle will bunch up a few inches below the shoulder, especially when the elbow is bent up (that is, when the biceps is contracted). There may be bruising associated with such a rupture as well.

SLAP lesions   This term is used to describe tears in the labrum of the glenohumeral joint. This circular cartilage is particularly susceptible to tears in active young people with minor instability of the glenohumeral joint. SLAP stands for superior labrum anterior posterior lesion, describing the common location of these injuries. They may occur as a result of repeated minor trauma or a single episode of trauma, as when the humerus is driven up against the glenoid. MRI or arthroscopy is required to determine how severe the lesion is since treatment differs for the four grades of injury. Pain relief, changes in activity, and rehabilitation may be enough but, especially in grades III and IV, surgical treatment may be required.

Glenohumeral arthritis　Arthritis of the glenohumeral joint occurs in various conditions. Long-standing rheumatoid arthritis very frequently causes some secondary OSTEOARTHRITIS here. GOUT occasionally occurs, and hydroxyapatite-related arthritis particularly affects the glenohumeral joint (see MILWAUKEE SHOULDER). INFECTIVE ARTHRITIS, NEUROPATHIC ARTHRITIS, and AVASCULAR NECROSIS of the humeral head are all rare but important causes of shoulder pain. Primary OSTEOARTHRITIS seldom affects the glenohumeral joint, and, if this is seen, investigations for a secondary cause such as CPPD or HEMOCHROMATOSIS should be done.

Subacromial bursitis　The head of the humerus and glenohumeral joint lie underneath the bony projection at the tip of the shoulder called the acromion. Separating them are the tendons of the rotator cuff and a bursa, the subacromial bursa. This is a thin envelope of tissue containing synovial cells that secrete a lubricating substance into the interior that allows the rotator cuff to move smoothly underneath the bony acromion. This bursa can become inflamed (subacromial bursitis) if there is impingement or increased pressure such as occurs in the rotator cuff syndrome. Less commonly bursitis may follow a fall onto the shoulder. A corticosteroid injection into the bursa is very helpful in settling the inflammation but must be combined with correction of the cause. This will most commonly be a rotator cuff syndrome or a disordered scapulohumeral rhythm. The latter indicates that the precise coordination between movement of the humerus and of the scapula has been lost.

Frozen shoulder　The condition commonly known as frozen shoulder is a painful limitation of shoulder movement in all directions. It is caused by capsulitis or inflammation of the capsule of the glenohumeral joint. The capsule shows an increase in fibrous tissue and shrinks, thus limiting movement of the joint. It affects about 2 percent of the population but is more common in association with certain other disorders. These include thyroid disease, tuberculosis, lung cancer, after a heart attack or stroke, and especially, diabetes. Some diabetics, 10–20 percent, will develop a frozen shoulder at some stage. Having a frozen shoulder on one side increases the risk of having it on the other side to about 10 percent. The frozen shoulder goes through three stages. The first stage is painful and lasts about three months. The second typically lasts for six months (there is less pain in this stage but worsening limitation of movement). In the third phase there is gradual lessening of pain and increase in movement. This process may take one to three years.

Acromioclavicular joint dislocation　The acromioclavicular joint is commonly affected by trauma in young people and osteoarthritis in older people. Pain is usually felt in a relatively small area over the joint, which is felt as a small bump and groove on top of the shoulder. Pain is usually made worse by bringing the arm across the chest under the chin. The joint may be dislocated by a fall onto the tip of the shoulder. Mountain biking, ice hockey, soccer, and rugby are frequently involved. There are six grades of dislocation. The first three grades reflect varying degrees of damage to the joint ligaments but with the end of the clavicle still either touching or very nearly touching the acromion. These are usually treated conservatively with pain relief and immobilization. Type III may require surgical treatment occasionally. When severe pain persists the end of the clavicle can be removed, and this often gives good pain relief with relatively little loss of function. In types IV to VI the end of the clavicle is displaced well away from its original position, and surgical intervention is required to restore the connection to the acromion.

Acromioclavicular joint arthritis　Osteoarthritis is quite common in the acromioclavicular joint. This may follow injury, may occur in isolation, or may be part of a generalized osteoarthritis. Pain is felt over the joint, which often develops marked bony swelling and tenderness. The pain is worst when raising the arm above shoulder height and when bringing it across the chest. X-rays will confirm the diagnosis. The shoulder complex should be carefully assessed and dysfunction in the rotator cuff and scapulohumeral rhythm addressed as far as possible. NSAIDs may help, and local heat and nonsteroidal creams may give temporary relief. Corticosteroid injections into the joint often give longer lasting relief and are particularly helpful before starting a shoulder rehabilitation program. Persistent pain that limits activity may require surgical removal of the end of the clavicle.

Osteolysis of the clavicle Occasionally either after an injury or following repeated minor stress, the bone of the end of the clavicle is resorbed. This is termed osteolysis. There is persistent pain and limitation of movement. X-rays will reveal the diagnosis by showing loss of bone at the end of the clavicle. This has become increasingly recognized in weight lifters presenting with severe shoulder pain and an apparently normal shoulder on physical examination. Rest or altering shoulder movements may result in considerable improvement and even regrowth of the bone. However, surgical removal of the end of the clavicle is sometimes required.

Glenohumeral joint instability Instability at the glenohumeral joint is increasingly recognized as an underlying cause of pain at the shoulder. It may follow trauma or be due to inherent looseness of the ligaments around the shoulder or widespread laxity as found in the HYPERMOBILITY SYNDROMES. Dislocation of the joint is the most obvious manifestation but lesser degrees of instability are now more frequently recognized. Instability of the glenohumeral joint is traditionally separated into anterior, posterior, and multidirectional. It can be further classified according to how it occurred and whether it is recurrent since this will impact on the treatment.

Shoulder dislocation Anterior dislocation is often caused by trauma, with the arm held away from the body such as might occur when falling to the side and putting one's hand out to soften the fall. Initial treatment is to relocate the joint and immobilize the arm. This dislocation is often accompanied by damage to the labrum and ligaments in front of and below the joint. Young athletes frequently require surgery to be able to return to their sport, while older, less active individuals do well with conservative treatment. Posterior dislocation is much less common and seldom requires surgery.

Multidirectional instability is not often due to trauma. Although it may first be diagnosed after a traumatic dislocation, multidirectional instability will more frequently cause other painful shoulder conditions. Especially common are rotator cuff syndrome and bicipital tendinitis (see above). Shoulder rehabilitation, usually a three- to four-month intensive exercise program, is the treatment of choice, although there are surgical techniques which may help if there is recurrent dislocation.

In a four-year study patients with nontraumatic shoulder dislocation had a good or excellent result approximately 90 percent of the time if their dislocation was posterior or multidirectional compared with only 45 percent with anterior dislocation. In traumatic dislocation by contrast only 36 percent of posterior dislocations and 13 percent of anterior dislocations did well without surgery. Recurrent dislocation is much more common in young people when the dislocation is anterior and if it is traumatic.

Scapular pain Pain underneath the scapula or shoulder blade together with a snapping or grinding sound can be very difficult to diagnose accurately. Occasionally there may be an obvious localized cause such as a bony outgrowth from an underlying rib. More often, however, it occurs with loss of scapulohumeral rhythm, and the pain comes from the soft tissues between the scapula and ribs. This is often called a bursitis. Because this area is relatively hidden from direct examination and imaging, being sure of the origin of the pain is difficult. Correcting faulty shoulder complex movements is the best treatment. The area underneath the scapula is sometimes injected, but there is a risk of puncturing the lung.

sicca syndrome See SJÖGREN'S SYNDROME.

sickle-cell disease (sickle-cell anemia) A genetic (inherited) disorder that results in an abnormal hemoglobin molecule and causes red blood cells to become fragile and sickle shaped. Sickle-cell disease can cause several musculoskeletal problems.

Sickle-cell disease is an autosomal recessive genetic disease. This means that someone has to inherit two abnormal genes to have the disease. People with only one abnormal gene have sickle-cell trait and usually have no clinical abnormalities. A change in a single base of the DNA code leads to a change in one amino acid of the hemoglobin chain. This hemoglobin S causes the red blood cells to be fragile, rupture easily, and sludge in small blood vessels.

Sickle-cell disease is more common in populations of African or Mediterranean ancestry. Approximately 8 percent of African Americans carry the sickle-cell gene and one in 400 has sickle-cell disease.

Symptoms and Diagnostic Path

The symptoms of sickle-cell disease start in childhood. Because their red blood cells break more easily, affected children are anemic and jaundiced. Jaundice refers to a yellow color of the skin and eyes caused by the accumulation of bilirubin, a pigment that is the end product of hemoglobin breakdown. Children with sickle-cell anemia are small and often have delayed puberty. Painful sickle-cell crises occur. These crises are often precipitated by an infection or dehydration and last several days. There is acute pain that is probably the result of an inadequate oxygen supply to deep tissues because sickled red blood cells sludge in small blood vessels.

Several musculoskeletal problems can occur in patients with sickle-cell disease.

Arthritis Acute, reversible arthralgia and arthritis are common during sickle-cell crises. More serious is chronic irreversible arthritis caused by bone infarcts in and around large joints such as the knees and hips. These infarcts cause acute bone pain, and large ones can cause AVASCULAR NECROSIS, particularly of the hip or shoulder.

Osteomyelitis and infective arthritis Patients with sickle-cell disease have a higher risk of developing OSTEOMYELITIS and INFECTIVE ARTHRITIS. Differentiating the symptoms of osteomyelitis from a sickle-cell crisis can be difficult. In many patients with sickle-cell disease the spleen becomes less efficient at eliminating certain bacteria, for example pneumococci and salmonellae, and infections with these organisms are common.

Bony deformities In sickle-cell disease the bone marrow is hyperactive, trying to overcome anemia. The hyperactive marrow can lead to deformities in the bones of the skull and spine. The skull becomes thickened with a prominent forehead. The vertebrae may become deformed, leading to spinal deformities.

Other musculoskeletal complications Acute painful swelling of a finger or toe (dactylitis) or the whole hand or foot can occur in infants. GOUT is more common in patients with sickle-cell disease because the high turnover of red blood cells leads to increased production of uric acid.

Diagnosis The diagnosis of sickle-cell disease is usually easy and based on the family history, clinical findings, and blood tests. Under a microscope the blood smear shows sickle-shaped cells. The diagnosis is confirmed by testing for hemoglobin S.

Treatment Options and Outlook

For most patients, treatment consists of avoiding sickle crises and adequate pain control when they do occur. The key to avoiding crises is prevention of infection. Children should receive all available immunizations and receive penicillin prophylaxis at least until the age of five years. Folic acid is given routinely as this helps the bone marrow to maintain a high rate of red cell production. Hydroxyurea is a drug that works indirectly by increasing the amount of fetal hemoglobin formed, and this reduces the frequency of crises in adults. Early use of antibiotics and blood transfusions are important aspects of treatment. A substance called poloxamer 188 that reduces the stickiness of sickle cells is currently undergoing trials. Blood transfusions have been shown to prevent strokes in at-risk patients and improve growth in patients receiving regular transfusions. It is also used before surgery to lower the very high rate of complications seen with surgery in sickle-cell disease. In a few highly selected children, it is possible to wipe out the patient's bone marrow and then restore it using an unaffected sibling's stem cells and thereby cure the patient of sickle-cell disease. This procedure has very significant dangers.

The prognosis for patients with sickle-cell disease has improved considerably in the past 30 years and the average life span now exceeds 50 years of age. Death is usually during a sickle crisis often related to an infection or due to organ failure, especially kidney failure.

silicone implants In the 1990s, there was public concern that silicone was associated with an increased risk of developing autoimmune disease that resulted in several lawsuits against companies that manufactured silicone for plastic surgery.

Without a doubt silicone can cause local inflammation. A fibrous scar forms around a breast implant. If the plastic container ruptures, releasing the silicone gel into the breast, tissue inflammation results. Consequently, most modern breast implants contain saline and not silicone. Whether silicone is associated with a risk of autoimmune disease is much more controversial.

In the early 1990s, a number of cases seemed to suggest that silicone implants increased the chances of developing scleroderma, SLE, fibromyalgia, and arthritis. These reports were difficult to interpret because the population group most likely to have a breast implant, women between the ages of 20 and 45 years, were also the group with the highest risk of developing autoimmune disease.

There were also concerns about nerve damage and cancer. Subsequent long-term studies and epidemiological surveys (i.e., studies looking at whole groups of women who have received breast implants rather than just reporting on those with symptoms) found no evidence of increased rheumatological or neurological disease. Several studies have in fact shown that women who had breast implants had fewer musculoskeletal problems than women who had other cosmetic surgery or the general population. Women having plastic surgery as a group are healthier and wealthier than the general population and live longer. Studies have confirmed this is true of women having breast implants as well. However at the height of the concern, Dow Corning Corporation, the largest manufacturer of silicone products, faced nearly 20,000 lawsuits and went into bankruptcy.

The U.S. government appointed the Institute of Medicine to investigate the dangers associated with breast implants in 1997. After examining all the available evidence, their report published in 1999, *Information for Women About the Safety of Silicone Breast Implants*, found no evidence to suggest either saline- or silicone gel–filled implants caused any systemic disease. They found that local complications including pain, rupture, and contractures around the implant causing disfigurement are the major risks associated with this type of surgery. After a period of not approving silicone gel implants, the FDA in 2006 approved both saline-filled and improved silicone gel–filled implants but

with certain conditions including a requirement to perform 10-year follow-up studies on all women receiving these implants. In 2007, 350,000 women had breast augmentation surgery in the United States, approximately 30 percent reconstructive and 70 percent cosmetic.

Sjögren's syndrome This is a common autoimmune disease characterized by dry mouth and eyes, arthritis, other organ involvement, and an increased risk of malignancy. The dry eyes and mouth were described over 100 years ago. However, it was only in 1933 that Sjögren, a Swedish ophthalmologist, described the connection with the arthritis and other manifestations. Although exact numbers are difficult to obtain, Sjögren's (pronounced sho-grins) syndrome is the second most common autoimmune rheumatic disease behind RHEUMATOID ARTHRITIS. It affects women nine times as often as men, and up to 2 million Americans may have Sjögren's syndrome. When occurring on its own it is called *primary* Sjögren's syndrome. However, a significant number of patients developing Sjögren's syndrome already have another autoimmune disease. It is then called *secondary* Sjögren's syndrome.

The characteristic feature of Sjögren's syndrome is reduced function of the glands that lubricate mucous membranes. This may occur in the eyes, mouth, throat, lungs, gut, or vagina. This is due in part to damage to these glands by an immune attack. Lymphocytes are attracted to the glands by CHEMOKINES. One of the most important chemokines here is called RANTES. The lymphocytes then accumulate in the gland and produce CYTOKINES such as IL-1 and TNF, which have further effects on the glandular cells as well as nerve function. This process leads to destruction of part of the gland but also interferes with the function, i.e., the secretion of lubricating fluid. Antibodies also interfere with important signals in the gland, reducing secretions without actually causing destruction.

While the processes of gland destruction are understood in some detail, how and why this process is initiated remain unclear.

Viruses are an attractive link. That is, evidence indicates that a viral infection could lead to persistence of the virus in the gland tissue. This would lead to an immune attack in the gland that, in genetically predisposed people, could become self-perpetuating. There has been evidence involving cytomegalovirus and Epstein-Barr virus, although not conclusively. In addition patients with HIV or HEPATITIS C infection can develop a syndrome very like primary Sjögren's syndrome. At present it is not clear whether hepatitis C initiates Sjögren's syndrome or merely causes similar but separate symptoms. Research into the possible role of two other retroviruses (HIV is a retrovirus), human retrovirus 5 and HTLV-1, in Sjögren's syndrome is ongoing.

Relatives of patients with Sjögren's syndrome have a higher-than-expected occurrence of both Sjögren's syndrome and autoimmune antibodies on blood testing (without having any disease). This suggests a familial susceptibility to the disease. Two genes, HLA-DR3 and HLA-B8, have been found more frequently than expected in Caucasian Sjögren's patients, and other genes may be important in particular racial groups.

Sjögren's patients characteristically overproduce antibodies and may develop very high levels in their blood. Some of these antibodies are auto-antibodies, i.e., they react against parts of the individual's own body. The most characteristic of these autoantibodies in Sjögren's syndrome are anti-Ro and anti-La antibodies, also called SSA and SSB (see Appendix II) antibodies (SS representing Sjögren's syndrome). Rheumatoid factor and so-called extractable nuclear antigens are common. Ro and La are examples of extractable nuclear antigens.

The overproduction of other antibodies is also common in Sjögren's syndrome. Some of these are monoclonal immunoglobulins (antibodies or parts of antibodies). This means that they are produced by one B cell and its progeny. B cells are the subset of lymphocytes that produce antibodies. While this finding is characteristic of a blood cell malignancy called multiple myeloma, it does not mean that Sjögren's patients with this abnormality have myeloma. However, these patients appear to be at higher risk of developing lymphoid tumors later on. Some of the excess immunoglobulins may also behave as CRYOGLOBULINS. There is clearly abnor-

mal control of B cells in Sjögren's syndrome, and those B cells found in affected glands are activated. It has been suggested that initially many different B cells are activated, producing an assortment of immunoglobulins, and that this may become fewer as time goes on, leading to monoclonal antibodies and later possibly the development of lymphoid tumors. Secondary Sjögren's syndrome may occur in association with rheumatoid arthritis, SYSTEMIC LUPUS ERYTHEMATOSUS (SLE), SCLERODERMA, MIXED CONNECTIVE TISSUE DISEASE, primary biliary cirrhosis, MYOSITIS, VASCULITIS, thyroid disease, or autoimmune hepatitis.

Symptoms and Diagnostic Path

Sjögren's syndrome may occur by itself, called primary Sjögren's, or in association with another autoimmune disease, called secondary Sjögren's. Unless otherwise mentioned, this discussion will be about primary Sjögren's syndrome. Secondary Sjögren's is similar, but separating out the effects of the two diseases is sometimes difficult. Sjögren's syndrome has a very slow onset, and it can take up to 10 years before being recognized. A very wide range of problems may occur apart from the well-recognized reduction in secretions. However, apart from the reduced secretions, arthritis, and RAYNAUD'S PHENOMENON, these are not common. General symptoms such as tiredness, muscle aches, joint pain without swelling, and low-grade fever are common and have often been present to some degree for years before the diagnosis is made.

Eyes The main tear-producing glands are under the upper outer eyelid. Since they are infiltrated with cells and antibodies they may enlarge, and the quantity and quality of the tears is reduced. Normally there is a thin tear film covering the front of the eye, protecting it from drying out as well as trapping dust particles. The tears are wiped over the eye by regular blinking and drain into the nasal passages through a small tube in the lower inner lid. The amount of tears produced can be measured by Schirmer's test. This involves hooking a strip of blotting paper over the lower eyelid. Although this is useful in diagnosis, the quality of the tears may be more important than the amount. In Sjögren's the mucin in the tears is reduced, making the film break up more easily as it covers the eye. Also the fat content may drop, allowing tears to evaporate quicker.

Loss of tear protection causes drying and irritation of the conjunctiva or outer layer of the eye. People often feel as though they have some grit in the eye and may become sensitive to light. The eye may appear red because of enlarged blood vessels. This is known as keratoconjunctivitis sicca and may also occur in other conditions. About 50 percent of patients feel they have dry eyes when the diagnosis is first made.

Mouth The salivary glands may be similarly involved. They quite often enlarge, and this may be intermittent. This enlargement is usually seen in both cheeks near the angle of the jaw, but just one side may enlarge at times. Reduced saliva leads to difficulty swallowing or talking for prolonged periods, such as a teacher or receptionist might be required to do. Taste may alter, and the mouth often feels generally sore. People who have smoked tend to have more severe symptoms. The saliva is often sticky and white. Studies show greater numbers of bacteria growing in the mouths of patients with Sjögren's. Dental caries are a major problem for almost all Sjögren's patients, and very conscientious care of the teeth is required.

Other reduced secretions Dryness at the back of the mouth and throat may extend into the airways. Hoarseness is common, and these patients are more susceptible to chest infections and obstructive airways disease. Loss of acid secretion in the stomach and reduced pancreatic secretions may occur. The latter may contribute to malabsorption of food and vitamins. Vaginal dryness is a common problem, and many patients complain of a dry skin.

Joints Half of all Sjögren's patients will develop arthritis, and many more will have joint pain without swelling. The arthritis may be the first manifestation of Sjögren's or appear only years after the diagnosis. Hands, shoulders, hips, knees, and feet are commonly affected.

Raynaud's phenomenon This occurs in about 40 percent of patients. Unlike in scleroderma, patients with Sjögren's syndrome seldom develop ulcers from reduced circulation.

Lungs Lung problems are common in Sjögren's syndrome but are only occasionally severe. A chronic cough and frequent sinus infections are most common. Occasionally this may lead to bronchiectasis (chronic lung infection) or obstructive airways disease. Interstitial lung disease, in which there is an autoimmune attack on the air spaces where gas is exchanged leading to scarring, is less common. Occasionally lymphomas develop in the lung (see below).

Heart Infants born to mothers with anti-Ro antibodies are at risk of developing heart block (see also NEONATAL LUPUS). This means that the electrical signal does not pass from the upper heart to the lower pumping chambers, and the infant's pulse will not respond to signals to speed up in response to the various stressors that require a faster heart rate. The intrinsic pulse rate without these signals may sometimes be too slow. Up to 15 percent of adult Sjögren's patients develop autonomic dysfunction affecting the heart. Here the nerves that speed up or slow down the heart are affected so that there is a poor blood pressure response to exertion or other stimuli. This may lead to weakness or fainting due to an inappropriately low blood pressure.

Gut Difficulty with swallowing due to dryness of the gullet (esophagus) is common. There may be a mild inflammation with reduced function of the lining of the stomach. This leads to low levels of acid being produced and can lead to vitamin B_{12} deficiency. Absorption of B_{12} requires it to bind to a small protein called intrinsic factor in the stomach. The production of intrinsic factor is reduced with long-standing inflammation. Clinically, apparent pancreatitis is very uncommon, but investigations have shown that mild pancreatic damage occurs in up to 25 percent of patients. Nearly a quarter of Sjögren's patients will have abnormal liver tests at some time. This may be due to cholangitis (inflammation of the bile ducts carrying bile to the gut). In addition a high percentage of patients with primary biliary cirrhosis (an autoimmune disease producing a similar disease to cholangitis) will develop secondary Sjögren's syndrome. Many other autoimmune disorders have been reported in association with Sjögren's syndrome. Some of these may lead to malabsorption, such as collagenous colitis, ULCERATIVE COLITIS, or a vasculitis, causing reduced blood supply to the gut.

Kidneys About one in 10 Sjögren's patients develops detectable kidney disease. The typical disease is called type I renal tubular acidosis. The kidney has difficulty getting rid of acid in the urine. This upsets the acid/base balance in the body and causes a low potassium level. It can also cause kidney stones and very unusually kidney failure. There are no kidney-related symptoms unless stones form. However, the biochemical abnormalities can cause marked weakness.

Vasculitis This affects up to one in 20 patients. It usually affects the skin but can occasionally affect other internal organs.

Nervous system Although uncommon, Sjögren's patients may get a peripheral neuropathy (decreased function of the nerves to the feet and hands). There is disagreement whether patients get more brain problems than the general population.

Thyroid Autoimmune thyroid disease occurs quite commonly in association with Sjögren's syndrome.

Lymphoproliferative disease Patients with Sjögren's syndrome are 30–40 times more likely to develop a lymphoma than the general population. Although this may sound very high, it should be remembered that lymphomas are rare diseases. These are quite often low-grade, including some that were previously called pseudolymphoma because pathologists were not sure they really were tumors. Studies show that 3 to 4 percent of Sjögren's patients will develop a lymphoma over 10 to 20 years, although this may be an overestimate as generally patients with more severe disease are followed up in hospital clinics.

Diagnosis Dry eyes, dry mouth, and intermittent swelling of the parotid glands strongly suggest Sjögren's syndrome. Strictly speaking this should be confirmed with a biopsy of the minor salivary glands (from inside the lower lip) showing typically increased collections of lymphocytes. However, in practice a positive anti-Ro (SSA) antibody with the typical clinical findings is often considered a firm diagnosis. While many Sjögren's patients will have a positive antinuclear antibodies (ANA) test (see Appendix II) this is not a good predictor of the diagnosis. It may indicate the presence of another disease such as SLE or it may be nonsignificant. There are many causes of dry mouth. Medications, espe-cially psychotherapeutic and antihypertensive ones, are common causes. Dehydration such as occurs in poorly controlled DIABETES causes a dry mouth, as do certain viral infections. Irradiation for tumors and hereditary problems with the salivary glands are rare causes. Viral infections, diabetes, and other conditions such as SARCOIDOSIS, ACROMEGALY, cirrhosis, bacterial infections, and tumors can all cause swelling of the salivary glands. The diagnosis of Sjögren's syndrome therefore should not be made too readily without considering these alternatives. FIBROMY-ALGIA patients commonly complain of dryness and have widespread pain, causing some difficulty in diagnosis. They will not, however, have a positive anti-Ro antibody or evidence of inflammation.

Secondary Sjögren's syndrome occurs in about 5 percent of patients with rheumatoid arthritis, although symptoms like dry eyes are much more common. Sjögren's syndrome is relatively easy to differentiate from rheumatoid arthritis clinically. This is much more difficult when secondary Sjögren's occurs in SLE, where salivary gland biopsy may be required to make this distinction.

A raised ESR and gamma globulin level reflecting the increased antibody production is very common. The C-reactive protein, however, is usually normal. In addition to the ANA and anti-Ro antibodies mentioned above, rheumatoid factor, parietal cell, thyroid, microsomal, mitochondrial, and smooth muscle antibodies are all found fairly frequently. A number of special tests are helpful in confirming reduced tear production. Schirmer's test involves putting a strip of filter paper over the eyelid and measuring the length of wetness after five minutes. Less than 5 mm indicates reduced tear secretion. If rose bengal stain is dropped into the eye of a patient with keratoconjunctivitis sicca, it stains the damaged cornea or conjunctiva and confirms this diagnosis. Another dye, fluorescein, can be used to measure tear break-up time. If this is too quick, it indicates a mucin or lipid abnormality. Measuring the rate of saliva flow (sialometry) is also possible, although many factors affect this and interpreting the result can be difficult. Scintigraphy, in which a radioactive dye is injected intravenously and the salivary gland uptake and appearance of dye in the mouth are measured, may be more accurate but is seldom performed.

Treatment Options and Outlook

Sjögren's syndrome is often a mild disease. The most appropriate approach is to treat the individual symptoms that cause trouble rather than a more generalized immunosuppressive approach as may be used in diseases like SLE. Obviously with the more severe manifestations, systemic immunosuppression will be required. This section will first discuss treatment of the more common local problems and then systemic treatment.

Dry eyes A wide variety of artificial eye drop solutions are available, and these are very useful for preventing symptoms. Since tears do drain away quite quickly, they need to be applied regularly. This may vary from every hour or two to twice a day, depending on how dry the eyes are. Thicker, more viscous preparations stay in the eye longer. These, however, cause blurring of vision, coat the eyelashes, and are best used at night. Most teardrop solutions contain a preservative, and it is possible to develop an allergy to this. In this case, preservative-free eyedrops can be used. Since they come in single-use containers, they are more expensive. The opening of the narrow duct that drains tears into the back of the nose can be plugged closed (punctual occlusion). This can sometimes lead to overflow tearing and therefore a temporary plug is usually trialed first. If keratoconjunctivitis sicca develops, corticosteroid-containing drops may be used but for only a week or two since there is a risk of cataracts or glaucoma developing. In severe keratoconjunctivitis there are several reports of the patient's own serum (blood with all the cells and clotting factors removed) being successfully used as eyedrops. Soft contact lenses can protect the cornea, although people with dry eyes often do not tolerate them well and the lenses may require regular wetting. Avoiding windy conditions and low humidity (indoors, fans, or air-conditioning especially) and wearing wraparound sunglasses also helps prevent excessive drying. CYCLOSPORINE is a powerful immunosuppressant primarily used in transplant medicine. A small amount instilled into the eye by a dropper twice a day has been shown to reduce the number of inflammatory cells in the tear glands and cause a modest improvement in dry eye symptoms. In trials so far it seems very safe. Blepharitis is inflammation or low-grade infection of the eyelids and is common in Sjögren's syndrome as well as the much more common rosacea or sebborrheic dermatitis. It needs to be distinguished from dry eyes as the cause of eye irritation, as it is treated differently (in the main by regular washing of the base of the eyelashes with warm water and a mild soap).

Dry mouth For symptomatic relief, chewing sugar-free gum is probably best. This stimulates saliva production. Lemon juice is also a potent natural saliva stimulant but can erode tooth enamel. Proprietary saliva substitutes are available, but most patients with mild symptoms prefer using sugar-free gum and carrying a water bottle for regular sips. It is important that these do not contain acid or sugar because Sjögren's patients are already at high risk of caries. Oral pilocarpine increases saliva in Sjögren's patients. The main difficulty is in getting the dose of pilocarpine right and avoiding the sweating, tremors, and diarrhea that go with too high a dose. CEVIMELINE has more specificity for the salivary gland receptors and is equally effective. It has similar side effects and should not be used by people with glaucoma or asthma. Dry foods are best avoided, and drinking water to assist swallowing is useful. Many patients have serious dental caries before Sjögren's is actually diagnosed, and progression can be very rapid. In addition to regular brushing and flossing, regular dental checks are recommended. A dentist with an interest in Sjögren's syndrome is preferable but may not be available in all localities. Application of a sodium fluoride varnish to the teeth by a dentist has been shown to slow down caries. Fluoride gel can also be applied to the teeth at night using plastic dental trays. Antibacterial rinses such as chlorhexidine are recommended, and a chlorhexidine varnish may soon be available.

Other dryness Lubricating gels are used for vaginal dryness and moisturizing creams for the skin.

Systemic therapy NSAIDs, corticosteroids in low doses, and HYDROXYCHLOROQUINE are helpful in treating the arthritis and fatigue. AZATHIOPRINE has been used for treating a range of systemic manifestations with some success, although a recent controlled study of moderate-dose azathioprine showed no benefit. Interstitial lung disease is usually treated with pulses of intravenous CYCLOPHOSPHAMIDE, and CYCLOSPO-RINE has also been found to be effective in a small number of patients. INTRAVENOUS IMMUNOGLOBU-LIN has been used with some success in treating the peripheral neuropathy of Sjögren's but is not standard therapy. Octreotide has been success-ful in treating pseudoobstruction of the bowel. Midodrane may help the tiredness due to low blood pressure and slow heart rate that can occur following damage to the autonomic nervous sys-tem (see above). Given the importance of B cells in the pathogenesis of Sjögren's syndrome, it is not surprising that emerging anti-B cell therapies are being trialed. A number of small case series have suggested that the B cell depleting biological, RITUXIMAB, improves symptoms and considerably reduces the number of lymphocytes in salivary glands. Several other agents are in the pipeline as well, but there are no controlled trials yet.

Other A herbal vitamin supplement called Longovital (Amarillo Biosciences) was found to increase salivary flow rate in a controlled trial. Acupuncture has produced improvement in symp-toms of dryness.

SLE See SYSTEMIC LUPUS ERYTHEMATOSUS.

sleep apnea (obstructive sleep apnea) A condi-tion in which a person, while asleep, has many episodes of stopped breathing. Patients with sleep apnea are fatigued and can be misdiagnosed as having FIBROMYALGIA.

Sleep apnea is due to an excess of soft tissue around the airway. While the patient is asleep the soft tissue at the back of the throat flops down and blocks the airway. The person does not breathe for a while, sometimes for 30 seconds or longer, and then wakes up for a second and gives a snort, starts breathing, and falls asleep without know-ing what happened. This can happen hundreds of time during the night so that the patient's sleep is very disturbed. Obesity, a thick neck, male sex, and drinking large amounts of alcohol at night all increase the risk of sleep apnea.

Symptoms and Diagnostic Path
The patient's bed partner is often first to notice the loud snoring and periods of stopped breath-ing while asleep. The patient is not refreshed in the morning and falls asleep during the day while performing usual day-to-day activities. Musculo-skeletal symptoms of arthralgia and myalgia are common, and sleep apnea can be mistaken for fibromyalgia.

The history from the patient's bed partner is classical, but to make the diagnosis a sleep study is performed. The patient spends a night in a sleep laboratory where breathing and sleep patterns are recorded.

Treatment Options and Outlook
Losing weight can improve the symptoms of sleep apnea in some patients, but most require continu-ous positive airway pressure (CPAP). This involves wearing a tightly fitting mask every night. CPAP is very effective, but many patients find it inconve-nient and stop. Surgery to reduce the amount of soft tissue at the back of the throat can be helpful in some patients. Patients with untreated sleep apnea are prone to work-related injuries and motor vehicle accidents because they are tired and fall asleep for a few seconds while performing a task. Sleep apnea elevates blood pressure, can cause an abnormal heart rhythm, and is associated with an increased risk of stroke and heart failure.

soft tissue arthritis–related problems This is a term used to describe a group of conditions affecting the soft tissues of the musculoskeletal system such as muscles, tendons, ligaments, their attachments to bone, as well as some nerve conditions. It there-fore excludes diseases primarily affecting bones and joints and by convention excludes true inflamma-tory disease even when this affects muscle or ten-dons. It is really a classification of convenience since it does not imply any causal or mechanistic link between the various conditions. These have largely been described elsewhere in this book as separate conditions. Broadly speaking, soft tissue problems can be seen as generalized or local. Generalized conditions cause symptoms in many parts of the body, local in only one or a small area.

Generalized Soft Tissue Arthritis–Related Problems
FIBROMYALGIA
HYPERMOBILITY SYNDROME

Local Soft Tissue Arthritis–Related Problems
ACHILLES TENDON DISORDERS
BURSITIS
CARPAL TUNNEL SYNDROME
EPICONDYLITIS
FOOT PAIN, some forms
GANGLION
Golfer's elbow/medial epicondylitis; see EPI-
 CONDYLITIS
HEEL PAIN, some forms
Housewife's knee; see PREPATELLAR BURSITIS
KNEE PAIN, some forms
Lateral epicondylitis/tennis elbow; see EPICONDYLITIS
OLECRANON BURSITIS
PLANTAR FASCIITIS
ROTATOR CUFF SYNDROME
Tarsal tunnel syndrome; see FOOT PAIN
TENDINITIS

The word *tendinitis* implies inflammation of the tendon and was first described as an entity in 1763, although no doubt it was felt long before then. Tendons join muscles to bone and transmit the pulling force of the muscle. They are composed of spirals of collagen that are wrapped into bundles forming a thick cord that is both strong and able to stretch. Because of the property of viscoelasticity, a sudden rapid muscle contraction will find the tendon relatively stiff while slower contractions allow greater stretch. With repeated stretching the tendon becomes more flexible. While this applies to all ages, maximum flexibility does slowly decrease with increasing age. Longer tendons or those subject to significant friction are enveloped in a synovial sheath that has two layers that allow sliding to take place with little friction. Not all tendons have a sheath. The tendon gets its blood supply from both its muscle and the surrounding sheath if it has one. It attaches to the bone at an enthesis, and inflammation here (enthesitis) is described under ANKYLOSING SPONDYLITIS and HEEL PAIN.

Inflammatory tendinitis can occur as part many conditions, including RHEUMATOID ARTHRITIS, ankylosing spondylitis, connective tissue diseases, psori-atic arthritis (see PSORIASIS AND PSORIATIC ARTHRITIS), TUBERCULOSIS, GOUT, and giant cell tumors of the tendon. Most tendinitis, however, is due to mechanical strain and occurs following excessive repetitive movement or repetitive movement without adequate training. Tendinitis may also follow more acute injury, especially if activities are resumed before adequate healing has taken place. Tendon malalignment leading to the tendon having to transmit force at an angle to the line of its fibers commonly causes tendinitis. Impaired blood supply and fluoroquinolone antibiotics (see DRUG-INDUCED RHEUMATIC DISEASE) are other causes. As a result of inflammation and scarring around the tendon, it can begin to stick or *trigger*. When this involves a tendon that curls a finger up, for example, the finger will be stuck in a curled position. Often, with a little extra force, it will suddenly flick straight (trigger finger). This can also occur with stenosing tenosynovitis, in which the tendon sheath tightens around the tendon. This is sometimes familial. Calcific tendinitis has a dramatic onset, with pain made worse by movement. It can be caused by calcium apatite crystals or CALCIUM PYROPHOSPHATE DIHYDRATE DEPOSITION DISEASE. Attacks are most common around the wrist, shoulder, and ankle.

Tendinitis is usually diagnosed by history and examination. If there is doubt or a possibility that there is a tear, then ultrasound is the best method to image tendons. It does, however, require an operator with experience in musculoskeletal ultrasound. MRI provides a good image of tendons and can also show up associated bone or joint problems. X-rays will reveal calcific tendinitis and may show associated arthritic changes.

The type of immune response, damage, and repair mechanisms will differ among the different forms of tendinitis and between short-lived or long-lasting (chronic) problems. Treatment has to be directed to each individual's situation. ICE and relative rest, for example using a wrist splint, are useful in settling the pain and swelling in most forms and in allowing healing to start. NSAIDs are effective but will seldom relieve pain to the extent that normal use is restored. This is a good thing since premature use is likely to lead to chronic tendinitis more often. If part of a generalized arthritis, better control of the disease as a whole may help.

In these situations, however, injection of a small amount of corticosteroid often resolves the inflammation. These injections must be given into the sheath surrounding the tendon and not the tendon itself. Despite the severity of inflammation in calcific tendinitis, there is a concern that corticosteroid injections may slow resolution. Corticosteroid injections are also the first-line treatment for tendons that are triggering. Surgery may be necessary if these fail. Surgery to remove the debris from within a tendon can also lead to healing of chronic tendinitis (see also TRIGGER FINGER, TROCHANTERIC BURSITIS; and WRIST PAIN, some forms).

spinal stenosis　A condition in which the spinal canal or nerve root canal does not provide adequate space for the spinal cord or nerve root to pass freely. Early reports of typical symptoms as well as operative findings date from the 1890s, well before the now more common disc protrusion was described. Spinal stenosis can affect the cervical spine (neck) or lumbar spine (lower back). The lumbar spine is affected much more often. Patients are generally aged between 45 and 65 years, but younger and older patients may be affected. Men develop spinal stenosis more frequently than women, especially in the lumbar spine.

At least at the lower back level, the cross section of the spinal canal can be seen as a somewhat rounded triangle with equal sides, the base against the vertebral body and the apex pointing backward toward the spine. Spinal stenosis can occur at three sites at any given level. It can occur within the central spinal canal down which the spinal cord passes. It can occur in the lateral recesses that are the angles at each side of the base of the triangle. The nerve root angles into the lateral recess before entering the nerve root canal and leaving the spine. Finally, spinal stenosis can occur within the nerve root canal. Most of this discussion will refer to central canal stenosis, although the degenerative changes may affect all three sites.

Degenerative spondylosis is the most common cause both in the neck and back. This starts with wear and tear changes to the intervertebral disc. To a certain degree these are normal aging events. As the disc loses height a greater load is put onto the two smaller facet joints behind the spinal canal, the disc acting as a large joint in front of the canal. As a response to this increased load, the facet joint capsule thickens, and small bony outgrowths (osteophytes) grow out from the edges of the joints. Similarly, a rim of extra bone growth develops around the lip of the vertebral body, thus narrowing the canal space from all sides. In addition the powerful ligament that runs down the length of the spinal canal, the ligamentum flavum, thickens. This can thicken from a normal 2–5 mm in width to 5–10 mm, causing significant narrowing of the canal and compressing the cord. Other degenerative changes may worsen the situation or, if severe, cause stenosis of their own accord. These include disc protrusion (see BACK PAIN), spondylolysis, and spondylolisthesis. Spondylolysis is a defect in the arch of bone from the vertebral body backward to the facet joints. Spondylolisthesis is the relative forward or backward movement of one vertebral body on another. In the presence of degenerative changes as described above spondylolisthesis can cause spinal stenosis with only 3–4 mm of movement. It seems likely that disturbance in the blood supply to the nerve root from compression of the very small arterioles surrounding the nerve plays a significant role in producing the symptoms of spinal stenosis.

People may have developmentally small spinal canals, and this is very common in people with achondroplastic dwarfism. Narrow canals have also been described in other families with no other bony problems. There is a range of canal width within the population, and those toward the narrow end of this range will be at greater risk of spinal stenosis.

There are a large number of rare causes of spinal stenosis. It may follow disc space infection, bony infection (osteomyelitis), tuberculosis of the spine, synovial cysts protruding into the canal and following trauma, or surgery. Excessive bone growth may also narrow the canal and cause compression. This can occur in PAGET'S DISEASE, ANKYLOSING SPONDYLITIS or DIFFUSE IDIOPATHIC SKELETAL HYPEROSTOSIS, and ACROMEGALY. GOUT and pseudogout (see CALCIUM PYROPHOSPHATE DIHYDRATE DEPOSITION DISEASE) have rarely been associated with spinal stenosis as has the development of benign fatty growths within the canal in people on long-term corticosteroids.

Symptoms and Diagnostic Path

The most typical symptom is a rather diffuse pain in the legs that comes on after walking a certain distance or on standing for a period. This is called neurogenic claudication. Patients have often noticed that the distance they are able to walk has gradually been getting less for some time before the pain starts. The pain is usually relieved by movements that bend the lower back forward slightly. This maneuver widens the spinal canal slightly. Patients with spinal stenosis often describe a vague numbness or weakness in the legs. There may be sciatic symptoms (pain in the area supplied by a nerve root) that are largely one-sided, but the claudication symptoms are usually felt in both legs. A long history of low-back pain is common.

Pain that radiates down the leg with tingling sensations and numbness and occurs in only certain positions is very common. These symptoms will often have preceded those of neurogenic claudication. The positions likely to bring it on are standing or bending backward. Occasionally patients with spinal stenosis may develop cauda equina symptoms due to compression of the lower few nerve roots. This can lead to incontinence of urine and feces, impotence, and loss of sensation in that part of the rear end that would be in contact with the saddle if one were riding a horse.

The findings on physical examination are often remarkably normal. Straight-leg raising is a maneuver that puts tension on the sciatic nerve to see if it is being trapped by, for example, a prolapsed disc. It also flexes the lower spine forward slightly and will therefore widen the spinal canal, relieving symptoms of spinal stenosis. If a patient therefore describes symptoms suggestive of sciatica but has very normal straight-leg raising, this should raise the possibility of spinal stenosis. In some patients there may be abnormal findings such as weakness and absent reflexes after walking but not after resting.

Cervical canal stenosis (in the neck) is less common but has largely similar causes. Because it affects the spinal cord much higher up, it will produce different symptoms. By far the most common presentation is with spasticity (abnormal stiffness of the limbs). Walking is experienced as difficult, and the patient is found to have abnormally brisk reflexes in both legs and arms, depending on exactly where in the cervical spine the compression occurs. Disturbance in rectal or bladder sphincter function may occur. Weakness of an arm occurs in one-third of affected people and weakness of both legs or legs and arms in 10 percent. There may be twitching and wasting of the muscles of the hand. Some patients describe a vague alteration in sensation, and loss of position sense may occur. Although cervical spondylosis is the common cause, neck pain is found in only a quarter of patients.

The diagnosis of spinal stenosis is often delayed. One reason is that the symptoms come on very slowly and may be quite vague at the start. Another is that even if there is a good history of nerve root symptoms, there may be no symptoms of nerve root impingement at rest. The lack of neck pain and the difficulty many patients have in describing what they feel is wrong can make cervical canal stenosis difficult to diagnose. Symptoms that are particularly helpful in suggesting the diagnosis include that the symptoms come on after walking a certain distance, that there is numbness and weakness associated with the pain, and that the claudication affects both legs and is relieved by slight forward bending of the lower back. Once the clinical diagnosis is made it should be confirmed with an MRI scan. This can demonstrate the typical degenerative bulging disc, bony enlargement of the facet joints, synovial cysts, and ligament enlargement. The canal may be unusually narrowed. Plain X-ray and CT scans are good at showing up bony lesions such as Paget's disease.

Treatment Options and Outlook

Nonoperative treatment NSAIDs are helpful with the pain and may help some of the leg symptoms as well. Exercises aimed at reducing the lumbar lordosis (curvature of the lower back) help to widen the canal and reduce symptoms. While a lordosis is normal in the lower back it has often become exaggerated, and even when not exaggerated a slight reduction can help. The therapist will determine if there is excessive anterior pelvic tilt and advise how to correct this. Abdominal strengthening exercises are a cornerstone but need to be combined with appropriate stretches. Injection of corticosteroids into the space surrounding the spinal cord has been used in lumbar canal stenosis but is not a proven therapy. Cycling is a good exercise for the lower legs since the lumbar spine naturally flexes forward during exercise. These measures should be tried in all patients with mild symptoms, in those without critical nerve problems, and in those in whom surgery is fraught with danger.

Operative treatment Severe spinal stenosis requires surgery. The main indications are intolerable pain, symptoms of the cauda equina syndrome, or neurological dysfunction that is getting worse. The aim of surgery is to enlarge the spaces that the spinal cord and nerve roots pass through while at the same time not removing so much bone that the spine becomes unstable. There are several surgical approaches to achieve this. With the standard single-level procedure, instability occurs in about 2 percent of patients, and therefore fusion of adjoining vertebrae is not routinely done. If there is associated degenerative spondylolisthesis (slippage of one vertebra on the other), then the risk of instability is high and fusion is performed. It may also be done when there is scoliosis. ARTHRODESIS may be done at a later stage for intractable pain or instability following surgery.

Outcome In some studies 80–85 percent of patients operated on have a good result. A good result is relief of pain and a return to the level of activity that existed before onset of spinal stenosis symptoms. However, in another study only 41 percent of patients were 50 percent or more satisfied with the results of surgery one year later, although most felt they had made the right decision to have surgery. If there is wasting of muscles or abnormal sphincter function, then some irreversible nerve damage has likely occurred and this may not recover. It is unlikely that patients will be able to perform significant lifting or walking tasks, and prolonged standing is likely to be uncomfortable. This should be considered in planning a return to work.

splints Splints are devices that provide support for a limb or joint. There are many types, and they are used for different reasons. Simple wrist or ankle sup-

ports, for example, may be bought over the counter and provide very little actual support. At the other extreme rigid splints can be used to immobilize a joint. Common reasons for using splints include:

- *Comfort* A firm, elasticized support can lend a degree of comfort to a painful wrist, for example. Some supports give a certain amount of warmth as well, which is also comforting.

- *Proprioception* A light elasticized ankle support, while providing virtually no physical support to the ankle, assists in the return to activity after an ankle sprain by improving proprioception. It increases the person's awareness of the ankle and its position in space. This is impaired by the ankle sprain and is one reason for sprains becoming recurrent.

- *Support* If movement is painful a splint that limits motion can protect a joint, e.g., a hinged knee splint that has metal strips up the sides so that side-to-side movement is minimized. This helps some patients with osteoarthritis of the knee.

- *Immobilization* After trauma or surgery it may be appropriate to immobilize a joint completely. This can often be achieved with a molded splint that wraps around one side of a joint and is held in place with bandages.

- *Range of Motion Treatment* Patients with painful joints naturally hold them in a position of comfort, and in time, they may lose the ability to straighten these joints because of tightening of the soft tissues. One technique to overcome this is to use progressive splinting. If, for example, a patient cannot straighten one knee, this joint is stretched as straight as possible and a plaster cast is molded to fit down the back of the leg in this position. At night the cast is strapped on and the patient sleeps with the leg as straight as possible. As the soft tissues stretch, more casts are molded to hold the leg a little straighter each time. This is most useful in children since their soft tissues stretch more easily.

- *Strengthening* Following hand surgery particularly, splints are constructed that allow controlled movement of the fingers against elastic resistance to aid in the rehabilitation while surgical healing is still taking place.

spondyloarthropathy   This term is used to describe a group of conditions characterized by chronic or ongoing inflammation of the axial skeleton. The axial skeleton consists of the spine and the large sacroiliac joints where the lower spine joins onto the pelvis. There are other characteristics that these diseases share to a varying degree. In most patients it is possible, at least after a year or two, to diagnose the specific disease, and they are therefore described separately in this book. The main spondyloarthropathies are

- ANKYLOSING SPONDYLITIS
- ENTEROPATHIC ARTHRITIS, including Crohn's disease, ulcerative colitis, and WHIPPLE'S DISEASE
- Psoriatic spondylitis; see PSORIASIS AND PSORIATIC ARTHRITIS
- REACTIVE ARTHRITIS
- Reiter's syndrome

In addition to the typical spinal involvement, the other features that are shared to a variable degree include

1. The presence of the HLA-B27 gene. This is discussed in the ankylosing spondylitis section since it is most closely associated with this disease. However, all the above conditions occur far more frequently in people carrying HLA-B27.
2. The tendency to develop an asymmetrical, lower-limb arthritis involving one to three joints typically. In addition to the axial arthritis, many patients will develop arthritis in an ankle and knee, for example, or a hip. This tends to be more common in those with reactive arthritis and psoriatic spondylitis.
3. Associated inflammatory eye disease.
4. An association with gut inflammation. Apart from the enteropathic arthritis that is by definition associated with a well-defined bowel disease, nonspecific bowel inflammation has been found in many patients with ankylosing spondylitis. In a significant number of people, reactive arthritis develops after a bowel infection.
5. Enthesitis, which is typical. Inflammation of the enthesis or specialized area where tendons and ligaments attach to bones is the pathological

hallmark of these diseases. The reason for this is not known.

Still's disease   See JUVENILE IDIOPATHIC ARTHRITIS.

stress fracture   A break that develops in bone because of fatigue failure rather than a sudden overwhelming force. This may occur in normal bone as a result of excessive forces or in abnormal bone as a result of everyday stresses. These are clearly different conditions, although the end result may look very similar.

Stress fractures in normal bone occur predominantly in athletes and soldiers. They result from forces applied repetitively to an area of bone. As a result of these forces remodeling of the bone occurs. This involves bone cells called osteoclasts eating away established bone followed by other bone cells called osteoblasts laying down new bone better able to withstand the forces being applied. This process is quite common in athletes. Those who develop a stress fracture are on one end of a spectrum where the osteoclastic activity is not followed by adequate repair. Predisposing factors include inadequate muscle strength or training beyond muscle exhaustion. Muscles normally contribute to the shock-absorbing capacity of the lower limb. When this is lost there is increased impact transmitted to bone. Stress fractures can also occur in the upper limbs, for example in baseball pitchers, simply due to the forces applied by muscle.

The most common cause of abnormal bones giving rise to stress fractures is OSTEOPOROSIS. Patients with RHEUMATOID ARTHRITIS and osteoporosis seem to be at particular risk of stress fractures. This may relate to the deformities many rheumatoid patients develop, leading to abnormal stresses being put on bones as well as the high use of CORTICOSTEROIDS. Other bone diseases such as OSTEOMALACIA, PAGET'S DISEASE, and alcohol abuse are well-recognized causes. Some patients with HYPERMOBILITY SYNDROME have bony fragility and develop stress fractures.

Symptoms and Diagnostic Path
Pain is the predominant symptom. This is often exquisite when force is applied across the fracture,

for example when standing or walking with a stress fracture in one of the leg bones. A few patients, however, have remarkably little pain and can continue to walk with a fracture through their hip bone. Since the bones are not displaced they are still able to take the person's weight. Typical sites of fracture in normal bones are the second metatarsal and tibia in athletes or soldiers. The metatarsal is the bone running down from the midfoot to the toe, and the fracture usually occurs nearer the toe. This is known as a march fracture. The area overlying the fracture is often slightly swollen, and pressing over it is extremely painful. The tibia (larger of the lower-leg bones) is more frequently affected in long-distance runners. The humerus or upper-arm bone may become involved in baseball pitchers.

In severe osteoporosis almost any bone may be involved, although some are more frequent. The lower end of the tibia, the neck of the femur (thighbone), and the outer part of the sacrum (lowest part of the spine) are typical areas in the lower half of the body. Ribs are often affected, and vertebral collapse in the spine may be seen as a stress fracture.

When a typical site is affected in an athlete the diagnosis is usually suspected immediately, often by the athlete. However, in a patient with active arthritis the lack of obvious trauma and presence of painful joints may lead to a stress fracture being overlooked initially. When it affects a long bone a very tender lump can often be felt at the fracture site. An X-ray will confirm the diagnosis but may not show the fracture early on. If the X-ray is negative, a technetium bone scan will show the lesion. CT and MRI scanning are also effective in demonstrating stress fractures but are seldom required. It is important to exclude osteomalacia, a bone disease caused by lack of calcium or vitamin D, and a pathological fracture caused by a tumor weakening the bone.

Treatment Options and Outlook

Relative rest and pain relief are required, and the fractures usually heal without specific treatment. For patients with a metatarsal fracture, for example, it is often adequate immobilization to wear a stiff shoe, although occasionally a plaster cast will be required. Attention to biomechanics and training schedules may be needed for athletes, and avoidance of running on hard surfaces or cambers is essential. In patients with osteoporosis or other bone disease, treatment of the underlying disease is obviously important.

CALCITONIN is effective in controlling the pain. This is given by injections under the skin and may cause flushing and diarrhea at the higher doses. The bisphosphonate group of drugs is also effective. These include PAMIDRONATE, ALENDRONATE, and RISEDRONATE. Most fractures heal within three to six months but may occasionally take longer.

Risk Factors and Preventive Measures

All the risk factors for osteoporosis and osteomalacia put individuals at risk of insufficiency fractures. Rheumatoid arthritis appears to put people at particular risk, probably because of the frequent biomechanical abnormalities, lack of fitness, and corticosteroid use. Patients on 5 mg a day or more of prednisolone or equivalent should be on osteoporosis prophylaxis treatment. People at risk of osteomalacia should be screened and treated with vitamin D. People over the age of 65 years should consider vitamin D and calcium supplementation even in the absence of obvious risk factors.

A family history or previous history of stress fracture increases the risk. Lack of fitness, eating disorders such as bulimia, having either flat or highly arched feet, and being female all increase the risk of a stress fracture in otherwise healthy people. Exercise programs should not be suddenly accelerated, and modification of the usual training regimen of female army recruits reduced the incidence of stress fractures. Taking the contraceptive pill in amennorrheic female athletes improves bone density.

Sweet's syndrome (acute febrile dermatosis) A rare condition described by Dr. R. D. Sweet in 1964, consisting of fever, a high white blood cell count, and a plaquelike skin rash. Sweet's syndrome is more common in women than men. Sweet's syndrome can cause arthritis and can be mistaken for Still's disease or VASCULITIS.

The cause of Sweet's syndrome is not known. It is associated with some cancers, particularly leukemia, infections, drugs such as lithium, connective tissue diseases such as RA and SLE, and inflammatory bowel disease, suggesting that an abnormal immune response is responsible. Approximately 20 percent of patients with Sweet's syndrome have an underlying malignancy, usually affecting the bone marrow.

Symptoms and Diagnostic Path

The characteristic symptoms of Sweet's syndrome are fever and rash. Fever and other systemic symptoms such as arthralgia, arthritis, myalgia, and conjunctivitis occur in most patients. Arthritis affects large joints such as knees, hips, wrists, and ankles but can also affect the fingers.

The rash of Sweet's syndrome usually consists of red plaques that are often tender. The plaques can be large, up to several inches in diameter, and can occur anywhere, including the face, arms, and trunk. Lesions on the legs can be mistaken for ERYTHEMA NODOSUM, which can occur with Sweet's syndrome.

The diagnosis of Sweet's syndrome is usually based on the appearance of the rash and a skin biopsy that shows dense infiltrates of neutrophils around blood vessels but no vasculitis. Laboratory tests usually show an elevated white blood cell count and ESR, but these can accompany inflammation of any cause and are not specific. In most patients extensive investigations have been performed to look for an infection before the diagnosis of Sweet's syndrome is made. Blood cultures and other tests for infection are negative.

Treatment Options and Outlook

Sweet's syndrome does not respond to antibiotics. Because an infection is usually the first diagnosis suspected, most patients with Sweet's syndrome usually receive several courses of antibiotics. A CORTICOSTEROID such as prednisone 1 mg/kg a day is effective and rapidly reduces symptoms. The dose of corticosteroid is tapered over about six weeks. NSAIDs can improve joint symptoms and fever. Sweets syndrome usually resolves completely but can relapse. Because Sweet's syndrome in adults can be the first sign of an underlying malignancy, a thorough physical examination and basic screening tests for malignancy should be performed.

Risk Factors and Preventive Measures

Sweet's syndrome occurs in association with and therefore presumably because of other medical conditions or medications in about 50 percent of people who get it. Apart from switching to an alternative medication if possible, these are obviously not preventable. Drugs implicated include lithium (for bipolar depression), furosemide (heart failure), cotrimoxazole and minocycline (antibiotics), and oral contraceptive agents. Both bacterial and viral infections are known to occasionally trigger Sweet's syndrome. Many autoimmune diseases have been associated with it, including RHEUMATOID ARTHRITIS, SLE, SJÖGREN'S SYNDROME, Crohn's disease, ulcerative colitis, and COMPLEMENT deficiency.

synovectomy The synovium is normally a thin layer of tissue surrounding most of the joints of the body and lies inside the tough joint capsule. In addition, synovial tissue lines tendons where they are subject to friction and is also found within bursas. Since cartilage has no blood supply of its own, the synovium secretes nutrients into the joint space for the cartilage. It also contains nerves that feed back information about the state of the joint. In many forms of inflammatory arthritis (see ARTHRITIS for definition) the synovium enlarges, becoming packed with white cells that promote inflammation. New blood vessels form and fluid leaks into the joint, carrying enzymes and CYTOKINES that cause damage to the cartilage as well as promoting more blood vessel growth and causing pain and swelling. To a certain degree this also happens in OSTEOARTHRITIS, although much less aggressively.

Because the white cells and all the proinflammatory molecules that they secrete enter by the synovial blood vessels, it seems logical that if the synovium is removed the arthritis will get better. Indeed this does happen, although it is not quite as simple as it once seemed. First the synovium will regrow, and second, removal of the synovium does not stop the cartilage from deteriorating. It may, however, dramatically relieve pain and swelling and improve function for months or years. There are two forms of synovectomy, surgical and radiochemical.

Surgical This involves opening the affected joint and stripping out as much synovium as possible. More and more this is being done by ARTHROSCOPY. Although this is a less invasive procedure, doing a complete synovectomy arthroscopically is difficult. Most synovectomies are done in patients with RHEUMATOID ARTHRITIS. It is particularly indicated when one or two large joints are not responding to adequate medical therapy. There is sometimes a lot of synovitis around the tendons since they cross the back of the wrist, and this can lead to damage and rupture of the tendons. A synovectomy here is valuable in preventing rupture. Synovectomy can sometimes relieve pain for up to 10 years, and about 70 percent of patients will have some benefit.

Patients with JUVENILE IDIOPATHIC ARTHRITIS of the pauciarticular type often have one or two troublesome joints. If these can be successfully treated with synovectomy, it may obviate the need to take potentially toxic medications. One study showed good pain relief in 70 percent of pauciarticular patients treated by synovectomy after seven years. In HEMOPHILIA, the large, swollen synovium may be a source of recurrent bleeding, and synovectomy can reduce the frequency of bleeds. However, synovectomy seems to cause a significant loss of movement in these patients. Surgical synovectomy is also the treatment of choice for a number of synovial diseases such as PIGMENTED VILLONODULAR SYNOVITIS, synovial chondromatosis (see KNEE PAIN), and rare synovial tumors.

Radiochemical This involves injecting a radioactive substance into the joint to damage the synovium by irradiation. The substance needs to be relatively safe, easy to handle, and remain in the joint. Although a number have been used over the years, yttrium 90 is now used by most centers. Because it is a radioactive treatment, the center needs to be licensed to do it. A few centers commonly undertake this treatment for a wide referral area. Large joints such as knees, hips, and ankles are most commonly treated in this way. Smaller joints in the hands were successfully treated in the past, but radioactive injection was shown to be no better than corticosteroid injections in these joints and is therefore no longer done.

synovial fluid See Appendix II.

systemic lupus erythematosus (SLE) A complex inflammatory disease potentially affecting many organs and systems in the body (e.g., neurological and cardiovascular). First described as a chronic skin condition in 1833, the *systemic* nature of SLE was recognized in 1872. The first of the laboratory tests demonstrating autoimmunity, the LE cell preparation, was discovered in 1948. Although no longer used, this has been replaced by several other tests that make the recognition of SLE and related diseases easier. Studies have shown SLE to affect between 12 and 50 people per 100,000 population in the United States and the developed world. Studies of a fairly rare disease that can range from mild to life threatening and predominantly affect very different organ systems (and therefore present to different types of specialists) are difficult. It is not clear, therefore, how much of the variation in these studies is real or due to the different approaches taken in doing the studies. SLE affects women more than men in a ratio of about seven to one. It affects African Americans more than Caucasians in the United States but is rare in black Africans living in Africa. Evidence also shows that SLE is more common in Chinese and Filipino people. Adding to the uncertainty of how many people suffer from SLE is the recent rise in self-diagnosis. A patient organization, the Lupus Foundation, ran a survey and found that 2.4 million people in the United States said that they had SLE. The U.S. government thought there were 239,000 people with SLE, and it seems likely that the true number is around half a million.

SLE is an autoimmune disease of unknown origin. The term *autoimmune* implies that the body's immune system behaves as though parts of the body itself were foreign and therefore initiates an inflammatory attack to damage or destroy those parts as it would to any other foreign antigen. Why it does this is unknown, but there are a number of theories. Very simply put, the immune system could respond to a foreign antigen that is very similar to a self-antigen. Once the foreign antigen (e.g., virus) is destroyed, the immune system mistakes the similar self-antigen for the foreign one and continues a chronic inflammatory attack. The same general theme could occur if the foreign antigen combined with a self-antigen or altered a self-antigen. In all these scenarios the immune system could start responding to other related self-antigens, a process known as antibody spreading. The initial recognition of a foreign or altered self-antigen can be by either circulating antibodies or lymphocytes known as T helper cells.

Although the initiating event remains theoretical, much is known about who is at risk of developing SLE and the abnormal immune processes that lead to tissue damage. Only the main issues will be touched here.

Genetics This clearly plays a role. There are many reports of identical twins developing SLE. Between 5 and 10 percent of relatives of SLE patients develop the disease. While the genetic contribution to SLE is clear, it is also complicated. A number of genes have been shown to be associated with an increased risk of developing SLE. However, they may have to act together with other genes either known or as yet unknown, or different genes may be important in different patients. People with the ancestral haplotype (grouping of genes passed down through millennia in one ancient family tree) HLA-A1, B8 (class I antigens) have long been known to be more likely than average to develop autoimmune conditions including SLE. The class II genes HLA-DR2 and DR3 are also found more frequently than expected in SLE patients. People having a null allele (i.e., a nonfunctional gene) for COMPLEMENT component C4 are at high risk of developing SLE. Genetic studies looking for an association between genes for specific molecules that play a significant role in immune processes and the development of SLE have thrown up a large number of such linkages. These include the genes for CYTOKINES TNF, IL-6, IL-10, IL-1Ra, and IL-10Ra; heat shock proteins; immunoglobulins or antibodies; complement receptors; and T cell receptors among others.

Sex hormones SLE occurs most frequently in young women, with a high female-to-male ratio between the ages of 15 and 65 years. However, the female-to-male ratio is 1 to 1 outside these years. This strongly suggests that estrogen plays a role in the development of SLE, but how it does so remains unknown.

Autoantibodies SLE is termed an immune complex disease. This implies that there is excessive formation of antibodies (directed against self in this case and therefore called autoantibodies) that clump together with antigen and deposit out in the tissues, where they cause inflammation. Once deposited out in tissue these immune complexes may bind to complement. Complement will release fragments (C3a and C5a) that attract inflammatory cells. These mononuclear phagocytes and polymorphonuclear leukocytes release substances that attract other cells, cause the blood vessels to become leaky, and also cause direct damage to the surrounding tissue. Platelets (the small blood cells that form clots) become activated and cause local thrombosis. Not all immune complexes are the same, and they will differ in their ability to initiate this cascade.

Many autoantibodies are tested for individually and have become important in various aspects of diagnosing and caring for patients with SLE. Some, such as the anti-DNA antibody, are named after the substance against which they are directed. The targets of others were not known when they were discovered, and they were named after the first patient they were described in, e.g., anti-Sm (for Smith), anti-Ro (SSA), and anti-La (SSB). Although the targets of these antibodies are now known, they retain the old names. The measurement of these autoantibodies may give different types of information:

1. *Assist in Making the Diagnosis* (see Appendix II) Almost all patients with SLE will have a positive ANA test. A negative test therefore makes SLE unlikely. Anti-Sm, anti-double-stranded DNA (dsDNA), and anti-ribosomal P protein antibodies, when present, make the diagnosis of SLE very likely, although they are not positive in all SLE patients. Antihistone antibodies (H2A, H2B) are found in a high proportion of DRUG-INDUCED LUPUS but are not found when hydralazine is the cause and seldom with minocycline. They are also found in other lupus patients occasionally, and the whole picture needs to be considered. High levels of anti-RNP antibodies suggest that the diagnosis is actually the OVERLAP SYNDROME.

2. *May Indicate Activity of the Disease* In some patients with a positive anti-dsDNA test, the level of the antibody rises before an increase in disease activity and may therefore indicate the need for increased monitoring or treatment. This has been more useful in patients with kidney disease than others. Unfortunately this has not proved to be a simple relationship, and other factors need to be taken into account.

3. *May Indicate an Increased Risk of Specific Complications* Anti-dsDNA antibodies are associated with an increased risk of developing kidney disease. Anti-Ro and anti-La antibodies are present in a subset of patients with subacute cutaneous lupus erythematosus and, if found in pregnant women, indicate a risk of the baby being born with heart block and a transient rash (see NEONATAL LUPUS). Antiribosomal P antibodies are very specific for SLE and indicate an increased risk of developing liver disease or a psychosis. Antiphospholipid antibodies (see ANTIPHOSPHOLIPID ANTIBODY SYNDROME) are associated with an increased risk of thrombosis, reduced platelet numbers, and recurrent fetal loss.

4. *May Cause Direct Damage* It should be pointed out that most antibodies measured in SLE do not cause direct damage. They may have no apparent function and have simply been found through careful research to give useful information, shown as above. Antibodies, however, may cause damage nonspecifically as immune complexes as described above, or they may directly attack tissues. The anti-dsDNA antibodies are certainly important in causing kidney inflammation. Although some are deposited there as immune complexes, others appear to bind to the glomerular basement membrane in the filtering part of the kidney. Some antibodies bind to lymphocytes and play a role in the disorganization of the immune system in SLE. Antibodies binding to the lining cells of blood vessels (endothelial cells) have been found and may cause some of the vascular problems by direct attack, although there are many other mechanisms.

5. *Are Useful for Research* Defining the types of antibody and their targets provide researchers with clues as to the cause and mechanisms of disease. Naturally occurring antibodies also lead researchers to make their own antibodies in the laboratory. These have proven to be a very powerful tool for unraveling immune and biochemical processes over the past 20 years.

Cellular immunity Lymphocytes are white cells that form a major part of the executive arm of the immune system (see IMMUNE RESPONSE). They are broadly divided into two groups, B cells and T cells. The B cells largely produce antibodies but can also recognize potentially harmful antigens and present them to the T cells. Some T cells (cytotoxic T cells) can attack and destroy other cells. These could be cancerous cells or normal cells infected with, for example, a virus. Other T cells, the T helper cells, recognize foreign antigens and stimulate both cytotoxic T cells and B cells to attack the foreign antigen. Other cells such as macrophages are also involved in this cellular immune system. A large number of abnormalities have been described in the cellular immune function of SLE patients, including reduced T cell numbers and function, reduced natural killer cell function, increased spontaneous activity of B cells, and increased responsiveness to T cell-secreted growth factors as well as abnormal accessory cell function. Many of these abnormalities may be a result of the chronic inflammatory process rather than the cause. The immune dysfunction in SLE is so widespread and complex that it is very difficult to tease out the importance and cause of the various findings.

Viruses An attractive hypothesis to explain many autoimmune diseases has for a long time been that someone is born with a genetic predisposition to respond abnormally to a particular immune stimulus. This person then meets the appropriate virus that switches on an immune response that becomes chronic and self-perpetuating. Studies looking for the implicated virus have a history of turning up exciting finds followed by disappointment with further research. More SLE patients than controls show evidence of previous infection with the Epstein-Barr virus (EBV), the cause of infectious mononucleosis or glandular fever. Cytomegalovirus has been found causing serious organ damage in SLE patients, but there is no good evidence that it's involved in the cause of

SLE. There are reports of SLE and SLE-like diseases developing after infection with human PARVOVIRUS B19. If this is a cause of SLE, though, then it is responsible for only a very few cases. Patients with HEPATITIS C infection often develop positive ANA tests and rarely develop an SLE-like disease. The relationship with polyomaviruses and retroviruses is also being investigated.

Complement Humans naturally form immune complexes as part of the response to many stimuli such as infections. There are, therefore, protective mechanisms to prevent immune complex-mediated disease. Complement is a series of proteins that work in a cascade to break large complexes up into smaller (and therefore more soluble) ones and to bind the complexes to other cells so that they can be removed from the blood. Deficiency of complement components C1, C2, and C4 are associated with a high risk of developing SLE, possibly due to the impaired ability to clear the blood of circulating immune complexes.

Tissue damage There may be, therefore, a direct inflammatory attack on tissues mediated through the mechanisms discussed above. Alternatively organ damage may occur because of loss of blood supply. This can occur as a result of an inflammatory reaction to immune complex deposits in the wall of the blood vessel or antiendothelial antibody-mediated attack leading to thrombosis of that blood vessel. In addition patients with the antiphospholipid syndrome are prone to developing noninflammatory thromboses. Antibodies acting in this way may cause chorea and widespread neurological dysfunction such as depression and cognitive impairment (see Symptoms below). In addition to these directly disease-related mechanisms of organ damage, SLE patients are also susceptible to drug-related adverse effects (see Treatment below) and multifactorial disease such as atherosclerosis (see Symptoms below).

Symptoms and Diagnostic Path

SLE is a very diverse disease. It may come on gradually over years or present as a life-threatening illness. Some patients have an annoying intermittent disease, while others have an inexorably progressive life- and organ-threatening disease. Most SLE patients will have nonspecific symptoms such as

fatigue, nausea, loss of weight, and less frequently, fever. One or more of these symptoms is usually present at the onset but does not differentiate SLE from many other conditions that could also cause this. The more specific lupus problems include:

Skin It is said that any rash can occur in SLE. However, a few are typical. The best known of these is the *butterfly* rash over the nose and cheeks. The red raised lesions are itchy or painful and made worse or brought on by exposure to sunlight. Similar rashes may occur on other Sun-exposed skin. Half of lupus patients are photosensitive. Not only does exposure to sunlight cause a rash, but it can also induce a flare of their disease in other organs. Subacute cutaneous lupus erythematosus (SCLE) is a distinct subset of lupus patients who develop raised papules or plaques that sometimes form circular lesions and typically wax and wane in different sun-exposed areas. They may have joint pain or arthritis but seldom any other manifestations of SLE. Typically they have a positive anti-Ro antibody. The skin lesions do not scar.

In contrast, discoid lupus lesions start as a papule or plaque, become thicker, and spread, leaving a central area of scarring. These typically occur on the cheeks but may affect other sun-exposed areas and the scalp, where they may cause permanent bald patches (alopecia). Discoid lupus lesions can occur as the main feature of DLE or as part of a more widespread SLE. Some of the other rashes that are common in SLE but occur in many other situations include panniculitis, alopecia, urticaria, mouth and nose ulcers, LIVEDO RETICULARIS, and vasculitic lesions (see VASCULITIS). Panniculitis is felt as a deep, tender nodule and consists of inflammatory cells surrounding an area of necrotic (dead) fat tissue. When alopecia is not associated with discoid lesions the hair usually grows back with successful treatment. Urticaria looks like hives and may be a manifestation of vasculitis.

Arthritis Arthralgia (joint pain) and arthritis (joint inflammation) affect more than 90 percent of SLE patients and are present at the time of diagnosis in over half. The arthritis affects the hands and wrists, knees, and hips most frequently but can affect any joint. Unlike rheumatoid arthritis, it does not erode away the cartilage and bone at the affected joints. However, a few patients do develop deformities of the fingers, called Jaccoud's arthritis. The tendons may also become inflamed (tenosynovitis) and occasionally rupture with very little force being applied. Some tendon ruptures are associated with inflammation while others may be related to corticosteroid therapy. INFECTIVE ARTHRITIS is more common in SLE than the general population. SLE is a well-known cause of AVASCULAR NECROSIS, and this should always be borne in mind if there is severe, unremitting hip pain.

Muscle disease   SLE is one of the connective tissue diseases that can cause polymyositis (see DERMATOMYOSITIS AND POLYMYOSITIS). However, a number of patients with SLE also suffer muscle pain and weakness without the diagnostic changes of polymyositis. A MYOPATHY frequently complicates long-term CORTICOSTEROID therapy at the doses that patients with severe lupus may require. This presents as painless weakness of largely shoulder and hip girdle muscles of very slow onset and is therefore quite often advanced before it is recognized. The muscle enzymes are normal. Muscle biopsy shows characteristic wasting of particular muscle fibers (type II) without any inflammation. Very occasionally long-term CHLOROQUINE or HYDROXYCHLOROQUINE therapy also produces a myopathy.

Kidney disease   This usually creeps up unnoticed by the patient until there is quite advanced disease. For this reason it is important to do regular blood and urine checks to look for early signs of kidney disease, especially if the anti-dsDNA is positive. The urine is abnormal if there is more than 0.5 g of protein in all the urine passed in 24 hours or more than five red cells and/or more than five white cells per high-power field on microscopy. Kidney biopsy can give further information about the type and stage of the disease. Excessive leaking of protein through the damaged filtration units of the kidney (glomeruli) may lead to the nephrotic syndrome (more than 3 g urinary protein per 24 hours). This leads to swelling of the legs and the collection of free fluid in the abdomen (ascites) and around the lungs (pleural effusions). Nephrotic patients are prone to infections and thromboses in both veins and arteries. More severe or prolonged inflammation that destroys the glomeruli reduces the number of filtering units available and leads to kidney failure. This can cause nausea,

loss of appetite, tiredness, itching, and in severe cases, diarrhea, drowsiness, coma, anemia, swelling, altered breathing, and fluid around the heart (pericarditis).

Neurological disease   Migraine and other headaches that tend to be resistant to painkillers are the most common neurological symptom in SLE. Generalized seizures or those confined to a single limb, for example, are characteristic but not common. Chorea is a jerky, sometimes complex movement disorder that can affect most parts of the body. It can occur in other diseases and in lupus is often associated with the presence of antiphospholipid antibodies. SLE patients may suffer strokes from vasculitis of the blood vessels in the brain or very similar problems from localized inflammation of the brain. Individual nerves, both those arising from the brain and those in the limbs, may be affected with diverse effects. The retinopathy (disease of the back of the eye) seen in SLE patients is quite characteristic. A peripheral neuropathy causing loss of feeling in the feet with or without weakness can occasionally occur. Also reported is a Guillain-Barré–like illness where progressive weakness starts in the legs and moves up the body a variable distance. If the muscles of respiration are affected the patient has to be put on a ventilator. However, as long as complications can be avoided, there is often an excellent recovery. Transverse myelitis is a devastating manifestation of SLE in which the spinal cord is affected, causing paralysis of the lower limbs, loss of feeling below the affected level, and loss of ability to control the bladder and bowel.

Long-term lupus patients may gradually develop neurocognitive problems including poor memory, problems with numbers, and speech difficulties. While this may be a result of some of the specific conditions listed above, lupus patients with no previous neurological problems may also be affected. A CT or MRI brain scan will often show thinning and shrinkage of the brain. Why this occurs is unclear, and no specific treatment is available.

Psychiatric disease   Psychosis can be a manifestation of SLE. It may also complicate treatment with corticosteroids (usually moderate or high doses). In the presence of both it is usual to reduce the corticosteroid dose and attribute the psychosis to SLE if it gets worse. Organic brain syndrome describes a state of impaired concentration and memory and possibly delirium in the absence of any possible cause other than SLE. Depression is common in lupus and has been associated with the antiribosomal P antibody. This suggests that the depression is actually caused by the lupus rather than a reaction to having a chronic debilitating disease. Patients with lupus have been shown to have cognitive impairment (reduced mental ability) more often than the general population. However, there is nothing specific or characteristic about these impairments.

Serositis The heart, lungs, and bowels each have a thin double layer of connective tissue surrounding them. This serves to separate them from the rest of the body and reduce friction between these moving internal organs and their protective bones and muscles. Normally there is a thin film of fluid between the two layers. Inflammation can cause considerable pain but may also be painless. When it involves the lining of the lungs this is termed pleuritis, the heart pericarditis and the bowel peritonitis. Excessive fluid collects between the layers and can be detected by chest X-ray or ultrasound examination and often by a careful examination. In SLE this collection is seldom large enough to compress the heart or lungs and interfere with their function but may occasionally do so. When this occurs the fluid must be drained off with some urgency.

Lung disease In addition to pleuritis lupus affects the lungs in a number of ways. Pneumonitis is caused by immune complex deposition in small blood vessels and the terminal air spaces of the lungs called alveoli. This is where gas exchange between air and blood takes place. Pneumonitis can be sudden and severe when it is difficult to differentiate from infection. It may also come on slowly with an irritating cough and shortness of breath during activities. Pulmonary hemorrhage is a rare but very serious occurrence, probably a result of vasculitis affecting blood vessels of the lung. PULMONARY HYPERTENSION may occur, although less frequently than in the CREST syndrome or SCLERODERMA. In SLE it is particularly important to consider secondary pulmonary hypertension due to emboli or infarcts. In late-stage disease a rare but serious complication known as *shrinking lung*

may occur. In this condition the chest X-ray is normal but the space occupied by the lungs becomes progressively smaller with the diaphragm moving up. The patient complains of increasing shortness of breath, and lung function tests show reduced lung volumes. Studies have shown abnormalities in both the chest wall and the diaphragm, but the exact cause can be difficult to determine.

Heart disease Myocarditis or inflammation of the muscle of the heart may occur along with MYOSITIS elsewhere (muscle disease) or in combination with pericarditis. The latter is usually painful and will lead to the diagnosis being suspected. If not accompanied by these other manifestations, myocarditis can be silent and present with established heart failure or heart rhythm abnormalities. Sophisticated testing suggests that it may be more common than suspected. Coronary artery disease will be discussed under atherosclerotic disease.

The heart valves may also be affected, leading to leaking valves, tight valves, or embolic events. Leaking valves impose a strain on the heart by requiring it to pump increased quantities of blood because a proportion leaks back. Tight valves that do not open adequately thereby place an increased strain on the pumping chamber of the heart (aortic valve) or inadequate filling of the left ventricle (mitral valve). Small collections of material may develop on the valves with pieces or emboli breaking off intermittently and lodging in blood vessels in the hands, feet, and brain particularly. Valve abnormalities are particularly associated with the presence of antiphospholipid antibodies.

Gastrointestinal disease Almost any part of the gastrointestinal tract from the mouth to the lower bowel may be affected by SLE. Mouth ulcers occur in roughly half of patients. Swallowing difficulties are usually due to the dryness of associated SJÖGREN'S SYNDROME, but poor muscle contraction and reflux of stomach contents similar to that in the CREST syndrome are also found. The most common stomach complaints are those related to NSAID use, but there is an association with atrophic gastritis and vitamin B_{12} deficiency.

SLE patients with abdominal pain may, of course, have any of the causes anybody else might have. However, it has been shown that if the SLE is active in a number of other areas it is much more likely that the abdominal pain is directly related to lupus rather than due to something else such as gallstones. Most severely ill patients with an acute abdomen and active lupus have an ischemic bowel (loss of blood supply) due to either vasculitis or a thrombosis. These patients need urgent surgery since they do not do well. SLE patients get bacterial overgrowth in the small bowel more frequently than expected. This causes bloating, diarrhea, constipation, and abdominal pain and is treated with broad-spectrum antibiotics. Chronic intestinal pseudo-obstruction is caused by dysfunction of the smooth muscle in the bowel wall and has been reported in many SLE patients. Protein-losing enteropathy (excessive protein is lost in the stools) and various forms of malabsorption are also rarely found. Many patients with CROHN'S DISEASE (a chronic inflammatory bowel disease) have positive ANA tests, but it is not clear that there is a true association between the two diseases. Pancreatitis is usually associated with alcohol or gallstones in the general population, and these may be factors in some lupus patients. However, some cases of pancreatitis in SLE patients appear to be due to the disease itself and some related to medication.

Liver disease The most common cause of liver abnormalities on blood testing are medications taken for the SLE. These were most often aspirin, NONSTEROIDAL ANTI-INFLAMMATORY DRUGS (NSAIDs), or AZATHIOPRINE. The liver is unusual in that in addition to its normal arterial supply it has a large vein bringing blood into it for detoxification, the portal vein, and a large vein taking blood out toward the heart, the hepatic vein. Thrombosis of either of these veins can occur, especially in the presence of the antiphospholipid syndrome. If the portal vein thromboses, there is a build up of pressure in the gut and swelling due to fluid in the peritoneal cavity (ascites). If the hepatic vein thromboses (Budd-Chiari syndrome), ascites also occurs, but in addition there will be liver damage. Hepatitis or inflammation of the liver occurs and is associated with anti-dsDNA and antiribosomal P antibodies. The differentiation between viral hepatitis, especially hepatitis C and SLE, can occasionally pose problems. SLE can cause a false-positive screening test for hepatitis C, and many patients with chronic hepatitis C develop positive ANA

and joint pain. In addition, alpha interferon, used in the treatment of hepatitis C, can occasionally induce SLE.

Blood system abnormalities Low white cell count (leukopenia) as well as neutropenia and lymphopenia are common in SLE itself but occasionally can be a side effect of immunosuppressive medication. Doing a bone marrow examination to differentiate between these causes may be necessary. Lymphopenia is usually associated with active lupus elsewhere. A low platelet count is common in SLE. Platelets are the smallest blood cells and initiate clotting in response to damage to a blood vessel. A few patients present with bleeding and very low platelets as the first manifestation of SLE. The platelet count can also vary with the activity of the disease, improving with successful treatment. Patients with antiphospholipid syndrome frequently have a low platelet count without having active inflammation. Anemia is common, and there are a number of possible causes. Chronic inflammation causes anemia as does kidney damage; blood may be lost into the gut; and SLE patients may develop autoimmune hemolytic anemia. This hemolytic anemia is due to antibodies directed against the red cells.

The spleen is involved in the body's normal processes for getting rid of immune complexes. It is probably for this reason that the spleen is frequently enlarged in lupus, although it can also be damaged and shrink. Many patients with lupus have enlarged lymph nodes at some time, and typically these fluctuate in size. Very occasionally tumors may develop in the spleen or lymph nodes.

Complement levels are low in active SLE due to increased consumption by immune complexes. Very rarely inherited low levels may be the cause of lupus.

Atherosclerotic disease Since improved treatment of SLE leads to increased life expectancy, atherosclerotic disease has become a more and more important cause of illness and death in lupus patients. A growing amount of evidence indicates that inflammation plays an important role in the initiation and progression of the fatty plaques that develop on the walls of blood vessels and finally lead to a manifestation of atherosclerosis. The four most common manifestations are myocardial infarction, stroke, peripheral vascular disease (poor circulation to the legs leading to dry gangrene in severe cases), and atherosclerotic kidney failure. Atherosclerosis is common in older individuals even if they do not have any risk factors. However, the presence of risk factors makes the disease present at a younger age and may make it more severe. Risk factors are additive in that the more a person has the greater the risk at, for example any given blood pressure or cholesterol level. The traditional risk factors are smoking, high blood pressure, raised cholesterol, and diabetes. Obviously SLE patients may also have these.

When the blood-vessel lining cells (endothelial cells) are activated they push signaling molecules called adhesion molecules, particularly ICAM-1 and E-selectin, through their walls to stick into the surface. White blood cells rolling by recognize these, activate, and stick onto the wall. Release of cytokines takes place and a low-grade inflammatory process is set up. Activation of the endothelial cells is induced by low-density lipoprotein (in patients with high cholesterol), advanced glycosylation end products (in diabetes), and also immune complexes, activated lymphocytes, and antiphospholipid antibodies. In this way SLE may be a powerful risk factor for atherosclerotic disease separate from more traditional risk factors. There may also be an effect through traditional risk factors in that lupus may cause high blood pressure. Treatment with corticosteroids may increase blood pressure, cause diabetes, worsen cholesterol, and make platelets more sticky than usual.

Although the mechanisms are not completely worked out, lupus patients are clearly at increased risk of atherosclerotic complications. Women between the ages of 35 and 44 years have a very low risk of myocardial infarction normally. However, women at these ages with SLE have a 50 times greater risk than those without. Even when all the traditional risk factors were controlled for (see CLINICAL TRIAL), SLE patients had a nearly five times greater risk of carotid atherosclerosis than controls. The carotid arteries take blood to the brain.

Pregnancy and SLE Women with SLE have special problems with pregnancy. This is not just in those with antiphospholipid antibody syndrome (see relevant section) but in many others as well. The remarks here relate mainly to SLE patients without the antiphospholipid syndrome. There is some disagreement about whether pregnancy makes lupus more active, but many people think it does. Certainly it does not improve in pregnancy as rheumatoid arthritis does. Patients with SLE who do get pregnant tend to have slightly more miscarriages, more premature deliveries, and babies with a lower birth weight than controls. Active kidney disease is a strong predictor of a poor outcome for the pregnancy. High blood pressure is a predictor of premature delivery and low-birth-weight babies (see PREGNANCY).

Patients with anti-Ro (SSA) antibodies may give birth to children with neonatal lupus (approximately one in four infants). This is caused by the mother's antibodies crossing the placenta and does not mean that the infant is going to have SLE. These infants have a characteristic rash, sometimes disturbed liver tests and an abnormal blood count, and most seriously but less commonly, heart block. In heart block the electrical conducting system is damaged so that impulses from the top half of the heart do not travel to the lower, pumping half, which therefore beats very slowly. The antibodies clear in a few weeks, and the blood, liver, and skin problems subside. However, the heart block may be permanent, and the majority of infants require a pacemaker. If mothers are shown to have the particular anti-Ro antibody, the risk of their child having heart block is about 12 percent. Women with anti-Ro antibodies also seem to have a higher miscarriage rate. This may be related to the heart block developing in utero.

Diagnosis Because SLE can present in so many different ways and affect so many different organs, patients with SLE can apparently have quite different diseases. One patient may have trouble with skin rashes and arthritis, another mainly kidney disease, and a third psychiatric problems, yet they all have SLE. So that the diagnosis of SLE is fairly consistent from place to place, the American College for Rheumatology (ACR) developed and refined criteria for classification of SLE. Currently the 1982 revised criteria are used. These are classification criteria and are therefore not essential for the diagnosis. However, if a patient did not meet four out of the 11 criteria, the evidence for SLE would have to be very good. For example, a patient may have typical kidney disease and positive ANA and anti-dsDNA tests and therefore have definite SLE despite fulfilling only three criteria. The 11 criteria include three typical rashes, mouth ulcers, arthritis, serositis, kidney disease, nervous system or psychiatric disorder, blood abnormalities, positive ANA, and one of several other immunological tests. Each criterion has clear definitions.

The diagnosis of SLE has become much easier with improved immunological testing over the past 15 years (see autoantibodies above). All patients should be checked for lupus anticoagulant and antiphospholipid syndrome on diagnosis and for any thromboses. Low white cell counts are common as is anemia and thrombocytopenia or low platelet count. Thrombocytopenia is particularly common in patients with the antiphospholipid syndrome. The ESR is usually raised in active disease and is a fairly reliable indicator of this, although it can also be raised due to a high protein level, kidney impairment, and other unrelated factors. The protein level is sometimes raised because of the excessive antibody formation. Low complement components C3 and C4 usually reflect increased use to solubilize immune complexes but may occasionally be the result of an inherited deficiency.

If central nervous system involvement is suspected, an MRI scan may be helpful, although it can be completely normal in lupus involving the nervous system. Newer magnetic resonance techniques such as quantitative magnetic resonance, magnetization transfer imaging, magnetic resonance spectroscopy, and diffusion-weighted imaging give further information in various ways but do not provide a diagnostic test. They are also not widely available, and conventional MRI remains the technique of first choice. A lumbar puncture is usually done as well. This may show increased cells or protein but may also be normal. A tracing of brain waves (EEG) is often abnormal but does not determine whether SLE is causing the abnormalities. Other organs are imaged as indicated by the patient's problems.

Treatment Options and Outlook

The treatment of SLE varies considerably from patient to patient and from time to time, according to which problems are active at any particular time. Some therapies need to be ongoing, but others are required only to settle a given manifestation and can then be discontinued. Since SLE can go into remission there will also be periods when no treatment is required. However, except in very mild disease, some form of ongoing monitoring is required since activity can flare at any time. A number of scoring systems have been developed to assess the disease activity in this disease that can affect different organs at different times. The best known is the systemic lupus erythematosus disease activity index or SLEDAI. This notes the presence or absence of 24 features of activity and weights them according to seriousness. The treatment of SLE is therefore very dependent on the particular manifestations and their severity. Much of this is highly specialized. This section will just give a brief overview of common treatments used, some of the newer developments, and then some comments on outcome.

General measures

- As mentioned above regular contact with a physician experienced in treating SLE is important to monitor both the disease and many of the therapies. Relying on symptoms is not sufficient since kidney disease and blood or liver disorders, for example, may cause no symptoms until well advanced. These are more usually picked up on laboratory testing.

- Sunlight is not only a frequent cause of rashes but also causes systemic illness. Any excessive sunlight should therefore be avoided and high-factor sun protection worn when exposed. Wearing hats and long sleeves is advisable when outdoors in summer. Sunlight coming through windows can also cause problems. There is a variation in photosensitivity, and some SLE patients are even sensitive to fluorescent light.

- Infections are common in patients with SLE and should be looked for whenever someone develops a fever. Antibiotic prophylaxis should be used for procedures on the teeth, bladder, or bowel in patients with heart valve abnormalities. An annual flu vaccine is advisable. If the spleen has been removed, vaccination against pneumococci is essential. This is usually done before the spleen is removed unless it is an emergency.

- Some of the drugs used in SLE are potentially toxic to the fetus, and effective contraception should be in place for women of childbearing age. Pregnancy in SLE should be carefully planned and treated as a high-risk pregnancy from the beginning (see PREGNANCY).

- Education leading to a better understanding of this rare and potentially severe disease is important in developing coping strategies. Information is obtained from the patient's physician, information booklets, and SLE patients support groups.

- No patient with SLE should smoke.

- No particular diet is required, but several factors are worth noting. Weight gain due to corticosteroids and the corticosteroids themselves can cause appreciable cholesterol increases, and appropriate diet may be required for this. Although there is some suggestion that fish oils reduce inflammation in SLE patients, this requires further trials to prove. Patients with SLE face many possible factors that lead to weak bones (OSTEOPOROSIS or OSTEOMALACIA), including chronic illness, corticosteroid use, and early menopause. Because sun avoidance is necessary for many, they may also become short of vitamin D (see osteomalacia). This should be checked for and supplemented if necessary.

- Vaccination with inactive or killed vaccines such as for influenza and pneumococcal infections is safe although somewhat less effective than in the general population. Live vaccines are avoided.

- Some radiotherapists are reluctant to treat patients with SLE who develop tumors for fear they will have exaggerated reactions to radiotherapy. Although limited by small numbers, most studies that have been done do not show any increased risk of adverse reactions.

Established treatments Many treatment strategies in SLE have been developed on an empiric basis (i.e., without understanding exactly how they work) and refined through controlled trials where possible. Being a rare disease, however, makes it difficult for many treatments to be studied in a controlled manner in enough patients. The following drugs have an accepted role in treating SLE:

- NSAIDs are commonly used for muscle, joint, or soft tissue pain and may be helpful for mild serositis. All the commonly used NSAIDs are effective, although some people respond better to one than to another. Patients with poor kidney function should take particular caution with using NSAIDs since they will be more than usually susceptible to the kidney-related side effects of these drugs. Noninfectious meningitis is a very rare adverse effect of NSAIDs, and SLE patients are said to be more prone to develop this than others, particularly with ibuprofen.

- Corticosteroids are the most frequently used drug in sudden flares of disease and, in adequate dosage, are effective in most forms of SLE. There are skin and eye preparations, preparations for injection into joints and soft tissues, and intravenous preparations for use in different situations. The particular form or preparation used is chosen to suit the purpose and resolve symptoms with the minimum total corticosteroid dose. Once the inflammation is settled the dose is usually reduced steadily to the minimum that will keep things under control. If control is not possible at a low dose, other agents will have to be added to avoid the long-term adverse effects of corticosteroids. Although extremely safe in the short term, corticosteroids have very significant long-term adverse effects. These are related to the total dose and length of treatment (see Corticosteroids in Appendix II).

- Antimalarials are very useful in treating skin manifestations as well as arthritis and help with the mild nonspecific symptoms such as fatigue and mild fever. HYDROXYCHLOROQUINE is most commonly used, but others include CHLOROQUINE and quinacrine. Patients on long-term hydroxychloroquine do have fewer flares. Rashes are not uncommon with hydroxychloroquine, but the most concerning adverse effect is the possible toxicity to the eye with long-term use. These drugs bind to some of the pigment at the back of the eye (retina) and can cause changes that lead to loss of vision. With low doses this is very unusual, but yearly eye checks by an ophthalmologist are advised. Fortunately the changes are visible before any loss of vision occurs, and no deterioration occurs if the drug is then stopped. There are concerns about toxicity to the fetus if the patient becomes pregnant, although a growing number of lupus patients have taken hydroxychloroquine during pregnancy (to control active disease) and have had normal healthy infants.

- AZATHIOPRINE is widely used in active SLE, especially when it is only possible to control inflammation with a relatively high dose of corticosteroids. When used in this situation, it lowers the number of flares, reduces the severity of illness, allows a lower dose of PREDNISONE to be used, and improves kidney function. These results were seen in a four year randomized, controlled study. As would be expected, showing these results in shorter trials is difficult. There is some disagreement about its effectiveness in inflammation of the kidney (nephritis). Azathioprine would generally not be the drug of first choice here, although it may be used later on in therapy or in patients with mild disease. Adverse effects include liver reactions and low blood counts, and regular monitoring blood tests are required for these to be picked up early. It seems likely that some tumors of the lymph nodes (non-Hodgkin's lymphomas) occur more frequently in patients on long-term azathioprine therapy, but this remains a very rare occurrence.

- CYCLOPHOSPHAMIDE is a potent immunosuppressive drug and has emerged as the drug of choice in severe kidney inflammation due to SLE. It is also commonly used in other life- or organ-threatening situations such as vasculitis or inflammatory nervous system lupus. It is usually best given as intermittent pulses of intravenous therapy. Common adverse effects include nausea and vomiting and there is always a drop in white cell count. Red cells and platelets may drop as well but usually with longer term treatment. Patients on cyclophosphamide are at increased risk of infections. Fertility may be affected. In men who wish to raise a family subsequently, it is possible to store sperm obtained prior to treatment. Young women about to undergo treatment with cyclophosphamide have been treated with the contraceptive pill to try to protect their ovaries. Now an agent called leuprolide can induce a prepubertal state, and in a nonrandomized trial has been shown to prevent ovarian failure in many but not all women undergoing treatment with cyclophosphamide. Irritation of the bladder may be severe if MESNA is not used to protect it. There is an increased risk of malignancy, usually after a number of years, and predominantly cancer of the bladder. Because of these serious potential adverse effects, cyclophosphamide is reserved for very serious disease and increasingly, courses are short with other agents being substituted once the disease is well controlled.

- METHOTREXATE has been less used in SLE than azathioprine. Some evidence does show that it is effective, especially for arthritis, rash, and serositis. Its use is similar to that in rheumatoid arthritis.

- DAPSONE is used occasionally for skin lesions, especially one called lupus profundus.

- INTRAVENOUS IMMUNOGLOBULIN (IVIG) is used in a number of autoimmune conditions, although its mechanism of action remains unclear. In SLE its main use is in the treatment of thrombocytopenia (low platelets).

- DANAZOL is a weak androgen (male hormone) that is useful in the treatment of thrombocytopenia. It must not be used in pregnancy or while breast-feeding. The chief adverse effects are hormonal, with disturbed menstrual cycle and sometimes male hormone effects such as excess hair growth. Occasionally liver tumors can develop with androgenic agents including danazol.

- Attention to risk factors for atherosclerosis is very important. Hypertension should be very well controlled, lipid profiles known and treated if necessary, prophylactic low-dose aspirin considered, especially if corticosteroids are being used, corticosteroid dose minimized, and homocysteine measured and controlled, especially in renal impairment. The antiphospholipid syndrome is a risk factor for thrombosis and needs treatment in its own right.

Newer and experimental approaches

- MYCOPHENOLATE MOFETIL is a newer immunosuppressant that has shown promise in early studies and is being investigated as a treatment for lupus nephritis. Mycophenolate mofetil is used in clinical practice as an alternative to azathioprine. In short- and medium-term studies treating lupus kidney disease, it has been shown to be equivalent in efficacy to cyclophosphamide with less toxicity but has not replaced cyclophosphamide yet as the long-term results are still not known.

- DHEA or dehydroepiandrosterone has achieved some popularity among patients with SLE. It is a weak androgen (male hormone). One randomized controlled trial has shown minor improvement in activity scores and fewer flares. The patients on DHEA also felt better overall. In a one-year trial, more than half the patients stopped taking DHEA, mostly because they either felt no better on it or they developed male hormone side effects, most commonly acne and increased facial and body hair. DHEA may have a beneficial effect on bone density, which is frequently a problem in SLE patients. A meta-analysis (i.e., combining the results of all suitable trials) did not find any benefit of women with SLE taking DHEA. Because DHEA is available over the counter, people have been taking a variety of doses, sometimes dictated more by cost than evidence. There is little information about the long-term side effects of DHEA.

- Bromocriptine has undergone a well-conducted randomized controlled study in SLE. It had been found that a number of SLE patients had raised prolactin. This is a hormone released in the brain that plays a major role in lactation but has also been found to have effects on the immune system. Although there were minor differences in the groups of patients, this study showed no real benefit of bromocriptine.

- CYCLOSPORINE was found to be effective in treating patients with severe kidney inflammation (nephritis) in whom either azathioprine or cyclophosphamide had not worked. This was not a controlled trial, however, and the role for cyclosporine is not yet clear. Cyclosporine was compared with prednisolone (a corticosteroid) and cyclophosphamide together in children with lupus nephritis. Although both groups did equally well from the kidney point of view, those on cyclosporine grew better. This was thought to be due to avoiding the stunting effects of corticosteroids in children. Concerns remain, however, about using conventional courses of cyclosporine in children.

- Stem cell or bone marrow transplantation (see BONE MARROW TRANSPLANTATION) have been used to treat a number of severe autoimmune diseases. In these procedures stem cells are first obtained from the patient or a compatible donor. The patient's bone marrow (the organ responsible for making all blood cells) is destroyed using very high doses of cyclophosphamide. Stem cell transplantation has now been used in over 100 patients with very severe SLE in Europe and the United States. While some patients actually go into a prolonged remission and others improve, a number do die as a result of the procedure. It remains therefore an expensive, high-risk procedure appropriate only for people with severe disease resistant to other treatments. In a variation of this a small group of very severe SLE patients have been treated with high doses of cyclophosphamide that all but destroys the bone marrow. However, the remaining cells grow back after about two weeks, and all patients in this group have improved, some quite dramatically. A number appear to relapse about three years after the procedure. This is a high-risk procedure and clearly appropriate only for people with severe disease resistant to other treatments.

- LEFLUNOMIDE, a relatively new drug that is well established in rheumatoid arthritis, has been tried at high doses in SLE. Some patients have responded well but others hardly at all, and its place in the treatment of SLE is not clear.

- RITUXIMAB is a B cell–depleting antibody that would be expected to have significant effects in SLE given the prominent role of B cells in this disease. Initially it was used in combination with cyclophosphamide but subsequently has been used with either mycophenolate mofetil or just corticosteroids. While some patients appear to do remarkably well, there have been a number of adverse effects including a rare condition known as progressive multifocal leukoencephalopathy. This is due to a reactivation of a virus and causes severe brain damage. It is important therefore to have results from randomized controlled trials to determine the best place for this new treatment. Other antibodies that interfere with B cell function are also being looked at.

- With the explosion of knowledge and rapid technological advances in immunology over the past 10–15 years, the possibility of using immunological methods to alter immune responses has arisen. Antibodies are made in response to antigens, usually part of an unwanted foreign particle. It has been known for some time that antigens given by certain routes in certain doses cause the immune system to accept them rather than produce an immune response against them (immune tolerance). This immune response would involve antibody production by B cells orchestrated by CD4 T cells. Therefore, if the antigen that was driving autoantibody production in SLE could be given in the right dose by the right route, perhaps the autoimmune process could be turned off. Although this rather simplifies things, a lot of research has been done over the past five years trying to develop a B cell toleragen (the antigen that could induce tolerance) or T cell vaccine that might achieve this. To date work has been done only in animals that develop lupus or with laboratory-grown cells. There are many problems. One is that although the molecule against which autoantibodies are directed may be known, e.g., DNA, the antigen is only a small fragment of that molecule. Finding the specific portion that is antigenic is difficult. This is compounded by there being more than one antigen.

Outcome The average survival of patients with SLE has improved in recent decades. More than 90 percent of patients survive five years from diagnosis, and more than 80 percent survive 10 years. Within that there is some variation. Younger patients do better than older patients, and higher levels of socioeconomic achievement also predict a better outcome. Those without organ-threatening disease or the antiphospholipid syndrome have virtually a normal life expectancy, whereas those with significant organ damage within the first year of diagnosis have a slightly reduced 10-year survival of 75 percent. Deaths tend to occur early, in the first five years, or late, after 15 or more years from diagnosis. The improvement in survival has come mainly from a reduction in the early deaths.

The three main causes of death in SLE patients are organ failure, infection, and cardiovascular disease. Organ failure chiefly involves kidney failure, central nervous system involvement, or multiorgan failure from severe, active SLE. Patients are at risk of infection by virtue of having SLE as well as from their immunosuppressive treatment. The most common sites of fatal infections are the lung, bladder, and joints. Most fatal infections are from bacteria that commonly cause infections in the rest of the population as well. High corticosteroid dose, immunosuppressive treatment, and a low white cell count are, however, risk factors for unusual or opportunistic infections. Cardiovascular disease leading to strokes, heart attacks, and impaired blood supply to the legs is made worse by the same things that affect everyone else (smoking, high blood pressure, etc.), but the disease clearly plays a major role as well.

Risk Factors and Preventive Measures
As the major risk factors are genetic and the female sex, these are clearly not preventable. Avoidance of ultraviolet light both from the sun and indoor fluorescent lighting for some very sensitive individuals is important in preventing flares of disease but the light does not cause it.

systemic sclerosis See SCLERODERMA.

tai chi chuan One of a group of therapies known as "mind-body" therapies. In tai chi chuan mythology the Taoist monk Chang Sanfeng created the movements that have become tai chi chuan based on a dream about a fight between a bird and a snake. This certainly gives a good image of the movements. It is the flowing from one pose to another, blending the eternal and ephemeral.

There are claims that it massages the inner organs, improving blood and lymph flow, increases energy flow, calms the mind and body, and opens joints. Controlled trials in these areas are few. A controlled trial shows that tai chi chuan does not make RHEUMATOID ARTHRITIS worse. There is interest in the prevention of falls (especially in older people), and controlled studies have shown improvement in balance and strength in people undertaking tai chi chuan for at least six months compared with control groups.

Takayasu's arteritis (pulseless disease) A type of VASCULITIS that affects large blood vessels. It affects women at least five times as often as men and usually starts between the ages of 10 and 40 years. Takayasu's arteritis occurs globally, but there are large geographic variations in frequency. It is common in India and Japan, but in the United States there are only approximately three new cases per million people a year.

Takayasu's arteritis affects large arteries such as the aorta and the blood vessels to the neck (carotid artery) and arms (subclavian arteries) and causes inflammation that leads to scarring and narrowing. The geographic differences in frequency led researchers to seek infectious or genetic causes, but so far no cause has been identified. In Japan a certain tissue type, HLA-Bw52 (see HLA) is associated with an increased risk of Takayasu's arteritis, but this is not the case everywhere. An autoimmune process may be involved because affected arteries are very inflamed and have a lot of white blood cells infiltrating their walls. Takayasu's arteritis occasionally occurs in patients who have SYSTEMIC LUPUS ERYTHEMATOSUS, ERYTHEMA NODOSUM, or INFLAMMATORY BOWEL DISEASE. The presence of antibodies to the inner lining layer of blood vessels, the endothelium, in some patients is an additional clue implicating autoimmunity as a cause. However, even if an autoimmune reaction is the cause, the triggers and mechanisms are not clear.

Symptoms and Diagnostic Path
Nonspecific systemic symptoms such as loss of weight, fatigue, athralgia, myalgia, and low-grade fever are common. High blood pressure is common if the disease affects the arteries to the kidneys. Later in the disease symptoms caused by inadequate blood supply to particular organs can occur. The pattern of these symptoms depends on the blood vessels and organs affected. For example, if Takayasu's arteritis affects blood vessels to the heart or brain, angina or stroke can occur. Inflammation at the base of the aorta often affects the aortic valve, causing it to leak and leading to heart failure. If the blood vessels to the arms or legs are affected, the patient may feel severe pain in the muscles during exercise. This happens because the blood supply to the exercising muscle is inadequate. This type of limb pain that comes on with exercise and disappears with rest is called claudication.

The diagnosis is made based on the physical findings and imaging of the arteries, usually by ARTERIOGRAPHY (see Appendix II). The American College of Rheumatology has published classification criteria that require three of the following six criteria:

- Onset of symptoms before the age of 40 years
- Claudication
- A decreased or absent pulse in one of the arteries in the arm
- A difference in blood pressure between the two arms
- A bruit over a large artery; a bruit is a blowing noise that can be heard with a stethoscope
- Narrowing of a large artery on arteriography that is not explained by atherosclerosis or another disease

Classification criteria were developed mainly for research purposes and are not always helpful in making the diagnosis in an individual patient.

Physical examination is very helpful because atherosclerosis is extremely rare in young women, the group most likely to develop Takayasu's arteritis. Therefore if there is no pulse in an artery in a young woman, the diagnosis should be suspected. Blood tests are not very helpful. The ESR (see Appendix II) is a nonspecific marker of infection or inflammation that is often elevated, particularly if the disease is active. Arteriography is usually performed and shows smooth narrowing of large arteries. In patients with narrowing caused by atherosclerosis the narrowing is much more irregular.

Treatment Options and Outlook

CORTICOSTEROIDS, initially in high doses, are used to control the disease. The dose of corticosteroid is tapered slowly. If this is not possible, another drug such as METHOTREXATE is added. It is difficult for physicians to know how active the disease is. Old, established scarring will not improve with aggressive therapy, but active inflammation will. The ESR can be a clue to how active the disease is. Performing arteriograms repeatedly is difficult because the procedure is invasive, requiring that an artery be punctured and dye injected into it. New MRI techniques are less invasive and have provided good images of arteries after dye is injected into a vein. These less invasive imaging techniques can easily

be repeated and may provide a way to evaluate the activity and progression of the disease.

Scarring and narrowing of arteries is permanent, and some patients require surgery to bypass a blocked artery. Alternatively a stent (a steel frame that expands and keeps the artery open) can be placed in the narrow segment of the artery. If the disease affects the aortic valve, heart surgery to replace the valve may be needed. Takayasu's arteritis is a chronic disease. The overall prognosis is good, and approximately 90 percent of patients are alive five years after diagnosis. Patients with progressive arterial disease or complications such as stroke or heart involvement have a worse prognosis.

Risk Factors and Preventive Measures

Although the distinct geographic differences in incidence of this disease suggest a physical cause, none has been found, and there are no known risk factors or preventive measures.

tarsal tunnel syndrome   See FOOT PAIN.

temporal arteritis   Also known as giant cell arteritis and cranial arteritis, this is an inflammatory disease affecting large- and medium-sized arteries, particularly around the head (see VASCULITIS). It is found throughout the world but appears to be more common in Caucasian people. It almost exclusively affects people over the age of 50 years and women three times as often as men. In the United States between 15 and 20 people in every 100,000 over the age of 50 get temporal arteritis each year.

The cause is unknown. Several families exist where more than one member has developed the disease. So-called clustering of the disease has also been observed in husband and wife, neighbors, friends, and small areas within a village. This suggests some factor in the environment may trigger the disease, but no obvious candidates exist. A number of viruses have been investigated as a possible cause without positive results. One report found a strong association with contact with pet birds, but this has not been confirmed. Large- and medium-sized arteries have an elastic layer in their walls, and it is here that the inflammatory attack seems to be concentrated. Lymphocytes, a few neutrophils, and the characteristic giant cells gather here to produce a granulomatous inflammation that affects blood vessels in patches. The wall of the artery is damaged, and it may clot off (thrombose). Arteries of the head and neck are particularly affected, but others may also be involved. These less frequently involved arteries are usually the aorta (the main blood vessel taking blood from the heart to the rest of the body) and its immediate branches. Interestingly the blood vessels within the brain are seldom affected, although the main supply vessel, the internal carotid artery, is very frequently involved as is its branch to the eye.

Symptoms and Diagnostic Path

General symptoms are common and may have been present for months before specific symptoms occur that allow a definite diagnosis to be made. These include fever, weight loss, tiredness, and loss of appetite. Headaches in someone with these symptoms are the most suggestive specific symptom. Headaches often begin early and may be very severe. They are most frequently felt over the temple and are often associated with tenderness of the scalp to even light touch. The arteries running up across the temple to supply the scalp (temporal arteries) may be swollen and tender and lack the normal pulsation of an artery.

As with most forms of vasculitis, the most devastating effects are those that result from thrombosis of an artery and the consequent loss of blood supply to a part of the body. In temporal arteritis blindness due to thrombosis of an artery taking blood to the eye (usually the central retinal artery) is the most feared thrombotic complication. Some eye symptoms occur in over 30 percent of patients, but actual loss of vision occurs in less than 10 percent. This is not always complete. However, complete, sudden, painless loss of vision is the most common form. If one eye is affected the other eye is at high risk.

Pain in the jaw on chewing sometimes accompanied by tingling of the tongue and loss of taste is very characteristic but not very common. Occasionally splitting of the wall of the aorta or even complete rupture can occur. When the larger arteries are narrowed by vasculitis, it is sometimes possible to hear the sound of irregular blood flow through these vessels (termed bruits, pronounced brooees). Usually this is heard by the doctor listening over the vessels with a stethoscope. When arteries of the head and neck are affected, the patient can sometimes hear these bruits. Temporal arteritis can also cause strokes, depression, confusion, deafness, and damage to the nerves to the feet and lower legs, although these are not common. Heart attacks have been described and liver function test abnormalities are common, although seldom serious. There is an association between temporal arteritis and POLYMYALGIA RHEUMATICA, but most patients with temporal arteritis do not have polymyalgia. Between 5 and 10 percent of patients with either temporal arteritis or polymyalgia have autoimmune thyroid disease. The thyroid disease usually precedes the temporal arteritis by some years.

If there are typical symptoms such as new headaches and jaw pain on chewing, the diagnosis is not difficult. However, these symptoms may be intermittent or not present in the early stages, and a patient may just present with mild fever and weight loss, for example. It is therefore important to consider temporal arteritis in patients over the age of 50 years with these nonspecific symptoms. All the arteries running over the scalp should be examined, not just the temporal arteries. The ESR is almost always raised. The most definitive test is to take a biopsy of an artery that is thickened and tender and show that there is granulomatous inflammation invading the wall of the vessel. A few patients have had a positive temporal artery biopsy but a normal ESR, but this is very unusual. There is often a nonspecific rise in the alpha globulins (a group of proteins in the blood) and in other markers of inflammation such as the C-reactive protein. These are not any more helpful than the ESR, however. Abnormal liver tests are common but not usually of any significance.

Treatment Options and Outlook

CORTICOSTEROIDS (usually prednisone) are the mainstay of treatment. They are effective in controlling the inflammation and preventing complications such as blindness if used correctly. However, the treatment usually needs to be continued for between two and three years, and there are significant side effects possible if prednisone is used for this length of time. Indeed, after the first three to four months, management of corticosteroid side effects becomes more difficult than management of the vasculitis. The principles of management include the following.

Adequate early treatment This is done to achieve control of the inflammation. For most people 40–60 mg of prednisone a day for the first month is the preferred dose. Lower doses or rapid reduction lead to relapse, and higher doses expose the patient to excessive amounts of prednisone that are unnecessary in the vast majority of patients. Higher doses are traditionally used in those patients with visual symptoms.

Prevention of early thrombosis Inflamed arteries are at risk of thrombosing. Corticosteroids cause alterations in the blood favoring thrombosis. There are numerous reports of patients with temporal arteritis going blind within 48 hours of starting prednisone therapy. While not proven it is possibly due to this increased risk of thrombosis. A treatment to prevent this is low-dose ASPIRIN therapy started at the same time or just before the prednisone. Two retrospective studies have shown that the incidence of loss of vision and other ischaemic (loss of blood supply) events were much less frequent in patients taking low-dose aspirin compared to those not taking it.

Prevent osteoporosis Many patients will be older women who are already at risk of postmenopausal osteoporosis. Corticosteroid therapy increases the rate of bone loss. Any at-risk individual starting long-term corticosteroid therapy should receive prophylaxis for at least the duration of therapy. This is best achieved with calcium and vitamin D supplements and a bisphosphonate such as ALENDRONATE, RISEDRONATE, or cyclical ETIDRONATE, although other agents are becoming available (see OSTEOPOROSIS). Hormone replacement therapy would not be a first-choice therapy here because of the slightly increased risk of thrombosis associated with its use.

Reduce the corticosteroid dose gradually The ideal rate of reduction is not known and will vary between patients. As a general guideline, gradual reduction to 10 mg a day of prednisone over the first four to six months is reasonable. The dose is then reduced more slowly, for example by 1 mg every one or two months if the patient remains in remission. Reducing the dose too rapidly increases the risk of relapse, and patients who relapse end up requiring greater amounts of prednisone. Patients vary in how rapidly the corticosteroid dose can be reduced. Monitoring both symptoms and the ESR is important when altering the dose.

Minimize the total dose of corticosteroids The number and frequency of adverse effects from the corticosteroids is proportional to the length of treatment and the total dose of corticosteroids. The above strategies will minimize the total dose and the common adverse effects.

A few patients will not be able to reduce their prednisone dose within a reasonable time frame without symptoms flaring. These patients may be treated with an immunosuppressive agent such as METHOTREXATE, AZATHIOPRINE, or even CYCLOPHOSPHAMIDE with success.

Temporal arteritis appears to be a self-limiting disease. If patients are able to come off therapy without any complications, they are likely to do very well. The early problems are largely related to the serious vascular disease and include blindness and strokes. The later problems are related to the corticosteroid therapy and include weight gain, vascular disease, osteoporosis, easy bruising, diabetes, and poor control of blood pressure.

Risk Factors and Preventive Measures

Although the occasional clustering of the disease in households or neighborhoods has sparked many investigations looking for a physical cause, none has been substantiated, and there are therefore no preventive measures possible.

tendinitis   See SOFT TISSUE ARTHRITIS–RELATED PROBLEMS.

tennis elbow   See EPICONDYLITIS.

thromboangiitis obliterans   See BUERGER'S DISEASE.

thrombocytopenia A low platelet count. Platelets play an important role in blood clotting, and the major problem caused by a low platelet count is an increased risk of bleeding. Paradoxically, some conditions that cause a low platelet count such as heparin-induced thrombocytopenia (HIT) and thrombotic thrombocytopenic purpura (TTP) increase the risk of clotting.

A low platelet count is usually the result of one of two processes, decreased production or increased destruction. Decreased production of platelets can occur with any condition that affects the bone marrow, the site of platelet production. An example is cancer that has spread to the bone marrow. Drugs, most often anticancer or immunosuppressive drugs, can suppress the bone marrow and decrease its ability to make platelets. For example, CYCLOPHOSPHAMIDE, a drug used to treat VASCULITIS and SYSTEMIC LUPUS ERYTHEMATOSUS (SLE), can cause thrombocytopenia as well as decrease the white blood cell count.

Increased destruction of platelets usually occurs through immune mechanisms. This often occurs as part of an autoimmune process, for example SLE, and the body forms antibodies against its own platelets. Another illness that causes the body to produce antiplatelet antibodies is idiopathic thrombocytopenic purpura (ITP), a rare condition of unknown cause that affects children more often than adults and can trigger severe thrombocytopenia. Antibodies against platelets can also develop in response to drugs. Many drugs such as sulfonamides, quinine, and quinidine can cause thrombocytopenia, but the best example is heparin-causing HIT.

Platelets filter through the spleen, and any condition that enlarges it can lead to increased destruction of platelets. This is one of the mechanisms contributing to thrombocytopenia in FELTY'S SYNDROME. Many infections, particularly viral infections, are associated with thrombocytopenia.

Symptoms and Diagnostic Path

Most patients do not have any symptoms until the platelet count is very low, often less than 20,000 per mm^3. The first symptom is usually purpura, a rash consisting of small, raised purple spots. Severe thrombocytopenia can cause blood to ooze from the nose and gums or bleeding from the bowel. HIT and TTP can be associated with the formation of blood clots and can, for example, cause stroke or thrombosis in a vein or artery.

There are two components, the diagnosis of thrombocytopenia, and the diagnosis of the underlying cause. Thrombocytopenia is diagnosed from a blood count (see CBC in Appendix II). It may be a specific finding on a diagnostic CBC ordered in a patient who has purpura or a chance finding on a CBC performed for some other reason.

When a diagnosis of thrombocytopenia is made, a careful history and physical examination will often reveal the cause. Mild thrombocytopenia is common in SLE. If a patient with rheumatoid arthritis has an enlarged spleen and thrombocytopenia, the diagnosis of Felty's syndrome is likely. A careful history will reveal exposure to drugs that can cause thrombocytopenia. If a patient is clotting rather than bleeding and has thrombocytopenia, it suggests a diagnosis of HIT, TTP, or ANTIPHOSPHOLIPID ANTIBODY SYNDROME.

Heparin-induced thrombocytopenia occurs in approximately 1 percent of people treated with the drug, usually about a week after treatment has been started. About 10 percent of these patients may develop arterial or venous clots. To prevent these complications, the diagnosis of HIT must be made early and treatment with heparin discontinued.

TTP is an unusual and serious syndrome consisting of thrombocytopenia, anemia due to increased breakdown of red blood cells (hemolysis), kidney failure, and CNS effects such as depressed level of consciousness. TTP was described by Dr. Eli Moschcowitz in 1924. TTP can follow infection or exposure to certain drugs such as ticlopidine and can occur in patients with autoimmune disease such as SLE.

Treatment Options and Outlook

Thrombocytopenia does not need treatment unless it is severe. If a drug is the cause, stopping the offending drug will often cure the problem. Severe autoimmune thrombocytopenia is often treated with high doses of corticosteroids. If that does not control the problem, other options are INTRAVENOUS IMMUNOGLOBULIN (IVIG), aggressive immunosuppression with cyclophosphamide, or removing the spleen (splenectomy). Platelet transfusions are seldom needed but may be required if a patient is actively bleeding. If a patient has an immunological cause for thrombocytopenia, the transfused platelets are rapidly destroyed and are not effective.

TTP is treated with PLASMAPHERESIS. Transfusion of platelets can be useful in an emergency, for example if someone has serious bleeding caused by severe thrombocytopenia, but is not useful for long-term treatment of TTP. Thrombocytopenia usually responds to treatment but can recur.

tissue type See HLA.

TNF antagonists See TUMOR NECROSIS FACTOR ANTAGONISTS.

torn cartilage See MENISCAL TEAR.

trigger finger The tendons that curl the fingers up into a fist are encased in a sheath as they run across the palm of the hand. They can become swollen and catch in this sheath, which often also constricts. This usually happens about a centimeter before the base of the finger and can result in the finger sticking in a curled up position as though pulling a trigger, hence the name trigger finger.

When occurring on its own, trigger finger usually results from repetitive grasping activities. The muscle involved is the flexor digitorum superficialis and lies in the forearm. Precipitating activities can occur in many situations, including driving for long periods, sport, hand work in industrial settings, massage, prolonged card playing (trigger thumb), horseback riding, and prolonged music practice. The three elements that predispose some people to developing trigger fingers are prolonged activity, poor technique, and increased muscle tension (as, for example, if driving is stressful and the steering wheel is tightly gripped for several hours at a time). Repeated trauma such as may occur with digging is another possible cause. People with widespread inflammatory arthritis such as RHEUMATOID ARTHRITIS are especially likely to develop trigger finger, often with very little or no obvious initiating factors. Prolonged playing of video games is a more recently described cause and may coexist with calluses and joint pain as the so-called arcade arthritis.

Symptoms and Diagnostic Path
The first symptom is often waking up in the morning and having pain and difficulty in straightening a finger. It will often flick straight suddenly as the tendon thickening or nodule squeezes through the narrowed part of the sheath. Sometimes it is necessary to use the other hand to pull the finger straight. Typically the triggering gets a little easier as the hand is used throughout the day.

The typical history and a competent examination are enough to make the diagnosis in the vast majority of patients. Ultrasound scanning is excellent at showing the tendon enlargement and triggering but is only occasionally necessary. DUPUYTREN'S CONTRACTURE and the cheiroarthropathy of DIABETES MELLITUS need to be excluded.

Treatment Options and Outlook
Management of trigger finger is divided into treatment to relieve symptoms and ways to avoid recurrence.

Treatment
- A light splint can be applied for six weeks, and this will result in two-thirds of patients being cured at one year.
- NSAIDs may be used in conjunction with splinting.
- Injection of CORTICOSTEROID along the tendon sheath is quicker and more effective and therefore the preferred treatment. Over 80 percent of patients are cured at one year following injection of corticosteroid. In addition, most patients who do not respond to splinting are cured by injection. The injection should be done by someone trained in this procedure and must not be given into the tendon.
- If these measures fail, surgical stripping of the sheath off the tendon is usually effective.

Outcome Corticosteroid injection provides pain relief in about five days and return to normal function in two weeks. With NSAIDs and splinting, return to normal function takes three to six weeks. When compared with surgery, patients having injection therapy had just as good results but returned to work an average of four weeks earlier than the surgical group.

Risk Factors and Preventive Measures

Repetitive grasping activities, especially if forceful or associated with trauma, are the main risk factors. Preventive measures include:

- The patient must be made aware of the activities that might play a role in causation. Getting expert advice on technique, for example in playing a musical instrument, may be important. Some limitation on the time spent doing these activities is also important in the first month or two after successful treatment.

- Wrapping a small amount of clingfilm or wearing a short "finger sock" around the proximal interphalangeal or middle joint of the affected finger improves awareness of movement and may help in the first two weeks after injection.

- Learning muscle relaxation techniques is important where excessive muscle tension is thought to have played a role.

- Wearing a quilter's glove may help those involved in repetitive movement.

trochanteric bursitis This bursa (see SOFT TISSUE ARTHRITIS–RELATED PROBLEMS) lies just behind the outer bony point of the hip bone, the greater trochanter. This may become inflamed, producing bursitis. Abnormality of the gait predisposes to this bursitis. This may be related to, for example, OSTEOARTHRITIS at the hip, being overweight, or muscle weakness around the pelvis. Another bursa overlying the tip of the greater trochanter can also become inflamed.

The pain from this bursitis is often worst when lying on the affected side at night or when setting off walking after a rest. There is a small area of marked tenderness about an inch behind and above the greater trochanter. Treatment involves injection of the bursa with CORTICOSTEROID and correction of any gait abnormality that might predispose to it.

It is likely that gluteal tendinitis is frequently misdiagnosed as trochanteric bursitis. A similar group of people are prone to develop this. Patients with both conditions should be encouraged to stretch the gluteal muscles with knee to chest stretches. The two conditions can be differentiated by ultrasound or MRI scanning but in practice this is seldom done.

tuberculosis (TB) An infectious disease caused by *Mycobacterium tuberculosis* that is spread from person to person by droplets that are coughed into the air. TB is a common disease worldwide, affecting millions of people. It is more common in developing countries. In the United States many cases occur in immigrants. The majority of people exposed to TB develop a primary infection that causes some lung inflammation and enlarged lymph nodes but then resolves. The infection then lies dormant, in most people forever, and does not cause disease. However, in some people the primary infection is not contained and spreads to the lungs, causing pulmonary TB, or to the brain, kidneys, and other organs. TB that has been dormant can reactivate many years after the primary infection. Any condition that suppresses the immune system such as HIV infection or treatment with CORTICOSTEROIDS or TUMOR NECROSIS FACTOR (TNF) ANTAGONISTS can cause TB to reactivate. TB affects the lungs primarily. The reason for describing it in this book is that it occasionally affects bones or joints.

TB is caused by an organism, *M. tuberculosis*. Infection spreads to other people from an infected person who has open TB. This means that the patient has lesions in the lung that are breaking down and releasing mycobacteria into the lung secretions. When a patient with open TB coughs, mycobacteria are launched into the air in microdroplets, and an uninfected person nearby can become infected by inhaling them. Outbreaks of TB can often be traced back to a single infected patient. People who have been exposed to TB in the past and developed a primary infection that was contained by the immune system are not infectious. Only a few people who are exposed to TB develop disease. It is uncertain why this happens. Genetic and social factors seem to play a role in determining whether the initial infection is contained. In some countries a vaccine called BCG (bacillus Calmette-Guérin) is used to prevent tuberculosis. BCG is a weaker strain of mycobacteria that does not usually cause disease in humans but stimulates the immune response to *M. tuberculosis.* More recently BCG has been used to treat bladder cancer by placing it into the bladder to stimulate the local immune response. Arthralgia (0.5–5 percent) and arthritis (less than 1 percent) can develop in patients treated for cancer using this vaccine (see DRUG-INDUCED RHEUMATIC DISEASE and REACTIVE ARTHRITIS).

Symptoms and Diagnostic Path

TB usually starts insidiously, causing fatigue, loss of energy, loss of weight, fever, and night sweats. If the lungs are the main site of infection, cough, sometimes producing blood, is prominent. Other organs such as lymph nodes, kidneys, and meninges (the lining of the brain) can be involved.

Musculoskeletal disease-caused TB is not common in the United States, but in developing countries it commonly causes spinal deformities. The most common musculoskeletal complication of TB is spine involvement, sometimes also called Pott's disease. The infection settles in a disc between two vertebrae and slowly expands to destroy the bone of the adjacent vertebrae. The bone collapses and the spine becomes deformed. If the infection affects the spinal cord, the legs may become paralyzed (paraplegia). The most common symptom of TB affecting the spine is back pain. TB can affect virtually any bone, but this is rare.

Tuberculosis affecting a joint causes chronic destructive arthritis, usually of one large joint such as the hip or knee. The affected joint is swollen and painful, but swelling is often more prominent than pain. Unlike INFECTIVE ARTHRITIS caused by bacterial infection that is very acute, tuberculous arthritis starts and progresses slowly over weeks and months. In addition to infecting and destroying a joint, tuberculosis can rarely cause a reactive arthritis. This is called Poncet's disease. Unlike tuberculous arthritis, Poncet's disease

affects many joints, is not destructive, and settles spontaneously.

A tuberculin skin test is used to diagnose previous exposure to TB. This is done by injecting a small amount of tuberculin protein under the skin and measuring the wheal a few days later. People who have not been exposed previously do not react, while those who have mount an immune response and form a wheal. A tuberculin skin test is useful in several situations. If someone is exposed to a patient with tuberculosis and is known to have had a negative skin test which then becomes positive, it indicates transmission of TB. A tuberculin skin test is also helpful in patients suspected of having TB. Most patients with active TB have a strongly positive tuberculin skin test. Unfortunately, a tuberculin skin test usually remains positive forever and most patients with inactive TB also have a positive test. This means that a positive test could be the result of exposure years ago, recent exposure, or active infection. Another limitation is that if a patient is severely ill or taking immunosuppressive drugs the test may be negative despite active infection.

Symptoms can provide a clue to diagnosis. TB should be suspected in every patient with a chronic cough and fever or unexplained weight loss and fever. The X-ray findings can also be helpful. TB typically causes scarring and small abscesses in the upper parts of the lungs. The presumptive diagnosis of TB is often made by finding the organisms in the sputum or another body fluid. These organisms stain in a particular way on slides prepared for microscopy and are termed *acid-fast bacilli* or AFBs. Some other mycobacteria are also acid-fast, and the definitive diagnosis is made when the organism is cultured, a process that can take several weeks. Molecular biology techniques that use polymerase chain reaction (PCR) to detect DNA specific for M. tuberculosis are much faster but are not widely available. Occasionally the diagnosis can be made only from a biopsy of affected tissue that shows changes that are typical for TB and are very different from other infections or cancer.

Diagnosing tuberculosis affecting bone or joints is more difficult. The clinical features provide some clues, as do the X-ray findings, which show destruction of bone, but a biopsy is usually needed.

Most patients with bone or joint TB do not have active pulmonary tuberculosis and are therefore not infectious.

Treatment Options and Outlook
The treatment of tuberculosis requires a combination of three drugs for at least six months. One such combination is rifampin, isoniazid, and pyrazinamide. Some tuberculosis organisms have become resistant to some of the common treatments. Patients with an infection caused by a resistant organism often need treatment with four drugs for longer than six months. Tuberculosis is cured if a patient takes the treatment correctly. Not completing the course of treatment is a common cause of failure to cure TB and facilitates the development of resistant organisms. One way to improve adherence to treatment is directly observed therapy (DOT). This involves health care workers physically observing a patient taking treatment twice a week. If someone develops a positive skin test but has no symptoms of infection treatment with a single drug, isoniazid is often prescribed to help the immune system contain the primary infection.

Risk Factors and Preventive Measures
The risk factor for acquiring new-onset tuberculosis is usually significantly close contact with someone with "open" or infectious tuberculosis. This may occur sporadically and unexpectedly but should be anticipated in high-risk situations. These include living and working in the third world and working with infectious patients in hospitals and in clinics attended by homeless or impoverished people (who have a higher incidence of tuberculosis and a longer delay before diagnosis and treatment). People exposed to these at-risk situations should be screened with a chest X-ray and tuberculin test and, if these suggest no previous contact with tuberculosis, they should be vaccinated with BCG. People working in very high-risk situations such as infectious diseases hospitals where tuberculosis patients are treated should have a regular screening program, usually annual chest X-rays.

The risk factor for reactivation of quiescent tuberculosis is anything that significantly weakens the immune system. These include very old age, cancer, and chronic infections, especially HIV and drugs that suppress the immune system. Antirheumatic drugs of importance in this regard include the TNF antagonists, CYCLOPHOSPHAMIDE, and AZATHIOPRINE. Screening for tuberculosis is routinely carried out before starting a TNF antagonist, and if this suggests previous exposure prophylactic treatment is usually given (see TUMOR NECROSIS FACTOR ANTAGONISTS).

tumor necrosis factor antagonists (TNF antagonists)
A class of drugs that blocks the inflammatory CYTOKINE tumor necrosis factor (TNF). These drugs were initially developed to treat severe sepsis, which is associated with very high levels of TNF, but they were not effective. Fortunately, later studies showed that ETANERCEPT and INFLIXIMAB were effective in patients with rheumatoid arthritis (RA) and have revolutionized its treatment. TNF antagonists are now also used to treat a wide range of other autoimmune and rheumatic diseases, including INFLAMMATORY BOWEL DISEASE, PSORIASIS, ANKYLOSING SPONDYLITIS, JUVENILE IDIOPATHIC ARTHRITIS, VASCULITIS, Still's disease, and BEHÇET'S DISEASE. They have been so successful that the market for TNF antagonists in the United States alone was $10 billion in 2007.

When they were first released, infliximab and etanercept seemed almost too good to be true. Clinical studies indicated they were very effective and had virtually no serious adverse effects. Information obtained after the drugs were marketed was also reassuring. For example, follow-up of patients who received etanercept in the early clinical trials found no increase in the rate of serious infection or cancer. However, wider use of TNF antagonists in the community soon generated reports of a range of adverse effects that have grown with increasing use.

Infections Individual clinical trials may not show an increase in rare adverse events. However, when several thousand patients taking part in different controlled trials were brought together in a meta-analysis, patients using a TNF antagonist were found to have roughly double the risk of getting infections as those patients on other DMARDs. Not all these infections are serious, but it was calculated that about one in 60 patients treated with a TNF antagonist will develop a serious infection.

A surprising number of these were found to be so-called granulomatous infections that are normally quite rare. The body forms granuloma to defend against organisms that it finds very difficult to destroy such as *Mycobacterium tuberculosis* (see TUBERCULOSIS), *Histoplasma capsulatum* (the cause of histoplasmosis), and *Coccidioides immitis* (coccidioidomycosis). To control the infection, these organisms are ingested by large cells, the macrophages, and surrounded by many other immune cells, forming a tight ball or granuloma. TNF is crucial in granuloma formation, and so blocking it causes difficulty in defending against these infections. More common bacteria remain the commonest causes of infection in these patients. In the southwestern United States, screening for coccidioidomycosis (chest X-ray and blood test) should be done before starting TNF antagonist treatment. Tuberculosis has become quite rare in developed countries. In the United States, between one in 2,000 and one in 3,000 individuals using TNF antagonists will develop tuberculosis, with greater numbers in countries such as Spain and Portugal where the background rate of tuberculosis is higher. It frequently affects organs other than the lungs and in these cases can be difficult to diagnose. Before starting a TNF antagonist all patients should be screened by history of tuberculous contact, chest X-ray, and skin test with tuberculin or one of the newer whole blood gamma-interferon tests. If these suggest latent tuberculosis, the patient should be treated before starting the TNF antagonist and carefully followed up. Mycobacteria other than tuberculosis also cause infections in TNF antagonist–treated patients with increased frequency.

The interaction between TNF antagonists and viral infections is less clear. Some viruses such as hepatitis B and C (see HEPATITIS) are often controlled rather than eliminated by the immune system, and reactivation of disease has been reported but clearly does not always occur. There are reports of HIV patients being successfully treated with TNF antagonists, but there are significant dangers in this and the need would have to be great. Limited data available at present suggest there is an increased risk of infection following orthopedic surgery in patients who continue their TNF antagonist. It

seems prudent therefore to stop it three weeks (for ETANERCEPT or ADALIMUMAB) and six weeks (for INFLIXIMAB) before invasive surgery. Live vaccines are contraindicated.

Malignancy Establishing whether a drug increases the incidence of cancer in patients with rheumatoid arthritis and similar diseases can be difficult for a number of reasons. One is that rheumatoid patients have a higher risk of malignancies by virtue of having the disease and those with more severe disease (who are more likely to receive TNF antagonists) are probably at even higher risk. These patients may also have received many other medications that confuse the issue. There is fairly consistent data that patients with rheumatoid arthritis have roughly double the risk of getting lymphoma than the general population (everybody of course has some risk). Some studies have suggested that the risk of lymphoma in people treated with adalimumab and infliximab is up to five times that of the general population and about three times for etanercept. There are, however, a number of well-done studies that show no increased risk. There are similar conflicting results from studies of other malignancies. One clear-cut exception seems to be when TNF antagonists are used in patients who have been treated with cyclophosphamide. Here the incidence of malignancies appears greatly increased, and this combination is not advisable. Like other immunosuppressants, TNF antagonists seem to increase the incidence of skin cancers, but not greatly.

Autoimmunity There are two types of autoimmunity the TNF antagonists can induce. The first is to stimulate the immune system to produce antibodies directed against the TNF antagonist itself, so-called neutralizing antibodies. The second is to induce an autoimmune disease. Neutralizing antibodies are quite frequent, especially with infliximab, which is only partly a human antibody. There is some evidence that the higher the neutralizing antibody levels the shorter the response to infliximab and that the concomitant use of an immunosuppressive drug such as methotrexate or azathioprine lowers the levels of antibodies. However, this is not a simple relationship. Although antibodies directed against adalimumab are less frequent, it is clear that their presence does predict a poor response.

Clinical trials show that about 10 percent of patients on etanercept and 60 percent on infliximab develop autoantibodies (i.e., antibodies directed against parts of the individual's own cells), usually ANA and anti-dsDNA. Only a very few patients have developed autoimmune disease however. These include DRUG-INDUCED LUPUS, PSORIASIS, VASCULITIS, and lung and eye disease.

Other   Skin reactions at the site of injection are common but seldom serious. Allergic reactions can occur, either of the immediate anaphylactic type or a delayed serum sickness type with sore muscles and joints and skin rash. Very rarely patients on TNF antagonists develop demyelinating disease where nerves start to dysfunction because they lose their fatty sheath. This can occur in the brain as happens with multiple sclerosis or elsewhere. Although initially thought a possible treatment for heart failure, a number of trials failed to prove this, and in fact those treated with a TNF antagonist did slightly worse. TNF antagonists should therefore be used with caution in the presence of heart failure. There are occasional reports of bone marrow failure. Psoriasis has occurred.

The price of TNF antagonists has caused controversy. To treat an average rheumatoid patient with a TNF antagonist costs more than $10,000 a year. At this price not every patient with RA can be treated. Besides, in some patients RA can be controlled with older drugs at a fraction of the price. So who should receive TNF antagonists? One argument is that early, effective treatment of RA will be cheaper in the long run because patients will be able to work and, in the long term, will not need expensive treatments such as joint replacement surgery. An alternative argument is that the expensive treatment should be reserved for patients who have not responded to traditional, cheaper DMARDs. Many HMOs take the second approach and require that a patient have failed treatment with several DMARDs before treatment with a TNF antagonist will be authorized. The costs of anti-TNF drugs may decrease over time when there is more competition in the marketplace. Even so, society will have to decide how to ration health care resources, even in societies not accustomed to the concept of rationing.

An important consideration is that although TNF antagonists are probably more effective than the gold standard drug for RA, methotrexate, they are not effective in every patient and do not cure RA. In the future tests will likely be developed to predict which patients are likely to respond to particular treatments (see PHARMACOGENETICS).

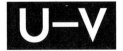

ulcerative colitis See INFLAMMATORY BOWEL DISEASE.

undifferentiated connective tissue disease See OVERLAP SYNDROME.

uveitis See EYE PROBLEMS.

vaccination When a virus or bacteria invades the body, the immune system recognizes small areas on the microbe as foreign. These are called antigenic determinants. As a result of this recognition the immune system is able to mount a response against the invading microbe and, hopefully, destroy it. Once the immune system has responded successfully to an infection, it retains a memory of the important antigenic determinants. This enables the immune system to mount another attack much more quickly and effectively should it come into contact with the same microbe again.

This natural ability is utilized in vaccination. By showing a person's immune system the important antigenic determinants of important disease-causing viruses and bacteria, it is possible to *pre-arm* the immune system and fully or at least partially protect the individual from that disease. This is usually done by killing the microbe and extracting parts that contain the important antigens. It can also be done by giving people an infection with a closely related but much less dangerous microbe than the one that is being protected against. In this way, vaccination has practically eradicated polio and diphtheria from the developed world. Tetanus and hepatitis B are much less common, and the fetal abnormalities caused by RUBELLA (German

measles) are theoretically completely preventable. Measles epidemics now occur every seven years rather than every second year as they did before vaccination. Several issues are relevant to the rheumatic diseases.

Immunosuppressed patients People on immunosuppressive treatment, especially potent drugs such as CYCLOPHOSPHAMIDE, AZATHIOPRINE, or high-dose CORTICOSTEROIDS, should not be given live vaccines. Although harmless to most people, these can cause serious illness in those without a competent immune system. Live vaccines include those against polio, measles, mumps, rubella, chicken pox, tuberculosis (BCG), typhoid, yellow fever, and the vaccinia vaccine against smallpox. These are not absolute contraindications. The use of live vaccines depends on the degree of immunosuppression and the importance of having the vaccine. Immunosuppressed patients may not respond very well to killed vaccines, but they will be safe.

Asplenia Patients who have no spleen are highly susceptible to infections with certain bacteria. In rheumatic disease patients the likely reason for not having a spleen is having it removed to treat resistant autoimmune THROMBOCYTOPENIA. Patients with SICKLE-CELL DISEASE are often effectively without a spleen because it has shrunken up due to loss of blood supply. Protecting against some of the infections these patients are at risk from is possible. Therefore, patients with sickle-cell disease and those about to have their spleen removed should be vaccinated against *Pneumococcus, Haemophilus* influenza type b, and *Meningococcus* before, not after, surgery.

Protection of immunosuppressed children It is important to vaccinate the relatives and close friends of children who are heavily immunosuppressed to lessen the risk of those children getting the common infectious diseases that could be devastating for them.

Musculoskeletal adverse reactions Local reactions to vaccination are common, and there are other less common adverse effects. Only musculoskeletal reactions will be discussed here. Oral polio vaccine quite commonly causes muscle aching. Rubella vaccine (usually given as part of the measles, mumps, rubella [MMR] vaccine) is well known to cause a short-lived arthritis (see rubella). Up to 15 percent of adult women get this arthritis after rubella vaccination but much fewer men or children. A few patients appear to have developed a longer lasting arthritis, but it is not yet clear whether this is related to the vaccine. Thrombocytopenia occurs in one in every 30,000 people vaccinated for rubella. Very rarely, OSTEOMYELITIS may follow BCG vaccination for tuberculosis and musculoskeletal symptoms following HEPATITIS B vaccination.

vasculitis Inflammation of blood vessels that damages arteries, veins, and the fine network of capillaries that joins them. The definition of vasculitis is deceptively simple but describes a vast range of diseases and symptoms. Vasculitis can mimic virtually any illness, and therefore, making the correct diagnosis can be difficult. Several illnesses can mimic vasculitis, for example cancer, infections, INFECTIVE ENDOCARDITIS, and CHOLESTEROL EMBOLI SYNDROME.

There are many different types and causes of vasculitis, and they are described in detail under their individual headings. The cause of most types of vasculitis is not known. Vasculitis typically affects several organs simultaneously. A rare type of vasculitis, CENTRAL NERVOUS SYSTEM VASCULITIS, affects only the central nervous system, most often the brain.

Kussmaul and Maier were probably the first to describe vasculitis in 1866. Then over decades physicians described different types of vasculitis. In 1952, Zeek classified vasculitis into different subtypes, based mainly on the size of the blood vessels affected. Unfortunately, there is a lot of overlap, and a particular type of vasculitis can affect different-sized vessels. Consequently, many other classifications evolved, but most rheumatologists still classify vasculitis into three groups based on the size of the vessels most often affected (see the table below).

Vasculitis affecting predominantly the small vessels of the skin is often called leukocytoclastic vasculitis, a name that describes its appearance under a microscope. The polymorphonuclear white blood cells that invade the blood vessel wall are often partially degenerated, and there is cellular debris present. The most prominent clinical feature is palpable purpura, a rash consisting of small, raised, purple spots. Leukocytoclastic vasculitis can occur with other rheumatic diseases, for example RHEUMATOID ARTHRITIS and SYSTEMIC LUPUS ERYTHEMATOSUS (see RHEUMATOID VASCULITIS).

Leukocytoclastic vasculitis is sometimes also called hypersensitivity vasculitis. More correctly this refers to vasculitis that is caused by a specific

THE PROPENSITY OF DIFFERENT TYPES OF VASCULITIS TO AFFECT BLOOD VESSELS OF PARTICULAR SIZE

Type of Vasculitis	Size of Vessel		
	Large	Medium	Small
Temporal arteritis	Often	Sometimes	Seldom
Takayasu's arteritis	Often	Sometimes	Seldom
Polyarteritis nodosa	Seldom	Often	Sometimes
Wegener's granulomatosis	Rare	Sometimes	Often
Churg-Strauss syndrome	Rare	Sometimes	Often
Leukocytoclastic vasculitis	No	Rare	Often

antigen, for example a viral infection or drug. Many drugs such as penicillins, sulfonamides, cephalosporins, thiazides, phenytoin, and captopril can cause vasculitis (see DRUG-INDUCED RHEUMATIC DISEASE). Similarly many infections have been associated with vasculitis, including HEPATITIS B, HEPATITIS C, HIV, Epstein-Barr virus, PARVOVIRUS, rubella, herpes virus, and many others.

Symptoms and Diagnostic Path

Vasculitis damages blood vessels and can impair the blood supply to organs and cause them to malfunction. Severe vaculitis can cause irreversible damage to tissues. At the site of damage in the vessel wall there is often overgrowth of endothelial cells and fibrous tissue, presumably a response to repair the damage. This can block the artery, particularly if the blood flowing through the narrow channel clots. The symptoms of vasculitis depend on the organs involved. Nonspecific complaints such as fever, loss of weight, arthralgia, and myalgia are common. Small-vessel vasculitis most often causes a rash consisting of small, raised, purple spots that can be felt as well as seen (palpable purpura). Other types of vasculitis cause symptoms that affect a range of organs. Temporal arteritis often causes headaches and may cause blindness. Wegener's granulomatosis often affects the upper respiratory tract, sinuses, lungs, and kidneys. Polyarteritis nodosa is more likely to affect nerves and kidneys. However, there is overlap of symptoms between different types of vasculitis. (See the table below.)

Diagnosing vasculitis can be difficult. The initial symptoms often suggest infection or cancer as possible diagnoses, but the constellation of symptoms and results of tests such as the ANTINEUTROPHIL CYTOPLASMIC ANTIBODY or ANCA (see Appendix II) lead to the correct diagnosis. For many types of vasculitis a biopsy of affected tissue is the most accurate way to make an unequivocal diagnosis. Because the treatment of vasculitis requires medications with potentially serious side effects, a correct diagnosis is important.

Treatment Options and Outlook

The treatment of different types of vasculitis varies and is described in detail under their individual entries. As a general principle, though, more severe vasculitis requires more aggressive treatment. If a drug or infection causes vasculitis that affects only the skin, specific treatment, other than stopping the offending drug, is seldom needed. Treatment of more severe vasculitis almost always involves immunosuppression with CORTICOSTEROIDS, often combined with CYCLOPHOSPHAMIDE or another immunosuppressant. The outcome of vasculitis varies and depends on how severe it is, how much organ damage has occurred before treatment, the response to treatment, and the severity of the side effects of treatment. Patients with kidney involvement leading to renal failure and vasculitis of the bowel leading to bleeding and gangrene have a worse prognosis.

viral arthritis   The most important viruses causing rheumatic disease have been discussed in separate sections in this book. These include HEPATITIS B, HEPATITIS C, PARVOVIRUS, RUBELLA, and HIV. Other viruses that may cause rheumatic symptoms will be briefly listed here. Viruses can cause arthritis by directly invading the joint, by forming complexes

APPROXIMATE FREQUENCY OF SYMPTOMS AND LABORATORY TESTS IN DIFFERENT TYPES OF VASCULITIS				
Symptom	Wegener's Granulomatosis	Churg-Strauss Syndrome	Polyarteritis Nodosa	Temporal Arteritis
Upper airway disease	95%	60%	No	No
Gastrointestinal vasculitis	5%	60%	70%	Rare
Nervous system affected	30%	15%	70%	Rare
Eosinophilia	Uncommon	Common	Uncommon	No
Elevated ESR	Common	Common	Common	Common
Positive ANCA	85% C-ANCA	70% P-ANCA	15% P-ANCA	No

with antibodies (see IMMUNE RESPONSE) that are then deposited in the blood vessels of joints and cause inflammation, or by surviving inside joint lining cells and thereby making them a target for the immune system. Viruses are usually only looked for directly in biopsy tissue from joints as part of a research project. The usual way of diagnosing viral arthritis is to find evidence of recent infection with the relevant virus in serial blood tests and make the reasonable assumption that the arthritis was caused by this infection.

Also known as arboviruses, *alphaviruses* are mosquito-borne viruses that have been known for many years to cause arthritis. Alphaviruses belong to the same family as rubella, the Togaviridae. O'nyong-nyong has recently become a problem in Uganda after disappearing for over 30 years. It causes a rash, fever, and arthritis.

Ross River virus in Australia and other South Pacific islands is probably the best known of the alphaviruses. There is fever and rash, and the arthritis affects mainly the hands, knees, and feet. Symptoms start about a week after being bitten by an infected mosquito. About 15 percent of infected people will get arthritis. Adults are more severely affected than children. In Australia, 5,000 cases a year occur, mostly during the summer months. Some people just get joint pain, but swelling of joints and tendons does occur and the arthritis may last up to six years. Barmah virus can cause a very similar disease and is found only in Australia. At least seven other mosquito-borne viruses in Australia are known to cause arthritis.

Pogosta disease, Ockelbo disease, and Karelin fever are all caused by related alphaviruses in northern Europe. Pogosta disease tends to cause epidemics every seven years and causes arthritis in over 90 percent of infected people. Another alphavirus, chikungunya, has caused a number of outbreaks in Southeast Asia in recent years. Unlike Ross River fever, chikungunya often causes a severe fever of sudden onset and the arthritis occasionally lasts for several years.

Mumps is a rare cause of arthritis. Most patients are young men. The arthritis may flit around or just affect one joint. There is often associated fever. The arthritis may last up to six months but does not cause lasting joint damage.

Adenovirus, a common cause of upper respiratory tract infections, has rarely caused an acute but short-lived arthritis.

Varicella-zoster, Epstein-Barr, Herpes simplex, and *cytomegalovirus* have all been associated with rare reports of arthritis.

Given the rarity with which the last six of these viruses cause arthritis, the occurrence of arthritis at the same time as or shortly after infection with one of them should always give rise to a careful consideration of another separate cause of the arthritis.

Risk Factors and Preventive Measures

The alphavirus-associated viral arthritides are only entirely avoided by not visiting the geographic areas mentioned above. If traveling to one of these areas, preventive measures against mosquito bites will have some effect. These include avoiding rural areas and the rainy season, not being outdoors in the evening, wearing long trousers and long-sleeved shirts, using insect repellent, and sleeping under a mosquito net. Mumps is prevented by routine vaccination with the measles, mumps, and rubella vaccine, and there are no effective preventive measures against the other viruses discussed in this section.

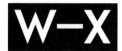

Wegener's granulomatosis A rare type of VASCU-LITIS that typically affects the sinuses, lungs, and kidneys. A limited form of the disease affecting only the lungs or upper respiratory tract can occur, but most such patients eventually develop kidney involvement. The features of the illness later named Wegener's granulomatosis were described by Dr. Heinz Klinger in 1931 and then by Friedrich Wegener in 1936. It occurs most often in young to middle-aged adults and affects one to three people in 100,000. Some studies have suggested a seasonal variation in frequency, with the disease more likely to occur in spring, but others have not confirmed this observation. Almost all patients with untreated Wegener's granulomatosis have died in a year, but modern drugs have improved the prognosis considerably.

The cause of Wegener's granulomatosis is not known. Research has focused on infection, genetics, environmental exposures, and autoimmunity as potential causes. No genetic or infectious cause has been identified. Some experts still believe that infection plays a major role because many relapses seem to occur after an infection, and eliminating bacteria from the nose with chronic antibiotic treatment has reduced the frequency of relapses in some studies. Exposure to silica dust, fumes, and pesticides has been associated with Wegener's granulomatosis in some studies, but many patients have no known exposure to any environmental toxin. In contrast to diseases like SLE where complexes of antibodies are deposited in affected tissues, in Wegener's granulomatosis there are few antibodies in tissues, and it is therefore sometimes called a pauci-immune vasculitis. However, many patients with Wegener's granulomatosis have ANTI-NEUTROPHIL CYTOPLASMIC ANTIBODIES or ANCA (see Appendix II). There are two types of ANCA: C-ANCA directed against proteinase 3 (PR3); and P-ANCA, usually directed against myeloperoxidase (MPO) (see Appendix II). It is not clear if ANCAs play a role in causing Wegener's. ANCAs are directed against neutrophils and may activate them and contribute to the damage to blood vessels and tissues that is typical of Wegener's granulomatosis. On the other hand, ANCAs may not play a direct part in causing disease but may be a response to tissue injury.

Symptoms and Diagnostic Path

Wegener's granulomatosis can affect virtually any organ and can mimic many illnesses. It usually starts gradually, with symptoms appearing over weeks or months. Some patients, though, have very rapid onset and progression of disease. Common initial symptoms affect the upper respiratory tract and lungs. Nonspecific complaints such as fever, loss of weight, arthralgia, and myalgia are common.

Upper respiratory tract The sinuses are often affected, causing sinus pain, persistent sinusitis, and a bloody or purulent discharge from the nose. Inflammation can cause the nasal cartilage to collapse so that the nose changes shape. The middle of the nose sinks, causing a *saddle deformity.* The ears are often affected, and patients have symptoms of pain, deafness, and discharge from the ear. Inflammation affecting the entrance to the airway can cause narrowing so that the flow of air into the lungs is restricted. Ulcers in the mouth and nose are common.

Lungs The lungs are affected in most patients, and symptoms such as coughing blood and shortness of breath are common. Most patients usually cough only small amounts of blood or blood-streaked sputum, but serious bleeding can occur.

Kidneys Wegener's granulomatosis damages the glomeruli that filter urine and can decrease renal function, causing the blood levels of CREATININE to rise (see Appendix II). If this is severe, it can cause kidney failure. The symptoms of renal failure are weakness, fatigue, itching, anemia, shortness of breath, and swelling of the legs. Most patients with Wegener's granulomatosis have an abnormal URINALYSIS (see Appendix II), but the small amounts of protein and blood in the urine do not cause symptoms.

Skin Wegener's granulomatosis, as do other types of vasculitis, typically causes a purpuric rash (small, purplish spots), but other rashes can occur.

Eyes Many patients develop eye inflammation. Wegener's granulomatosis can affect the eyes, causing scleritis (see EYE PROBLEMS) or inflammation of the area behind the eye, pushing it forward (proptosis). Inflammatory tissue behind the eye can destroy the eye, the bony cavity containing it, and the muscles that move the eye and is sometimes referred to as a pseudotumor.

Diagnosis Diagnosing Wegener's granulomatosis can be difficult because early in the illness many of the symptoms are not specific. For example, differentiating the sinus symptoms caused by Wegener's granulomatosis from those caused by other illnesses can be impossible, but clues to the diagnosis are persistent or recurrent attacks of sinusitis that cause destruction of tissues in the nose. Usually the diagnosis is suspected because of the unusual constellation of symptoms.

Blood tests A positive C-ANCA is found in 80–90 percent of patients with active Wegener's granulomatosis. The most common target for C-ANCAs is proteinase-3 (PR3), an enzyme found in neutrophils. A positive test can sometimes occur in patients with lymphoma, cancer, infection, and other types of vasculitis. A positive C-ANCA (PR3) in a patient with classical features of Wegener's granulomatosis confirms the diagnosis, and some clinicians believe that a biopsy to make an unequivocal diagnosis is not required in this situation. The level of C-ANCA has been studied as a way to monitor disease activity and predict relapses, but the results have been conflicting.

Other blood tests are not helpful in making the diagnosis but are useful for monitoring the effects of the disease and its treatment. The creatinine level is used to monitor kidney function and the white blood cell count to prevent cyclophosphamide toxicity.

Upper respiratory tract The sinuses are often affected on an X-ray or CT scan. A biopsy of sinus tissue sometimes shows changes typical of Wegener's but more often changes of chronic inflammation.

Lungs The lungs are affected in most patients, and the X-ray typically shows patches of inflammation that may be nodular and have small cavities in the center. A biopsy of lung tissue is the most accurate way of making the diagnosis. Biopsies performed with a bronchoscope passed through the nose under local anesthesia have a very low yield, and an open lung biopsy is needed. This involves surgery through the chest wall. The biopsy shows vasculitis with neutrophils invading and destroying the walls of small and medium-sized blood vessels and granulomas, which are palisades of cells surrounding a central area of dead tissue.

Kidneys A urinalysis is often abnormal showing blood and protein. The creatinine level may be elevated if kidney function is affected. Patients taking cyclophosphamide need regular urine monitoring to detect bladder inflammation (cystitis). If the kidneys are involved, a biopsy can be performed. It often shows patchy inflammation of the glomeruli that are surrounded with crescents of inflammatory cells. This finding is not specific and can occur when other autoimmune diseases affect the kidney. However, a kidney biopsy can be helpful, particularly if a lung biopsy is considered too risky.

Skin If there is a rash, a skin biopsy may show vasculitis.

Treatment Options and Outlook

Regular contact with a physician experienced in treating vasculitis is important to monitor both the disease and many of the therapies. Some of the complications of vasculitis such as kidney failure cause no symptoms until well advanced, and regular monitoring of laboratory tests is important.

Infections are common in patients with vasculitis, particularly those taking immunosuppressive drugs, and should be looked for whenever a patient develops a fever. An annual flu vaccine is advisable, and vaccination against pneumococcus is recommended.

Many of the drugs used to treat vasculitis can be harmful to the fetus. Therefore, women of child-bearing age should use effective contraception (see PREGNANCY).

Education that leads to a better understanding of this rare and often severe disease is important in developing coping strategies. Information can be obtained from physicians, information booklets, and patient support groups.

Patients with vasculitis should not smoke. Vasculitis damages small blood vessels. Smoking causes small vessels to constrict, increasing the chance that they will block up completely.

Most patients with significant ear, sinus, lung, kidney, or eye disease will benefit from seeing physicians specializing in these respective subspecialties.

Established treatments   Before treatment was available, patients with Wegener's granulomatosis survived an average of six months. Treatment with corticosteroids increased this to 12 months. In the 1970s, Dr. A. Fauci and his colleagues at the National Institutes of Health (NIH) developed a treatment program that resulted in improved long-term survival to better than 80 percent.

CYCLOPHOSPHAMIDE, a potent immunosuppressive drug, is the anchor of the NIH treatment program. The standard treatment for Wegener's is daily cyclophosphamide combined with a corticosteroid such as prednisone, both given as tablets (see Appendix I). Several studies have examined alternative treatments that cause fewer side effects. One such program uses monthly intravenous cyclophosphamide, as is done for SLE. Intravenous cyclophosphamide does cause fewer side effects than tablets but does not seem as effective at keeping the disease in remission. Cyclophosphamide, administered intravenously or by mouth, can have serious side effects. Nausea, vomiting, and a drop in the white cell count are common. Red cell and platelet counts may also decrease but usually with long-term treatment. Patients on cyclophosphamide have a greater risk of infection. A range of common and OPPORTUNISTIC INFECTIONS occurs in 40–70 percent of patients. Factors that increase the risk of infection are high doses of corticosteroids and a low white blood cell count. *Pneumocystis*

carinii pneumonia (PCP) is a preventable, serious opportunistic infection that can complicate treatment. The risk is highest during the initial phase of treatment, and some physicians prescribe antibiotics to prevent this infection.

Fertility may be affected. The risk of sustained ovarian failure and infertility after treatment with cyclophosphamide has ranged from 11–59 percent. The risk may be lower with IV pulse cyclophosphamide regimens than oral regimens, but the difference is not great. Cyclophosphamide also reduces the sperm count in men. Thus if the clinical situation allows, sperm or ova can be banked before starting treatment with cyclophosphamide in order to preserve future fertility. Several strategies to preserve fertility have been tried. Young women about to undergo treatment with cyclophosphamide have been treated with the contraceptive pill to try to protect their ovaries, but the results of these studies were mixed. Early results from studies using a drug called leuprolide are more promising. Cyclophosphamide has significant long-term side effects. These are related to the total dose and length of treatment. CHLORAMBUCIL is sometimes used for patients who are unable to take cyclophosphamide.

CORTICOSTEROIDS are initially used in high doses with cyclophosphamide to control inflammation and induce remission. Once the inflammation has settled the dose is reduced steadily to the minimum compatible with disease control. Corticosteroids have significant long-term side effects. These are related to the total dose and length of treatment (see Appendix I).

METHOTREXATE has been used to treat Wegener's and is effective, although probably not quite as effective as cyclophosphamide, for inducing and maintaining remission. In order to avoid the risks of long-term cyclophosphamide, many rheumatologists will substitute weekly oral methotrexate for cyclophosphamide if a patient has been in remission for a few months and is doing well.

AZATHIOPRINE is an alternative to methotrexate for maintaining remission.

Trimethoprim/sulfamethoxazole is an antibiotic (trade name: Septra) that has been used to treat Wegener's limited to the upper respiratory tract. In patients with disease affecting many organs it may decrease long-term disease activity in the upper airways.

INTRAVENOUS IMMUNOGLOBULIN (IVIG) is occasionally added to the treatment of patients who are severely affected and not responding to standard drugs.

Newer and experimental approaches   The combination antibiotic trimethoprim/sulfamethoxazole (TMP/SMX) has been used for mild Wegener's for many years, often with corticosteroids. In the absence of infection, however, it has very little effect and should not be used in patients with serious disease. The high doses used are also not compatible with methotrexate. MYCOPHENOLATE MOFETIL appears to be effective in maintaining patients in remission, although the studies are very small so far. The TUMOR NECROSIS FACTOR antagonist ETANERCEPT has not been found to be useful in maintaining remission. When INFLIXIMAB was added to other drugs to improve control it was effective, but there were significant serious side effects, and it cannot be recommended. There are reports of RITUXIMAB effectively inducing remission, but further studies are required.

Outcome   The usual treatment plan has two stages, to induce remission and then to maintain it. Most rheumatologists use high doses of corticosteroids with cyclophosphamide to induce remission, but some use corticosteroids and methotrexate in patients with milder disease. The dose of corticosteroid is decreased, and then methotrexate or less often azathioprine is substituted in place of cyclophosphamide to maintain remission. With modern treatment most patients with Wegener's go into remission after several months of treatment. The goal then is to sustain remission for at least six months and then slowly taper treatment. About half of patients with Wegener's relapse and need a second or multiple courses of treatment. The prognosis is worst in patients with severe lung or kidney disease.

Risk Factors and Preventive Measures

There are no known risk factors or preventive measures for Wegener's granulomatosis.

Whipple's disease   When Whipple first described this disease in 1907, he described a rod-shaped organism and wondered whether this might cause the disease. It took another 85 years to prove him correct. Whipple's disease is rare and is found mostly in middle-aged Caucasian men, often farmers or those with some involvement in farming. The disease affects many parts of the body, especially joints, gut, and skin.

For many years it was known that there were rod-shaped objects in the lining of the small bowel of patients with Whipple's disease that showed up with a particular stain known as PAS. Evidence steadily accumulated that this was an infection causing the disease. However, it was impossible to grow the putative bacterium to prove that it was actually an organism. With advancing technology, it eventually became possible, in 1992, to use polymerase chain reaction (PCR) to prove that it was a bacterium. The bacterium is called *Tropheryma whippelii*. It has been shown to be present in many organs in affected people. Growing the organism in artificial media has since become possible, although this is still very difficult and the PCR test is used for diagnosis.

Symptoms and Diagnostic Path

Over 80 percent of patients with Whipple's disease get arthritis. This usually precedes the other symptoms by five to eight years. Large joints are involved most commonly, especially the wrists, knees, and ankles. Hips, shoulders, and elbows may be affected, but smaller joints would be unusual. The typical arthritis causes attacks of joint pain and swelling occurring in different joints, sometimes lasting only six hours and sometimes days. It may, however, become ongoing when it is often confused with RHEUMATOID ARTHRITIS. It does not, however, cause erosive damage to the joints like rheumatoid arthritis does. Less frequently it may also affect the spine.

Often the appearance of diarrhea, abdominal pain, and weight loss results in the diagnosis being made. Chest pain due to pleurisy occurs. Involvement of the heart is less common, frequently affecting the valves when it is involved. Lymph nodes may be enlarged. Darkish discoloration of the skin, rashes, thyroid involvement, and occasionally kidney involvement are other features. The brain may be affected with confusion, poor memory, loss of interest, and a form of dementia.

The characteristic arthritis and absence of other causes may lead to a small bowel biopsy being done to show the typical PAS-positive material. However, only after other symptoms appear is the diagnosis often considered and biopsies done. In most studies the diagnosis is made only about six years after the first symptoms. PAS-positive material can sometimes be seen in joint fluid that is removed. However, this stain will be done only if the diagnosis is suspected. It is now possible to identify the organism using PCR. This has been successful in joint fluid, lymph nodes, and surgically removed joint lining as well as small bowel biopsies. It is hoped that with the recent culture of *Tropheryma whippelii,* more widely available and user-friendly tests will be developed to look for evidence of infection with this unusual organism. X-rays do not show any erosive destructive changes as they do in rheumatoid arthritis, which is the most commonly confused diagnosis. They may, however, show loss of joint space (cartilage), especially at the wrists and hips.

Treatment Options and Outlook

Whipple's disease was always fatal until antibiotics were shown to be effective. Somewhere between 70 and 90 percent of patients can now be cured with an adequate course of antibiotics. Antibiotics that penetrate the brain should be used in case there is some undetected infection there that reactivates once treatment is stopped. The brain has a special barrier (the blood-brain barrier) that means not all molecules that get into the bloodstream can get into the brain, and this includes some antibiotics. A currently recommended treatment plan is as follows:

1. Start with a two-week course of streptomycin 1 g per day and benzylpenicillin 1.2 million units per day.
2. Follow this with a one- to two-year course of trimethoprim and sulfamethoxazole (cotrimoxazole, trade name: Septra) 960 mg twice daily.

With this treatment the diarrhea will usually stop within a week and joint pain within a month. The patient will put on weight and feel generally better within the first few months, but neurological problems such as confusion and poor memory may take longer to improve. Although a very rare disease, Whipple's disease is very exciting since it is an example of scientific advances leading to the understanding and cure of a previously fatal multisystem disease.

Risk Factors and Preventive Measures

Tropheryma whippelii is related to bacteria called Actinomycetes found in the soil. This and the fact that over 80 percent of patients are men, 30 percent farmers, and most of the others with occupational exposure to soil suggest that the infection is contracted from repeated exposure to working with soil. This is not however known for sure. The preponderance of men of European origin also suggests a genetic susceptibility or inability to eradicate the infection. The disease is so rare that there is no practical preventive measure.

wrist pain   Pain in the wrist can be caused by a problem in any of the tissues in that area, most often bones, joints, tendons, and nerves. Pain caused by problems in the fingers and hand can sometimes be difficult to differentiate because severe inflammation of the hand can cause swelling and pain that extends up to the wrist.

Bones   Trauma causing bruising or a fracture is a common cause of wrist pain. A clue to the diagnosis is that the pain and swelling follow a traumatic event and there is intense tenderness directly over the painful area. The patient usually remembers an injury, particularly one that involved falling with the arm outstretched. Such an injury is the most common cause of a fracture at the end of the radius and ulna, the bones of the lower arm, called a Colles' fracture. Other common injuries are dislocation of the lunate and fracture of the scaphoid or hammate, small bones that form part of the wrist. An X-ray provides the diagnoses, and treatment is to return the bones to their original position and immobilize the wrist in a cast until healed. Treatment may require surgery. Occasionally the diagnosis of fractured scaphoid is missed or the correct diagnosis is made but the fracture does not heal, termed nonunion of the scaphoid. This can cause chronic wrist pain months or years after the initial trauma that caused the fracture and usually requires surgical repair.

Keinbock's disease, also called avascular necrosis of the lunate, is a rare condition that causes chronic wrist pain and swelling, usually in young adults. An X-ray shows deformity and, later, increased sclerosis (denser and therefore whiter on the X-ray) and collapse of the lunate, a small bone in the wrist. Surgery is usually needed to repair the damage, stabilize the wrist, and prevent later osteoarthritis.

Joints The joints of the wrist can be divided into three groups:

1. Joints between the lower end of the radius and ulna and the small bones of the wrist
2. Joints between the small bones of the wrist (the carpal joints)
3. Joints between the metacarpals, the raylike bones between the wrist and the fingers, and the small joints of the wrist (the carpometacarpal joints)

Virtually any type of inflammatory or non-inflammatory arthritis can affect the wrist (see ARTHRITIS) but RHEUMATOID ARTHRITIS, JUVENILE IDIOPATHIC ARTHRITIS, and pseudogout (see CALCIUM PYROPHOSPHATE DIHYDRATE DEPOSITION DISEASE) are common causes of wrist arthritis. OSTEOARTHRITIS typically affects the first carpometacarpal joint, the joint where the base of the thumb meets the wrist.

Tendons The tendons that flex the wrist and fingers run across the front of the wrist, and those that extend them run across the back of it. Inflammation of tendons (see TENDINITIS) can cause wrist pain. One of the most common is DE QUERVAIN'S TENOSYNOVITIS. This typically causes pain and sometimes swelling close to the lower end of the radius, the bone on the thumb side of the arm.

Nerves Pressure on a nerve as it passes through a narrow space can damage it. The usual symptoms are pain, numbness, and tingling. Entrapment of nerves in the arm usually causes symptoms that affect the fingers and hand. In CARPAL TUNNEL SYNDROME, though, symptoms are often poorly localized and can affect the wrist.

X-rays   See Appendix II.

APPENDIXES

APPENDIX I
DRUGS USED TO TREAT ARTHRITIS AND RELATED CONDITIONS

Please note that the side effects and precautions discussed below are not complete. Common side effects and particular precautions are discussed to promote safe, intelligent use of medications. If you have concerns that are not mentioned below and for additional information, you should consult the package insert and your doctor or pharmacist.

abatacept (Trade name: Orencia) Abatacept is a specially designed protein that decreases the immune response by preventing two types of cells, T-lymphocytes and antigen-presenting cells, from interacting and stimulating each other. Therefore, abatacept is sometimes called a "co-stimulation modulator." Abatacept is infused intravenously and acts as a DMARD in RA and is being tested in other rheumatic conditions.

Side effects There is limited long-term information. Common: Cough, respiratory infections, and exacerbations of chronic obstructive pulmonary disease. Uncommon: Infections (some serious) are more frequent in patients receiving abatacept. Requires intravenous injection, and minor reactions such as fever, chills, rash, and itching during or after infusion occur in 2–9 percent of people. Serious allergy (anaphylaxis) is rare. The combination of abatacept with other biological immunosuppressants (e.g., etanercept, anakinra, infliximab) is usually avoided because it increases the risk of infection.

acetaminophen (Trade names: Acephen, Aceta, Apacet, Panadol, Tylenol, and others) An analgesic (painkiller) used to treat pain of mild-to-moderate intensity. Acetaminophen is also an antipyretic and reduces fever, but it has little effect on inflammation. Acetaminophen causes fewer serious gastrointestinal side effects than NSAIDs and is recommended as the drug of first choice for osteoarthritis. However, many patients find that an NSAID controls osteoarthritis pain more effectively.

Side effects In therapeutic doses acetaminophen seldom causes serious side effects. Nausea occurs but is not related to damage to the gut. Allergy and rash are rare. Liver damage has occurred, usually when doses larger than that prescribed have been taken or if the drug is taken with concurrent alcohol consumption. In overdose fatal liver failure can occur.

acetaminophen with narcotics such as codeine/hydrocodone/oxycodone/propoxyphene

- **acetaminophen with codeine** (Trade names: Tylenol with codeine)
- **acetaminophen with hydrocodone** (Trade names: Lortab, Lorcet, Vicodin)
- **acetaminophen with oxycodone** (Trade names: Percocet, Roxicet, Tylox)
- **acetaminophen with propoxyphene** (Trade names: Darvocet–50, Darvocet–100)

A combination of acetaminophen and a narcotic is prescribed for pain of moderate-to-severe intensity that has not responded to treatment with acetaminophen or an NSAID.

Side effects In therapeutic doses acetaminophen seldom causes side serious effects. Nausea occurs but is not related to damage to the gut. Allergy and rash are rare. Liver damage has occurred, usually when doses of acetaminophen larger than the prescribed dose have been taken. In overdose fatal liver failure can occur. The narcotic component of combination analgesics frequently causes minor side effects, including nausea, vomiting, constipation, dizziness, and lightheadedness. Allergic reactions resulting in rash or bronchospasm are uncommon. Addiction can occur. Propoxyphene, alone and in combination, is banned in some countries because the risk of serious side effects is considered to outweigh its efficacy as a painkiller.

Aciphex   See RABEPRAZOLE.

Actemra   See TOCILIZUMAB.

Actonel   See RISEDRONATE.

adalimumab   (Trade name: Humira) A specially designed protein to block the effects of tumor necrosis factor (TNF), a proinflammatory cytokine. Adalimumab is a fully human monoclonal antibody that binds to TNF, blocking its effects, and acts a DMARD in RA. Adalimumab is also used to treat psoriasis, psoriatic arthritis, ankylosing spondylitis, and Crohn's disease.

Side effects   The side effects are likely to be similar to those of other drugs that block TNF and have been on the market longer. Common: Requires subcutaneous injection and minor skin injection reactions resulting in redness and itching around the injection site can occur. Approximately 5 to 10 percent of patients receiving anti-TNF drugs will develop a positive antinuclear antibody (ANA) test, raising the concern that they may increase the risk of autoimmune diseases such as SLE. So far this has not been a common problem. Uncommon: The risk of infections (sometimes serious) such as pneumonia is increased. Rare: Case reports or small series of patients developing diabetes, cancer, lymphoma, VASCULITIS, SLE-like autoimmune disease, multiple sclerosis–like demyelinating disorders, liver disease, hematological abnormalities including aplastic anemia, severe allergy, meningitis and infection with TUBERCULOSIS, atypical

mycobacteria, aspergillosis, histoplasmosis, listeria, and reactivation of hepatitis B have been reported in patients receiving TNF antagonists. TNF antagonists may increase mortality in patients with heart failure.

alendronate   (Trade name: Fosamax) A bisphosphonate used to treat and prevent osteoporosis and to treat Paget's disease.

Side effects   Mild gastrointestinal symptoms with nausea, indigestion, and constipation are common. Difficulty swallowing, vomiting, erosive esophagitis (ulcers in the esophagus), and allergic reactions are rare.

Bisphosphonates are inconvenient because they need to be taken on an empty stomach, first thing in the morning, with a full glass of water. To prevent the tablet refluxing back up the esophagus, the patient should remain upright for at least an hour after taking the tablet. Bisphosphonates are very poorly absorbed, and therefore after taking the tablet the patient cannot eat or drink anything other than water for at least 30 minutes. Most manufacturers have produced a tablet that can be taken once a week that is much more convenient than a daily dose. Osteonecrosis of the jaw occurs when an area of the jawbone such as a tooth socket does not heal and leaves the bone exposed; this can occur rarely in patients receiving bisphosphonates, usually intravenous bisphosphonates used to treat cancer.

allopurinol   (Trade names: Lopurin, Zyloprim) Decreases production of uric acid by inhibiting xanthine oxidase, a key enzyme in the pathway leading to uric acid. Allopurinol is used to prevent future attacks of gout, particularly in patients with recurrent attacks of gout, uric acid kidney stones, or deposits of uric acid in the soft tissues (tophi).

Side effects   Common: Mild allergic rash. Uncommon: Can precipitate an acute attack of gout when treatment is started. To prevent this, many physicians also prescribe an NSAID or colchicine for a few months. An allergic reaction called the *allopurinol hypersensitivity syndrome* causes severe rash, often with blisters and peeling, and impaired kidney and liver function. This is very rare. Factors that increase the risk for the allopurinol hypersensitivity syndrome include impaired kidney function and diuretic therapy. Bone marrow suppression is rare but occurs frequently if allopurinol is prescribed with standard doses of azathioprine (trade name: Imuran) or mercaptopurine (trade name: Purinethol). Allopurinol inhibits the breakdown of these anticancer drugs; they should therefore be avoided or used in much smaller doses than usual.

Ambien   See ZOLPIDEM.

amitriptyline   (Trade names: Elavil, Endep, Enovil) A tricyclic antidepressant, a class of drug commonly used to treat depression, chronic pain, or fibromyalgia.
   Side effects   Common: Sleepiness. Because of this effect, tricyclics with sedative side effects are often used to improve sleep. The sedative effects can persist, resulting in unwanted sleepiness during the day. This often becomes less pronounced with continued use. Anticholinergic side effects such as dry mouth and eyes, blurred vision, constipation, and slowness or difficulty passing urine can occur, particularly when treatment is started, but tolerance to these side effects may also develop. Uncommon: Postural hypotension resulting in dizziness when standing up suddenly, tremor, nausea, confusion, sexual dysfunction, GI symptoms, paradoxical stimulation rather than sedation, bone marrow suppression, abnormal liver function tests, seizures, hair loss, and heart rhythm problems.

anakinra   (Trade name: Kineret) An interleukin-1 receptor antagonist, anakinra is a specially designed protein that binds to the interleukin-1 receptor and blocks the effects of the proinflammatory cytokine interleukin-1. Anakinra acts as a DMARD in RA and is being tested in other rheumatic conditions such as Still's disease and gout.
   Side effects   Few serious adverse effects occur, but there is limited long-term information. Common: Requires subcutaneous injection and minor

skin injection, reactions resulting in redness and itching around the injection site are common. The neutrophil count decreases modestly in 5–10 percent of patients and markedly in 0.3 percent of patients receiving anakinra. Uncommon: Infections (sometimes serious) are twice as frequent in patients receiving anakinra than placebo. Serious infections (7 percent) and a serious decrease in the neutrophil count (3 percent) were more common when anakinra was combined with etanercept. That combination is usually avoided.

Anaprox   See NAPROXEN.

Ansaid   See FLURBIPROFEN.

antimalarials   See HYDROXYCHLOROQUINE AND CHLOROQUINE PHOSPHATE.

Arcoxia   See ETORICOXIB.

Aredia   See PAMIDRONATE.

Arthrotec   See DICLOFENAC.

artificial tears   (Trade names: Artificial Tears, Bion Tears, Cellufresh, Hypotears, Isopto Alkaline, Isopto Plain, Isopto Tears, Just Tears, Nature's Tears, Ocucoat, Ocucoat PF, Refresh, Refresh Plus, Tears Naturelle, Tears Naturelle II, Tears Naturelle Free, Ultra Tears, and many others) Eye drops or ointments are used to protect eyes against dryness. Many contain hydroxypropyl methylcellulose, or a similar chemical, that retains liquid. Artificial tears are used to treat dry eyes that are often part of Sjögren's syndrome and many other autoimmune diseases.
   Side effects   Common: Mild blurring of vision. Uncommon: Irritation of the eye by preparations containing a preservative. This may be due to an allergic response to the preservative and can be

overcome by switching to a nonpreservative-containing preparation.

Ascriptin   See CHOLINE SALICYLATE.

aspirin   (Trade names: Anacin, Ascriptin, A.S.A, Bayer Aspirin, Bufferin, Easprin, Ecotrin, Zorprin, and many others) A nonsteroidal anti-inflammatory drug (NSAID) that inhibits cyclooxygenase (COX-1 and COX-2) enzymes, decreasing the formation of inflammatory mediators such as prostaglandins. Aspirin is prescribed for three major reasons.

1. Analgesic and anti-inflammatory effects: Aspirin is used to treat pain and inflammation caused by many rheumatic and nonrheumatic conditions, including rheumatoid arthritis, osteoarthritis, rheumatic fever, Still's disease (also known as juvenile idiopathic arthritis), and Kawasaki disease. NSAIDs do not affect the progression of arthritis.
2. Antipyretic effects: Aspirin reduces fever.
3. Antithrombotic effects: Aspirin, by irreversibly inhibiting COX-1, reduces platelet aggregation, the initial step in the formation of blood clots. Aspirin is widely used to treat and prevent myocardial infarction and stroke. In patients with the anticardiolipin antibody syndrome, aspirin is prescribed to reduce the risk of thrombosis.

Side effects   Common: GI symptoms such as indigestion or heartburn and fluid retention with ankle edema. Less common: Peptic ulcers with or without complications such as perforation, gastrointestinal obstruction, or bleeding. Risk factors for complicated peptic ulcers caused by NSAIDs are age older than 65 years, previous peptic ulcer or bleeding ulcer, and cotreatment with a corticosteroid. NSAIDs can increase blood pressure, impair kidney function, and cause abnormal liver function tests (usually mild), rashes, ringing in the ears, and a feeling of lightheadedness. Uncommon: Serious allergy to NSAIDs can result in anaphylaxis with bronchospasm, urticaria, and angioedema. Reye's syndrome is a rare condition that causes liver failure and coma in children treated with aspirin for a viral illness.

auranofin   (Trade name: Ridaura; also known as oral gold) A disease-modifying antirheumatic drug (DMARD) most often prescribed to treat rheumatoid arthritis and occasionally used to treat psoriatic arthritis.

Side effects   Common: Diarrhea, gas and cramping, itching, skin rash, mouth ulcers, and protein in the urine. Uncommon: Serious allergic reactions such as a generalized skin rash with peeling, bone marrow suppression resulting in a low white cell count or low platelet count, hepatitis, peripheral neuropathy, fever, and lung inflammation.

azathioprine   (Trade name: Imuran) An anticancer drug that interferes with DNA synthesis, particularly in cells regulating the immune system. Azathioprine is metabolized to active products including 6-mercaptopurine, a related anticancer drug. Smaller doses of azathioprine are used to treat rheumatic diseases other than cancer, and the mode of action is more immunoregulatory as opposed to the cell destruction of cancer chemotherapy. Azathioprine is used as a disease-modifying antirheumatic drug (DMARD) to treat rheumatoid arthritis, usually in patients unable to tolerate other DMARDs. It is also commonly used to treat systemic lupus erythematosus, dermatomyositis or polymyositis, vasculitis, and other connective tissue diseases.

Side effects   Common: GI symptoms such as vomiting, diarrhea and nausea, and mild increases in liver enzymes. Uncommon: Dose-related bone marrow suppression can result in a decrease in the white blood cell and platelet count. A genetic variation in an enzyme, thiopurine methyl transferase (TPMT), slows the metabolism of azathioprine and increases sensitivity to the drug substantially. The homozygous form (both strands of DNA affected) of the gene associated with impaired TPMT activity occurs in approximately 1 in 300 people. Genetic testing for the gene is becoming available. If standard doses of azathioprine (trade name: Imuran) or mercaptopurine (trade name: Purinethol) are prescribed with allopurinol (trade name: Zyloprim), severe adverse effects, particularly bone marrow suppression, are likely because allopurinol inhibits the breakdown of these drugs. Mouth ulcers, rash, herpes zoster (shingles) (caused by reactivation of the chicken pox virus), and an increased risk of infection occur. The range of infections is wide, including not only usual organisms but also unusual ones. Pancreatitis, severe hepatitis, severe lung inflammation, and serious allergic reactions are rare. Azathioprine may cause a small increase in the risk of some malignancies such as lymphoma and leukemia.

Azulfidine See SULFASALAZINE.

Benemid See PROBENECID.

Bextra See VALDECOXIB.

Boniva See IBANDRONATE.

bosentan (Trade name: Tracleer) A drug that blocks endothelin, a powerful vasoconstrictor, thus dilating blood vessels, particularly in the lung. Used to treat pulmonary hypertension.
Side effects Common: Abnormal liver function tests (frequent monitoring of liver function tests is needed), headache, flushing, edema, anemia. Rare: serious allergy, liver failure, cirrhosis of the liver.

Butazolidin See PHENYLBUTAZONE.

calcitonin (Trade names: Cibacalcin (human), Miacalcin (salmon)) A hormone that slows the resorption of bone. Calcitonin is used to treat and prevent osteoporosis and to treat Paget's disease. Calcitonin nasal spray is used to treat and prevent osteoporosis.
Side effects Common: Calcitonin injections can cause flushing, headache, nausea, diarrhea,

redness at the injection site, and less often, an allergic rash or hypocalcemia (low blood calcium level). The flushing, nausea, and diarrhea can sometimes be overcome by reducing the dose. Nasal calcitonin seldom causes side effects other than mild nasal irritation.

calcium

- **calcium carbonate** (Trade names: Alka-Mints, Calci-Chew, Caltrate, Os-Cal, Oyst-Cal 500, Rolaids Calcium Rich, Titralac, Tums, Tums E-X, and many others)
- **calcium citrate** (Trade name: Citracal)
- **calcium lactate** Generic
- **calcium phosphate dibasic** Generic

Calcium supplements are used to prevent and treat osteoporosis.
Side effects Common side effects are a chalky taste and constipation. Calcium supplements rarely cause hypercalcemia (a high blood calcium level) or kidney stones.

capsaicin (Trade names: Zostrix, Capsin, Theragen, Trixaicin, Capsagel) An analgesic cream or ointment. Developed from hot chilies, capsaicin may deplete nerves that conduct pain signals of an important neurotransmitter, substance P. Capsaicin is used to decrease joint pain, most often that caused by osteoarthritis. Capsaicin is also used to treat neuralgia (nerve pain) associated with diabetes or occurring after herpes zoster (shingles).
Side effects Common: A burning sensation when initially applied (this decreases with chronic use), skin irritation, and severe pain and a burning sensation if inadvertently applied to eyes, broken skin, or genital organs.

carisoprodol (Trade names: Rela, Soma) A muscle relaxant used to treat painful muscle spasm and fibromyalgia.
Side effects Common: Drowsiness. Less common: Flushing, nausea, vomiting, feeling light-

headed, central nervous system stimulation, shakiness, and rash. Uncommon: Addiction, bone marrow suppression, and allergy resulting in swelling of the face or tongue.

Celebrex   See CELECOXIB.

celecoxib   (Trade name: Celebrex) A nonsteroidal anti-inflammatory drug (NSAID) that inhibits the cyclooxygenase-2 (COX-2) enzyme, decreasing the formation of inflammatory mediators such as prostaglandins. Celecoxib is selective for COX-2 and has little effect on COX-1 and therefore does not inhibit platelet aggregation. NSAIDs are used to treat pain and inflammation due to many causes and for arthritis-related pain caused by rheumatoid arthritis, osteoarthritis, and bursitis. NSAIDs do not affect the progression of arthritis.

Side effects   Common: GI symptoms, usually indigestion or heartburn and fluid retention with ankle edema. Less common: Peptic ulcers with or without complications such as perforation, gastrointestinal obstruction, or bleeding. Risk factors for complicated peptic ulcers caused by NSAIDs are age older than 65 years, previous peptic ulcer or bleeding ulcer, and cotreatment with a corticosteroid. The risk of peptic ulcers and their complications is lower with selective COX-2–inhibiting NSAIDs, such as celecoxib, than nonselective NSAIDs. NSAIDs can increase blood pressure, impair kidney function, and cause abnormal liver function tests (usually mild), rashes, ringing in the ears, and a feeling of lightheadedness. Uncommon: Serious allergy to NSAIDs can result in anaphylaxis with bronchospasm, urticaria, and angioedema. Patients allergic to sulfonamides may have a higher risk of allergy. NSAIDs, particularly those that are more selective COX-2 inhibitors, are associated with an increased risk of heart attack and stroke.

Cellcept   See MYCOPHENOLATE MOFETIL.

certolizumab pegol   (Trade name: Cimzia) A specially designed protein that acts as an antibody against tumor necrosis factor (TNF), a pro-inflammatory cytokine. Certolizumab has molecules of polyethylene glycol (PEG) added that protect it from destruction and thus allow it to remain in the body longer. Certolizumab is approved in the United States for the treatment of Crohn's disease and rheumatoid arthritis.

Side Effects   There is limited long-term information but the side effects are likely to be similar to those of other drugs that block TNF and have been on the market longer. Common: Requires subcutaneous injection, and minor skin injection reactions resulting in redness and itching around the injection site can occur. Approximately 5 to 10 percent of patients receiving anti-TNF drugs will develop a positive antinuclear antibody (ANA) test, raising the concern that they may increase the risk of autoimmune diseases such as SLE. So far this has not been a common problem. Uncommon: The risk of infections (sometimes serious) such as pneumonia is increased. Rare: Case reports or small series of patients developing diabetes, cancer, lymphoma, VASCULITIS, SLE-like autoimmune disease, multiple sclerosis–like demyelinating disorders, liver disease, hematological abnormalities including aplastic anemia, severe allergy, meningitis, and infection with TUBERCULOSIS, atypical mycobacteria, aspergillosis, histoplasmosis, listeria, and reactivation of hepatitis B have been reported in patients receiving TNF antagonists. TNF antagonists may increase mortality in patients with heart failure.

cevimeline   (Trade name: Evoxac) A drug that stimulates the cholinergic nerves to salivary glands, increasing the production of saliva, and used to treat the symptom of dry mouth that often occurs in patients with Sjögren's syndrome.

Side effects   Common: Sweating, dizziness, headache, blurred vision, a runny or blocked nose, and GI problems such as nausea and diarrhea.

chlorambucil   (Trade name: Leukeran) An anticancer drug that interferes with the formation of DNA, particularly in white blood cells, and modulates the immune system. Smaller doses of chlorambucil are used to treat rheumatic problems than are used to treat cancer. Side effects are less common with these lower doses. Chlorambucil is seldom prescribed but is sometimes used to suppress the immune system in patients who cannot take cyclophosphamide. Cyclophosphamide (and chlorambucil) are used to treat vasculitis, lupus affecting vital organs such as the brain and kidney, autoimmune eye disease, and Behçet's disease.

Side effects Common: Bone marrow suppression with a decrease in the white cell count and/or platelet count. Less common: Rash, GI symptoms (nausea, vomiting, and diarrhea), and mouth ulcers. Herpes zoster (shingles), caused by reactivation of the chicken pox virus, and risk of infection are increased. The range of infections is wide, including those caused by common organisms and also unusual ones. Uncommon: Confusion, seizures, changes in menstrual cycle and infertility, lung fibrosis, severe hepatitis, fever, and increased risk of cancer.

chloroquine See HYDROXYCHLOROQUINE AND CHLOROQUINE SULFATE.

choline magnesium salicylate (Trade name: Trilisate) A nonsteroidal anti-inflammatory drug (NSAID) belonging to a subgroup called nonacetylated salicylates that differs from other NSAIDs in that it is a weak inhibitor of cyclooxygenase (COX) enzymes that decrease the formation of inflammatory mediators such as prostaglandins. NSAIDs are used to treat pain and inflammation due to many causes and for arthritis-related pain caused by rheumatoid arthritis, osteoarthritis, and bursitis. NSAIDs do not affect the progression of arthritis.

Side effects Common: GI symptoms, usually indigestion or heartburn, and fluid retention with ankle edema. Less common: Peptic ulcers with or without complications such as perforation, gastrointestinal obstruction, or bleeding. Risk factors for complicated peptic ulcers caused by NSAIDs are age older than 65 years, previous peptic ulcer or bleeding ulcer, and cotreatment with a corticosteroid. Nonacetylated salicylates are salicylates like aspirin, but their different chemical structure makes them behave more like COX-2-selective NSAIDs, so they do not inhibit platelet aggregation significantly and are less likely to cause serious GI complications. NSAIDs can increase blood pressure, impair kidney function, and cause abnormal liver function tests (usually mild), rashes, ringing in the ears, and a feeling of lightheadedness. Uncommon: Serious allergy to NSAIDs can result in anaphylaxis with bronchospasm, urticaria, and angioedema.

choline salicylate (Trade name: Arthropan) A nonsteroidal anti-inflammatory drug (NSAID) belonging to a subgroup called nonacetylated salicylates that differs from other NSAIDs in that it is a weak inhibitor of cyclooxygenase (COX) enzymes that decrease the formation of inflammatory mediators such as prostaglandins. NSAIDs are used to treat pain and inflammation due to many causes and for arthritis-related pain caused by rheumatoid arthritis, osteoarthritis, and bursitis. NSAIDs do not affect the progression of arthritis.

Side effects Common: GI symptoms, usually indigestion or heartburn, and fluid retention with ankle edema. Less common: Peptic ulcers with or without complications such as perforation, gastrointestinal obstruction, or bleeding. Risk factors for complicated peptic ulcers caused by NSAIDs are age older than 65 years, previous peptic ulcer or bleeding ulcer, and cotreatment with a corticosteroid. Nonacetylated salicylates are salicylates like aspirin, but their different chemical structure makes them behave more like COX-2–selective NSAIDs, so they do not inhibit platelet aggregation significantly and are less likely to cause serious GI complications. NSAIDs can increase blood pressure, impair kidney function, and cause abnormal liver function tests (usually mild), rashes, ringing in the ears, and a feeling of lightheadedness. Uncommon: Serious allergy to NSAIDs can result in anaphylaxis with bronchospasm, urticaria, and angioedema.

chondroitin sulfate See GLUCOSAMINE AND CHONDROITIN SULFATE.

cimetidine (Trade name: Tagamet) A histamine type 2 receptor antagonist (H_2-receptor antagonist or H$_2$-blocker) that decreases acid production by the stomach and is used to treat indigestion, reflux esophagitis, and peptic ulcers. H$_2$-receptor antagonists, except in high doses, do not provide adequate protection against NSAID-induced peptic ulcers.

Side effects H$_2$-receptor antagonists are generally well tolerated and have few adverse effects. Common: Minor, transient symptoms such as dizziness, headache, and diarrhea. Uncommon: Increased breast tissue with swelling in men (gynecomastia), rash, hepatitis, and myopathy. Cimetidine, because it inhibits liver enzymes that metabolize some drugs, increases the concentrations of several drugs, including warfarin, theophylline, phenytoin, quinidine, propranolol, and tricyclic antidepressants.

Cimzia   See CERTOLIZUMAB.

cisapride   (Trade name: Propulsid) Stimulates GI motility by increasing the concentrations of a chemical messenger, acetylcholine, in the bowel wall. Cisapride is occasionally used to improve GI motility in patients with scleroderma. It was used to treat GERD (gastroesophageal reflux disease), but rare, serious side effects have resulted in restricted use. It is no longer available on the general market in the United States.

Side effects Common: Rash, stomach cramps, diarrhea, and increased intestinal gas. Less common: Nervousness, vomiting, and drowsiness. Rare: A serious, sometimes fatal, heart rhythm problem called torsades de pointes. This usually occurred when cisapride was taken in overdose or with another drug that slowed its metabolism. Many drugs block the enzyme that breaks down cisapride, leading to high concentrations and the potential for fatal arrhythmias.

Clinoril   See SULINDAC.

codeine   (Codeine is usually prescribed as a generic or as a combination analgesic. See ACETAMINOPHEN WITH NARCOTICS.) It is a narcotic analgesic that decreases pain by acting through specific opiate receptors in the brain and is used to treat moderate-to-severe pain not controlled by acetaminophen or an NSAID. Codeine is occasionally prescribed to suppress cough.

Side effects Common: Nausea, vomiting, constipation, poor appetite, dizziness, feeling lightheaded, and sleepiness. Uncommon: Feeling nervous or agitated, sleeping badly, an allergic reaction with urticarial rash (hives) or bronchospasm, confusion, feeling high, and addiction.

colchicine   (Colchicine was usually prescribed as a generic but in 2009 the FDA gave three-year marketing exclusivity to the manufacturer of the brand name Colcrys) It suppresses inflammation in acute gout, probably by altering white blood cell migration to areas of inflammation. Colchicine is used to suppress and treat acute attacks of gout and also to treat familial Mediterranean fever.

Side effects Common: Dose-related nausea, vomiting, diarrhea, and stomach cramps. Less common: Decreased appetite and mild hair loss. Uncommon: Neuropathy, myopathy, rash, bone marrow suppression, hepatitis, and decreased sperm count.

collagen   (Trade names: None) Also known as chicken collagen. Collagen is a potential treatment for rheumatoid arthritis but has been ineffective in most clinical trials. The theory underlying the use of collagen is similar to the concept of allergy shots with low doses of allergen desensitizing allergic responses. Collagen taken by mouth was thought to make the immunologically active cells in the wall of the gut tolerant to collagen and thus tolerant to the patient's collagen, a major component of joints and connective tissue. There are ongoing studies, but the evidence so far does not support a role for collagen treatment in rheumatoid arthritis.

corticosteroids
Trade names

Tablets:	**prednisone:** Deltasone, Orasone
	methylprednisolone: Medrol
	dexamethasone: Dexone

Injections: **methylprednisolone:** SoluMedrol
hydrocortisone: Solu-Cortef
dexamethasone: Decadron

Intra-
articular
injections:
methylprednisolone acetate: Depo-Medrol
triamcinolone: Aristocort, Aristo-span, Kenalog

Corticosteroids are also called glucocorticoids or sometimes just steroids. They are related to cortisone, a stress hormone produced by the adrenal gland, and differ from anabolic steroids used by some athletes to increase muscle strength. Corticosteroids, acting through glucocorticoid receptors found on most cells, suppress the immune response. Various preparations are used to treat rheumatic diseases.

- Tablets: High doses of oral corticosteroids, often in combination with another immunosuppressant, are prescribed to control vasculitis, SLE affecting organs such as kidneys or the brain, and dermatomyositis or polymyositis. After the illness is controlled the doses of corticosteroids are tapered. Many patients with rheumatoid arthritis (RA) take low doses of corticosteroids, usually in combination with a DMARD, to help suppress inflammation. Acute inflammation in a joint (for example in RA) or in other organs (for example pleurisy caused by SLE) can be treated with corticosteroid tablets, initially in high doses and then tapering rapidly (sometimes referred to as a *dose pack*).

- Injections: Very high doses of pulse corticosteroids are administered intravenously in situations where the need for treatment is urgent, such as vasculitis or SLE threatening life or an organ.

- Intra-articular injections: In rheumatoid arthritis, other types of inflammatory arthritis, and osteoarthritis, a long-acting depot corticosteroid is injected into a swollen joint to suppress inflammation. Long-acting depot corticosteroids are also injected into bursas to treat bursitis or near a tendon to treat tendinitis.

Side effects of intra-articular injections The local injection of a long-acting steroid into a joint exposes the individual to a low systemic dose of corticosteroid that seldom causes adverse effects other than occasionally aggravating pain and swelling for a day or two. An injection of a corticosteroid directly into a tendon can weaken it and lead to rupture. There is concern, mainly theoretical, that repeated intra-articular corticosteroid injections could damage cartilage. Therefore, the number of injections into any one joint is kept to a minimum. Side effects such as bleeding or infection in the injected joint are rare and result from the injection itself, rather than the corticosteroid.

Side effects of oral and injected corticosteroids The frequency and severity of side effects are dose related; high doses invariably cause side effects, but low doses do so less often. Side effects include osteoporosis, hypertension, diabetes, cataracts, myopathy, increased appetite and weight gain, low serum potassium concentration, cushingoid features (fat redistribution resulting in a moon-shaped face and obesity), increased skin fragility and bruising, emotional lability, insomnia, depression, feeling lightheaded, and an increased white blood cell count. Corticosteroids increase the risk of infections. These can be regular infections, such as pneumonia, but can also be less common infections, such as tuberculosis. Avascular necrosis is uncommon.

cuprimine See PENICILLAMINE.

cyclobenzaprine (Trade name: Flexeril) A muscle relaxant used to treat painful muscle spasm and, less often, fibromyalgia.

Side effects Common: Drowsiness is common, and because of this, cyclobenzaprine is often taken at night to improve sleep. Anticholinergic side effects such as dry mouth and eyes, blurred vision, constipation, and slowness or difficulty passing urine are common, particularly when treatment is started. Tolerance to these side effects may develop. Nausea, confusion, and stomach upset can occur. Paradoxical stimulation, rather than sedation, is uncommon.

Rare: Hepatitis, allergy, and heart rhythm disturbances.

cyclophosphamide (Trade names: Cytoxan, Neosar) An anticancer drug that interferes with DNA synthesis, particularly in cells regulating the immune system. Smaller doses of cyclophosphamide are used to treat rheumatic diseases other than cancer with a mode of action that is more immunoregulatory as opposed to cell destruction as in cancer chemotherapy. Cyclophosphamide is used to treat systemic lupus erythematosus, vasculitis, and other serious connective tissue diseases. Cyclophosphamide is prescribed as either a daily tablet or a monthly intravenous injection. The monthly intravenous regimen is preferred for the treatment of systemic lupus erythematosus and the daily oral dose for the treatment of vasculitis.

Side effects The side effects of cyclophosphamide are related to the dose, duration, and route of treatment. The risk of infection is greater when it is administered in doses that result in a marked decrease in the white blood cell count. The risk of secondary malignancies increases with duration of exposure. Common: Nausea, vomiting, bone marrow suppression resulting in low white blood cell count or thrombocytopenia, and ovarian failure resulting in premature menopause and infertility. Cyclophosphamide is metabolized to acrolein, a bladder irritant that frequently causes cystitis (bladder inflammation), and occasionally hemorrhagic cystitis (i.e., with blood in the urine). MESNA is a drug that is often prescribed with IV injections of cyclophosphamide to protect the bladder. Herpes zoster (shingles), caused by reactivation of the chicken pox virus, and an increased risk of infection, particularly if the patient is also receiving high doses of corticosteroids, can occur. The range of infections is wide, including those caused by common organisms and unusual ones. Infertility due to ovarian failure is common. Monthly intravenous administration rarely causes bladder problems and is associated with a slightly lower frequency of ovarian failure and infections than daily oral administration. Uncommon: Lung inflammation, hepatitis, allergy, and delayed side effects such as increased frequency of bladder cancer, skin cancer, and leukemia.

cyclosporine (cyclosporin, cyclosporin A) (Trade names: Sandimmune, Neoral) Two preparations containing the identical drug—cyclosporine—are available. Neoral is a newer, microemulsion preparation that is more completely and reproducibly absorbed than the older preparation, Sandimmune. Cyclosporine is an immunosuppressive drug whose main use is to prevent rejection after organ transplantation. It also acts as a DMARD in RA and is sometimes prescribed for other indications such as psoriasis and psoriatic arthritis, dermatomyositis, Behçet's disease, SLE, and autoimmune eye inflammation not responding to standard treatments. Cyclosporine decreases the production of the cytokine interleukin-2 (IL-2). This, and effects on other mediators, suppress the immune response.

Side effects Common: Nausea, vomiting, intestinal gas, cramps, diarrhea, increased hair growth, a small increase in blood pressure, tremor, headache, muscle cramps, decreased kidney function, increased serum potassium and uric acid, and decreased serum magnesium concentrations. Uncommon: Hypertrophy of the gums, gout, seizures, infection, and allergic reactions.

Cymbalta   See DULOXETINE.

Cytotec   See MISOPROSTOL.

Cytoxan   See CYCLOPHOSPHAMIDE.

danazol (Trade name: Danocrine) A mild androgen (male hormone) that decreases the frequency of attacks in hereditary angioedema and increases the platelet count in autoimmune thrombocytopenia. The mechanism of action in autoimmune diseases is unclear, but it increases the synthesis of complement, a group of proteins that clear antigen/antibody complexes (see COMPLEMENT). It is also used to treat endometriosis and fibrocystic breast disease.

Side effects Common: Abnormal liver function tests and androgenic effects such as acne, increased facial and body hair, irregular menstrual cycles, bleeding between monthly cycles, weight gain, and fluid retention. Uncommon: Hepatitis, pancreatitis, thrombocytopenia, low white blood cell count, and raised intracranial pressure.

Danocrine   See DANAZOL.

dapsone   (Trade name: Avlosulfon) A sulfone drug similar in structure to sulfonamide (sulfa) antibiotics. The most common indication is leprosy, but it is also occasionally used to treat severe skin problems caused by systemic or discoid lupus erythematosus, leukocytoclastic vasculitis, and pyoderma gangrenosum.
   Side effects   Common: Rash and GI symptoms. Dapsone can cause dose-related hemolysis (breakdown of red blood cells) and anemia, particularly but not exclusively in individuals with a hereditary deficiency of the enzyme glucose-6 phosphate dehydrogenase (G-6PD). A dose-related increase in the concentrations of methemoglobin, a type of hemoglobin that does not carry oxygen well, resulting in a dusky or bluish skin color, occurs. Uncommon: Low white blood cell count, severe allergic skin rash, and hepatitis.

Darvocet   See ACETAMINOPHEN WITH PROPOXYPHENE.

Daypro   See OXAPROZIN.

Demerol   See MEPERIDINE.

denosumab   Also known as AMG162, denosumab is a monoclonal antibody synthesized to block the effects of receptor activator of nuclear factor kappa B ligand (RANK ligand), a factor that stimulates bone resorption. Denosumab was approved by the Food and Drug Administration as a treatment for osteoporosis. The drug increases bone density and reduces the risk of fractures. Little is known about its side effects, but most monoclonal antibodies that are injected intravenously can cause minor infusion reactions (chills, itching, rash, dizziness) and rarely serious allergy. Denosumab may increase the risk of infections.

Depen   See PENICILLAMINE.

DepoMedrol   See CORTICOSTEROIDS.

Desyrel   See TRAZODONE.

dexamethasone   See CORTICOSTEROIDS.

DHEA (dehydroepiandrosterone)   (Available in health food stores in the form of natural products/food supplements) DHEA is a precursor hormone secreted by the adrenal gland that is converted to the androgenic (male) hormones androstenedione, testosterone, and androsterone and the estrogenic (female) hormone estradiol. In limited clinical studies DHEA resulted in a small decrease in the corticosteroid requirements in patients with mild SLE and an increase in bone density. It is also promoted as an antiaging hormone with little scientific support.
   Side effects   Common: Androgenic side effects such as acne, greasy hair, and increased body and facial hair are more common in women; estrogenic side effects such as breast growth and tenderness are more common in men. Because DHEA is classified as a food supplement and not a drug, it has not undergone rigorous safety or efficacy testing, and knowledge about the long-term responses of malignancies such breast and prostate cancer that are hormone responsive are unknown.

diclofenac   (Trade names: Cataflam [immediate release], Voltaren [enteric coated, extended release], Arthrotec [diclofenac plus misoprostol]) A nonsteroidal anti-inflammatory drug (NSAID) that inhibits cyclooxygenase (COX-1 and COX-2) enzymes, decreasing the formation of inflammatory mediators such as prostaglandins. Arthrotec combines diclofenac with misoprostol, a drug that protects against peptic ulcers. NSAIDs are used to treat pain and inflammation resulting from a variety of causes. Common indications are rheumatoid arthritis, osteoarthritis, Still's disease (also known as juvenile idiopathic arthritis), gout, ankylosing spondylitis, and bursitis. NSAIDs do not affect the progression of arthritis.

Side effects   For the side effects of the misoprostol component of Arthrotec, see MISOPROSTOL. Common: GI symptoms, usually indigestion or heartburn and fluid retention with ankle edema. Less common: Peptic ulcers with or without complications such as perforation, gastrointestinal obstruction, or bleeding. Risk factors for complicated peptic ulcers caused by NSAIDs are age older than 65 years, previous peptic ulcer or bleeding ulcer, and treatment with a corticosteroid. NSAIDs can increase blood pressure, impair kidney function, and cause abnormal liver function tests (usually mild), rashes, ringing in the ears, and a feeling of lightheadedness. Uncommon: Serious allergy to NSAIDs can result in anaphylaxis with bronchospasm, urticaria, and angioedema. NSAIDs are associated with an increased risk of heart attack and stroke.

Didronel   See ETIDRONATE.

diflunisal   (Trade name: Dolobid) A nonsteroidal anti-inflammatory drug (NSAID) that inhibits cyclooxygenase (COX-1 and COX-2) enzymes, decreasing the formation of inflammatory mediators such as prostaglandins. NSAIDs are used to treat pain and inflammation, resulting from a variety of causes. Common indications are rheumatoid arthritis, osteoarthritis, gout, ankylosing spondylitis, and bursitis. NSAIDs do not affect the progression of arthritis.

Side effects   Common: GI symptoms, usually indigestion or heartburn, and fluid retention with ankle edema. Less common: Peptic ulcers with or without complications such as perforation, gastrointestinal obstruction, or bleeding. Risk factors for complicated peptic ulcers caused by NSAIDs are age older than 65 years, previous peptic ulcer or

bleeding ulcer, and treatment with a corticosteroid. NSAIDs can increase blood pressure, impair kidney function, and cause abnormal liver function tests (usually mild), rashes, ringing in the ears, and a feeling of lightheadedness. Uncommon: Serious allergy to NSAIDs can result in anaphylaxis with bronchospasm, urticaria, and angioedema. NSAIDs are associated with an increased risk of heart attack and stroke.

Disalcid   See SALSALATE.

Dolobid   See DIFLUNISAL.

doxepin   (Trade name: Sinequan) A tricyclic antidepressant, a class of drug commonly used to treat depression, chronic pain, and fibromyalgia.

Side effects   Common: Sleepiness, and because of this sedative antidepressants are often used to improve sleep. The sedative effects can persist, resulting in unwanted sleepiness during the day. Anticholinergic side effects such as dry mouth and eyes, blurred vision, constipation, and slowness or difficulty passing urine can occur, particularly when treatment is started, but tolerance to these side effects may develop. Uncommon: Postural hypotension resulting in dizziness when standing up suddenly, tremor, nausea, confusion, sexual dysfunction, GI symptoms, paradoxical stimulation rather than sedation, bone marrow suppression, abnormal liver function tests, seizures, hair loss, and heart rhythm problems.

doxycycline   See MINOCYCLINE.

duloxetine   (Trade name: Cymbalta) An antidepressant, a class of drug commonly used to treat depression, anxiety, chronic pain due to nerve damage, and fibromyalgia.

Side effects   Common: Nausea, sleepiness, fatigue, decreased appetite, insomnia, blurred vision. Uncommon: Postural hypotension resulting in dizziness when standing up suddenly, liver toxicity, increased risk of suicide, tremor, nausea, confusion, sexual dysfunction, seizures, increased blood pressure, and palpitations.

Duragesic   See FENTANYL.

Easprin   See ASPIRIN.

Ecotrin   See ASPIRIN.

Elavil   See AMITRIPTYLINE.

Enbrel   See ETANERCEPT.

epoprostenol   (Trade Name: Flolan) A synthesized form of prostacyclin, a powerful natural vasodilator that dilates blood vessels, particularly in the lung. Used intravenously to treat pulmonary hypertension.
   Side effects   Common: headache, flushing, edema, nausea, chest pain, jaw pain, low blood pressure, dizziness, and nervousness. Uncommon: muscle pain, palpitations, vomiting, and allergy. Epoprostenol is infused intravenously continuously; side effects such as infection can occur from the IV catheter. If the drug infusion is stopped suddenly, the pressure in the pulmonary arteries can rebound and increase.

esomeprazole   (Trade name: Nexium) A proton pump inhibitor (a class of drugs also known as PPIs) that decreases gastric acid production and is used to treat and prevent peptic ulcers and gastroesophageal reflux (GERD), common side effects of NSAIDs.
   Side effects   Proton pump inhibitors seldom cause side effects. Uncommon: Constipation, rash, dizziness, diarrhea, abdominal pain, and elevated liver enzymes.

etanercept   (Trade name: Enbrel) A specially designed protein to block the effects of tumor necrosis factor (TNF), a proinflammatory cytokine. Etanercept consists of two receptors for TNF coupled together. TNF binds to the false receptors on etanercept and not the real receptors. In other words, etanercept acts as a decoy and mops up TNF before it binds to the real receptors where it would activate inflammation. Etanercept acts as a DMARD in RA and is also used to treat juvenile idiopathic arthritis (JIA) psoriatic arthritis, and ankylosing spondylitis.
   Side effects   Few adverse effects occur but there is limited long-term information. Common: It requires subcutaneous injection, and minor skin injection reactions resulting in redness and itching around the injection site are common. Approximately 5–10 percent of patients receiving etanercept will develop a positive antinuclear antibody (ANA) test, raising the concern that etanercept may increase the risk of autoimmune diseases such as SLE. So far this has not been a common problem, but the long-term effects are not yet known. Uncommon: The risk of infections (sometimes serious) such as pneumonia is increased. Rare: Case reports or small series of patients developing diabetes, cancer, lymphoma, VASCULITIS, SLE-like autoimmune disease, multiple sclerosis-like demyelinating disorders, liver disease, hematological abnormalities including aplastic anemia, severe allergy, meningitis and infection with TUBERCULOSIS, atypical mycobacteria, aspergillosis, histoplasmosis, listeria, and reactivation of hepatitis B have been reported in patients receiving TNF antagonists. TNF antagonists may increase mortality in patients with heart failure.

etidronate   (Trade name: Didronel, also known as Disodium Etidronate, Sodium Etidronate). A bisphosphonate used to treat and prevent osteoporosis and to treat Paget's disease.
   Side effects   Common: Mild gastrointestinal symptoms with nausea, indigestion, and constipation. Uncommon: Allergic rash, fever, poor mineralization of bone, and hypocalcemia. Bisphosphonates are inconvenient because they need to be taken on an empty stomach with a full glass of water. To prevent the tablet refluxing back up the esophagus, the patient must stay upright for

at least an hour. Bisphosphonates are very poorly absorbed, and therefore after taking the tablet the patient cannot eat or drink anything other than water for at least 30 minutes. Etidronate is seldom used to treat osteoporosis because there is evidence that alendronate and risedronate (other bisphosphonates) prevent osteoporotic fractures more effectively. Osteonecrosis of the jaw occurs when an area of the jawbone such as a tooth socket does not heal and leaves the bone exposed; this can occur rarely in patients receiving bisphosphonates, usually intravenous bisphosphonates used to treat cancer.

etodolac   (Trade name: Lodine) A nonsteroidal anti-inflammatory drug (NSAID) that inhibits cyclooxygenase (COX-1 and COX-2) enzymes, decreasing the formation of inflammatory mediators such as prostaglandins. Because etodolac tends more toward a COX-2-blocking effect, it may cause less GI side effects than nonselective NSAIDs. NSAIDs are used to treat pain and inflammation, resulting from a variety of causes. Common indications are rheumatoid arthritis, osteoarthritis, gout, ankylosing spondylitis, and bursitis. NSAIDs do not affect the progression of arthritis.

Side effects Common: GI symptoms, usually indigestion or heartburn, and fluid retention with ankle edema. Less common: Peptic ulcers with or without complications such as perforation, gastrointestinal obstruction, or bleeding. Risk factors for complicated peptic ulcers caused by NSAIDs are age older than 65 years, previous peptic ulcer or bleeding ulcer, and treatment with a corticosteroid. NSAIDs can increase blood pressure, impair kidney function, and cause abnormal liver function tests (usually mild), rashes, ringing in the ears, and a feeling of lightheadedness. Uncommon: Serious allergy to NSAIDs can result in anaphylaxis with bronchospasm, urticaria, and angioedema. NSAIDs are associated with an increased risk of heart attack and stroke.

etoricoxib   (Trade name: Arcoxia) A nonsteroidal anti-inflammatory drug (NSAID) that inhibits the cyclo-oxygenase-2 (COX-2) enzyme, decreasing the formation of inflammatory mediators such as prostaglandins. Etoricoxib is selective for COX-2 and has little effect on COX-1 and therefore does not inhibit platelet aggregation. NSAIDs are used to treat pain and inflammation due to many causes, and for arthritis-related pain caused by rheumatoid arthritis, osteoarthritis, and bursitis. NSAIDs do not affect the progression of arthritis. Etoricoxib is approved for use in Europe but not in the United States.

Side effects Common: GI symptoms, usually indigestion or heartburn and fluid retention with ankle edema. Less common: Peptic ulcers with or without complications such as perforation, gastrointestinal obstruction, or bleeding. Risk factors for complicated peptic ulcers caused by NSAIDs are age older than 65 years, previous peptic ulcer or bleeding ulcer, and treatment with a corticosteroid. The risk of peptic ulcers and their complications is lower with selective COX-2 inhibiting NSAIDs, such as etoricoxib, than nonselective NSAIDs. NSAIDs can increase blood pressure, impair kidney function, and cause abnormal liver function tests (usually mild), rashes, ringing in the ears, and a feeling of lightheadedness. Uncommon: Serious allergy to NSAIDs can result in anaphylaxis with bronchospasm, urticaria, and angioedema. NSAIDs, particularly COX-2 selective drugs, increase the risk of heart attack and stroke.

Evista   See RALOXIFENE.

Evoxac   See CEVIMELINE.

famotidine   (Trade name: Pepcid) A histamine type 2 receptor antagonist (H_2-receptor antagonist or H_2-blocker) that decreases acid production by the stomach and is used to treat indigestion, reflux esophagitis, and peptic ulcers. H_2-receptor antagonists, except in high doses, do not provide adequate protection against NSAID-induced peptic ulcers.

Side effects H_2-receptor antagonists are generally well tolerated. Common: Minor, transient symptoms such as dizziness, headache, and diarrhea. Uncommon: Rash and hepatitis.

febuxostat (Trade name: Uloric) Decreases production of uric acid by inhibiting xanthine oxidase, a key enzyme in the synthesis of uric acid. Febuxostat is used to prevent future attacks of gout, particularly in patients with recurrent attacks of gout, uric acid kidney stones, or deposits of uric acid in the soft tissues (tophi).

Side effects Common: mild rash. Uncommon: increased liver function tests, nausea, and can precipitate an acute attack of gout when treatment is started. To prevent this many physicians also prescribe an NSAID or colchicine for a few months. Bone marrow suppression can occur if febuxostat is prescribed with standard doses of azathioprine (Trade name: Imuran) or mercaptopurine (Trade name: Purinethol). Febuxostat inhibits the metabolism of these anticancer drugs, and therefore unless much smaller doses than usual of azathioprine or mercaptopurine are prescribed, bone marrow suppression is likely. In some clinical trials, a slightly higher risk of heart attack and stroke was seen with febuxostat compared to allopurinol.

Feldene See PIROXICAM.

fenoprofen (Trade name: Nalfon) A nonsteroidal anti-inflammatory drug (NSAID) that inhibits cyclooxygenase (COX-1 and COX-2) enzymes, decreasing the formation of inflammatory mediators such as prostaglandins. NSAIDs are used to treat pain and inflammation, resulting from a variety of causes. Common indications are rheumatoid arthritis, osteoarthritis, gout, ankylosing spondylitis, and bursitis. NSAIDs do not affect the progression of arthritis.

Side effects Common: GI symptoms, usually indigestion or heartburn, and fluid retention with ankle edema. Less common: Peptic ulcers with or without complications such as perforation, gastrointestinal obstruction, or bleeding. Risk factors for complicated peptic ulcers caused by NSAIDs are age older than 65 years, previous peptic ulcer or bleeding ulcer, and treatment with a corticosteroid. NSAIDs can increase blood pressure, impair kidney function, and cause abnormal liver function tests (usually mild), rashes, ringing in the ears, and a feeling of lightheadedness. Uncommon: Serious allergy to NSAIDs can result in anaphylaxis with bronchospasm, urticaria, and angioedema. NSAIDs are associated with an increased risk of heart attack and stroke.

fentanyl (Trade names: Duragesic, Sublimaze) A strong narcotic analgesic used to treat severe pain not controlled by acetaminophen, an NSAID, or by weaker narcotics, such as codeine or hydrocodone. Narcotics do not affect inflammation but decrease pain by acting through specific opiate receptors in the brain. When used for intractable pain, fentanyl is applied to the skin in a patch that works over 72 hours. Heat, due to either a fever or local application to the patch, should be avoided since it increases absorption and may result in an overdose.

Side effects Common: Nausea, vomiting, constipation, decreased appetite, dizziness, lightheadedness, sedation, and low blood pressure. Uncommon: Allergy resulting in an urticarial rash or bronchospasm, confusion, agitation, insomnia, euphoria, addiction, and suppression of respiration.

Flexeril See CYCLOBENZAPRINE.

Flolan See EPOPROSTENOL.

fluoxetine (Trade name: Prozac) An antidepressant of the selective serotonin reuptake inhibitor (SSRI) type, a class of drug commonly used to treat depression, chronic pain, and fibromyalgia.

Side effects Common: Anxiety, dizziness, insomnia, dry mouth, and GI side effects such as nausea and diarrhea. Uncommon: Tremor, confusion, rash, sexual dysfunction, sedation, and allergy.

flurbiprofen (Trade name: Ansaid) A nonsteroidal anti-inflammatory drug (NSAID) that inhibits cyclooxygenase (COX-1 and COX-2) enzymes, decreasing the formation of inflammatory mediators such as prostaglandins. NSAIDs are used to treat pain and inflammation, resulting from a variety of causes. Common indications are rheumatoid arthritis, osteoarthritis, gout, ankylosing spondylitis, and bursitis. NSAIDs do not affect the progression of arthritis.

Side effects Common: GI symptoms, usually indigestion or heartburn, and fluid retention with ankle edema. Less common: Peptic ulcers with or without complications such as perforation, gastrointestinal obstruction, or bleeding. Risk factors for complicated peptic ulcers caused by NSAIDs are age older than 65 years, previous peptic ulcer or bleeding ulcer, and treatment with a corticosteroid. NSAIDs can increase blood pressure, impair kidney function, and cause abnormal liver function tests (usually mild), rashes, ringing in the ears, and a feeling of lightheadedness. Uncommon: Serious allergy to NSAIDs can result in anaphylaxis with bronchospasm, urticarial rash and angioedema. NSAIDs are associated with an increased risk of heart attack and stroke.

folic acid (folate) (Trade name: Folvite and many generic preparations) A vitamin used to protect against the side effects of methotrexate such as mouth ulcers, nausea, and changes in blood count. Folic acid is the precursor of folinic acid, which blocks the effects of methotrexate.

Side effects Uncommon: Rash, flushing, and neuropathy in people who are deficient in vitamin B_{12}. In high doses, folic acid can decrease the therapeutic efficacy of methotrexate.

folinic acid (Leucovorin, Tetrahydrofolate) (Trade name: Wellcovorin) A vitamin used to protect against the side effects of methotrexate such as mouth ulcers, nausea, and changes in blood count. Folinic acid blocks the effects of methotrexate.

Side effects Uncommon: Rash, flushing, and neuropathy in people who are deficient in vitamin B_{12}. In high doses, folinic acid can decrease the therapeutic efficacy of methotrexate. Folinic acid is a vitamin.

Forteo See TERIPARATIDE.

Fosamax See ALENDRONATE.

gabapentin (Trade name: Neurontin) An anticonvulsant (antiseizure drug) that is also used to treat chronic pain, particularly painful neuropathy. Gabapentin is structurally similar to the inhibitory central nervous system neurotransmitter gamma-aminobutyric acid (GABA), but this may not explain its mechanism of action, which is uncertain.

Side effects Uncommon: Sleepiness, dizziness, double vision, loss of balance, fatigue, low white blood cell count, and GI symptoms.

gammaglobulin (intravenous immune globulin, IVIG) (Trade names: Gamimune, Gammagard, Iveegam, Polygam, Sandoglobulin) An immunoglobulin or protein produced by the body to fight infection. Gammaglobulin is most often used as replacement therapy for patients who, usually because of an inherited problem, do not make enough gammaglobulin. Gammaglobulin is also used to treat idiopathic thrombocytopenic purpura (ITP) (see THROMBOCYTOPENIA), KAWASAKI DISEASE, and rare types of nerve damage such as chronic inflammatory demyelinating polyneuropathy. Gammaglobulin has also sometimes been used to treat some autoimmune problems, such as SLE, dermatomyositis, vasculitis, and RA, that are not responding to standard treatments, but the evidence supporting these indications is limited.

Side effects Common: Flushing, increased heart rate, chills, and shortness of breath during the infusion. Uncommon: Low blood pressure, serious allergic reactions, and aseptic meningitis. Gammaglobulin is made from pooled human blood products, and despite extensive precautions, there is a potential risk of transmitting a viral infection.

glucosamine and chondroitin sulfate (Available as many dietary supplement preparations in health food stores) Glucosamine and chondroitin sulfate are substances found in the joints that, with other raw materials, form the constituents of cartilage. Some clinical trials, not always of rigorous design, suggest that glucosamine is approximately as effective as an NSAID in the treatment of osteoarthritis. The mechanism of action is unclear, and it may not be a simple case of replacing the raw materials that make up cartilage but rather an anti-inflammatory mechanism. Large controlled clinical trials are under way.

Side effects Few, but studies are limited.

gold, oral See AURANOFIN.

gold injections (injectable gold) (Trade names: Solganal, an aurothioglucose gold preparation; Myochrysine [discontinued]; and Aurolate, a gold sodium thiomalate preparation) Gold is a disease-modifying antirheumatic drug (DMARD) used to treat rheumatoid arthritis and occasionally psoriatic arthritis. The mechanism of action is uncertain.

Side effects Common: Itching, skin rash, mouth ulcers, a metallic taste, and proteinuria. Uncommon: A severe skin rash with peeling, other serious allergic reactions, bone marrow suppression resulting in low white blood cell count or thrombocytopenia, hepatitis, peripheral neuropathy, fever, and lung inflammation. A *nitritoid reaction,* characterized by feeling flushed and lightheaded immediately after a gold injection, is unpleasant but is not a true allergic reaction.

golimubab (Trade name: Simponi) This is a new anti-TNF (tumor necrosis factor) blocker approved by the FDA in 2009. It is given monthly by injection under the skin. Its uses and side effects are likely similar to older drugs in this class (etanercept, adalimumab).

Humira See ADALIMUMAB.

hyaluronan injections (viscosupplements, hyaluronic acid) Several types of hyaluronan injections are available (Trade names: Hyalgan, Synvisc, Orthovisc, Euflexxa, Supartz). Viscosupplement injections are used to treat osteoarthritis of the knee. Their mechanism of action is uncertain. Hyaluronic acid is a component of normal joint fluid that improves viscosity and shock absorption. Initially viscosupplements injected into an arthritic joint were thought to replace the lubricant hyaluronic acid. However, the residence time of hyaluronan in the joint is much shorter than the duration of clinical benefit. Therefore, other mechanisms, probably anti-inflammatory, are likely.

Side effects Common: Knee inflammation resulting in pain and swelling and injection site irritation. Uncommon: Any intra-articular injection has a small risk of introducing an infection. Allergic reactions can occur.

hyaluronate See HYALURONAN INJECTIONS.

hydrocodone See ACETAMINOPHEN WITH NARCOTICS.

hydrocortisone See CORTICOSTEROIDS.

hydroxychloroquine and chloroquine phosphate (antimalarials) (Trade names: Plaquenil—hydroxychloroquine—and Aralen—chloroquine) Drugs used to treat malaria (antimalarials) that were found to act as disease-modifying antirheumatic drugs (DMARDs) in rheumatoid arthritis and to improve skin and joint symptoms in SLE. Antimalarials are also occasionally used to treat psoriatic arthritis but can cause a flare of the skin disease. Their mechanism of action is not known.

Side effects Common: Headache, blurred vision, and mild GI symptoms such as indigestion and nausea can occur. Uncommon: Two ocular side effects occur. The first is small flecks in the clear layer over the lens of the eye, the cornea. The second, toxicity to the retina, is rare but can cause irreversible loss of vision. Other uncommon side effects are skin rashes, sometimes with hyperpigmentation, myopathy, cardiomyopathy, dizziness or deafness, and neuropathy.

ibandronate (Trade name: Boniva) A bisphosphonate used to treat and prevent osteoporosis.

Side effects Mild gastrointestinal symptoms with nausea, indigestion, and constipation are common. Difficulty swallowing, vomiting, erosive esophagitis (ulcers in the esophagus), and allergic reactions are rare. Osteonecrosis of the jaw occurs when an area of the jawbone such as a tooth socket does not heal and leaves the bone exposed; this can occur rarely in patients receiving bisphosphonates, usually intravenous bisphosphonates used to treat cancer.

Bisphosphonates are inconvenient because they need to be taken first thing in the morning with a full glass of water. To prevent the tablet refluxing back up the esophagus the patient cannot go back to bed. Bisphosphonates are very poorly absorbed and therefore after taking the tablet the patient cannot eat or drink anything other than water for at least 30 minutes. Ibandronate can be taken once a month.

ibuprofen (Trade names: Advil, Genpril, Ibuprin, Motrin, Nuprin) A nonsteroidal anti-inflammatory drug (NSAID) that inhibits cyclooxygenase (COX-1 and COX-2) enzymes, decreasing the formation of inflammatory mediators such as prostaglandins. NSAIDs are used to treat pain and inflammation resulting from a variety of causes. Common indications are rheumatoid arthritis, osteoarthritis, gout, ankylosing spondylitis, and bursitis. NSAIDs do not affect the progression of arthritis.

Side effects Common: GI symptoms, usually indigestion or heartburn and fluid retention with ankle edema. Less common: Peptic ulcers with or without complications such as perforation, gastrointestinal obstruction, or bleeding. Risk factors for complicated peptic ulcers caused by NSAIDs are age older than 65 years, previous peptic ulcer or bleeding ulcer, and treatment with a corticosteroid. NSAIDs can increase blood pressure, impair kidney function, and cause abnormal liver function tests (usually mild), rashes, ringing in the ears, and a feeling of lightheadedness. Uncommon: Serious allergy to NSAIDs can result in anaphylaxis with bronchospasm, urticaria, and angioedema. NSAIDs are associated with an increased risk of heart attack and stroke.

iloprost (Trade Name: Ventavis) A synthesized form of prostacyclin, a powerful natural vaso-dilator that dilates blood vessels, particularly in the lung. Used by inhalation to treat pulmonary hypertension.

Side effects Common: headache, flushing, edema, nausea, chest pain, jaw pain, low blood pressure, dizziness, nervousness. Uncommon: muscle pain, palpitations, vomiting, and allergy.

imipramine (Trade name: Tofranil) A tricyclic antidepressant, a class of drug commonly used to treat depression, chronic pain, and fibromyalgia.

Side effects Common: Sleepiness, and because of this sedative tricyclics are often used to improve sleep. The sedative effects can persist, resulting in unwanted sleepiness during the day. Anticholinergic side effects such as dry mouth and eyes, blurred vision, constipation, and slowness or difficulty passing urine can occur, particularly when treatment is started, but tolerance to these side effects may develop. Uncommon: Postural hypotension resulting in dizziness when standing up suddenly, tremor, nausea, confusion, sexual dysfunction, GI symptoms, paradoxical stimulation rather than sedation, bone marrow suppression, abnormal liver function tests, seizures, hair loss, and heart rhythm problems.

Imuran See AZATHIOPRINE.

Indocin See INDOMETHACIN.

indomethacin (Trade name: Indocin) A nonsteroidal anti-inflammatory drug (NSAID) that inhibits cyclooxygenase (COX-1 and COX-2) enzymes, decreasing the formation of inflammatory mediators such as prostaglandins. NSAIDs are used to treat pain and inflammation, resulting from a variety of causes. Common indications are rheumatoid arthritis, osteoarthritis, gout, ankylosing spondylitis, and bursitis. NSAIDs do not affect the progression of arthritis.

Side effects Common: GI symptoms, usually indigestion or heartburn, and fluid retention with ankle edema. Less common: Peptic ulcers with or without complications such as perforation, gastrointestinal obstruction, or bleeding. Risk factors for complicated peptic ulcers caused by NSAIDs are age older than 65 years, previous peptic ulcer or bleeding ulcer, and treatment with a corticosteroid. NSAIDs can increase blood pressure, impair kidney function, and cause abnormal liver function tests (usually mild), rashes, ringing in the ears, and a feeling of lightheadedness. Uncommon: Serious allergy to NSAIDs can result in anaphylaxis with bronchospasm, urticaria, and angioedema. NSAIDs are associated with an increased risk of heart attack and stroke.

infliximab (Trade name: Remicade) A specially designed protein to block the effects of tumor necrosis factor (TNF), a proinflammatory cytokine. Infliximab is a monoclonal antibody that binds to TNF, blocking its effects. Infliximab acts as a DMARD in RA and is also used to treat juvenile idiopathic arthritis (JIA), psoriatic arthritis, ankylosing spondylitis, and Crohn's disease. Limited data support the use of anti-TNF therapy in vasculitis.

Side effects Common: Requires intravenous administration and minor reactions during the infusion include fever, chills, rash, and itching. These infusion reactions are seldom serious. Approximately 5–10 percent of patients receiving infliximab will develop a positive antinuclear antibody (ANA) test, raising the concern that it may increase the risk of autoimmune diseases such as SLE. So far, this has not been a problem, but the long-term effects are not yet known. Uncommon: Infliximab is used with methotrexate to treat RA. The combination of infliximab and methotrexate can cause a mild elevation of the liver enzyme tests more often than methotrexate alone does. Uncommon: The risk of infections (sometimes serious) such as pneumonia is increased. Rare: Case reports or small series of patients developing diabetes, cancer, lymphoma, VASCULITIS, SLE-like autoimmune disease, multiple sclerosis-like demyelinating disorders, liver disease, hematological abnormalities including aplastic anemia, severe allergy, meningitis, and infection with TUBERCULOSIS, atypical mycobacteria, aspergillosis, histoplasmosis, listeria, and reactivation of hepatitis B have been reported in patients receiving TNF antagonists. TNF antagonists may increase mortality in patients with heart failure.

intravenous immunoglobulin (IVIG) See GAMMAGLOBULIN.

Kenalog See CORTICOSTEROIDS.

ketoprofen (Trade names: Orudis, Oruvail) A nonsteroidal anti-inflammatory drug (NSAID) that inhibits cyclooxygenase (COX-1 and COX-2) enzymes, decreasing the formation of inflammatory mediators such as prostaglandins. NSAIDs are used to treat pain and inflammation, resulting from a variety of causes. Common indications are rheumatoid arthritis, osteoarthritis, gout, ankylosing spondylitis, and bursitis. NSAIDs do not affect the progression of arthritis.

Side effects Common: GI symptoms, usually indigestion or heartburn, and fluid retention with ankle edema. Less common: Peptic ulcers with or without complications such as perforation, gastrointestinal obstruction, or bleeding. Risk factors for complicated peptic ulcers caused by NSAIDs are age older than 65 years, previous peptic ulcer or bleeding ulcer, and treatment with a corticosteroid. NSAIDs can increase blood pressure, impair kidney function, and cause abnormal liver function tests (usually mild), rashes, ringing in the ears, and a feeling of lightheadedness. Uncommon: Serious allergy to NSAIDs can result in anaphylaxis with bronchospasm, urticaria, and angioedema. NSAIDs are associated with an increased risk of heart attack and stroke.

ketorolac (Trade name: Toradol) A nonsteroidal anti-inflammatory drug (NSAID) that inhibits cyclooxygenase (COX-1 and COX-2) enzymes, decreasing the formation of inflammatory mediators such as prostaglandins. NSAIDs are used to treat pain and inflammation, resulting from a variety of causes. Ketorolac is designed to treat acute pain, for example postoperative pain, for a few days and should not be used chronically.

Side effects Common: GI symptoms, usually indigestion or heartburn, and fluid retention with ankle edema. Less common: Peptic ulcers with or without complications such as perforation, gastrointestinal obstruction, or bleeding. Risk factors for complicated peptic ulcers caused by NSAIDs are age older than 65 years, previous peptic ulcer or bleeding ulcer, and treatment with a corticosteroid. NSAIDs can increase blood pressure, impair kidney function, and cause abnormal liver function tests (usually mild), rashes, ringing in the ears, and a feeling of lightheadedness. Uncommon: Serious allergy to NSAIDs can result in anaphylaxis with bronchospasm, urticaria, and angioedema. NSAIDs are associated with an increased risk of heart attack and stroke.

Kineret   See ANAKINRA.

lansoprazole   (Trade name: Prevacid) A proton pump inhibitor (a class of drugs also known as PPIs) that decreases gastric acid production and is used to treat and prevent peptic ulcers and gastroesophageal reflux (GERD), common side effects of NSAIDs.
   Side effects Proton pump inhibitors seldom cause side effects. Uncommon: Constipation, rash, dizziness, diarrhea, abdominal pain, and elevated liver enzymes.

leflunomide   (Trade name: Arava) A disease-modifying antirheumatic drug (DMARD) most often prescribed to treat rheumatoid arthritis and occasionally psoriatic arthritis. Leflunomide alters the immune response, particularly in lymphocytes, by blocking an enzyme, dihydrorotate dehydrogenase, important for the formation of pyrimidines, components of DNA. Leflunomide can damage the developing fetus in pregnant animals. Women of childbearing potential taking leflunomide require adequate contraception, and the drug is avoided in pregnancy. Because it is cleared very slowly from the body over months or years, women of childbearing potential who stop taking leflunomide are treated with a course of cholestyramine (trade name: Questran), a resin that binds leflunomide in the gut and helps to clear it from the body.
   Side effects Common: Rash, mild increase in liver enzymes, loose or frequent bowel motions, diarrhea, and other GI problems such as cramps, nausea, and very occasionally vomiting. Uncommon: Hair thinning, loss of weight, infections, low white blood cell count, and neuropathy.

Lodine   See ETODOLAC.

Lortab   See ACETAMINOPHEN WITH NARCOTICS.

lumiracoxib   (Trade name: Prexige) A nonsteroidal anti-inflammatory drug (NSAID) that inhibits the cyclo-oxygenase-2 (COX-2) enzyme, decreasing the formation of inflammatory mediators such as prostaglandins. Lumiracoxib is selective for COX-2 and has little effect on COX-1 and therefore does not inhibit platelet aggregation. NSAIDs are used to treat pain and inflammation due to many causes and for arthritis-related pain caused by rheumatoid arthritis, osteoarthritis, and bursitis. NSAIDs do not affect the progression of arthritis. Lumiracoxib has been withdrawn from the market in most countries because of serious liver toxicity. It was never marketed in the United States.

Lyrica   See PREGABALIN.

magnesium choline salicylate   See CHOLINE MAGNESIUM SALICYLATE.

meclofenamate sodium   (Trade name: Meclomen) A nonsteroidal anti-inflammatory drug (NSAID) that inhibits cyclooxygenase (COX-1 and COX-2) enzymes, decreasing the formation of inflammatory mediators such as prostaglandins. NSAIDs are used to treat pain and inflammation resulting from a variety of causes. Common indications are rheumatoid arthritis, osteoarthritis, gout, ankylosing spondylitis, and bursitis. NSAIDs do not affect the progression of arthritis.

Side effects   Common: GI symptoms, usually indigestion or heartburn, and fluid retention with ankle edema. Less common: Peptic ulcers with or without complications such as perforation, gastro-intestinal obstruction, or bleeding. Risk factors for complicated peptic ulcers caused by NSAIDs are age older than 65 years, previous peptic ulcer or bleeding ulcer, and treatment with a corticosteroid. NSAIDs can increase blood pressure, impair kidney function, and cause abnormal liver function tests (usually mild), rashes, ringing in the ears, and a feeling of lightheadedness. Uncommon: Serious allergy to NSAIDs can result in anaphylaxis with bronchospasm, urticaria, and angioedema. NSAIDs are associated with an increased risk of heart attack and stroke.

Meclomen   See MECLOFENAMATE SODIUM.

meperidine (meperidine hydrochloride, pethidine) (Trade name: Demerol) A strong narcotic analgesic used to treat severe pain not controlled by acet-aminophen, an NSAID, or by weaker narcotics, such as codeine or hydrocodone. Narcotics do not affect inflammation but decrease pain by acting through specific opiate receptors in the brain.

Side effects   Common: Nausea, vomiting, constipation, decreased appetite, dizziness, lightheadedness, sedation, and low blood pressure. Uncommon: Allergy resulting in an urticarial rash or bronchospasm, confusion, agitation, insomnia, euphoria, seizures, addiction, and suppression of respiration.

mesna   (Trade name: Mesnex) A compound rich in sulfhydryl (—SH) groups that bind acrolein and other metabolites of cyclophosphamide (trade name: Cytoxan) in the urinary tract and prevents cyclophosphamide-induced bladder toxicity.

Side effects   Common: A bad taste in the mouth, headache, diarrhea, nausea, and muscle pain. Uncommon: An allergic rash or urticaria.

methocarbamol   (Trade names: Delaxin, Marbaxin, Robaxin, Robomol) A muscle relaxant used to treat painful muscle spasm and fibromyalgia.

Side effects   Common: Drowsiness, dizziness. Uncommon: Flushing, nausea, rash, bone marrow suppression, and allergic reactions.

methotrexate (MTX)   (Trade names: Folex, Rheumatrex) An anticancer drug that is used in low doses, usually administered once a week, as a disease-modifying antirheumatic drug (DMARD) for rheumatoid arthritis (RA), psoriatic arthritis, and juvenile idiopathic arthritis and to treat systemic lupus erythematosus, dermatomyositis or polymyositis, vasculitis, and other connective tissue diseases. Methotrexate is the gold-standard DMARD against which new drugs to treat RA are compared. In patients requiring high doses of corticosteroids to control an autoimmune problem, the addition of methotrexate may allow lower doses to be used, a so-called steroid-sparing effect. Methotrexate blocks an enzyme, dihydrofolate reductase, important in synthesizing the active form of the vitamin folic acid. This effect accounts for the anti-cancer effects of methotrexate but is probably not the most important mechanism of action of methotrexate in arthritis, where increased release of a chemical mediator, adenosine, may play a role.

Side effects   Common: Mouth ulcers, nausea, and mild increases in liver enzymes. Folic acid, a vitamin, decreases the frequency of minor side effects. Uncommon: Vomiting, increased number of rheumatoid nodules, fatigue, photosensitivity, hair thinning, hepatitis, liver cirrhosis, pneumonitis (also known as *methotrexate lung*), bone marrow suppression, and increased risk of infection. Rare: Increased risk of some cancers such as lymphoma.

Miacalcin   See CALCITONIN.

milnacipran   (Trade name: Savella) An antidepressant used to treat fibromyalgia.

Side effects   Common: Headache, constipation, nausea, fatigue, insomnia, sweating, increase in blood pressure and heart rate. Uncommon: vomiting, liver toxicity, increased risk of suicide, sexual dysfunction, seizures, increased risk of bleeding, palpitations.

minocycline (Trade name: Minocin) A tetracycline antibiotic used as a disease-modifying antirheumatic drug (DMARD) to treat rheumatoid arthritis. The mechanism of action in RA is unknown and may involve inhibition of enzymes such as matrix metalloproteinases, effects unrelated to its antibiotic actions.

Side effects Common: Diarrhea, nausea, and photosensitivity. Tetracyclines are avoided in children because they cause discoloration of the permanent teeth. Uncommon: Dizziness, rash, sometimes with dark discoloration of the skin (hyperpigmentation), and reversible DRUG-INDUCED LUPUS.

misoprostol (Trade name: Cytotec) A drug structurally similar to a prostaglandin. NSAIDs, particularly the nonselective ones that inhibit both COX-1 and COX-2, decrease the formation of prostaglandins that stimulate inflammation and also those that protect against peptic ulcers. Misoprostol protects against NSAID-induced peptic ulceration by acting as a prostaglandin replacement.

Side effects Common: Diarrhea and stomach cramps. If used during pregnancy, misoprostol causes abnormalities of the unborn baby and can cause abortion. Uncommon: Nausea, vomiting, headache, and allergy.

morphine (Trade name: Kadian, MS Contin, Oramorph SR, Roxanol) A strong narcotic analgesic used to treat severe pain not controlled by acetaminophen, an NSAID, or by weaker narcotics, such as codeine or hydrocodone. Narcotics do not affect inflammation but decrease pain by acting through specific opiate receptors in the brain.

Side effects Common: Nausea, vomiting, constipation, decreased appetite, dizziness, lightheadedness, sedation, and low blood pressure. Uncommon: Allergy resulting in an urticarial rash or bronchospasm, confusion, agitation, insomnia, euphoria, addiction, and suppression of respiration.

Motrin See IBUPROFEN.

mycophenolate mofetil (mycophenolic acid) (Trade name: CellCept) An immunosuppressive drug whose main use is to prevent rejection after organ transplantation. Mycophenolate suppresses the immune system by interfering with DNA synthesis by blocking the formation of purines (building blocks for DNA), particularly in cells such as lymphocytes. Rheumatologists use mycophenolate to treat systemic lupus erythematosus and as maintenance treatment to keep vasculitis in remission. In patients requiring high doses of corticosteroids to control an autoimmune problem, mycophenolate treatment may allow lower doses of corticosteroids to be used, acting as a steroid-sparing agent.

Side effects Common: GI symptoms such as vomiting, diarrhea, stomach pain, and nausea. Uncommon: Bone marrow suppression, allergic reactions, mild increases in liver enzymes, herpes zoster, and increased risk of infection, skin cancer, and lymphoma.

myochrysine See GOLD INJECTIONS.

nabumetone (Trade name: Relafen) A nonsteroidal anti-inflammatory drug (NSAID) that inhibits cyclooxygenase (COX-1 and COX-2) enzymes, decreasing the formation of inflammatory mediators such as prostaglandins. NSAIDs are used to treat pain and inflammation resulting from a variety of causes. Common indications are rheumatoid arthritis, osteoarthritis, gout, ankylosing spondylitis, and bursitis. NSAIDs do not affect the progression of arthritis.

Side effects Common: GI symptoms, usually indigestion or heartburn, and fluid retention with ankle edema. Less common: Peptic ulcers with or without complications such as perforation, gastrointestinal obstruction, or bleeding. Risk factors for complicated peptic ulcers caused by NSAIDs are age older than 65 years, previous peptic ulcer or bleeding ulcer, and treatment with a corticosteroid. NSAIDs can increase blood pressure, impair kidney function, and cause abnormal liver function tests (usually mild), rashes, ringing in the ears, and a feeling of lightheadedness. Uncommon: Serious allergy to NSAIDs can result in anaphylaxis with bronchospasm, urticaria, and angioedema. NSAIDs are associated with an increased risk of heart attack and stroke.

Nalfon See FENOPROFEN.

Naprelan See NAPROXEN.

Naprosyn See NAPROXEN.

naproxen (Trade names: Aleve, Anaprox, Naprosyn; controlled-release [slow-release] naproxen: Naprelan) A nonsteroidal anti-inflammatory drug (NSAID) that inhibits cyclooxygenase (COX-1 and COX-2) enzymes, decreasing the formation of inflammatory mediators such as prostaglandins. NSAIDs are used to treat pain and inflammation resulting from a variety of causes. Common indications are rheumatoid arthritis, osteoarthritis, gout, ankylosing spondylitis, and bursitis. NSAIDs do not affect the progression of arthritis.
   Side effects Common: GI symptoms, usually indigestion or heartburn, and fluid retention with ankle edema. Less common: Peptic ulcers with or without complications such as perforation, gastrointestinal obstruction, or bleeding. Risk factors for complicated peptic ulcers caused by NSAIDs are age older than 65 years, previous peptic ulcer or bleeding ulcer, and treatment with a corticosteroid. NSAIDs can increase blood pressure, impair kidney function, and cause abnormal liver function tests (usually mild), rashes, ringing in the ears, and a feeling of lightheadedness. Uncommon: Serious allergy to NSAIDs can result in anaphylaxis with bronchospasm, urticaria, and angioedema. NSAIDs are associated with an increased risk of heart attack and stroke. Naproxen, because of its strong antiplatelet effects, may be less likely to do this.

Neoral See CYCLOSPORINE.

Neurontin See GABAPENTIN.

Nexium See ESOMEPRAZOLE.

nitroglycerin ointment (nittropaste) (Trade names: Nitro-Bid Ointment, Nitrol Ointment) A vasodilator that dilates arteries and veins and is most often used to dilate the arteries in the heart in the treatment of angina. Nitroglycerin ointment is also used in people with RAYNAUD'S PHENOMENON and SCLERODERMA to improve the blood supply to the tips of the fingers.
   Side effects Common: Flushing, dizziness, and headache.

nizatidine (Trade name: Axid) A histamine type 2 receptor antagonist (H_2-receptor antagonist or H_2-blocker) that decreases acid production by the stomach and is used to treat indigestion, reflux esophagitis, and peptic ulcers. H_2-receptor antagonists, except in high doses, do not provide adequate protection against NSAID-induced peptic ulcers.
   Side effects H_2-receptor antagonists are generally well tolerated and have few adverse effects. Common: Minor, transient symptoms such as dizziness, headache, and diarrhea. Uncommon: Rash and hepatitis.

Norflex See ORPHENADRINE CITRATE.

nortriptyline (Trade names: Aventyl Hydrochloride, Pamelor) A tricyclic antidepressant, a class of drug commonly used to treat depression, chronic pain, and fibromyalgia.
   Side effects Common: Dizziness, drowsiness, headache, anticholinergic side effects such as dry mouth and eyes, blurred vision, constipation, and slowness or difficulty passing urine can occur, particularly when treatment is started, but tolerance to these side effects may develop. Uncommon: Postural hypotension resulting in dizziness when standing up suddenly, tremor, nausea, confusion, sexual dysfunction, GI symptoms, paradoxical stimulation rather than sedation, bone marrow suppression, abnormal liver function tests, seizures, hair loss, and heart rhythm problems.

omeprazole (Trade name: Prilosec) A proton pump inhibitor (a class of drugs also known as PPIs) that decreases gastric acid production and is used to treat and prevent peptic ulcers and gastro-esophageal reflux (GERD)—common side effects of NSAIDs.

Side effects Proton pump inhibitors seldom cause side effects. Uncommon: Constipation, rash, dizziness, diarrhea, abdominal pain, and elevated liver enzymes.

Orencia   See ABATACEPT.

orphenadrine citrate (Trade name: Norflex) A muscle relaxant used to treat painful muscle spasms and fibromyalgia.

Side effects Common: Drowsiness or dizziness and anticholinergic symptoms such as dry eyes, dry mouth, blurred vision, constipation, and particularly in men with prostate problems, difficulty passing urine. Less common: Flushing, nausea, and rash.

Orudis   See KETOPROFEN.

Oruvail   See KETOPROFEN.

Os-cal   See CALCIUM.

oxaprozin (Trade name: Daypro) A nonsteroidal anti-inflammatory drug (NSAID) that inhibits cyclooxygenase (COX-1 and COX-2) enzymes, decreasing the formation of inflammatory mediators such as prostaglandins. NSAIDs are used to treat pain and inflammation resulting from a variety of causes. Common indications are rheumatoid arthritis, osteoarthritis, gout, ankylosing spondylitis, and bursitis. NSAIDs do not affect the progression of arthritis.

Side effects Common: GI symptoms, usually indigestion or heartburn, and fluid retention with ankle edema. Less common: Peptic ulcers with or without complications such as perforation, gastrointestinal obstruction, or bleeding. Risk factors for complicated peptic ulcers caused by NSAIDs are age older than 65 years, previous peptic ulcer or bleeding ulcer, and treatment with a corticosteroid. NSAIDs can increase blood pressure, impair kidney function, and cause abnormal liver function tests (usually mild), rashes, ringing in the ears, and a feeling of lightheadedness. Uncommon: Serious allergy to NSAIDs can result in anaphylaxis with bronchospasm, urticaria, and angioedema. NSAIDs are associated with an increased risk of heart attack and stroke.

oxycodone (Trade names: Roxicodone, OxyContin [a controlled-release or slow-release preparation]; trade names of oxycodone in combination preparations with acetaminophen include Percocet, Roxicet, Tylox [see ACETAMINOPHEN WITH NARCOTICS] and those with aspirin include Percodan, Roxiprin.) A narcotic analgesic that decreases pain by acting through specific opiate receptors in the brain and that is used to treat moderate-to-severe pain not controlled by acetaminophen or an NSAID.

Side effects Common: Nausea, vomiting, constipation, poor appetite, dizziness, feeling lightheaded, and sleepiness. Uncommon: Feeling nervous or agitated, sleeping, an allergic reaction with urticarial rash (hives) or bronchospasm, confusion, feeling "high," addiction, and suppression of respiration.

oxycodone with acetaminophen (Trade names: Percocet, Roxicet, Tylox) See ACETAMINOPHEN WITH NARCOTICS.

OxyContin   See OXYCODONE.

Pamelor   See NORTRIPTYLINE.

pamidronate (Trade name: Aredia) A bisphosphonate used to treat Paget's disease. It is also effective in treating osteoporosis but is not commonly used for this purpose since it has to be given by intravenous infusion.

Side effects Common: Pamidronate is administered as an intravenous infusion and can cause inflammation at the infusion site (thrombophlebitis). Uncommon: Fever, nausea, diarrhea, aching bones, rash, a low white blood cell, and low plasma concentrations of calcium, phosphate, and magnesium. Osteonecrosis of the jaw occurs when an area of the jawbone such as a tooth socket does not heal and leaves the bone exposed; this can occur rarely in patients receiving bisphosphonates, usually intravenous bisphosphonates used to treat cancer.

pantoprazole (Trade name: Protonix) A proton pump inhibitor (a class of drugs also known as PPIs) that decreases gastric acid production and is used to treat and prevent peptic ulcers and gastroesophageal reflux (GERD), common side effects of NSAIDs.

Side effects Proton pump inhibitors seldom cause side effects. Uncommon: Constipation, rash, dizziness, diarrhea, abdominal pain, and elevated liver enzymes.

paroxetine (Trade name: Paxil) An antidepressant, a class of drug commonly used to treat depression, chronic pain, and fibromyalgia.

Side effects Common: Dizziness, insomnia or drowsiness, dry mouth, and GI side effects such as nausea and diarrhea. Uncommon: Tremor, confusion, rash, sexual dysfunction, sedation, allergy, anticholinergic side effects such as blurred vision, constipation, and slowness or difficulty passing urine.

penicillamine (d-penicillamine) (Trade names: Cuprimine, Depen) A chelating agent that binds metals such as copper and lead and acts as a disease-modifying antirheumatic drug (DMARD) in RA and is sometimes used to treat scleroderma. In the treatment of RA, penicillamine has largely been replaced by drugs with fewer side effects.

The evidence supporting a role for penicillamine in scleroderma is weak. The mechanism of action in RA is unknown.

Side effects Common: Rash, itching, urticaria, a metallic taste, and proteinuria. Uncommon: Allergic reactions, bone marrow suppression resulting in low white blood cell count or thrombocytopenia, glomerulonephritis, hepatitis, optic nerve inflammation, myopathy, fever, drug-induced lupus, and myasthenia gravis.

Percocet See ACETAMINOPHEN WITH NARCOTICS.

phenylbutazone (Trade names: Butazolidin, Butazone) A nonsteroidal anti-inflammatory drug (NSAID) that inhibits cyclooxygenase (COX-1 and COX-2) enzymes, decreasing the formation of inflammatory mediators such as prostaglandins. Phenylbutazone has a reputation for being more effective than other NSAIDs for treating the symptoms of ankylosing spondylitis. Because of its propensity for causing bone marrow suppression, it is not generally available. Phenylbutazone is used only to treat pain in patients with ankylosing spondylitis that has not responded to other NSAIDs.

Side effects Common: GI symptoms, usually indigestion or heartburn, and fluid retention with ankle edema. Less common: Peptic ulcers with or without complications such as perforation, gastrointestinal obstruction, or bleeding. Risk factors for complicated peptic ulcers caused by NSAIDs are age older than 65 years, previous peptic ulcer or bleeding ulcer, and treatment with a corticosteroid. NSAIDs can increase blood pressure, impair kidney function, and cause abnormal liver function tests (usually mild), rashes, ringing in the ears, and a feeling of lightheadedness. Uncommon: Serious allergy to NSAIDs can result in anaphylaxis with bronchospasm, urticaria, and angioedema. Phenylbutazone can rarely cause bone marrow suppression or failure.

pilocarpine (Trade name: Salagen) A drug that stimulates the cholinergic nerves to salivary glands, increasing the production of saliva. It is used to treat the symptom of dry mouth that often occurs in patients with Sjögren's syndrome.

Side effects   Common: Sweating, dizziness, headache, blurred vision, a runny or blocked nose, passing urine more often, feeling flushed, and GI problems such as nausea or diarrhea.

piroxicam   (Trade name: Feldene) A nonsteroidal anti-inflammatory drug (NSAID) that inhibits cyclooxygenase (COX-1 and COX-2) enzymes, decreasing the formation of inflammatory mediators such as prostaglandins. NSAIDs are used to treat pain and inflammation resulting from a variety of causes. Common indications are rheumatoid arthritis, osteoarthritis, gout, ankylosing spondylitis, and bursitis. NSAIDs do not affect the progression of arthritis.

Side effects   Common: GI symptoms, usually indigestion or heartburn, and fluid retention with ankle edema. Less common: Peptic ulcers with or without complications such as perforation, gastrointestinal obstruction, or bleeding. Risk factors for complicated peptic ulcers caused by NSAIDs are age older than 65 years, previous peptic ulcer or bleeding ulcer, and treatment with a corticosteroid. NSAIDs can increase blood pressure, impair kidney function, and cause abnormal liver function tests (usually mild), rashes, ringing in the ears, and a feeling of lightheadedness. Uncommon: Serious allergy to NSAIDs can result in anaphylaxis with bronchospasm, urticaria, and angioedema. NSAIDs are associated with an increased risk of heart attack and stroke.

Plaquenil   See   HYDROXYCHLOROQUINE   AND PHOSPHATE.

prednisolone   See CORTICOSTEROIDS.

prednisone   See CORTICOSTEROIDS.

pregabalin   (Trade name: Lyrica) Used to treat pain due to nerve damage and fibromyalgia.

Side effects   Common: Weight gain, tremor, sleepiness, edema, insomnia. Uncommon: Postural hypotension resulting in dizziness when standing up suddenly, liver toxicity, increased muscle enzymes, nausea, confusion, sexual dysfunction, seizures, increased blood pressure, and palpitations. Rare: serious allergy.

probenecid   (Trade names: Benemid, Probalan) A uricosuric that lowers serum uric acid levels by increasing uric acid excretion in the urine and is used to prevent attacks of gout.

Side effects   Common: Headache and GI symptoms such as nausea and, less often, vomiting. Uncommon: Rash, itching, allergic reactions, precipitation of an acute attack of gout, and bone marrow suppression.

Propulsid   See CISAPRIDE.

prosorba column (Protein A Immunoadsorption Column)   (Trade name: Prosorba Column) Production of Prosorba Column ceased in 2006. Blood is drawn from the patient, passed through the prosorba column, and reinjected into the patient, a process known as apheresis. The prosorba column was used to treat RA not responding to other treatments and to treat idiopathic thrombocytopenic purpura (ITP) (see THROMBOCYTOPENIA). The column contains a protein (protein A) from a common type of bacterium (staphylococcus) and acts as a filter, removing proteins that promote RA or ITP from the blood passing through it.

Side effects   Common: Apheresis (removing blood, filtering it, and returning it to the patient), whether using the prosorba column or not, often causes minor side effects of short duration such as joint pain, fatigue, nausea, rash, low blood pressure, flushing, dizziness, tingling, fever, and chills. Uncommon: Many patients with autoimmune diseases have small fragile veins, and obtaining venous access for apheresis can be a problem. CRYOGLOBULINEMIA has been described.

Protonix   See PANTOPRAZOLE.

proton pump inhibitors See ESOMEPRAZOLE, LANSOPRAZOLE, OMEPRAZOLE, PANTOPRAZOLE, and RABEPRAZOLE.

Prozac See FLUOXETINE.

rabeprazole (Trade name: Aciphex) A proton pump inhibitor (a class of drugs also known as PPIs) that decreases gastric acid production and is used to treat and prevent peptic ulcers and gastro-esophageal reflux (GERD), common side effects of NSAIDs.

Side effects Proton pump inhibitors seldom cause side effects. Uncommon: Constipation, rash, dizziness, diarrhea, abdominal pain, and elevated liver enzymes.

raloxifene (Trade name: Evista) A selective estrogen receptor modulator (SERM) that acts on estrogen receptors in bone without stimulating those in the breast or uterus. Raloxifene is used to treat and prevent osteoporosis in postmenopausal women, and clinical trials are underway examining its role in the prevention of breast cancer in high-risk individuals.

Side effects Common: Hot flashes and leg cramps. Uncommon: Blood clots in veins (deep vein thrombosis).

ranitidine (Trade name: Zantac) A histamine type 2 receptor antagonist (H_2-receptor antagonist or H_2-blocker) that decreases acid production by the stomach and is used to treat indigestion, reflux esophagitis, and peptic ulcers. H_2-receptor antagonists, except in high doses, do not provide adequate protection against NSAID-induced peptic ulcers.

Side effects H_2-receptor antagonists are generally well tolerated and have few adverse effects. Common: Minor, transient symptoms such as dizziness, headache, and diarrhea. Uncommon: rash and hepatitis.

rasburicase (Trade names: Elitek, Fasturtec) Rasburicase is a manufactured enzyme that breaks down uric acid, the substance that crystallizes to form gout crystals. Rasburicase is approved to prevent the formation of large amounts of uric acid that can occur when some types of cancer are treated. It is being tested as a treatment for refractory gout, but it is immunogenic and stimulates the body to make antibodies against it, resulting in allergy and decreased efficacy.

Side effects There is limited long-term information. Common: Requires intravenous injection and minor injection reactions such as itching, chills, skin rash, and dizziness are common. Uncommon: Serious allergic reactions (anaphylaxis), an abnormal type of hemoglobin in red blood cells (methemoglobinemia), and a low white blood cell count.

Reclast See ZOLEDRONIC ACID.

Relafen See NABUMETONE.

Remicade See INFLIXIMAB.

Remodulin See TREPROSTINIL.

Rheumatrex See METHOTREXATE.

Ridaura See AURANOFIN.

risedronate (Trade name: Actonel) A bisphosphonate used to treat and prevent osteoporosis and to treat Paget's disease.

Side effects Mild gastrointestinal symptoms with nausea, indigestion, and constipation are common. Difficulty swallowing; vomiting and allergic reactions are rare.

Bisphosphonates are inconvenient because they need to be taken on an empty stomach with a full glass of water. To prevent the tablet refluxing back up the esophagus, the patient must remain upright for an hour afterward. Bisphosphonates are very poorly absorbed, and therefore after taking the tablet the patient cannot eat or drink anything other than water for at least 30 minutes. Most manufacturers have produced a tablet that can be taken once a week to reduce the inconvenience. Osteonecrosis of the jaw occurs when an area of the jawbone such as a tooth socket does not heal and leaves the bone exposed; this can occur rarely in patients receiving bisphosphonates, usually intravenous bisphosphonates used to treat cancer.

Rituxan See RITUXIMAB.

rituximab (Trade names: Rituxan, MabThera) A monoclonal antibody that targets B lymphocytes. Rituximab is a specially designed protein that acts as an antibody to a cell marker called CD20 on B-lymphocytes. Rituximab reduces the B-cell count and thus suppresses the immune response. It is used to treat lymphoma and rheumatoid arthritis, and many studies are examining its use in other autoimmune diseases such as SLE, polymyositis, and cryoglobulinemia.

Side effects There is limited long-term information. Common: Requires intravenous injection and minor injection reactions such as itching, rash, chills, and dizziness are common. Uncommon: Infections (sometimes serious), heart failure, abnormal heart rhythm, serious allergic reactions (anaphylaxis, severe skin rashes), low white cell count, reactivation of hepatitis B, and a viral infection of the brain called progressive multifocal leukoencephalopathy (PML).

Robaxin See METHOCARBAMOL.

rofecoxib (Trade name: Vioxx) A nonsteroidal anti-inflammatory drug (NSAID) that inhibits the cyclooxygenase-2 (COX-2) enzyme, decreasing the formation of inflammatory mediators such as prostaglandins. Rofecoxib is selective for COX-2 and has little effect on COX-1, and therefore it does not inhibit platelet aggregation. Rofecoxib was withdrawn from the market because of an increased risk of heart attack and stroke.

Salagen See PILOCARPINE.

salsalate (Trade names: Argesic-SA, Disalcid, Salflex) A nonsteroidal anti-inflammatory drug (NSAID) belonging to a subgroup called nonacetylated salicylates that differs from other NSAIDs in that it is a weak inhibitor of cyclooxygenase (COX) enzymes that decrease the formation of inflammatory mediators such as prostaglandins. NSAIDs are used to treat pain and inflammation due to many causes and for arthritis-related pain caused by rheumatoid arthritis, osteoarthritis, and bursitis. NSAIDs do not affect the progression of arthritis.

Side effects Common: GI symptoms, usually indigestion or heartburn, and fluid retention with ankle edema. Uncommon: Peptic ulcers with or without complications such as perforation, gastrointestinal obstruction, or bleeding. Risk factors for complicated peptic ulcers caused by NSAIDs are age older than 65 years, previous peptic ulcer or bleeding ulcer, and treatment with a corticosteroid. Nonacetylated salicylates are salicylates like aspirin, but their different chemical structure makes them behave more like COX-2-selective NSAIDs so that they do not inhibit platelet aggregation significantly and are less likely to cause serious GI complications. NSAIDs can increase blood pressure, impair kidney function, and cause abnormal liver function tests (usually mild), rashes, ringing in the ears, and a feeling of lightheadedness. Serious allergy to NSAIDs can result in anaphylaxis with bronchospasm, urticaria, and angioedema.

Sandimmune See CYCLOSPORINE.

Savella See MILNACIPRAN.

sertraline (Trade name: Zoloft) An antidepressant, a class of drug commonly used to treat depression, chronic pain, and fibromyalgia.

Side effects Common: Dizziness, insomnia or drowsiness, dry mouth, and GI side effects such as nausea and diarrhea. Uncommon: Tremor, confusion, rash, sexual dysfunction, sedation, and allergy.

Simponi   See GOLIMUMAB.

Solganal   See GOLD INJECTIONS.

Soma   See CARISOPRODOL.

sucralfate   (Trade name: Carafate) An aluminum sucrose sulfate that binds to damaged areas of the stomach, coats them, and protects against peptic ulcer.

Side effects   Sucralfate has few side effects. Common: Constipation.

sulfasalazine (5-aminosalicylic acid [5 ASA] plus sulfapyridine)   (Trade names: Azulfidine, Azulfidine EN-tabs) A combination of a sulfonamide antibiotic and a poorly absorbed salicylate that acts as a disease-modifying antirheumatic drug (DMARD) in RA. It is also used for other types of inflammatory arthritis such as juvenile idiopathic arthritis (JIA), Reiter's syndrome, ankylosing spondylitis, and psoriatic arthritis. Sulfasalazine is also used to treat inflammatory bowel disease, occurring with or without arthritis.

Side effects   Common: Rash and GI symptoms such as nausea, vomiting, diarrhea, and cramps. Uncommon: Fever, low white blood cell count, bone marrow suppression, a peeling skin rash, hepatitis, drug-induced lupus, photosensitivity, temporary decrease in sperm count, and anemia.

sulfinpyrazone   (Trade name: Anturane) A uricosuric that lowers serum uric acid levels by increasing uric acid excretion in the urine and that is used to prevent attacks of gout.

Side effects   Common: GI symptoms such as nausea and cramps, less often vomiting. Uncommon: Rash, itching, an allergic reaction, bringing on an attack of gout, bone marrow suppression problems, hepatitis, and proteinuria.

sulindac   (Trade name: Clinoril) A nonsteroidal anti-inflammatory drug (NSAID) that inhibits cyclooxygenase (COX-1 and COX-2) enzymes, decreasing the formation of inflammatory mediators such as prostaglandins. NSAIDs are used to treat pain and inflammation resulting from a variety of causes. Common indications are rheumatoid arthritis, osteoarthritis, gout, ankylosing spondylitis, and bursitis. NSAIDs do not affect the progression of arthritis.

Side effects   Common: GI symptoms, usually indigestion or heartburn, and fluid retention with ankle edema. Less common: Peptic ulcers with or without complications such as perforation, gastrointestinal obstruction, or bleeding. Risk factors for complicated peptic ulcers caused by NSAIDs are age older than 65 years, previous peptic ulcer or bleeding ulcer, and treatment with a corticosteroid. NSAIDs can increase blood pressure, impair kidney function, and cause abnormal liver function tests (usually mild), rashes, ringing in the ears, and a feeling of lightheadedness. Uncommon: Serious allergy to NSAIDs can result in anaphylaxis with bronchospasm, urticaria, and angioedema. NSAIDS are associated with an increased risk of heart attack and stroke.

Synvisc (Hylan GF 20)   See HYALURONAN INJECTIONS.

tacrolimus (FK506)   (Trade name: Prograf) An immunosuppressive drug whose main use is to prevent rejection after organ transplantation. Tacrolimus is under evaluation for the treatment of RA and appears to be similar to cyclosporine in its mechanism of action and side effects.

teriparatide   (Trade name: Forteo) A synthesized parathyroid hormone that is injected to treat osteoporosis.

Side effects   Common: muscle cramps, increased blood calcium concentration. Uncommon: chest pain, rash, itching, irritation at the site of injection, dizziness.

tetracyclines   See MINOCYCLINE.

thalidomide (Trade name: Thalomid) Thalidomide is a sleeping tablet that was taken off the market in 1961 when it was recognized that it caused birth defects. Recently thalidomide has been investigated (under strict control) for the treatment of mouth ulcers in patients with HIV, mouth and genital ulcers in Behçet's disease, and skin rashes of SLE or discoid LE that have not responded to other treatments. Thalidomide alters the immune response perhaps by decreasing tumor necrosis factor (TNF) production and the formation of new blood vessels (angiogenesis).

Side effects Common: Thalidomide causes serious birth defects if taken during pregnancy. Nerve damage, which can be painful, severe, and permanent; sleepiness; constipation; rash; headaches; and edema are common. Uncommon: Low white blood cell count.

tocilizumab (Trade name: Actemra) A specially designed protein that acts as an antibody against interleukin-6 (IL-6), a pro-inflammatory cytokine. Tocilizumab is approved in Europe for the treatment of rheumatoid arthritis and was approved by the Food and Drug Administration in the United States in 2010.

Side effects There is limited long-term information, but the side effects are likely to be similar to those of other drugs that block the inflammatory response. Common: Requires intravenous injection and minor injection reactions such as itching, chills, rash, and dizziness are common. Concentrations of cholesterol and triglycerides can increase. Uncommon: Infections (sometimes serious). Increased liver function tests and hypertension.

Tolectin See TOLMETIN.

tolmetin (Trade name: Tolectin) A nonsteroidal anti-inflammatory drug (NSAID) that inhibits cyclooxygenase (COX-1 and COX-2) enzymes, decreasing the formation of inflammatory mediators such as prostaglandins. NSAIDs are used to treat pain and inflammation resulting from a variety of causes. Common indications are rheu-matoid arthritis, osteoarthritis, gout, ankylosing spondylitis, and bursitis. NSAIDs do not affect the progression of arthritis.

Side effects Common: GI symptoms, usually indigestion or heartburn, and fluid retention with ankle edema. Less common: Peptic ulcers with or without complications such as perforation, gastro-intestinal obstruction, or bleeding. Risk factors for complicated peptic ulcers caused by NSAIDs are age older than 65 years, previous peptic ulcer or bleeding ulcer, and treatment with a corticosteroid. NSAIDs can increase blood pressure, impair kidney function, and cause abnormal liver function tests (usually mild), rashes, ringing in the ears, and a feeling of lightheadedness. Uncommon: Serious allergy to NSAIDs can result in anaphylaxis with bronchospasm, urticaria, and angioedema. NSAIDs are associated with an increased risk of heart attack and stroke.

Toradol See KETOROLAC.

Tracleer See BOSENTAN.

tramadol (Trade name: Ultram) A narcotic analgesic that decreases pain by acting through specific opiate receptors in the brain and that is used to treat moderate-to-severe pain not controlled by acetaminophen or an NSAID.

Side effects Common: Nausea, vomiting, constipation, poor appetite, dizziness, feeling lightheaded, and sleepiness. Uncommon: Feeling nervous or agitated, sleeping badly, seizures, an allergic reaction with urticarial rash (hives) or bronchospasm, confusion, feeling high, and addiction.

trazodone (Trade name: Desyrel) An antidepressant, a class of drug commonly used to treat depression, chronic pain, and fibromyalgia.

Side effects Common: Dizziness, drowsiness, dry mouth, and GI side effects such as nausea and diarrhea. Uncommon: Tremor, confusion, rash, sexual dysfunction, sedation, allergy, anticholinergic side effects such as blurred vision, constipation, and slowness or difficulty passing urine.

treprostinil (Trade Name: Remodulin) A synthesized form of prostacyclin, a powerful natural vasodilator that dilates blood vessels, particularly in the lung. Used by continuous infusion (usually under the skin) to treat pulmonary hypertension.

Side effects Common: Irritation and pain at the site of the subcutaneous infusion, headache, flushing, edema, nausea, chest pain, jaw pain, low blood pressure, dizziness, nervousness. Uncommon: Muscle pain, palpitations, vomiting, and allergy. If the drug infusion is stopped suddenly the pressure in the pulmonary arteries can rebound and increase.

Trilisate See CHOLINE MAGNESIUM SALICYLATE.

tumor necrosis factor (TNF) antagonists See ADALIMUMAB; ETANERCEPT; INFLIXIMAB; GOLIMUMAB; CERTOLIZUMAB.

Tums See CALCIUM.

Tylenol See ACETAMINOPHEN.

Tylenol #3 See ACETAMINOPHEN WITH NARCOTICS.

Tylox See ACETAMINOPHEN WITH NARCOTICS.

Uloric See FEBUXOSTAT.

Ultram See TRAMADOL.

valdecoxib (Trade name: Bextra) A nonsteroidal anti-inflammatory drug (NSAID) that inhibits the cyclooxygenase-2 (COX-2) enzyme, decreasing the formation of inflammatory mediators such as prostaglandins. Valdecoxib is selective for COX-2 and has little effect on COX-1. Therefore it does not inhibit platelet aggregation. Valdecoxib was withdrawn from the market because of increased risk of serious allergic reactions.

venlafaxine (Trade name: Effexor) An antidepressant, a class of drug commonly used to treat depression, chronic pain, and fibromyalgia.

Side effects Common: Dizziness, insomnia or drowsiness, dry mouth, and GI side effects such as nausea and diarrhea. Uncommon: Tremor, confusion, rash, sexual dysfunction, sedation, allergy, anticholinergic side effects such as blurred vision, constipation, and slowness or difficulty passing urine.

Ventavis See ILOPROST.

Vicodin See ACETAMINOPHEN WITH NARCOTICS.

Vioxx See ROFECOXIB.

Voltaren See DICLOFENAC.

Zantac See RANITIDINE.

zoledronic acid (zoledronate) (Trade name: Reclast) A bisphosphonate that is injected intravenously to treat osteoporosis, Paget's disease, and high blood calcium concentrations in patients with some types of cancer.

Side effects Common: Itching, chills, joint and muscle aching, and flulike symptoms are common. Uncommon: palpitations, nausea, rash, edema, low blood calcium concentration. Rare: Osteonecrosis of the jaw occurs when an area of the jawbone such as a tooth socket does not heal and leaves the bone exposed; this can occur rarely in patients receiving bisphosphonates, usually intravenous bisphosphonates used to treat cancer. Inflammation of the eye and atrial fibrillation are rare.

zolpidem (Trade name: Ambien) A hypnotic (sleeping pill) used to improve sleep in conditions such as fibromyalgia. Zolpidem binds to the same receptors in the brain that drugs such as diazepam (trade name: Valium) and other benzodiazepines bind to causing sleepiness.

Side effects Common: Sleepiness, feeling hungover the next day, and headache. Uncommon: Dizziness, allergy, mental stimulation, confusion, and forgetfulness.

Zorprin See ASPIRIN.

Zostrix See CAPSAICIN.

Zyloprim See ALLOPURINOL.

APPENDIX II
COMMON LABORATORY AND DIAGNOSTIC TESTS

Interpreting Laboratory Tests

It is important to recognize that the *normal range* for most laboratory tests is not rigid but is statistically defined. The cutoff between *normal* and *abnormal* for many tests is calculated mathematically, usually so that the bottom 2.5 percent and the top 2.5 percent of people tested are designated abnormally high or low. This means that an abnormal laboratory result does not automatically imply that someone has a disease. In fact, for uncommon diseases such as SLE, there are many more healthy people with an abnormal ANA test than there are patients with SLE.

alkaline phosphatase Similar forms of this enzyme are found in liver and bone. An elevated alkaline phosphatase level is found in patients with liver disease, particularly conditions such as gallstones that obstruct the flow of bile. Any condition that causes bone to turn over more rapidly, for example a fracture or PAGET'S DISEASE, will also elevate the alkaline phosphatase level. If it is unclear if the source of an elevated alkaline phosphatase level is bone or liver, a bone-specific alkaline phosphatase can be measured.

Alkaline phosphatase is a standard component of most liver function tests (see LFTs), and an elevated alkaline phosphatase in an otherwise healthy patient is a common finding. This may be the first manifestation of Paget's disease.

angiogram See ARTERIOGRAPHY.

anticardiolipin antibody See ANTIPHOSPHOLIPID ANTIBODY.

anticentromere antibody Autoantibodies are antibodies directed against molecules within human cells, on the cell surface, or in blood or other fluids. Many of them give useful information because they are associated with particular diseases or manifestations of disease. The anticentromere antibody has been found in 60–95 percent of patients with CREST syndrome or limited SCLERODERMA. However, the test is not very specific, and it is also found in a small number of patients with diffuse scleroderma and other conditions.

anti-cyclic citrullinated protein (anti-CCP) This recently described antibody test has become widely used and has partially replaced RHEUMATOID FACTOR in the investigation of polyarthritis. The test has gone through a number of refinements and currently a third-generation test is being used by many laboratories. When used as an aid to the diagnosis of RHEUMATOID ARTHRITIS, it has been shown to be as sensitive but more specific than rheumatoid factor. In a review of many studies, anti-CCP was found to be 68 percent sensitive, i.e., 68 percent of people with rheumatoid arthritis had a positive test. This is similar to rheumatoid factor. However it had a 95 percent specificity, which means that 95 percent of people with a range of other diseases had a negative test. This is more specific than rheumatoid factor.

When patients first develop a polyarthritis, it is often not characteristic enough to make a definite diagnosis, and it is then termed undifferentiated arthritis. It would be useful if a blood test could assist in the diagnosis at this early stage, and although not perfect, anti-CCP is the best predictor of rheumatoid arthritis at present. In this situation, a positive test means the individual is about 25 times more likely to develop rheumatoid arthritis than any other form of arthritis and a negative test means rheumatoid arthritis is about 25 times less likely. Patients with a positive anti-CCP test have more severe disease with a greater chance of joint damage than those with a negative test regardless of their rheumatoid factor result. However they have a lower risk of getting rheumatoid manifestations other than arthritis (e.g., lungs or vasculitis) than those with positive rheumatoid factor. Very few patients with connective tissue diseases have a positive anti-CCP, but nearly half of those with PALINDROMIC RHEUMATISM do.

antineutrophil cytoplasmic antibody (ANCA)   In 1982, an autoantibody that reacted against the cytoplasm of neutrophils was discovered. Over the subsequent 20 years the clinical implications of antineutrophil cytoplasmic antibodies have become clearer. There are two common types of antibodies, C-ANCA and P-ANCA, named because of their different staining patterns. C-ANCAs stain the whole cytoplasm, whereas P-ANCAs cause staining around the nucleus (perinuclear). The most common target for C-ANCA is proteinase-3 (PR3), an enzyme found in neutrophils. P-ANCAs have several targets, but the antibodies associated with rheumatic diseases are often directed against an enzyme, myeloperoxidase (MPO).

A positive C-ANCA is found in 80–90 percent of patients with active WEGENER'S GRANULOMATOSIS. A positive test can sometimes occur in patients with lymphoma, cancer, infection, and other types of vasculitis such as CHURG-STRAUSS SYNDROME. A positive C-ANCA (PR3) in a patient with classical features of Wegener's granulomatosis confirms the diagnosis. Some clinicians believe that if the C-ANCA is positive, a biopsy to prove the diagnosis unequivocally is not required. The level of C-ANCA has been studied as a way to monitor disease activity and predict relapses in Wegener's granulomatosis. The results have been conflicting.

A positive P-ANCA test, particularly with MPO antibodies, is found in approximately 60 percent of patients with Churg-Strauss syndrome or microscopic polyangiitis. A positive P-ANCA is also found in patients with INFLAMMATORY BOWEL DISEASE.

antinuclear antibody (ANA)   Autoantibodies are antibodies directed against molecules within human cells, on the cell surface, or in blood or other fluids. Antinuclear antibodies are directed against components of the nucleus, the part of the cell that contains DNA, and can be detected by a blood test. The ANA test can have different patterns, depending on how the nuclei of the cells stain in the laboratory. These are homogeneous or diffuse, speckled, nucleolar, and peripheral or rim. They are not specific for any illness, but some patterns occur more frequently with certain conditions. For example, a homogenous pattern is more common in patients with SLE.

The ANA test is positive in many patients with connective tissue diseases, some infections, and a few normal people. It is commonly used as a screening test for the connective tissue diseases, but although it is very sensitive (i.e., most patients with a connective tissue disease will have a positive test), it is not very specific (i.e., many other people without disease will also have a positive test). A positive test therefore needs to be interpreted with caution in conjunction with the clinical findings.

Almost all patients (99 percent) with SYSTEMIC LUPUS ERYTHEMATOSUS have a positive ANA test, as do 90 percent of SCLERODERMA patients, over 80 percent of those with SJÖGREN'S SYNDROME, and less frequently those with DERMATOMYOSITIS AND POLYMYOSITIS (60 percent), RHEUMATOID ARTHRITIS (50 percent), WEGENER'S GRANULOMATOSIS and other forms of vasculitis, infections such as HEPATITIS C and PARVOVIRUS, and patients taking certain drugs, for example hydralazine. The ANA test is by definition always positive in DRUG-INDUCED LUPUS. Approximately 5 percent of the normal population will have a positive ANA test, although usually at a low level.

antiphospholipid antibody   Antiphospholipid antibodies were first recognized as causing a false-positive test result in early blood tests for syphilis. These antibodies are often asymptomatic and do not always result in complications. When complications such as thrombosis occur in patients who have persistently elevated levels of antiphospholipid antibodies, this is termed the ANTIPHOS-PHOLIPID ANTIBODY SYNDROME. Approximately 3 percent of healthy people have antiphospholipid antibodies, but these are often transiently positive and not associated with disease. Treatment with some drugs, for example chlorpromazine, quinidine, and hydralazine, can cause antiphospholipid antibodies. These drug-induced antiphospholipid antibodies, and those found in association with HIV infection, are seldom associated with thrombosis.

The term lupus anticoagulant was coined when it was recognized that some patients with SLE had antibodies that apparently acted as anticoagulants in the laboratory by prolonging tests of blood clotting such as the Russell viper venom time or activated partial thromboplastin time. However, the term lupus anticoagulant turned out to be a misnomer because the anticoagulant effects occur only in the test tube. These patients in fact have an increased risk of blood clots, rather than excessive bleeding that would be the expected if the antibody acted as an anticoagulant. It was also a misnomer because many people who had a positive lupus anticoagulant test did not have lupus. The antiphospholipid antibody syndrome and the lupus anticoagulant syndrome are now known to be related, and some patients who have an antiphospholipid antibody also have a positive lupus anticoagulant test. However, the overlap is not perfect, and sometimes one test is positive and the other negative. Both tests are associated with an increased risk of thrombosis.

Antiphospholipid antibodies bind to a substance called cardiolipin and are often measured as anticardiolipin antibodies, which may be of the IgG, IgM, or IgA subtype. The IgG and IgM subtypes are most often associated with the antiphospholipid antibody syndrome. The results from different laboratories have been standardized and are usually reported as GPL units for IgG and MPL units for IgM. Low levels (less than 20 GPL or MPL units) of anticardiolipin antibodies can occur with an acute infection and are not associated with blood clots.

arteriography (angiogram)   An X-ray that shows blood vessels. To obtain clear images of blood vessels, a dye that shows up on X-ray is injected into an artery. An arteriogram is usually performed when a blocked artery is suspected. For example, a coronary arteriogram is often performed in patients with angina to see which artery in the heart is blocked and how severe the obstruction is. Arteriograms of abdominal and renal blood vessels are often performed in patients with POLY-ARTERITIS NODOSA. To inject dye into the arteries of the heart, gut, or kidney, a thin plastic tube (catheter) is threaded up through the large artery in the groin (femoral artery). Newer techniques such as magnetic resonance angiography (MRA) are less invasive because the dye can be injected into a peripheral vein rather than directly into the artery.

arthrocentesis   See JOINT ASPIRATION.

biopsy   The process of removing a small sample of tissue to examine it under the microscope or culture it. A biopsy is usually performed when the diagnosis is not clear or when it is vital to make the correct diagnosis. A tissue sample can be obtained from virtually any organ. However, if the disease affects many organs, the biopsy is taken from the most accessible site that is likely to provide the answer. For example, a skin biopsy is much easier to obtain than a lung biopsy.

Biopsies are also performed to determine how severely a disease has affected an organ. For example, kidney biopsies are often performed in patients with SLE not to make the diagnosis of SLE but to provide information that helps determine what is the best treatment.

One of the problems with performing a biopsy is that only a small piece of tissue is obtained. This piece may not be representative of the whole and can therefore sometimes provide misleading information.

bone scan   See RADIONUCLIDE BONE SCAN.

CBC (complete blood count)   The CBC is a blood test that includes measurements of the white blood cell count, platelet count, and hemoglobin or hematocrit (also known as crit).

The white blood cells fight infection. Different types of white blood cell have different functions. Very important for fighting infection are the neutrophils, also known as polymorphs or sometimes just polys. If the neutrophil count is very low, less than 500 per mL (neutropenia), the risk of serious bacterial infection is high. The most common cause of severe neutropenia is cancer chemotherapy or bone marrow transplantation.

Eosinophils are another type of white blood cell. They are elevated in patients who have an allergy, vasculitis, cancer, a parasitic infection, or a rare disease such as EOSINOPHILIA MYALGIA SYNDROME.

Platelets are important for blood clotting. If a person has too few platelets (see THROMBOCYTOPENIA), wounds can ooze or bleed.

The hemoglobin and hematocrit are closely related and measure the number and health of red blood cells. Hemoglobin is the protein in red blood cells that enables them to carry oxygen, and the hematocrit measures the volume of red blood cells. If the hemoglobin and hematocrit are low, a person is anemic. There are many causes of anemia. It can be caused by genetic conditions, decreased availability of raw materials, and increased loss or destruction or decreased production of red blood cells.

Genetic causes of anemia   One of the most common genetic causes of anemia in the United States is SICKLE-CELL DISEASE. Other genetic causes of anemia are rare and usually diagnosed in childhood.

Decreased availability of raw materials   Iron, folate, vitamin B$_{12}$ and several other vitamins and minerals are needed for the body to make hemoglobin. If a person has a poor diet or has a gut problem such as CELIAC DISEASE and is unable to absorb one or more of these nutrients, anemia will result.

Increased loss or destruction of red blood cells   Any cause of bleeding will cause anemia when the loss exceeds the ability of the body to make new red blood cells. Slow invisible blood loss, usually from the bowel, is more common than the dramatic loss of large amounts of blood. Red blood cells are destroyed in the spleen, and any cause of an enlarged spleen can cause anemia.

Decreased production of red blood cells   Blood cells are manufactured in the bone marrow, and any disease or drug that affects the marrow can decrease production. Immunosuppressive drugs such as CYCLOPHOSPHAMIDE can cause anemia, as can any disease that invades the bone marrow directly.

One of the most common types of anemia is called anemia of chronic disease. This type of anemia occurs in patients with RA, SLE, and other chronic inflammatory or infective diseases. The mechanism is not clear, but it is thought that chronic disease affects the bone marrow's ability to make red blood cells.

All patients with poor kidney function are anemic. This is because the kidneys make a hormone called erythropoietin that stimulates red blood cell production. Low levels of this hormone also contribute to anemia of chronic disease.

A CBC is usually checked regularly if a person is taking medicines like METHOTREXATE, CYCLOPHOSPHAMIDE, AZATHIOPRINE, GOLD, PENICILLAMINE, and SULFASALAZINE because they can sometimes lower the white cell count or the platelet count. A CBC may also be checked occasionally if a patient is taking an NSAID regularly. This is useful to do this because if the patient suddenly becomes anemic, it may be an early warning of bleeding from a stomach problem caused by the NSAID.

creatine kinase (CK)   Also called creatine phosphokinase or CPK, this enzyme leaks out of injured or inflamed muscle into the bloodstream. CK leaks out of both heart and skeletal muscle and can be measured with a blood test. Elevated levels occur with a heart attack and with many illnesses that affect muscle. The types of CK released from heart and skeletal muscle can be distinguished by measuring subtypes.

Creatine kinase is elevated in approximately 95 percent of patients with DERMATOMYOSITIS AND POLYMYOSITIS. The test is useful both for helping make the diagnosis and for judging response to treatment. Any muscle injury, for example an intramuscular injection, will cause the CK to rise. Unless the injury is severe, these elevations are minor and transient. Massive increases in CK are seen in patients with severe muscle injury due to RHABDOMYOLYSIS.

creatinine   A person's kidney function can be checked by measuring the creatinine level in a blood test. It rises if the kidneys are not working well. A close watch is kept on the creatinine concentration if someone is taking a drug like CYCLO-SPORINE that can decrease kidney function. The creatinine level is usually checked from time to time in patients who are taking an NSAID, because occasionally NSAIDs can decrease kidney function. The body gets rid of METHOTREXATE in the urine, so the creatinine level is usually monitored from time to time in patients who are taking methotrexate. A more exact measure of kidney function is the creatinine clearance, but this requires that urine be collected for 24 hours, something that is difficult to achieve reliably.

CRP (C-reactive protein)   See ESR AND CRP.

cryoglobulins   These are abnormal immuno-globulins that precipitate when blood is cooled to less than 37°C and that redissolve on warming. The type of immunoglobulin found is used to classify the type of CRYOGLOBULINEMIA. Within each class of immunoglobulin, antibodies may be produced by one B lymphocyte and its progeny (monoclonal) or many different unrelated lymphocytes (polyclonal). In type I cryoglobulinemia, there is one monoclonal immunoglobulin, usually IgM. In type II, there is both polyclonal IgG and monoclonal IgM (usually RHEUMATOID FACTOR), and in type III, both polyclonal IgG and polyclonal IgM. Type I cryoglobulinemia is usually caused by Waldenstrom's macroglobulinemia, lymphoma, or multiple myeloma. Types II and III cryoglobulinemia, together referred to as mixed cryoglobulinemia, may be associated with chronic infection with hepatitis viruses B and C, lymphoma, chronic lymphocytic leukemia, myeloma, and autoimmune diseases such as rheumatoid arthritis, Sjögren's syndrome, systemic sclerosis, and SLE. In some patients there

is no apparent cause, and this is termed *essential* mixed cryoglobulinemia.

Special preparations are needed to draw a blood sample to test for the presence of cryoglobulins. Blood should be taken in prewarmed syringes and given directly to the laboratory. The amount of abnormal cryoglobulin protein is sometimes measured as a *cryocrit*—expressed as a percent. The cryocrit does not correlate very well with the severity of symptoms but is a guide to how a patient is responding to treatment.

CT (computed tomography)   CT, also called computerized axial tomography (CAT), is an X-ray test that provides computer-generated images of bones, organs, and soft tissues. MRI usually provides better images of muscles, tendons, and joints than CT, but CT is often preferred when disease of the chest, abdomen, or brain is suspected. Modern computer programs can manipulate the X-ray information obtained to provide three dimensional pictures of bones and joints that may help in planning difficult surgery. Sometimes in order to obtain better definition between normal and abnormal tissue, a contrast dye is injected. This dye can cause allergies, particularly if it contains iodine, and can also affect kidney function, particularly in patients who already have decreased kidney function. CT scans expose patients to a small amount of radiation and are therefore avoided during pregnancy.

DEXA (dual-energy X-ray absorptiometry)   A test used to measure bone density and thus to screen for and diagnose OSTEOPOROSIS. In addition to DEXA there are several other ways bone density can be measured. These include quantitative computerized tomography (QCT) and quantitative ultrasound, but DEXA is the most widely used technique. A DEXA test is similar to an X-ray in that it is painless and quick, but it exposes the patient to much less radiation than a standard X-ray. A DEXA report usually provides information about bone density at two sites where osteoporotic fractures are common, the spine and hip. The results are reported as a T score and a Z score.

The T score represents the relationship between a person's bone density and that of an average young adult. If the T score is -2 it means that the person's bone density is two standard deviations below average. All people are not all exactly the same, and a standard deviation is a statistical measurement of the normal spread for any measurement, be it weight, height, or bone density. For anything measured, height, weight, or bone density, only 2.5 percent of people will fall below two standard deviations from the average. The risk of fracture almost doubles for a decrease in bone density of one standard deviation (i.e., a T score of -1). A T score above -1 is regarded as normal; a score between -1 and -2.5 is called osteopenia (some loss of bone mass), and a T score of -2.5 and below is considered diagnostic for osteoporosis. A T score of -2.5 was selected, somewhat arbitrarily, as the bone density score at which the risk of fracture was increased enough for all patients to be treated for osteoporosis. Most techniques for measuring bone density report the result as both a T score and a Z score. The Z score represents how far a person's score is from the average of other people of the same age and sex. The Z score is not as useful as the T score for deciding when a person needs treatment. However, if a patient has osteoporosis with a low T score, for example -3.0, and a low Z score, for example below -1.5, this indicates that the osteoporosis is likely to be caused by factors other than simple aging.

Guidelines from the National Osteoporosis Foundation and other authoritative bodies generally recommend that a DEXA scan to screen for osteoporosis be performed in all postmenopausal women older than 65 years, in women who have had a fracture, and in patients who have risk factors for osteoporosis such as corticosteroid use.

DNA antibodies   Autoantibodies are antibodies directed against molecules within human cells, on the cell surface, or in blood or other fluids. The role autoantibodies play and their diagnostic value vary. Many are simply markers of disease, while others appear to play a direct role in causing disease. Anti-DNA antibodies give diagnostic and prognostic information and cause disease manifestations. Three types of anti-DNA antibodies can be detected. If not otherwise qualified, the term usually refers to anti-double-stranded DNA antibodies (also termed anti-dsDNA). The anti-dsDNA antibodies give diagnostic information in that if a patient has a positive test, he or she is very likely to have SLE. That is, a positive test is very specific for SLE (see Glossary for explanation of specificity). About 60 percent of SLE patients are anti-dsDNA positive. These patients are at an increased risk of developing kidney disease. It is likely that complexes of DNA and anti-DNA antibodies play an important role in causing glomerulonephritis, although other factors are involved.

The levels of anti-dsDNA antibodies fluctuate and tend to be higher when the disease is more active. They can be used to follow the course of the illness in individual patients. Attempts have been made to predict relapses of SLE by following the level of anti-DNA at regular levels. Although rising levels do seem to predict relapse in a few patients, this has not proved reliable enough for general use.

echocardiogram   An ultrasound test of the heart. The first test performed to assess the structure and function of the heart is usually ultrasound because it is noninvasive, does not expose patients to radiation, and is painless, quick, and relatively inexpensive. Ultrasound is an excellent tool for assessing the structure of all three layers of the heart—the pericardium (outer lining layer), myocardium (heart muscle), and endocardium (heart valves). It can diagnose a pericardial effusion (fluid in the pericardium), abnormalities of heart valves causing them to leak, and abnormal vegetations due to infection (see INFECTIVE ENDOCARDITIS) or other causes such as ANTIPHOSPHOLIPID ANTIBODY SYNDROME. An echocardiogram provides useful information about how well the heart is pumping, measured as an ejection fraction. It can also be used to estimate the pressure on the right side of the heart (see PULMONARY HYPERTENSION).

There are two types of echocardiogram, transthoracic and transesophageal. A transthoracic involves the operator moving a transducer (a flat probe about the size and shape of a pack of cigarettes) on the front of the chest. The patient is awake, and there is no pain or discomfort. A transesophageal echocardiogram is performed by passing a small probe down the esophagus (food pipe or gullet) and obtaining images from a position much closer to the heart. A transesophageal echocardiogram is similar to having an upper GI endoscopy performed. Having a tube passed through the mouth and down the esophagus is uncomfortable and makes patients gag and retch. Therefore the procedure is usually done under a sedative. The transesophageal method provides a much clearer view of the heart valves and is preferred if infective endocarditis is suspected.

electromyography (EMG) An electromyogram can be a useful test for confirming muscle disease and for showing which muscles are involved. It involves inserting a very fine needle into a muscle and measuring the electrical activity, both spontaneous and on attempted contraction of the muscle. In DERMATOMYOSITIS AND POLYMYOSITIS typical findings of muscle irritability and low-amplitude, disordered impulses are found in 90 percent of patients early in the disease but less frequently later or in severely affected muscles. The test can also be useful for diagnosing other problems that affect muscles such as MYASTHENIA GRAVIS. The height of the signal reflects the response, and in myasthenia after repeated electrical stimulation the response decreases in amplitude.

Nerve conduction studies are often performed at the same time as an EMG to check that a nerve problem is not the cause of muscle weakness. Nerve conduction studies are performed by placing two electrodes on the skin along a nerve. One electrode produces an impulse, felt as a small shock, and the other records the signal. The strength of the signal and the time it takes to travel between two points provides information about the function of the nerve. Nerve conduction studies are useful for diagnosing conditions such as CARPAL TUNNEL SYNDROME.

An EMG and nerve conduction studies cause some discomfort. The insertion of needles into muscles can be painful, and the small shocks administered to study nerves are uncomfortable.

ESR and CRP The ESR (erythrocyte sedimentation rate, also known as *sed rate*) and the CRP (C-reactive protein) are two different blood tests that are both nonspecific markers of inflammation. The ESR and CRP often, but not always, go up with infection or inflammation and come down with successful treatment.

The ESR is performed by taking a fresh blood sample and measuring how far the red blood cells settle in one hour in a thin, 100 mm long column of blood in a glass tube. When there is inflammation the proteins present in the blood help the red cells stick together and they sink faster. CRP is a protein that can be measured in stored blood and is therefore more convenient to measure.

The ESR and CRP can be elevated in any type of inflammatory arthritis, autoimmune disease, infection, or cancer. An elevated level therefore often indicates the presence of one of these conditions, but the finding is not specific and does not indicate a particular diagnosis. The symptoms of TEMPORAL ARTERITIS and POLYMYALGIA RHEUMATICA can be vague, and an elevated ESR is a useful clue to those diagnoses. A normal ESR does not exclude the presence of an inflammatory disorder. However, an elevated ESR in a patient in whom a noninflammatory diagnosis such as FIBROMYALGIA is suspected is a useful indicator that the diagnosis may be incorrect.

The ESR increases a little as people age and is also elevated by anemia, whatever the cause.

HLA-B27 The HLA-B antigens are molecules that human cells express on their surface. In Caucasian populations, approximately 10 percent of people have the HLA-B27 gene. The frequency of this gene varies widely in other populations. It almost never occurs in the Black African population living in the sub-Saharan desert but is found in as many as 50 percent of Haida Indians in Canada. The presence of HLA-B27 increases the likelihood of the diagnosis of ANKYLOSING SPONDYLITIS (AS) in patients of Caucasian extraction. Because approximately 10 percent of healthy people have the HLA-B27 gene, this test is of limited diagnostic value both in patients with features typical of AS and in those with poorly characterized back pain.

joint aspiration The fluid removed from within joints by inserting a needle into the joint and drawing the fluid into a syringe is frequently helpful in diagnosing the type of arthritis. Once fluid has been aspirated, therapeutic substances (usually corticosteroids) may be injected via the same needle. This is discussed under the various forms of arthritis where appropriate. Aspiration of synovial fluid is critical to the diagnosis and treatment of INFECTIVE ARTHRITIS, important in diagnosing GOUT and other types of arthritis caused by crystals (see ARTHRITIS), bleeding into the joint as in HEMOPHILIA or ligament rupture, and helpful in differentiating inflammatory from noninflammatory arthritis. Occasionally it may allow diagnosis of rare joint diseases such as AMYLOIDOSIS. Important aspects of the fluid include the following:

Appearance Normal synovial fluid is clear and either colorless or pale yellow. It is also very viscous. With increasing inflammation the number of white cells suspended in the fluid increases, typically making it turbid in REACTIVE ARTHRITIS, cloudy in gout, and like thin pus in established infection. Viscosity decreases with inflammation. This can be crudely estimated by dropping a thin string of fluid from the needlepoint. The longer the string of fluid is before breaking off, the greater the viscosity. Blood staining may be from the trauma of the needle but, if uniform, probably indicates bleeding within the joint. Bleeding into a joint may be found in trauma, destructive types of arthritis, especially gout or pseudogout (see CALCIUM PYROPHOSPHATE DIHYDRATE DEPOSITION DISEASE), hemophilia, anticoagulation, and PIGMENTED VILLONODULAR SYNOVITIS. Occasionally a fat layer is seen on top of the blood aspirated from a joint, and this indicates the presence of a fracture within the joint space. Small white bodies in the fluid (called rice bodies) are found in severe inflammatory arthritis, most frequently RHEUMATOID ARTHRITIS.

Cell count The number of cells counted under a microscope is used to separate effusions caused by inflammatory and noninflammatory types of arthritis. By convention, less than 2,000 cells per mL is noninflammatory and more is inflammatory. The type of cell present may also give information. For example, if more than 90 percent of the cells are polymorphonuclear cells, then gout or infective arthritis is very likely, while increasing numbers of lymphocytes are seen in rheumatoid arthritis.

Polarized light microscopy If arthritis caused by crystals is suspected, fresh fluid should be examined under a polarizing microscope. Urate crystals that cause gout can be confidently identified in this way, although other crystals frequently need further tests for positive identification. Although a relatively straightforward procedure, a good technique and fresh fluid are required for reliable results. Apart from the classical needle-shaped urate crystals found in gout, other crystals that may be seen include CPPD crystals, cholesterol crystals, corticosteroid crystals (from injections), or talc crystals from the injector's gloves.

Microbiology A Gram's stain is usually done immediately if infection is suspected. This can either show the type of organism present or sometimes positively identify it. The fluid is also cultured or put into a broth or onto an agar plate that is conducive to bacteria growing. This is inspected over the next five days to see if organisms are growing. These can then be further examined to identify them and predict which antibiotics will be most effective. For unusual organisms such as TUBERCULOSIS, special procedures and prolonged culture have to be undertaken. Therefore, if the diagnosis is not suspected, the organism will not be found.

Special stains These are occasionally performed for specific purposes such as looking for amyloid material (Congo red stain) or hydroxyapatite crystals (alizarin red).

La See SSA AND SSB.

LFTs (liver function tests) No single test provides a good measure of liver function and a panel of tests that measures different aspects of liver function, is used. Most LFT panels measure bilirubin, ALKALINE PHOSPHATASE, albumin, total protein, AST (aspartate aminotransferase), and ALT (alanine aminotransferase) concentrations.

Bilirubin levels are increased in patients who have an increased rate of breakdown of red blood cells (see SICKLE-CELL DISEASE) or obstruction to the flow of bile in the liver. Albumin is one of the proteins made in the liver. A low concentration can be due to inability of the liver to make enough, either because dietary intake of the raw materials needed is poor (i.e., malnutrition) or because of liver disease. Another cause of a low albumin concentration is excessive loss of protein in the urine, as occurs with nephrotic syndrome. The concentration of total protein also decreases in situations where albumin does. An elevated total protein concentration occurs when increased amounts of protein, usually immunoglobulins, are made. This can happen in many chronic inflammatory conditions such as RA and SLE (see IMMUNE RESPONSE) and a wide range of proteins is produced from different cell lines, sometimes called a polyclonal increase in protein. Certain malignancies of B cells such as multiple myeloma cause one type of cell to proliferate and produce a single protein, called a monoclonal gammopathy.

AST and ALT are enzymes that increase when liver cells are damaged. This can be caused by drugs, infection (see HEPATITIS), malignancy, and autoimmune disease. LFTs, particularly AST and ALT, are monitored regularly in everyone taking METHOTREXATE and LEFLUNOMIDE. This is done because by keeping a careful check on the LFTs the risk of serious liver problems is reduced. LFTs, are also checked occasionally in people taking NSAIDs, AZATHIOPRINE, and other medicines because they can cause liver problems.

lumbar puncture A test performed to obtain a sample of cerebrospinal fluid (CSF), the fluid that surrounds the brain and spinal cord. CSF is obtained by inserting a needle, usually in the area of the lower back, into the space around the spinal cord and draining a few teaspoonfuls of fluid. CSF is usually crystal clear and has very few cells and a low protein content. Inflammation caused by VASCULITIS or cancer, for example, or infection caused by meningitis can raise the protein and cell content of CSF. The organism causing meningitis can often be isolated from the CSF in patients with meningitis.

lupus anticoagulant See ANTIPHOSPHOLIPID ANTIBODY.

magnetic resonance imaging (MRI) MRI even more than CT imaging has revolutionized the way in which diseases and structural abnormalities are assessed and diagnosed. The implications for rheumatic diseases and orthopedic conditions have been profound. With the use of MRI, it is now possible to obtain a three-dimensional image of almost any part of the body down to the detail of the shape and size of blood vessels. The initial information is obtained by getting images of thin, transverse slices through the area of interest. Once this information has been obtained it can be manipulated by the computer software to give considerable additional information and many different views. Top of the line machines can show real-time movement. Manipulation of the signal can give information about the qualities of the tissues being scanned, for example whether or not they are inflamed.

The phenomenon of nuclear magnetism is ingeniously exploited to provide this wealth of information. Atoms with an uneven number of protons or neutrons in their nuclei have a magnetic moment. Hydrogen, present in water and fat, is the most important atom in MRI. The magnetic moments are normally directed randomly. These moments are aligned by applying a magnetic field across the area of interest. This alignment is then disturbed by a radio-frequency pulse of known frequency, duration, and angle. After this radio-frequency pulse the moments (usually called spins) will realign with the magnetic field. This realignment is termed relaxation and will be accompanied by the emission of radio-frequency energy. An antenna coil is used to pick up these emissions. Hundreds of these projections are acquired for each slice. The computer then reconstructs this information into a visible image using complex formulas.

MRI provides excellent images of soft tissues and is therefore useful in studying muscles, tendons, ligaments, joints, and other soft tissues such as brain. Although not demonstrating bone structure as well as CT scanning, it will show inflammatory bone lesions better. MRI is not generally used to image lungs or bowel, but virtually any other body part may be imaged. In most situations excellent contrast can be achieved without using any contrast material (dye), thus avoiding injections and possible reactions. When contrast material is required, such as when examining tumors, gadolinium is used. The ability to show increased water content of tissues (and therefore likely inflammation) is invaluable in certain situations in rheumatic diseases. There is no radiation and MRI has been used safely in pregnancy, although it is still avoided in this situation unless absolutely necessary.

Gadolinium-based dyes have generally been considered very safe. However in recent years, it has become apparent that a small number of patients, especially those with poor kidney function, get an unusual reaction called nephrogenic systemic fibrosis. This condition has similarities to systemic sclerosis. For this reason, the less stable of the gadolinium dyes have been banned in Europe and Japan, and many units now routinely measure the creatinine level in at-risk patients before doing an MRI scan with contrast. Scans without contrast are of course safe. Patients with poor kidney function can still undergo a scan with contrast, but there must be a very important reason for using the dye and the patient must understand the risk.

Because time is needed to acquire the information to build up images, movement by the patient is a common cause of poor images. Very powerful magnets are used, and therefore all metal objects need to be removed both for patient safety and to prevent interference with the images. Older metal surgical clips may contraindicate MRI. Modern clips and heart valve prostheses can usually be scanned without danger, although this should be checked in each case. Pacemakers will be affected by the magnetic field and special precautions need to be taken. The metal in orthopedic implants does not usually cause a problem.

nailfold microscopy This test examines the loops of capillaries at the base of the nail using a powerful magnifying glass or an ophthalmoscope. Abnormal loops of capillaries occur in patients with connective tissue diseases such as scleroderma and SLE. If there is also loss of capillaries, sometimes termed *capillary dropout*, then the patient is more likely to have scleroderma. Most patients with primary RAYNAUD'S PHENOMENON do not develop an auto-

immune disease, but a few do, and abnormal findings on nailfold microscopy are more common in those patients.

radionuclide bone scan This imaging technique involves injecting a radioactive substance into the patient's vein and then passing a gamma camera over the patient, sometimes at a number of time points, to see where the substance has localized. It has been known since the 1920s that some radioactive substances would localize in bone if injected intravenously. Many of the early substances, however, were either unstable or too toxic. Technetium-99m-labeled phosphates were introduced in the 1970s and refined over the next few years into the technetium-labeled diphosphonates, MDP and HDP, used today. The major factors that determine how much technetium is taken up by bone are blood flow through the bone and osteoblastic activity (new bone formation). Areas where there is increased blood flow or osteoblastic activity will show up as *hot spots*. Further information can be gained by taking repeated images to look at the movement of the tracer over time. These radioactive agents are fairly weak, very stable, and almost completely excreted in four hours.

Technetium scans are extremely sensitive in showing any bony injury or lesion from fractures to tumors and from conditions such as PAGET'S DISEASE and osteomyelitis. It also shows both osteoarthritis and inflammatory arthritis (see ARTHRITIS). However, the scans lack the detail of CT or MRI scans. While being very sensitive for abnormalities, radionuclide bone scans do not always allow the nature of the abnormality to be determined. They are particularly useful for demonstrating STRESS FRACTURES and insufficiency fractures in OSTEOPOROSIS, where X-rays are frequently normal in the early stages. They are ideal for looking for metastatic bony deposits in patients with cancer since the whole body is easily scanned in one procedure. They will demonstrate AVASCULAR NECROSIS much earlier than X-rays although not earlier than MRI. They are also used to localize areas of deep or diffuse pain that can then be examined in more detail with MRI or CT scanning.

rheumatoid factor   Rheumatoid factor is an antibody directed against immunoglobulin. The rheumatoid factor measured by most laboratories is an IgM antibody directed against IgG. Rheumatoid factor is usually measured to aid the diagnosis of RA. The frequency of a positive rheumatoid factor test in patients with RA is approximately 70 percent but varies in different studies. A positive rheumatoid factor test can also occur in patients with SLE (approximately 25 percent), other autoimmune diseases, and infections such as INFECTIVE ENDOCARDITIS and HEPATITIS, cancer, and in approximately 5–10 percent of healthy people. This means that it is not a good screening test and that a positive test is not diagnostic for RA. However, it is useful, particularly early in the disease, because patients with early RA who have a positive rheumatoid factor will tend to develop more severe disease. A positive test may therefore help in the decision about how aggressively to treat a patient. Patients who have complications of rheumatoid arthritis affecting organs other than the joints, for example rheumatoid nodules or lung or eye disease, almost always have a positive test.

The amount of rheumatoid factor present can be measured in different ways but is often expressed as a titer, a measure of how much a patient's serum can be diluted and the test still be positive (for example 1:40 or 1:640). A high titer, for example 1:640, is much more likely to occur in RA and is rare in healthy people. Changes in the titer of rheumatoid factor are not useful for monitoring the course of RA, and there is no reason to perform the test repeatedly.

Ro   See SSA AND SSB.

Scl-70   Approximately 50 percent of patients with diffuse SCLERODERMA develop antibodies against a protein called topoisomerase-I (also called Scl-70). This test is positive is less than 5 percent of patients with other autoimmune diseases and is seldom positive in healthy people. Therefore, a negative Scl-70 test does not exclude the diagnosis of diffuse scleroderma, but a positive test suggests that it is the likely diagnosis.

SSA and SSB   These antibodies, also termed anti-Ro (SSA for SJÖGREN'S SYNDROME A) and anti-La (SSB for Sjögren's syndrome B) are antinuclear antibodies found in patients with primary Sjögren's syndrome (75 percent), SLE (50 percent), and other autoimmune diseases. Anti-Ro antibodies occur more often than anti-La, and most patients with anti-La antibodies also have anti-Ro. Rarely patients with SLE have a negative ANA test and a positive test for anti-Ro antibodies. Women with anti-Ro/SSA and anti-La/SSB antibodies have an increased chance of delivering children with NEONATAL LUPUS and an abnormal heart rhythm called congenital heart block. In patients with SLE, the presence of anti-SSA and anti-SSB antibodies is associated with increased photosensitivity and a rash known as subacute cutaneous lupus. The test is most often performed in pregnant women with SLE, women who have given birth to a child with heart block, and patients in whom the diagnosis of primary Sjögren's syndrome is suspected.

synovial fluid analysis   See JOINT ASPIRATION.

ultrasound   At the simplest level, ultrasound consists of placing a probe against the patient's skin. The probe then emits a pulse of sound and receives and records its echo or echoes. Sound waves bounce off tissue interfaces (e.g., the interface between fat and tendon) particularly well and will also reflect the homogeneity (sameness) of a tissue. Sound waves do not pass easily through solid material such as bone, and therefore, gallstones and kidney stones will cast an *echo-free shadow* behind them. A special type of ultrasound has been developed to measure the density of bones. Many developments have occurred in ultrasound over the past three decades, and it is now a very sophisticated method of imaging the body. Of all forms of imaging, ultrasound is most dependent on the ultrasonographer. In addition to interpreting the images obtained the ultrasonographer has to use the probe to interrogate the area of interest.

Advantages of ultrasound compared with other musculoskeletal imaging techniques are that it is quick, widely available, noninvasive, and fairly cheap. It is also very effective when used as a guide to needle placement when taking a biopsy or aspirating a collection of fluid. In musculoskeletal practice, ultrasound is most frequently used to assess tendons. It demonstrates tendinitis, tears, and complete rupture very accurately. At the shoulder, for example, it can also show that the ROTATOR CUFF tendons are bunching up as the arm is lifted, thus confirming mechanical impingement. In many countries it has become the imaging modality of choice at the shoulder. Ultrasound is extremely effective at demonstrating BURSITIS from any cause. Increasingly ultrasound is being used to demonstrate joint effusions, and a few rheumatologists even have portable machines in their offices to extend their examination of joints. Ultrasound is particularly helpful in demonstrating effusions in joints that are difficult to assess clinically such as shoulders, hips, and wrists. If, for example, septic arthritis were suspected in a hip joint, the absence of an effusion on ultrasound would virtually exclude that diagnosis. Although not good at imaging, bone ultrasound can show signs very suggestive of OSTEOMYELITIS.

uric acid   The uric acid level in a blood test is often elevated in patients with GOUT but is often mistakenly thought to be a diagnostic test for gout. The blood urate levels are not very useful in making the diagnosis during an acute attack of gout. Many people with mildly raised urate levels will never develop gout, and 40 percent of people with acute gout will have a normal level during the attack. Most of this second group will, however, have a raised uric acid level later when the attack has settled. The best way to diagnose gout is to identify uric acid crystals in synovial fluid (see JOINT ASPIRATION).

urinalysis   A urinalysis is a urine test to detect blood, glucose (sugar), and protein, all of which should be negative. Urine is usually tested using a dipstick with small squares that change color in the presence of blood, sugar, or protein. Some dipsticks also detect nitrite and leukocyte ester-ase—substances that indicate the presence of a urinary infection. If the test for blood or protein is positive, the urine is examined under a microscope and further tests performed to identify the cause. A positive test for glucose usually indicates a diagnosis of DIABETES MELLITUS. However, some healthy people without diabetes have an abnormally low threshold for spilling glucose into the urine.

There are many causes of an abnormal urinalysis, but the most common ones are menstrual blood, infections of the bladder and urinary tract, drugs, kidney stones, tumors, and autoimmune diseases affecting the kidney. Drugs such as cyclophosphamide can damage the bladder and cause blood in the urine, and gold and penicillamine can cause glomerulonephritis so that protein leaks into the urine.

X-rays   Also known as radiography, X-ray images are often used to diagnose bone and chest diseases. X-rays, a type of radiation, pass through the body, but different tissues absorb them differently. Tissues that absorb well, such as bone appear white on the image. Those that do not absorb much, such as air, appear black. X-rays are very useful for diagnosing abnormalities of bones and joints but not very useful for lesions in soft tissues such as muscles. X-rays are used to help with the diagnosis and monitoring of many rheumatic diseases. The typical X-ray changes of RHEUMATOID ARTHRITIS and GOUT for example, differ, and this can be very useful for making the correct diagnosis. Many patients with early arthritis have normal X-rays because at this stage most of the damage occurs in the cartilage, a tissue that does not show up well on X-rays other than as space between bones. There is a lot of research trying to use MRI, which provides much more detailed images of soft tissues such as cartilage, to diagnose early arthritis and measure its response to treatment. The advantages of X-rays are that the test is quick, relatively cheap, widely available, and easy to perform. The disadvantages are that it exposes patients to a small dose of radiation, and is therefore avoided in pregnant women, and that it does not provide much detail about soft tissues.

APPENDIX III
USEFUL ARTHRITIS-RELATED WEB SITES

Only a few resources are listed. An extensive guide is available on the Arthritis Foundation's Web site. Click on "disease center" and there, alphabetically, are all the rheumatic diseases with helpful links and addresses. Remember, medical information on the Internet is not always accurate and readers should evaluate information critically.

General Arthritis or Health-Related Sites

The American College of Rheumatology (ACR)
http://www.rheumatology.org/

This Web site is mainly for health professionals but there is a patient information page. The ACR does not answer medical questions about specific treatments, diagnoses, or symptoms. Fact Sheets: *What Is a Rheumatologist?*, *The Role of the Advanced Practice Nurse*, *The Role of the Registered Nurse*, *The Role of the Occupational Therapist*, *The Role of the Physical Therapist*, *The Role of the Social Worker*, *The Role of Interdisciplinary Team Management*, *The Role of the Psychologist*, and *The Role of the Rheumatologist* are available online as is disease-specific information about most common rheumatic conditions and links to useful sites including organizations in countries outside the United States.

The Arthritis Foundation
http://www.arthritis.org/

This site is an outstanding resource for patients with arthritis and their families. The organization provides books and brochures for patients with arthritis, referrals to rheumatologists in an area, and publishes a magazine, *Arthritis Today*. Call toll-free 800-283-7800 or go to the Web site.

The Web site has extensive information that is clearly written about all aspects of arthritis including surgery and drugs. The popular *Drug and Supplement Guides* are available. Other areas covered include financial planning, exercise, tips for living with arthritis, travel, marriage and dating, alternative therapies, and specific rheumatic diseases.

MedicineNet
http://www.medterms.com/script/main/hp.asp

This is a comprehensive Web site that has a medical dictionary, descriptions of arthritis-related and other illnesses, as well as information about medications and laboratory tests.

MedlinePlus Health Information
http://medlineplus.gov/

This Web site provides an excellent resource. It is produced by the National Library of Medicine and has information from the National Institutes of Health and other sources covering many illnesses. There are also directories of hospitals and physicians, a medical encyclopedia and dictionaries, health information in Spanish, as well as information about drugs and links to clinical trials. There is no advertising and the site does not endorse any products. There is a link to MEDLINE, the computerized, searchable database of medical literature.

National Institute of Arthritis and Musculo-skeletal and Skin Diseases
http://www.niams.nih.gov/index.htm

This site provides unbiased health information regarding a range of musculoskeletal illnesses.

New York Online Access to Health (NOAH)
http://www.noah-health.org/english/illness/
    arthritis/

This site provides information on a very large number of topics aimed at patients. You will probably have to spend some time finding exactly what you need.

Well Aware
http://www.well-aware.co.uk

A Web site based in the United Kingdom that provides information about medical conditions, drugs, and complementary therapies. The site is comprehensive and the information is concise and written in plain English. You have to log in, but it is free. The site does have advertising.

Yahoo! Health
http://health.yahoo.com/

This site has three major subdivisions: an encyclopedia, a drug index, and health centers. The arthritis and pain health center has descriptions of rheumatic illnesses and links that provide information about laboratory tests.

Resource Sites Devoted to Specific Topics

Alexander Technique
The Alexander Technique
http://www.life.uiuc.edu/jeff/alextech.html

The American Society for the Alexander Technique
http://www.alexandertech.org

Ankylosing Spondylitis
Spondylitis Association of America
http://www.spondylitis.org

Behçet's Disease
Behçet's Organization Worldwide
http://www.behcets.org

Chiropractic Medicine
The American Chiropractic Association
http://www.amerchiro.org

Dietary Supplements
Food and Drug Administration Center for Food
    Safety and Applied Nutrition
http://www.cfsan.fda.gov/~dms/ds-savvy.html

MedlinePlus Health Information Vitamin and Mineral Supplements
http://www.nlm.nih.gov/medlineplus/vitaminand
    mineralsupplements.html

National Center for Complementary and Alternative Medicine
http://www.nccam.nih.gov/

Eosinophilia Myalgia Syndrome
National Eosinophilia Myalgia Syndrome Network
http://www.nemsn.org/

Fibromyalgia
American Fibromyalgia Syndrome Association
http://www.afsafund.org/

Fibromyalgia Network
http://www.fmnetnews.com/

FRAX
WHO fracture risk analysis
http://www.shef.ac.uk/FRAX/

Gulf War Syndrome
Office of the Special Assistant for Gulf War Illnesses
http://www.gulflink.osd.mil/

Hypermobility
The Hypermobility Syndrome Association (United
    Kingdom)
http://www.hypermobility.org/

Inflammatory Bowel Disease
Crohn's & Colitis Foundation of America
http://www.ccfa.org/

Juvenile Rheumatoid Arthritis
MedlinePlus Health Information Juvenile Rheumatoid Arthritis
http://www.nlm.nih.gov/medlineplus/
    juvenilerheumatoidarthritis.html

The Nemours Foundation
http://kidshealth.org/kid/health_problems/bone/
    juv_rheum_arthritis.html

Occupational Therapy
American Occupational Therapy Association
http://www.aota.org/index.asp

Osteoporosis
National Osteoporosis Foundation
http://www.nof.org/

Paget's Disease
The Paget Foundation
http://www.paget.org/

Pain
American Pain Foundation
http://www.painfoundation.org/

American Pain Society
http://www.fmnetnews.com/

Podiatry
American Podiatric Medical Association
http://www.apma.org/

Podiatry Encyclopedia
http://www.curtin.edu.
au/curtin/dept/physio/podiatry/encyclopedia/

Podiatry Forum
http://www.podiatrychannel.com/

Polymyositis
Myositis Association of America
http://www.myositis.org/

Pulmonary Hypertension
Pulmonary Hypertension Association
http://www.phassociation.org/

Psoriatic Arthritis
National Psoriasis Foundation
http://www.psoriasis.org/

Raynaud's Phenomenon
Raynaud's Association
http://www.raynauds.org/

Reflex Sympathetic Dystrophy
Reflex Sympathetic Dystrophy Syndrome Association of America
http://www.rsds.org/

Rheumatoid Arthritis
Rheumatoid Arthritis Information Network
http://www.healthtalk.com/rain/

Sarcoidosis
National Sarcoidosis Resource Center
http://www.nsrc-global.net/

Scleroderma
Scleroderma Foundation
http://www.scleroderma.org/

Sjögren's Syndrome
Sjögren's Syndrome Foundation
http://www.sjogrens.org

Systemic Lupus Erythematosus
Lupus Foundation of America
http://www.lupus.org/

Wegener's Granulomatosis
Wegener's Granulomatosis Support Group
http://www.wgsg.org/

GLOSSARY

Common abbreviations and medical terms.

ACR   American College of Rheumatology. An organization representing rheumatologists in the United States to promote research, education, and training of professionals and patients (see Appendix III for Web site address).

acromioclavicular joint   A joint in front of the shoulder between the clavicle (collarbone) and acromion.

acromion (acromion process)   The upper and outermost part of the scapula (shoulder blade) that lies above the shoulder joint socket and protects it.

acute   An event that happens suddenly and usually lasts only a short time. The opposite of acute is chronic.

adhesion molecules   Intercellular adhesion molecule (ICAM) and vascular cell adhesion molecule (VCAM) are examples of receptors on cells that allow them to attach to each other, an important initial part of the immune response.

allele   Alternative variants of a gene that can occur at a particular locus.

alternative medicine (complementary medicine)   Unconventional medicines or treatments that are not part of mainstream Western medicine. Examples include ACUPUNCTURE, BEE VENOM, COPPER BRACELET, MAGNETS, HOMEOPATHY, herbal supplements, and the ALEXANDER TECHNIQUE.

ANA   Antinuclear antibody test (see Appendix II).

analgesic   Pain reliever.

anemia   A low level of hemoglobin in the blood. Hemoglobin is the protein in red cells that carries oxygen. Severe anemia can cause dizziness, fatigue, and lack of energy. Very severe anemia can cause heart failure (see CBC in Appendix II).

angioedema   Swelling of the face, tongue, or throat, usually caused by an allergic reaction, angiotensin-converting enzyme (ACE) inhibitors (a class of drugs used to lower blood pressure), or rarely by hereditary or acquired abnormalities of the complement cascade (see COMPLEMENT). Angioedema occurs more often in patients with SLE or other autoimmune diseases.

angiogram   An X-ray of blood vessels (see ARTERIOGRAPHY in Appendix II).

antibody   Proteins made by white blood cells called lymphocytes. Antibodies can bind to markers, called antigens, and neutralize or destroy cells or microorganisms that the immune system recognizes as foreign or harmful.

anti-CCP antibodies   Antibodies to cyclic citrullinated peptides that are effective in diagnosing rheumatoid arthritis.

anticoagulant   A substance that prevents blood from clotting. Two drugs often used for this purpose are heparin and warfarin.

antigen   The target that an antibody recognizes and to which it binds. Antigens bind to specific receptors on T cells and B lymphocytes and activate them.

arteriogram   An X-ray of blood vessels (see ARTERIOGRAPHY in Appendix II).

arthralgia   Painful joints without swelling or warmth.

arthritis   Pain in a joint with signs of inflammation such as swelling, warmth, and decreased movement. There are many causes of arthritis (see ARTHRITIS).

AS   ANKYLOSING SPONDYLITIS.

aspiration   Removing fluid, usually from a joint, by drawing it out through a needle attached to a syringe.

autoimmune disease   A condition in which the immune system, for reasons that are poorly understood, makes antibodies against its own cells, and this inappropriate immune response damages the body.

biopsy   The removal of a small sample of tissue, for example, skin, kidney, or lung, so that it can be examined by a histopathologist to aid diagnosis or predict prognosis more accurately (see Appendix II).

bone marrow suppression   Bone marrow cells, precursors of the formed elements of blood, are sensitive to many immunosuppressive and anticancer drugs. Bone marrow suppression results in a decrease in the cellular components of blood—platelets, leukocytes (white blood cells), and erythrocytes (red blood cells).

bone spur   A small outgrowth of new bone usually caused by osteoarthritis. Most bone spurs do not cause symptoms and are not important. However, if new bone is formed by the vertebrae and narrows a canal that carries a nerve, it can cause pressure on the nerve and pain and numbness in parts of the body served by that nerve.

Bouchard's nodes   Bony nodules over the proximal interphalangeal (PIP) joints of the fingers caused by osteoarthritis. The nodules can be painful if they are bumped, and they decrease the flexibility of the PIP joint. No effective treatment is available.

bursas   Small sacs lined with synovial cells that are found close to joints and tendons. Their function is to facilitate smooth movement of tissues and to act as shock absorbers. Bursas can become inflamed (see BURSITIS).

camptodactyly   An inherited condition in which the little finger slowly becomes more and more bent at the PIP. It affects girls twice as often as boys and starts within the first 10 years of life. Both hands are affected in 70 percent of patients. It must be distinguished from DUPUYTREN'S CONTRACTURE, and no treatment is required.

cardiomyopathy   Degeneration of heart muscle that can be caused by viral infection, drugs, some autoimmune diseases, and other muscle or heart diseases.

CBC   Complete blood count (see Appendix II).

chronic   A condition that lasts for a long time, usually years. The opposite of chronic is acute.

CK   Creatine kinase (see Appendix II).

CNS   Central nervous system.

copper bracelet   Copper worn in contact with the skin, either as a bracelet or a disc, is an alternative remedy that many people use to treat arthritis. It appears to be safe, but there is no good evidence showing that it is effective.

COX   Cyclooxygenase, an enzyme regulating the formation of prostaglandins (see CYCLOOXYGENASE).

CPK   Creatine phosphokinase (see CREATINE KINASE in Appendix II).

CRP   C-reactive protein (see Appendix II).

CT   Computed tomography (see Appendix II).

deep-vein thrombosis (DVT)   Formation of a blood clot in a deep vein, most often in the leg. The clot can break off and eventually lodge in a blood vessel in the lung—known as a pulmonary embolus. Predisposing factors for development of a DVT are immobilization, for example bed rest, and an increased propensity for blood to clot—a hypercoagulable state—for example the ANTIPHOSPHOLIPID ANTIBODY SYNDROME.

DEXA   Dual-energy X-Ray absorptiometry (see Appendix II).

DIP   See distal interphalangeal.

distal interphalangeal (DIP)   The joints closest to the ends of the fingers.

DJD   Degenerative joint disease—another term for OSTEOARTHRITIS.

DVT   See deep-vein thrombosis.

echocardiography   Also known as an *echo*. An ultrasound of the heart used to obtain images of cardiac chambers and valves and to estimate heart muscle function and intracardiac pressures (see Appendix II).

edema   Accumulation of fluid in the soft tissues.

effusion   Swelling of a joint caused by an increase in the amount of synovial fluid present.

ELISA   Enzyme-linked immunosorbent assay.

enthesopathy   Inflammation at the point where tendons join bone (enthesis). This is a common symptom of ANKYLOSING SPONDYLITIS, REITER'S SYNDROME, and the SPONDYLOARTHROPATHIES.

eosinophil   A type of white blood cell usually present in low numbers. An increase in the numbers of eosinophils is called eosinophilia and is typically caused by asthma, other allergic reactions, drugs, infection with intestinal parasites, cancer, or VASCU-LITIS.

ESR Erythrocyte sedimentation rate, also known as *sed rate*. A nonspecific blood test that measures inflammation (see ESR in Appendix II).

fascia Deep connective tissue made up mostly of collagen. Fascia lies below the skin, forming part of the subcutaneous tissues, and in deeper tissues separates muscles and tissue planes.

fasciitis Inflammation of the fascia.

FDA Food and Drug Administration, a body of the U.S. government that regulates food and drugs.

generic Drugs have two names, a brand name that the manufacturer chooses for marketing and a generic name that represents the chemical constituent of the drug. For example, acetaminophen is the generic name of a well-known analgesic. Several different brands (Tylenol, Panadol, and others) all contain the identical drug—acetaminophen.

GI Gastrointestinal as in *GI side effects*, pertaining nonspecifically to any or all of the gut from mouth to anus.

glomerulonephritis Inflammation of the glomeruli, areas of the kidney where blood is filtered to form urine.

hematuria Blood in the urine. This may be *frank hematuria*, which is visible to the naked eye, or *microscopic hematuria*, which is detected by dipstick testing or microscopy.

hemoglobin The protein in red blood cells that binds and transports oxygen.

hemolysis Breakdown of red blood cells.

hepatitis Inflammation of the liver resulting in elevated blood levels of alanine aminotransferase (ALT) and aspartate aminotransferase (AST) enzymes. Hepatitis can be acute and may resolve completely or may be chronic and can lead to liver scarring or cirrhosis. There are many causes of hepatitis, the commonest being viral infection, drugs, alcohol, and autoimmune disease.

HLA Human leukocyte antigen—molecules on the surface of cells that help present antigen to T cell.

hyperpigmentation Darkening of the skin.

hypertension High blood pressure.

idiopathic A condition in which the cause is not known.

idiosyncratic Something that occurs unpredictably in some individuals only. For example, hepatitis can be an idiosyncratic side effect of a drug. This means that only a few people will develop hepatitis when taking that drug, and who these people are cannot be predicted.

immunocompromised A situation in which a person's immune system is not able to respond adequately to organisms and therefore increases the risk of infection. Immunosuppression is a frequent cause.

immunosuppression Suppression of the immune system. This can occur as a result of uncommon genetic conditions that impair antibody formation or other components of the IMMUNE RESPONSE. More often immunosuppression is induced by the administration of drugs that suppress components of the immune system. Immunosuppression is often part of the therapy for autoimmune diseases. Because immunological response to foreign organisms is also impaired, such therapy increases the risks of infection. Therefore immunosuppressive treatment is always a balance between achieving adequate suppression to control the disease and avoiding too much that will allow infections to occur.

incidence The number of people in a population that are diagnosed with a condition for the first time within a given period of time. Incidence is usually expressed as the number diagnosed per 1,000 or 100,000 population per year.

infarct Death of tissue when the blood supply is cut off or is inadequate, often because of a clot in a blood vessel (artery). Examples are stroke (cerebral infarct) and heart attack (myocardial infarct).

inflammation A tissue response resulting from infection, trauma, autoimmune disease and many other noxious stimuli. Inflammation is characterized by tissue warmth, redness, swelling, and pain.

intra-articular In or into a joint, as in an *intra-articular injection*.

lesion An abnormality, usually one than can be seen directly or by using an imaging technique.

leukopenia   Low total white blood cell count. A decrease in isolated cell populations may occur, for example lymphopenia and neutropenia.

LFTs   Liver function tests (see Appendix II).

ligament   Dense fibrous tissue that connects bones.

livedo reticularis   A reddish, purple lacy rash found on the insides of the arms and legs that is associated with antiphospholipid antibody syndrome and cholesterol emboli syndrome.

locus   The position on a chromosome where a particular gene is found.

lymphocyte   A type of white blood cell that contributes to the immune response. T lymphocytes (also called T cells) attack cells directly and control other elements of the immune response, and B lymphocytes (also called B cells) produce antibodies.

macrophage   A type of cell, derived from monocytes circulating in the blood system, found in tissues and that ingests or engulfs foreign substances. It also secretes many CYTOKINES that influence other aspects of the immune response.

MCP   See metacarpophalangeal.

metacarpophalangeal (MCP)   The joints forming the first row of knuckles closest to the wrist.

metatarsophalangeal (MTP)   The joints at the base of the toes where they join the raylike bones of the foot (metatarsals).

monarthritis   Arthritis affecting one joint.

monocyte   A white blood cell formed in the bone marrow that enters the bloodstream and migrates into tissues, where it becomes a macrophage.

morbidity   The consequences of an illness.

MRI   Magnetic resonance imaging (see Appendix II).

MTP   See metatarsophalangeal.

myalgia   Muscle pain or achiness.

myopathy   Weakness and degeneration of muscle without associated inflammation.

myositis   Inflammation in a muscle, often associated with an increase in the concentrations of muscle enzymes measured in a blood test.

narcotics   Strong analgesics that are related to morphine and are potentially addictive.

nephrotic syndrome   A syndrome caused by a heavy leak of protein into the urine. The features are heavy proteinuria, edema affecting the legs and sometimes the face, and a low concentration of protein in the blood. Many serious kidney problems, for example glomerulonephritis, can cause nephrotic syndrome.

neuropathy   Nerve damage that may alter sensation or movement in an organ or limb.

neutrophil   A type of white blood cell that directly ingests bacteria, antigens, or debris through the process of phagocytosis. Neutrophils circulate and move rapidly to areas of infection or injury. They are the major cell type found in pus. They are also known as segmented cells (segs), polymorphonuclear leukocytes (polys or PMNs), or granulocytes.

NSAID   Nonsteroidal anti-inflammatory drug.

OA   Osteoarthritis.

osteophyte   A small spur of new bone close to a joint. Osteophytes are typically found in OSTEOAR-THRITIS.

pauciarticular arthritis   Arthritis affecting a few joints, usually four or less.

pericarditis   Inflammation of the pericardium, a membranous sac that encloses the heart.

peritonitis   Inflammation of the peritoneum, the thin tissuelike membrane that lines the abdominal cavity.

photosensitivity   Increased skin sensitivity to sunlight and other sources of ultraviolet light.

PIP   See proximal interphalangeal.

placebo   A Latin word meaning *I shall please.* Used to describe a drug or treatment that is considered to be inactive. A placebo is often used to treat one group of patients in a clinical trial to see if a new treatment is more effective.

pleural effusion   A collection of fluid in the space between two layers of pleura, thin membranes that encase the lungs. Fluid with a low protein content is a transudate and collects in conditions associated with fluid overload such as heart failure. Fluid with a high protein content is called an exudate and collects in inflammatory conditions such as rheumatoid arthritis affecting the pleura or as a result of a malignancy in the lung.

pleurisy Inflammation of the pleura, the thin tissuelike membrane layer around the lungs.

pneumonitis Lung inflammation.

polyarticular Affecting many joints.

prevalence The total number of people in a population who are affected by a condition (newly diagnosed and previously diagnosed) at any given time. Prevalence is usually expressed as a percentage.

prognosis An estimate of the likely outcome of an illness.

proteinuria Protein in the urine.

proximal interphalangeal (PIP) The joints forming the knuckles in the middle of the fingers.

RA Rheumatoid arthritis.

range of motion The range through which a joint can move.

remission An illness or process is inactive and no fresh damage is occurring.

resect To remove surgically.

rheumatism An old-fashioned lay term for aches and pains in and around joints.

rheumatoid factor A blood test that is often positive in patients with rheumatoid arthritis (see Appendix II).

rheumatology The study of arthritis and arthritis-related problems.

sacroiliac joint (SI joint) Two sacroiliac joints join the spine to the pelvis. These joints are most often affected in ANKYLOSING SPONDYLITIS.

sensitivity The proportion of people with a disease who have a positive test. For example, the antinuclear antibody (ANA) test (see Appendix II) is very sensitive and is positive in 95 percent of patients with SLE. A test that is both sensitive and specific is most helpful. See specificity below.

SERM Selective estrogen receptor modulator, a class of drugs that has some of the effects of estrogen in some tissues. For example, RALOXIFENE has estrogenic effects on bone but antiestrogenic effects on breast tissue.

SLE Systemic lupus erythematosus.

specificity The proportion of people without disease who have a negative test result. In other words, if a test is positive, how strongly does it suggest the diagnosis of a particular disease? A test that has many false positive results is not very specific. For example, the antinuclear antibody (ANA) test (see Appendix II), although sensitive, is not very specific for SLE, and a positive test is found in many healthy people. A test that is both sensitive and specific is most helpful.

spondylitis Inflammation of the vertebrae of the spine.

strain Injury to soft tissues such as tendons and ligaments caused by biomechanical imbalance, trauma, or overuse.

synovial fluid The fluid lining the joint cavity.

synovitis Inflammation of a joint.

synovium The thin layer of membranelike tissue that lines many joints and tendons.

tendon A fibrous cord that joins muscle to bone.

thrombocytopenia A low platelet count.

urticaria An raised, lumpy, itchy allergic skin rash commonly known as hives.

WBC See white blood cells.

white blood cells (WBC) One of the cellular components of blood. White blood cells (also called leukocytes) initiate and regulate the immune response. The main types of white blood cells are neutrophils (also called granulocytes), lymphocytes, monocytes, and eosinophils. These cells circulate in the blood but can localize in tissues where inflammation is present.

BIBLIOGRAPHY

Alarcon, G. S. 1992. Arthritis due to tuberculosis, fungal infections, and parasites. *Current Opinion in Rheumatology* 4, no. 4:516–519.

Albano, S. A.; E. Santana-Sahagun; and M. H. Weisman. 2001. Cigarette smoking and rheumatoid arthritis. *Seminars in Arthritis & Rheumatism* 31, no. 3:146–159.

Alehtaha, D., and J. S. Smolen. 2002. Laboratory testing in rheumatoid arthritis patients taking disease-modifying antirheumatic drugs: Clinical evaluation and cost analysis. *Arthritis & Rheumatism* 47, no. 2:181–188.

Allcock, R. J.; J. J. O'Sullivan; and P. A. Corris. 2001. Palliation of systemic sclerosis-associated pulmonary hypertension by atrial septostomy. *Arthritis & Rheumatism* 44, no. 7:1,660–1,662.

American College of Rheumatology Subcommittee on Rheumatoid Arthritis Guidelines. 2002. Guidelines for the management of rheumatoid arthritis: 2002 Update. *Arthritis & Rheumatism* 46, no. 2:328–346.

Arnson, Y.; D. Amital; L. Fostick; et al. 2007. Physical activity protects male patients with post-traumatic stress disorder from developing severe fibromyalgia. *Clinical and Experimental Rheumatology* 25, no. 4:529–533.

Bach, D. S. 2009. Perspectives on the American College of Cardiology/American Heart Association guidelines for the prevention of infective endocarditis. *Journal of the American College of Cardiology* 53, no. 20:1,852–1,854.

Badesch, D. B.; V. F. Tapson; M. D. McGoon; et al. 2000. Continuous intravenous epoprostenol for pulmonary hypertension due to the scleroderma spectrum of disease. A randomized, controlled trial. *Annals of Internal Medicine* 132, no. 6:425–434.

Bakker, E. W.; A. P. Verhagen; E. Van Trijffel; et al. 2009. Spinal mechanical load as a risk factor for low back pain: a systematic review of prospective cohort studies. *Spine* 15, no. 34: E281–293.

Barnett, M. L.; J. M. Kremer, Sr.; D. O. Clegg; et al. 1998. Treatment of rheumatoid arthritis with oral type II collagen. Results of a multicenter, double-blind, placebo-controlled trial. *Arthritis & Rheumatism* 41, no. 2:290–297.

Barrett, J. H.; P. Brennan; M. Fiddler; and A. Silman. 2000. Breast-feeding and postpartum relapse in women with rheumatoid and inflammatory arthritis. *Arthritis & Rheumatism* 43, no. 5:1,010–1,015.

Bartley, J. 2008. Prevalence of vitamin D deficiency among patients attending a multidisciplinary tertiary pain clinic. *New Zealand Medical Journal* 121, no. 1,286:57–62.

Bell, J. A., and A. Burnett. 2009. Exercise for the primary, secondary and tertiary prevention of low back pain in the workplace: a systematic review. *Journal of Occupational Rehabilitation* 19, no. 1:8–24.

Benedict, N.; A. Seybert; M. A. Mathier. 2007. Evidence-based pharmacological management of pulmonary hypertension. *Clinical Therapeutics* 29, no. 10: 2,134–2,153.

Bennett, M. L.; J. M. Jackson; J. L. Jorizzo; et al. 2000. Pyoderma gangrenosum. A comparison of typical and atypical forms with an emphasis on time to remission. Case review of 86 patients from 2 institutions. *Medicine* 79, no. 1:37–46.

Berezne, A.; B. Ranque; D. Valeyre; et al. 2008. Therapeutic strategy combining intravenous cyclophosphamide followed by oral azathioprine to treat worsening interstitial lung disease associated with systemic sclerosis: a retrospective multicenter open-label trial. *Journal of Rheumatology* 35, no. 6:1,064–1,072.

Berman, A.; P. Cahn; H. Perez; et al. 1999. Human immunodeficiency virus infection associated arthritis: clinical characteristics. [see comments.]. *Journal of Rheumatology* 26, no. 5:1,158–1,162.

Berman, B. M.; J. P. Swyers; and J. Ezzo. 2000. The evidence for acupuncture as a treatment for rheumatologic conditions. *Rheumatic Diseases Clinics of North America* 26, no. 1:103–115.

Bernatsky, S.; J. F. Bolvin; L. Joseph; et al. 2006. Mortality in systemic lupus erythematosus. *Arthritis and Rheumatism* 54, no. 8:2,550–2,557.

Bingham, S.; D. Veale; U. Fearon; et al. 2002. High-dose cyclophosphamide with stem cell rescue for severe rheumatoid arthritis: Short-term efficacy correlates with reduction of macroscopic and histologic synovitis. *Arthritis & Rheumatism* 46, no. 3:837–839.

Boers, M.; A. C. Verhoeven; H. M. Markusse. 1997. Randomised comparison of combined step-down prednisolone, methotrexate and sulphasalazine with sulphasalazine alone in early rheumatoid arthritis. *Lancet* 350, no. 9,074:309–318.

Bolster, M. B., and R. M. Silver. 1999. Assessment and management of scleroderma lung disease. *Current Opinion in Rheumatology* 11, no. 6:508–513.

Bongers, E. M.; M. C. Gubler; N. V. Knoers. 2002. Nail-patella syndrome. Overview on clinical and molecular findings. *Paediatric Nephrology* 17, no. 9:703–712.

Borenstein, D. G. 2001. Epidemiology, etiology, diagnostic evaluation, and treatment of low back pain. *Current Opinion in Rheumatology* 13, no. 2:128–134.

Brandt, K. D.; S. A. Mazzuca; B. P. Katz; et al. 2005. Effects of doxycycline on progression of osteoarthritis: results of a randomized, placebo-controlled, double blind trial. *Arthritis and Rheumatism* 52, no. 7: 1,956–1,959.

Brissot, P.; M. B. Troadec; E. Bardou-Jacquet; et al. 2008. Current approach to hemochromatosis. *Blood Review* 22, no. 4:195–210.

Broderick, J. E. 2000. Mind-body medicine in rheumatologic disease. *Rheumatic Diseases Clinics of North America* 26, no. 1:161–176.

Burt, R. K.; Y. Loh; W. Pearce; et al. 2008. Clinical applications of blood-derived and marrow-derived stem cells for nonmalignant diseases. *Journal of the American Medical Association* 299, no. 8:925–936.

Buskila, D. 2000. Hepatitis C–associated arthritis. *Current Opinion in Rheumatology* 12, no. 4:295–299.

———. Fibromyalgia, chronic fatigue syndrome, and myofascial pain syndrome. *Current Opinion in Rheumatology* 13, no. 2:117–127.

Calabrese, L. H. 1991. Vasculitis and infection with the human immunodeficiency virus. *Rheumatic Diseases Clinics of North America* 17, no. 1:131–147.

Calabrese, L. H.; G. F. Duna; and J. T. Lie. 1997. Vasculitis in the central nervous system. *Arthritis & Rheumatism* 40, no. 7:1,189–1,201.

Callen, J. P. 1998. Pyoderma gangrenosum. *Lancet* 351, no. 9,102:581–585.

Campion, E. W. 1992. Desperate diseases and plasmapheresis. *New England Journal of Medicine* 326, no. 21:1,425–1,427.

Carter, J. D. 2005. Treatment of polychondritis with a TNF antagonist. *Journal of Rheumatology* 32, no. 7:1,413.

Cassidy, J. T. 1999. Medical management of children with juvenile rheumatoid arthritis. *Drugs* 58, no. 5:831–850.

Chan, F. K; V. W. Wong; B. Y. Suen; et al. 2007. Combination of a cyclo-oxygenase inhibitor and a proton pump inhibitor for prevention of recurrent ulcer bleeding in patients at very high risk: a double blind randomized trial. *Lancet* 369, no. 9,573:1,621–1,626.

Chariot, P.; E. Ruet; F. J. Authier; Y. Levy; and R. Gherardi. 1994. Acute rhabdomyolysis in patients infected by human immunodeficiency virus. *Neurology* 44, no. 9:1,692–1,696.

Cilliers, A. M. 2006. Rheumatic fever and its management. *British Journal of Medicine* 333, no. 7,579:1,153–1,156.

Cines, D. B., and V. S. Blanchette. 2002. Immune thrombocytopenic purpura. *New England Journal of Medicine* 346, no. 13:995–1,008.

Clark, W. F.; G. A. Rock; N. Buskard; et al. 1999. Therapeutic plasma exchange: An update from the Canadian Apheresis Group. *Annals of Internal Medicine* 131, no. 6:453–462.

Clegg, D. O.; D. J. Reja; C. L. Harris; et al. 2006. Glucosamine, chondroitin and the two in combination for painful knee osteoarthritis. *New England Journal of Medicine* 354, no. 8: 795–808.

Coates, L. C.; R. R. Anderson; O. Fitzgerald; et al. 2008. Clues to the pathogenesis of psoriasis and psoriatic arthritis from imaging: a literature review. *Journal of Rheumatology* 35, no. 7: 1,438–1,442.

Cohen, M. D., and A. Abril. 2001. Polymyalgia rheumatica revisited. *Bulletin on the Rheumatic Diseases* 50, no. 8:1–4.

Cohen, S.; E. Hurd; J. Cush; et al. 2002. Treatment of rheumatoid arthritis with anakinra, a recombinant human interleukin-1 receptor antagonist, in combination with methotrexate: Results of a twenty-four-week, multicenter, randomized, double-blind, placebo-controlled trial. *Arthritis & Rheumatism* 46, no. 3:614–624.

Crosbie, D.; C. Black; L. McIntyre; et al. 2007. Dehydroepiandrosterone for systemic lupus erythematosus. *Cochrane Database of Systematic Reviews* 17, no. 4: CD005114.

Cuellar, M. L. 1998. HIV infection-associated inflammatory musculoskeletal disorders. *Rheumatic Diseases Clinics of North America* 24, no. 2:403–421.

Cush, J. J.; A. F. Kavanaugh; N. J. Olsen; et al. 1999. *Rheumatology: Diagnosis and Therapeutics.* Baltimore: Williams and Wilkins.

Daikh, B. E., and M. M. Holyst. 2001. Lupus-specific autoantibodies in concomitant human immunodeficiency virus and systemic lupus erythematosus: Case report and literature review. *Seminars in Arthritis & Rheumatism* 30, no. 6:418–425.

Delmas, P. D. 2002. Treatment of postmenopausal osteoporosis. *Lancet* 359, no. 9,322:2,018–2,026.

Delmas, P. D., and P. J. Meunier. 1997. The management of Paget's disease of bone. *New England Journal of Medicine* 336, no. 8:558–566.

Derry, S., and Y. K. Loke. 2000. Risk of gastrointestinal hemorrhage with long-term use of aspirin: meta-analysis. *BMJ* 321, no. 7,270:1,170–1,171.

Deyo, R. A. 2002. Diagnostic evaluation of LBP: Reaching a specific diagnosis is often impossible. *Archives of Internal Medicine* 162, no. 13:1,444–1,447.

Deyo, R. A., and J. N. Weinstein. 2001. Low back pain. *New England Journal of Medicine* 344, no. 5:363–370.

Dixon, T.; P. Mitchell; T. Beringer; et al. 2006. An overview of the prevalence of 25-hydroxy-vitamin D inadequacy among elderly patients with or without fragility fracture in the United Kingdom. *Current Medical Research and Opinion* 22, no. 2:405–415.

Donahue, K. E.; G. Gartlehner; D. E. Jonas; et al. 2008. Systematic review: comparative effectiveness and harms of disease-modifying medications for rheumatoid arthritis. *Annals of Internal Medicine* 148, no. 2:124–134.

Drenth, J. P., and J. W. van der Meer. 2001. Hereditary periodic fever. *New England Journal of Medicine* 345, no. 24:1,748–1,757.

Eastell, R. 1998. Treatment of postmenopausal osteoporosis. *New England Journal of Medicine* 338, no. 11:736–746.

Eisenberg, S.; I. Aksentijevich; Z. Deng; D. L. Kastner; and Y. Matzner. 1998. Diagnosis of familial Mediterranean fever by a molecular genetics method. *Annals of Internal Medicine* 129, no. 7:539–542.

Eleftheriou, D., and P. A. Brogan. 2009. Vasculitis in children. *Best Practise and Research in Clinical Rheumatology* 23, no. 3:309–323.

Erhardt, A.; A. Sagir; L. Guillevin; E. Neuen-Jacob; and D. Haussinger. 2000. Successful treatment of hepatitis B virus associated polyarteritis nodosa with a combination of prednisolone, alpha-interferon and lamivudine. *Journal of Hepatology* 33, no. 4:677–683.

Espinoza, L. R.; J. L. Aguilar; C. G. Espinoza; et al. 1991. Characteristics and pathogenesis of myositis in human immunodeficiency virus infection—distinction from azidothymidine-induced myopathy. *Rheumatic Diseases Clinics of North America* 17, no. 1:117–129.

Evans, J. M., and G. G. Hunder. 2000. Polymyalgia rheumatica and giant cell arteritis. *Rheumatic Diseases Clinics of North America* 26, no. 3:493–515.

Fain, O.; M. Hamidou; P. Cacoub; et al. 2007. Vasculitides associated with malignancies: analysis of 60 patients. *Arthritis and Rheumatism* 57, no. 8:1,473–1,480.

Felson, D. T.; Y. Zhang; M. T. Hannan; et al. The incidence and natural history of knee osteoarthritis in the elderly. The Framingham Osteoarthritis Study. *Arthritis & Rheumatism* 38, no. 10:1,500–1,505.

Fiechtner, J. J., and R. R. Brodeur. 2000. Manual and manipulation techniques for rheumatic disease. *Rheumatic Diseases Clinics of North America* 26, no. 1:83–96.

FitzGerald, G. A., and C. Patrono. 2001. The coxibs, selective inhibitors of cyclooxygenase-2. *New England Journal of Medicine* 345, no. 6:433–442.

Font, C.; O. Miro; E. Pedrol; et al. 1996. Polyarteritis nodosa in human immunodeficiency virus infection: Report of four cases and review of the literature. *British Journal of Rheumatology* 35, no. 8:796–799.

Fox, R. I.; M. Stern; and P. Michelson. 2000. Update in Sjögren syndrome. *Current Opinion in Rheumatology* 12, no. 5:391–398.

Furst, D. E. 2002. Stem cell transplantation for autoimmune disease: Progress and problems. *Current Opinion in Rheumatology* 14, no. 3:220–224.

Furst, D. E.; E. C. Keystone; F. C. Breedveld; et al. 2001. Updated consensus statement on tumor necrosis factor blocking agents for the treatment of rheumatoid arthritis and other rheumatic diseases (April 2001). *Annals of the Rheumatic Diseases* 60 Suppl 3:iii2–iii5.

Gabel, G. T. 1999. Acute and chronic tendinopathies at the elbow. *Current Opinion in Rheumatology* 11, no. 2:138–143.

Gabriel, S. E. 2001. The epidemiology of rheumatoid arthritis. *Rheumatic Diseases Clinics of North America* 27, no. 2:269–281.

Garfinkel, M., and H. R. Schumacher, Jr. 2000. Yoga. *Rheumatic Diseases Clinics of North America* 26, no. 1:125–132.

Gartlehner, G.; R. A. Hansen; B. L. Jonas; et al. 2008. Biologics for the treatment of juvenile idiopathic arthritis: a systematic review and critical analysis of the evidence. *Clinical Rheumatology* 27, no. 1:67–76.

George, J. N.; M. A. el Harake; and G. E. Raskob. 1994. Chronic idiopathic thrombocytopenic purpura. *New England Journal of Medicine* 331, no. 18:1,207–1,211.

George, J. N.; G. E. Raskob; S. R. Shah; et al. 1998. Drug-induced thrombocytopenia: A systematic review of published case reports. *Annals of Internal Medicine* 129, no. 11:886–890.

Gertz, M. A.; M. Q. Lacy; and A. Dispenzieri. 1999. Amyloidosis: Recognition, confirmation, prognosis, and therapy. *Mayo Clinic Proceedings* 74, no. 5:490–494.

Gladman, D. D.; P. J. Mease; C. T. Richlin; et al. 2007. Adalimumab for long-term treatment of psoriatic arthritis: 48-week data from the adalimumab effectiveness in psoriatic arthritis trial (2007). *Arthritis and Rheumatism* 56, no. 2:476–488.

Gloth, M. J., and A. M. Matesi. 2001. Physical therapy and exercise in pain management. *Clinics in Geriatric Medicine* 17, no. 3:525–535.

Goldenberg, D. L. 1999. Fibromyalgia syndrome a decade later: What have we learned? *Archives of Internal Medicine* 159, no. 8:777–785.

Goldenberg, D.; M. Mayskiy; C. Mossey; et al. 1996. A randomized double blind crossover trial of fluoxetine and amitriptyline in the treatment of fibromyalgia. *Arthritis and Rheumatism* 39, no. 11:1,852–1,859.

Gonzalez-Lopez, L.; J. I. Gamez-Nava; G. Jhangri. 2000. Decreased progression to rheumatoid arthritis or other connective tissue diseases in patients with palindromic rheumatism treated with antimalarials. *Journal of Rheumatology* 27, no. 1:41–46.

Guillevin, L. 1999. Virus-associated vasculitides. *Rheumatology* 38, no. 7:588–590.

Guzman, J.; R. Esmail; K. Karjalainen; et al. 2001. Multidisciplinary rehabilitation for chronic low back pain: Systematic review. *BMJ* 322, no. 7,301:1,511–1,516.

Hadler, N. M. 2000. Chiropractic. *Rheumatic Diseases Clinics of North America* 26, no. 1:97–102.

Hansmann, Y. 2009. Treatment and prevention of Lyme disease. *Current Problems in Dermatology* 37:111–129.

Hertzman, P. A.; D. J. Clauw; L. D. Kaufman; et al. 1995. The eosinophilia-myalgia syndrome: Status of 205 patients and results of treatment 2 years after onset. *Annals of Internal Medicine* 122, no. 11:851–855.

Hertzman, P. A.; H. Falk; E. M. Kilbourne; S. Page; and L. E. Shulman. 1991. The eosinophilia-myalgia syndrome: *The Los Alamos Conference. Journal of Rheumatology* 18, no. 6:867–873.

Himeno, M.; N. Tsugawa; A. Kuwabara; et al. 2009. Effect of vitamin D supplementation in institutionalized elderly. *Journal of Bone and Mineral Metabolism* (E-pub, ahead of print).

Hoffman, G. S. 1997. Treatment of Wegener's granulomatosis: Time to change the standard of care? *Arthritis & Rheumatism* 40, no. 12:2,099–2,104.

Hoffman, G. S.; M. C. Cid; D. B. Hellmann; et al. 2002. A multicenter, randomized, double-blind, placebo-controlled trial of adjuvant methotrexate treatment for giant cell arteritis. *Arthritis & Rheumatism* 46, no. 5:1,309–1,318.

Hoffman, G. S.; G. S. Kerr; R. Y. Leavitt; et al. 1992. Wegener granulomatosis: An analysis of 158 patients. *Annals of Internal Medicine* 116, no. 6:488–498.

Hoffman, G. S.; R. Y. Leavitt; G. S. Kerr; and A. S. Fauci. 1992. The treatment of Wegener's granulomatosis with glucocorticoids and methotrexate. *Arthritis & Rheumatism* 35, no. 11:1,322–1,329.

Huatuco, E. M.; E. L. Durigon; F. L. Lebrun; et al. 2008. Seroprevalence of human parvovirus B19 in a suburban population in São Paulo, Brazil. *Rev Saude Publica* 42, no. 3:443–449.

Hume, P.; W. Hopkins; K. Rome; et al. 2008. Effectiveness of foot orthoses for treatment and prevention of lower limb injuries: a review. *Sports Medicine* 38, no. 9: 759–779.

Hurwitz, S. R. 1996. Case management study: Heel pain in the adult. *Bulletin on the Rheumatic Diseases* 45, no. 4:1–3.

Ilowite, N. T. 2002. Current treatment of juvenile rheumatoid arthritis. *Pediatrics* 109, no. 1:109–115.

Jain, N., and K. Hennessey. 2009. Hepatitis B vaccination coverage among U.S. adolescents, National Immunization Survey—Teen (2006). *Journal of Adolescent Health* 44, no. 6:561–567.

Janowsky, E. C.; L. L. Kupper; and B. S. Hulka. 2000. Meta-analyses of the relation between silicone breast implants and the risk of connective-tissue diseases. *New England Journal of Medicine* 342, no. 11:781–790.

Janssen, N. M., and M. S. Genta. 2000. The effects of immunosuppressive and anti-inflammatory medications on fertility, pregnancy, and lactation. *Archives of Internal Medicine* 160, no. 5:610–619.

Jonas, W. B.; K. Linde; and G. Ramirez. 2000. Homeopathy and rheumatic disease. *Rheumatic Diseases Clinics of North America* 26, no. 1:117–123.

Kanis, J. A.; E. V. McCloskey; H. Johansson; et al. 2008. Case finding for the management of osteoporosis with FRAX-assessment and intervention thresholds for the UK. *Osteoporosis International* 19, no. 10: 1,395–1,408.

Kaptchuk, T. J. 2002. Acupuncture: Theory, efficacy, and practice. *Annals of Internal Medicine* 136, no. 5:374–383.

Katz, J. N., and B. P. Simmons. 2002. Clinical practice. Carpal tunnel syndrome. *New England Journal of Medicine* 346, no. 23:1,807–1,812.

Kemler, M. A.; G. A. Barendse; M. van Kleef; et al. 2000. Spinal cord stimulation in patients with chronic reflex sympathetic dystrophy. *New England Journal of Medicine* 343, no. 9:618–624.

Kerr, G. S.; C. W. Hallahan; J. Giordano; et al. 1994. Takayasu arteritis. *Annals of Internal Medicine* 120, no. 11:919–929.

Kerrison, C.; J. E. Davidson; A. G. Cleary; et al. 2004. Pamidronate in the treatment of childhood SAPHO syndrome. *Rheumatology* 43, no. 10:1,246–1,251.

Khan, M. A. 2002. Update on spondyloarthropathies. *Annals of Internal Medicine* 136, no. 12:896–907.

Kirwan, J. R. 2001. Systemic low-dose glucocorticoid treatment in rheumatoid arthritis. *Rheumatic Diseases Clinics of North America* 27, no. 2:389–403.

Klinger, G.; Y. Morad; C. A. Westall; et al. 2001. Ocular toxicity and antenatal exposure to chloroquine or hydroxychloroquine for rheumatic diseases. *Lancet* 358, no. 9,284:813–814.

Klings, E. S.; N. S. Hill; M. H. Ieong; et al. 1999. Systemic sclerosis-associated pulmonary hypertension: Short- and long-term effects of epoprostenol (prostacyclin). *Arthritis & Rheumatism* 42, no. 12:2,638–2,645.

Klippel, J. H. 1997. Systemic lupus erythematosus: Demographics, prognosis, and outcome. *Journal of Rheumatology—Supplement* 48:67–71.

Koren, G.; A. Pastuszak; and S. Ito. 1998. Drugs in pregnancy. *New England Journal of Medicine* 338, no. 16:1,128–1,137.

Kremer, J. M. 1997. Safety, efficacy, and mortality in a long-term cohort of patients with rheumatoid arthritis taking methotrexate: Followup after a mean of 13.3 years. *Arthritis & Rheumatism* 40, no. 5:984–985.

Kremer, J. M.; G. S. Alarcon; R. W. Lightfoot Jr.; et al. 1994. Methotrexate for rheumatoid arthritis. Suggested guidelines for monitoring liver toxicity. American College of Rheumatology. *Arthritis & Rheumatism* 37, no. 3:316–328.

Kremer, J. M.; G. S. Alarcon; M. E. Weinblatt; et al. 1997. Clinical, laboratory, radiographic, and histopathologic features of methotrexate-associated lung injury in patients with rheumatoid arthritis: A multicenter study with literature review *Arthritis & Rheumatism* 40, no. 10:1,829–1,837.

Langford, C. A. 2001. Treatment of polyarteritis nodosa, microscopic polyangiitis, and Churg-Strauss syndrome: Where do we stand? *Arthritis & Rheumatism* 44, no. 3:508–512.

———. 2001. Wegener granulomatosis. *American Journal of the Medical Sciences* 321, no. 1:76–82.

Lauer, G. M., and B. D. Walker. 2001. Hepatitis C virus infection. *New England Journal of Medicine* 345, no. 1:41–52.

Lee, D. M., and M. E. Weinblatt. 2001. Rheumatoid arthritis. *Lancet* 358, no. 9,285:903–911.

Leighton, C. 2001. Drug treatment of scleroderma. *Drugs* 61, no. 3:419–427.

Leventhal, L. J. 1999. Management of fibromyalgia. *Annals of Internal Medicine* 131, no. 11:850–858.

Levine, J. S.; D. W. Branch; and J. Rauch. 2002. The antiphospholipid syndrome. *New England Journal of Medicine* 346, no. 10:752–763.

Lunardi, C.; C. Bason; M. Leandri; et al. 2002. Autoantibodies to inner ear and endothelial antigens in Cogan's syndrome. *Lancet.* 360, no. 9,337:915.

Maddison, P. J.; D. A. Isenberg; P. Woo; and D. N. Glass. 1998. *Oxford Textbook of Rheumatology* 2nd edition. New York: Oxford University Press.

Mader, J. T.; D. Mohan; and J. Calhoun. 1997. A practical guide to the diagnosis and management of bone and joint infections. *Drugs* 54, no. 2:253–264.

Mader, R. 2005. Current therapeutic options in the management of diffuse idiopathic skeletal hyperostosis. Expert opinion. *Pharmacotherapy* 6, no. 8:1,313–1,318.

Malhotra, A., and D. P. White. 2002. Obstructive sleep apnoea. *Lancet* 360, no. 9,328:237–245.

Mankin, H. J. 1992. Nontraumatic necrosis of bone (osteonecrosis). *New England Journal of Medicine* 326, no. 22:1,473–1,479.

Martimo. K. P.; J. Verbeek; J. Karppinen; et al. 2008. Effect of training and lifting equipment for preventing back pain lifting and handling: systematic review. *British Medical Journal* 336, no. 7,641: 429–431.

May, K. P.; S. G. West; M. R. Baker; and D. W. Everett. 1993. Sleep apnea in male patients with the fibromyalgia syndrome. *American Journal of Medicine* 94, no. 5:505–508.

Mayes, M. D. 2000. Photopheresis and autoimmune diseases. *Rheumatic Diseases Clinics of North America* 26, no. 1:75–81.

McGonagle, D.; P. G. Conaghan; and P. Emery. 1999. Psoriatic arthritis: A unified concept twenty years on. *Arthritis & Rheumatism* 42, no. 6:1,080–1,086.

McGonagle, D.; S. Reade; H. Marzo-Ortega; et al. 2001. Human immunodeficiency virus associated spondyloarthropathy: Pathogenic insights based on imaging findings and response to highly active antiretroviral treatment. *Annals of the Rheumatic Diseases* 60, no. 7:696–698.

Medina, P. J.; J. M. Sipols; and J. N. George. 2001. Drug-associated thrombotic thrombocytopenic purpura-hemolytic uremic syndrome. *Current Opinion in Hematology* 8, no. 5:286–293.

Meeker, W. C., and S. Haldeman. 2002. Chiropractic: A profession at the crossroads of mainstream and alternative medicine. *Annals of Internal Medicine* 136, no. 3:216–227.

Merkel, P. A. 1999. Rheumatic disease and cystic fibrosis. *Arthritis & Rheumatism* 42, no. 8:1,563–1,571.

Meyer, U. A. 2000. Pharmacogenetics and adverse drug reactions. *Lancet* 356, no. 9,242:1,667–1,671.

Mitchell, H.; M. B. Bolster; and E. C. LeRoy. 1997. Scleroderma and related conditions. *Medical Clinics of North America* 81, no. 1:129–149.

Moake, J. L. 2002. Thrombotic microangiopathies. *New England Journal of Medicine* 347, no. 8:589–600.

Moreland, L. W.; J. E. Brick; R. E. Kovach; et al. 1988. Acute febrile neutrophilic dermatosis (Sweet syndrome): A review of the literature with emphasis on musculoskeletal manifestations. *Seminars in Arthritis & Rheumatism* 17, no. 3:143–153.

Moriguchi, M.; C. Terai; H. Kaneko; et al. 2001. A novel single-nucleotide polymorphism at the 5'-flanking region of SAA1 associated with risk of type AA amyloidosis secondary to rheumatoid arthritis. *Arthritis & Rheumatism* 44, no. 6:1,266–1,272.

Moseley, J. B.; K. O'Malley; N. J. Petersen; et al. 2002. A controlled trial of arthroscopic surgery for osteoarthritis of the knee. *New England Journal of Medicine* 347, no. 2:81–88.

Nadelman, R. B.; J. Nowakowski; D. Fish; et al. 2001. Prophylaxis with single-dose doxycycline for the prevention of Lyme disease after an Ixodes scapularis tick bite. *New England Journal of Medicine* 345, no. 2:79–84.

Nadelman, R. B., and G. P. Wormser. 1998. Lyme borreliosis. *Lancet* 352, no. 9,127:557–565.

Nangaku, M.; T. Miyata; and K. Kurokawa. 1999. Pathogenesis and management of dialysis-related amyloid bone disease. *American Journal of the Medical Sciences* 317, no. 6:410–415.

Natelson, B. H. 2001. Chronic fatigue syndrome. *JAMA: Journal of the American Medical Association* 285, no. 20:2,557–2,559.

Neves, O.; C. M. Stein; C. Thornton; I. Gangaidzo; and J. E. Thomas. 1991. Rhabdomyolysis associated with human immunodeficiency virus (HIV) infection. *Central African Journal of Medicine* 37, no. 11:387–388.

Newman, J. H.; L. Wheeler; K. B. Lane; et al. 2001. Mutation in the gene for bone morphogenetic protein receptor II as a cause of primary pulmonary hypertension in a large kindred. *New England Journal of Medicine* 345, no. 5:319–324.

Newman, L. S.; C. S. Rose; and L. A. Maier. 1997. Sarcoidosis. *New England Journal of Medicine* 336, no. 17:1,224–1,234.

O'Dell, J. R. 2002. Treating rheumatoid arthritis early: A window of opportunity? *Arthritis & Rheumatism* 46, no. 2:283–285.

Olin, J. W. 2000. Thromboangiitis obliterans (Buerger's disease). *New England Journal of Medicine* 343, no. 12:864–869.

Ortmann, R. A., and J. H. Klippel. 2000. Update on cyclophosphamide for systemic lupus erythematosus. *Rheumatic Diseases Clinics of North America* 26, no. 2:363–375.

Ostensen, M. 1999. Sex hormones and pregnancy in rheumatoid arthritis and systemic lupus erythematosus. *Annals of the New York Academy of Sciences* 876:131–143.

Ostensen, M., and R. Ramsey-Goldman. 1998. Treatment of inflammatory rheumatic disorders in pregnancy: What are the safest treatment options? *Drug Safety* 19, no. 5:389–410.

Parkin, J., and B. Cohen. 2001. An overview of the immune system. *Lancet* 357, no. 9,270:1,777–1,789.

Patkar, A. A.; P. S. Masand; P. Manelli; et al. 2007. A randomized controlled trial of controlled rease paroxetine in fibromyalgia. *American Journal of Medicine* 120, no. 5:448–454.

Petri, M. 1994. Systemic lupus erythematosus and pregnancy. *Rheumatic Diseases Clinics of North America* 20, no. 1:87–118.

———. 1998. Pregnancy in SLE. *Baillieres Clinical Rheumatology* 12, no. 3:449–476.

Petri, M., D. Spence; L. R. Bone; and M. C. Hochberg. 1992. Coronary artery disease risk factors in the Johns Hopkins Lupus Cohort: Prevalence, recognition by patients, and preventive practices. *Medicine* 71, no. 5:291–302.

Pinals, R. S. 1994. Polyarthritis and fever. *New England Journal of Medicine* 330, no. 11:769–774.

Pincus, T.; R. H. Brooks; and L. F. Callahan. 1994. Prediction of long-term mortality in patients with rheumatoid arthritis according to simple questionnaire and joint count measures. *Annals of Internal Medicine* 120, no. 1:26–34.

Pincus, T., and T. Sokka. 2001. Quantitative target values of predictors of mortality in rheumatoid arthritis as possible goals for therapeutic interventions: An alternative approach to remission or ACR20 responses? *Journal of Rheumatology* 28, no. 7:1,723–1,734.

Pincus, T. and C. M. Stein. 1999. ACR 20: Clinical or statistical significance? *Arthritis & Rheumatism* 42, no. 8:1,572–1,576.

Pincus, T.; C. M. Stein; and F. Wolfe. 1997. "No evidence of disease" in rheumatoid arthritis using methotrexate in combination with other drugs: A contemporary goal for rheumatology care? *Clinical & Experimental Rheumatology* 15, no. 6:591–596.

Pisetsky, D. S., and E. W. St. Clair. 2001. Progress in the treatment of rheumatoid arthritis. *JAMA: Journal of the American Medical Association* 286, no. 22:2,787–2,790.

Podolsky, D. K. 2002. Inflammatory bowel disease. *New England Journal of Medicine* 347, no. 6:417–429.

Pradhan, E. K.; M. Baumgarten; P. Langenberg; et al. 2007. Effect of mindfulness based stress reduction in rheumatoid arthritis patients. *Arthritis and Rheumatism* 57, no. 7:1,134–1,142.

Prins, J. B.; J. W. van der Meer; G. Bleijenberg. 2006. Chronic fatigue syndrome. *Lancet* 367, no. 9,507:346–355.

Puechal, X. 2001. Whipple disease and arthritis. *Current Opinion in Rheumatology* 13, no. 1:74–79.

Pyasta, R. T., and R. S. Panush. 1999. Common painful foot syndromes. *Bulletin on the Rheumatic Diseases* 48, no. 10:1–4.

Rao, J. K.; N. B. Allen; and T. Pincus. 1998. Limitations of the 1990 American College of Rheumatology classification criteria in the diagnosis of vasculitis. *Annals of Internal Medicine* 129, no. 5:345–352.

Raynauld, J. P. 1997. Cardiovascular mortality in rheumatoid arthritis: How harmful are corticosteroids? *Journal of Rheumatology* 24, no. 3:415–416.

Reid, S.; T. Chalder; A. Cleare; et. 2000. Chronic fatigue syndrome. *BMJ* 320, no. 7,230:292–296.

Reveille, J. D. 2000. The changing spectrum of rheumatic disease in human immunodeficiency virus infection. *Seminars in Arthritis & Rheumatism* 30, no. 3:147–166.

Rho, R. H.; R. P. Brewer; T. J. Lamer; and P. R. Wilson. 2002. Complex regional pain syndrome. *Mayo Clinic Proceedings* 77, no. 2:174–180.

Rhodes, J. M. 1996. Cholesterol crystal embolism: An important "new" diagnosis for the general physician. *Lancet* 347, no. 9,016:1,641.

Richards, R. N. 2008. Side effects of short-term corticosteroids. *Journal of Cutaneous Medicine and Surgery* 12, no. 2:77–81.

Robinson, W. H.; M. C. Genovese; and L. W. Moreland. 2001. Demyelinating and neurologic events reported in association with tumor necrosis factor alpha antagonism: By what mechanisms could tumor necrosis factor alpha antagonists improve rheumatoid arthritis but exacerbate multiple sclerosis? *Arthritis & Rheumatism* 44, no. 9:1,977–1,983.

Roden, D. M., and A. L. George, Jr. 2002. The genetic basis of variability in drug responses. *Nature Reviews. Drug Discovery* 1, no. 1:37–44.

Rose, S.; M. A. Young; and J. C. Reynolds. 1998. Gastrointestinal manifestations of scleroderma. *Gastroenterology Clinics of North America* 27, no. 3:563–594.

Roses, A. D. 2000. Pharmacogenetics and the practice of medicine. *Nature* 405, no. 6,788:857–865.

Rosner, I. A.; C. G. Burg; J. J. Wisnieski; et al. 1993. The clinical spectrum of the arthropathy associated with hidradenitis suppurativa and acne conglobata. *Journal of Rheumatology* 20, no. 4:684–687.

Rowe, P. C.; H. Calkins; K. DeBusk; et al. 2001. Fludrocortisone acetate to treat neurally mediated hypotension in chronic fatigue syndrome: A randomized controlled trial. *JAMA: Journal of the American Medical Association* 285, no. 1:52–59.

Rubin, L. J. 1997. Primary pulmonary hypertension. *New England Journal of Medicine* 336, no. 2:111–117.

Rubin, L. J.; D. B. Badesch; R. J. Barst; et al. 2002. Bosentan therapy for pulmonary arterial hypertension. *New England Journal of Medicine* 346, no. 12:896–903.

Ruddy, S.; E. D. Harris; and C. B. Sledge. 2000. *Kelley's Textbook of Rheumatology,* 6th edition. Philadelphia: W.B. Saunders.

Sakane, T.; M. Takeno; N. Suzuki; and G. Inaba. 1999. Behçet's disease. *New England Journal of Medicine* 341, no. 17:1,284–1,291.

Salvarani, C.; F. Cantini; L. Boiardi; and G. G. Hunder. 2002. Polymyalgia rheumatica and giant-cell arteritis. *New England Journal of Medicine* 347, no. 4:261–271.

Samuels, J.; I. Aksentijevich; Y. Torosyan; et al. 1998. Familial Mediterranean fever at the millennium. Clinical spectrum, ancient mutations, and a survey of 100 American referrals to the National Institutes of Health. *Medicine* 77, no. 4:268–297.

Sapadin, A. N., and R. Fleischmajer. 2002. Treatment of scleroderma. *Archives of Dermatology* 138, no. 1:99–105.

Sare, G. M.; L. J. Gray; P. M. Bath. 2008. Association between hormone replacement therapy and subsequent arterial and venous vascular events: a meta-analysis. *European Heart Journal* 29, no. 16:2,031–2,041.

Sawitzke, A. D.; H. Shi; M. F. Finco; et al. 2008. The effect of glucosamine and/or chondroitin sulphate on the progression of knee osteoarthritis: a report from the glucosamine/chondroitin intervention trial. *Arthritis and Rheumatism* 58, no. 10: 3,183–3,191.

Scheiman. J. M.; N. D. Yeomans; N. J. Talley; et al. 2006. Prevention of ulcers by esomeprazole in at risk patients using nonselective NSAIDs and COX-2 inhibitors. *American Journal of Gastroenterology* 101, no. 4:701–710.

Schott, G. D. 2001. Reflex sympathetic dystrophy. *Journal of Neurology, Neurosurgery & Psychiatry* 71, no. 3:291–295.

Schwartzman, R. J. 2000. New treatments for reflex sympathetic dystrophy. *New England Journal of Medicine* 343, no. 9:654–656.

Sergent, J. S. 1983. Extrahepatic manifestations of hepatitis B infection. *Bulletin on the Rheumatic Diseases* 33, no. 6:1–6.

Shojania, K. 2000. Rheumatology: 2. What laboratory tests are needed? *CMAJ: Canadian Medical Association Journal* 162, no. 8:1,157–1,163.

Singh, G.; O. Wu; P. Langhorne; et al. 2006. Risk of acute myocardial infarction with nonselective nonsteroidal anti-inflammatory drugs: a meta-analysis. *Arthritis Research & Therapy* 8, no. 5:R153.

Smith, J. R., and J. T. Rosenbaum. 2002. Management of uveitis: A rheumatologic perspective. *Arthritis & Rheumatism* 46, no. 2:309–318.

Smith, J. W. 1990. Infectious arthritis. *Infectious Disease Clinics of North America* 4, no. 3:523–538.

Smith, K. G.; R. B. Jones; S. M. Burns; et al. 2006. Long-term comparison of Rituximab treatment for refractory systemic lupus erythematosus and vasculitis:

remission, relapse and re-treatment. *Arthritis and Rheumatism* 54, no. 9:2,970–2,982.

Sokka, T.; H. Kautiainen; T. Mottonen; and P. Hannonen. 1999. Work disability in rheumatoid arthritis 10 years after the diagnosis. *Journal of Rheumatology* 26, no. 8:1,681–1,685.

Sokka, T., and T. Pincus. 2001. Markers for work disability in rheumatoid arthritis. *Journal of Rheumatology* 28, no. 7:1,718–1,722.

Solomon, D. H. 2005. Selective cyclooxygenase 2 inhibitors and cardiovascular events. *Arthritis and Rheumatism* 52, no. 7:1,968–1,978.

St. Clair, E. W., and R. M. McCallum. 1999. Cogan's syndrome. *Current Opinion in Rheumatology* 11, no. 1:47–52.

Steere, A. C. 2001. Lyme disease. *New England Journal of Medicine* 345, no. 2:115–125.

Stein, C. M. 2001. *Arthritis Medicines A–Z: A Doctor's Guide to Today's Most Commonly Prescribed Arthritis Drugs.* New York: Crown.

Stein, C. M.; N. Brown; D. E. Vaughan; et al. 1998. Regulation of local tissue-type plasminogen activator release by endothelium-dependent and endothelium-independent agonists in human vasculature. *Journal of the American College of Cardiology* 32, no. 1:117–122.

Stein, C. M. and P. Davis. 1996. Arthritis associated with HIV infection in Zimbabwe. *Journal of Rheumatology* 23, no. 3:506–511.

Stein, C. M., and T. Pincus. 1999. Placebo-controlled studies in rheumatoid arthritis: Ethical issues. *Lancet* 353, no. 9,150:400–403.

Stein, C. M.; T. Pincus; D. Yocum; et al. 1997. Combination treatment of severe rheumatoid arthritis with cyclosporine and methotrexate for forty-eight weeks: An open-label extension study. The Methotrexate-Cyclosporine Combination Study Group. *Arthritis & Rheumatism* 40, no. 10:1,843–1,851.

Stein, C. M., and J. E. Thomas. 1991. Behçet's disease associated with HIV infection. *Journal of Rheumatology* 18, no. 9:1,427–1,428.

Steinfeld, R.; R. M. Valente; and M. J. Stuart. 1999. A commonsense approach to shoulder problems. *Mayo Clinic Proceedings* 74, no. 8:785–794.

Stollerman, G. H. 1997. Rheumatic fever. *Lancet* 349, no. 9,056:935–942.

Stone, J. H.; G. S. Hoffman; P. A. Merkel; et al. 2001. A disease-specific activity index for Wegener's granulomatosis: Modification of the Birmingham Vasculitis Activity Score. International Network for the Study of the Systemic Vasculitides (INSSYS). *Arthritis & Rheumatism* 44, no. 4:912–920.

Sule, S. D., and F. M. Wigley. 2000. Update on management of scleroderma. *Bulletin on the Rheumatic Diseases* 49, no. 10:1–4.

Tashkin, D. P.; R. Elashoff; P. J. Clements; et al. 2007. Effects of one-year treatment with cyclophosphamide on outcomes at two years in scleroderma lung disease. *American Journal of Critical Care Medicine* 176, no. 10:952–953.

Tatsis, E.; A. Schnabel; W. L. Gross. 1998. Interferon-alpha treatment of four patients with Churg-Strauss Syndrome. *Annals of Internal Medicine* 129, no. 5:370–374.

Thamsborg, G; A. Florescu; P. Oturai; et al. 2005. Treatment of knee osteoarthritis with pulsed electromagnetic fields: a randomized double blind placebo controlled study. *Osteoarthritis Cartilage* 13, no. 7:575–581.

Thomsen, H. S.; P. Marckmann; V. B. Loqaqer. 2008. Update on nephrogenic systemic fibrosis. *Magnetic Resonance Imaging Clinics of North America* 16, no. 4: 551–560.

Totemchokchyakarn, K., and G. V. Ball. 1997. Sarcoid arthropathy. *Bulletin on the Rheumatic Diseases* 46, no. 3:3–5.

Trock, D. H. 2000. Electromagnetic fields and magnets. Investigational treatment for musculoskeletal disorders. *Rheumatic Diseases Clinics of North America* 26, no. 1:51–62.

Tugwell, P.; T. Pincus; D. Yocum; M. Stein; O. Gluck; G. Kraag; R. McKendry; J. Tesser; P. Baker; and G. Wells. 1995. Combination therapy with cyclosporine and methotrexate in severe rheumatoid arthritis. The Methotrexate-Cyclosporine Combination Study Group. *New England Journal of Medicine* 333, no. 3:137–141.

Tugwell, P.; G. Wells; J. Peterson; et al. 2001. Do silicone breast implants cause rheumatologic disorders? A systematic review for a court-appointed national science panel. *Arthritis & Rheumatism* 44, no. 11:2,477–2,484.

Tyndall, A. and EBMT/EULAR International Data Base. 2001. Autologous hematopoietic stem cell transplantation for severe autoimmune disease with special reference to rheumatoid arthritis. *Journal of Rheumatology* 28, Suppl. 64:5–7.

Tyndall, A., and T. Koike. 2002. High-dose immunoablative therapy with hematopoietic stem cell support in the treatment of severe autoimmune disease: current status and future direction. *Internal Medicine* 41, (8):608–12.

Uhl, T. L., and J. A. Madaleno. 2001. Rehabilitation concepts and supportive devices for overuse injuries of the upper extremities. *Clinics in Sports Medicine* 20, no. 3:621–639.

Urowitz, M. B.; D. D. Gladman; M. Abu-Shakra; and V. T. Farewell. 1997. Mortality studies in systemic lupus erythematosus. Results from a single center. III. Improved survival over 24 years. *Journal of Rheumatology* 24, no. 6:1,061–1,065.

Van Doornum, S.; G. McColl; and I. P. Wicks. 2002. Accelerated atherosclerosis: An extraarticular feature of rheumatoid arthritis? *Arthritis & Rheumatism* 46, no. 4:862–873.

Van Herck, K.; A. Vorsters; P. Van Damme. 2008. Prevention of viral hepatitis (B and C) reassessed. *Best Practise and Research in Clinical Gastroenterology* 22, no. 6:1,009–1,029.

Vassilopoulos, D., and L. H. Calabrese. 1998. Rheumatologic manifestations of HIV-1 and HTLV-1 infections. *Cleveland Clinic Journal of Medicine* 65, no. 8:436–441.

———. 2002. Hepatitis C virus infection and vasculitis: Implications of antiviral and immunosuppressive therapies. *Arthritis & Rheumatism* 46, no. 3:585–597.

Vergne, P.; P. Bertin; C. Bonnet; et al. 2000. Drug-induced rheumatic disorders: Incidence, prevention and management. *Drug Safety* 23, no. 4:279–293.

Violante, F. S.; T. J. Armstrong; C. Fiorentina; et al. 2007. Carpal tunnel syndrome and manual work: a longitudinal study. *Journal of Occupational and Environmental Medicine* 49, no. 11:1,189–1,196.

Vogel, V. G.; J. P. Costantino; D. L. Wickerham; et al. 2006. Effects of tamoxifen v. raloxifene on the risk of developing invasive breast cancer and other disease outcomes: the NSABP study of tamoxifen and raloxifene (STAR)P-2 trial. *Journal of the American Medical Association* 295, no. 23:2,727–2,741.

Walker, A. M.; D. Funch; N. A. Dreyer; et al. 1993. Determinants of serious liver disease among patients receiving low-dose methotrexate for rheumatoid arthritis. *Arthritis & Rheumatism* 36, no. 3:329–335.

Walport, M. J. 2001. Complement. First of two parts. *New England Journal of Medicine* 344, no. 14:1,058–1,066.

———. 2001. Complement. Second of two parts. *New England Journal of Medicine* 344, no. 15:1,140–1,144.

Ward, M. M.; J. P. Leigh; and J. F. Fries. 1993. Progression of functional disability in patients with rheumatoid arthritis. Associations with rheumatology subspecialty care. *Archives of Internal Medicine* 153, no. 19:2,229–2,237.

Ward, M. M.; E. Pyun; and S. Studenski. 1995. Causes of death in systemic lupus erythematosus. Long-term followup of an inception cohort. *Arthritis & Rheumatism* 38, no. 10:1,492–1,499.

Weinblatt, M. E.; J. M. Kremer; A. D. Bankhurst; et al. 1999. A trial of etanercept, a recombinant tumor necrosis factor receptor: Fc fusion protein, in patients with rheumatoid arthritis receiving methotrexate. *New England Journal of Medicine* 340, no. 4:253–259.

Wener, M. H.; R. J. Johnson; E. H. Sasso; and D. R. Gretch. 1996. Hepatitis C virus and rheumatic disease. *Journal of Rheumatology* 23, no. 6:953–959.

White, B.; W. C. Moore; F. M. Wigley; et al. 2000. Cyclophosphamide is associated with pulmonary function and survival benefit in patients with scleroderma and alveolitis. *Annals of Internal Medicine* 132, no. 12:947–954.

Wigley, F. M. 2002. Raynaud's Phenomenon. *New England Journal of Medicine* 347, no. 13:1,001–1,008.

Wolfe, F.; J. J. Cush; J. R. O'Dell; et al. 2001. Consensus recommendations for the assessment and treatment of rheumatoid arthritis. *Journal of Rheumatology* 28, no. 6:1,423–1,430.

Wolfe, F.; D. M. Mitchell; J. T. Sibley; et al. 1994. The mortality of rheumatoid arthritis. *Arthritis & Rheumatism* 37, no. 4:481–494.

Wolfe, F.; J. R. O'Dell; A. Kavanaugh; et al. 2001. Evaluating severity and status in rheumatoid arthritis. *Journal of Rheumatology* 28, no. 6:1,453–1,462.

Wolfe, F.; Q. Rehman; N. E. Lane; and J. Kremer. 2001. Starting a disease modifying antirheumatic drug or a biologic agent in rheumatoid arthritis: Standards of practice for RA treatment. *Journal of Rheumatology* 28, no. 7:1,704–1,711.

Yanagi, T.; T. Matsumura; R. Kamekura; et al. 2007. Relapsing polychondritis and malignant lymphoma: is polychondritis paraneoplastic? *Archives of Dermatology* 143, no. 1:89–90.

Yassi, A. 1997. Repetitive strain injuries. *Lancet* 349, no. 9,056:943–947.

———. 2000. Work-related musculoskeletal disorders. *Current Opinion in Rheumatology* 12, no. 2:124–130.

Yocum, D. E.; W. L. Castro; and M. Cornett. 2000. Exercise, education, and behavioral modification as alternative therapy for pain and stress in rheumatic disease. *Rheumatic Diseases Clinics of North America* 26, no. 1:145–159.

Ytterberg, S. R. 1999. Viral arthritis. *Current Opinion in Rheumatology* 11, no. 4:275–280.

Zemer, D.; M. Pras; E. Sohar; et al. 1986. Colchicine in the prevention and treatment of the amyloidosis of familial Mediterranean fever. *New England Journal of Medicine* 314, no. 16:1,001–1,005.

Zuckner, J. 1994. Drug-related myopathies. *Rheumatic Diseases Clinics of North America* 20, no. 4:1,017–1,032.

INDEX

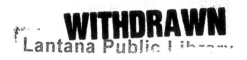